Lecture Notes in Electrical Engineering

Volume 269

For further volumes:
http://www.springer.com/series/7818

Shaozi Li · Qun Jin · Xiaohong Jiang
James J. (Jong Hyuk) Park
Editors

Frontier and Future Development of Information Technology in Medicine and Education

ITME 2013

Volume 3

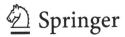

Editors
Shaozi Li
Cognitive Science
Xiamen University
Xiamen
People's Republic of China

Qun Jin
Networked Information Systems Lab,
  Human Informatics and Cognitive
  Sciences
Waseda University
Waseda
Japan

Xiaohong Jiang
School of Systems Information Science
Future University Hakodate
Hakodate, Hokkaido
Japan

James J. (Jong Hyuk) Park
Department of Computer Science and
  Engineering
Seoul National Universityof Science and
  Technology (SeoulTech)
Seoul
Korea, Republic of South Korea

ISSN 1876-1100 ISSN 1876-1119 (electronic)
ISBN 978-94-007-7617-3 ISBN 978-94-007-7618-0 (eBook)
DOI 10.1007/978-94-007-7618-0
Springer Dordrecht Heidelberg New York London

Library of Congress Control Number: 2013948373

© Springer Science+Business Media Dordrecht 2014
This work is subject to copyright. All rights are reserved by the Publisher, whether the whole or part of the material is concerned, specifically the rights of translation, reprinting, reuse of illustrations, recitation, broadcasting, reproduction on microfilms or in any other physical way, and transmission or information storage and retrieval, electronic adaptation, computer software, or by similar or dissimilar methodology now known or hereafter developed. Exempted from this legal reservation are brief excerpts in connection with reviews or scholarly analysis or material supplied specifically for the purpose of being entered and executed on a computer system, for exclusive use by the purchaser of the work. Duplication of this publication or parts thereof is permitted only under the provisions of the Copyright Law of the Publisher's location, in its current version, and permission for use must always be obtained from Springer. Permissions for use may be obtained through RightsLink at the Copyright Clearance Center. Violations are liable to prosecution under the respective Copyright Law.
The use of general descriptive names, registered names, trademarks, service marks, etc. in this publication does not imply, even in the absence of a specific statement, that such names are exempt from the relevant protective laws and regulations and therefore free for general use.
While the advice and information in this book are believed to be true and accurate at the date of publication, neither the authors nor the editors nor the publisher can accept any legal responsibility for any errors or omissions that may be made. The publisher makes no warranty, express or implied, with respect to the material contained herein.

Printed on acid-free paper

Springer is part of Springer Science+Business Media (www.springer.com)

Message from the ITME 2013 General Chairs

ITME 2013 is the 5th International Symposium on IT in Medicine and Education. This conference took place in July 19–21, 2013, in Xining, China. The aim of the ITME 2013 was to provide an international symposium for scientific research on IT in Medicine and Education. It was organized by Qinghai University, Future University Hakodate, Xiamen University, Shandong Normal University. ITME 2013 is the next event in a series of highly successful international symposia on IT in Medicine and Education, ITME-12 (Hokkaido, Japan, August 2012), ITME-11 (Guangzhou, China, December 2011), ITME-09 (Jinan, China, August 2009), ITME-08 (Xiamen, China, December 2008).

The papers included in the proceedings cover the following topics: IT Application in Medicine Education, Medical Image Processing and compression, e-Health and e-Hospital, Tele-medicine and Tele-surgery, Standard in Health Informatics and cross-language solution, Computer-Aided Diagnostic (CAD), Health informatics education, Biomechanics, modeling and computing, Digital Virtual Organ and Clinic Application, Three Dimension Reconstruction for Medical Imaging, Hospital Management Informatization, Construction of Medical Database, Medical Knowledge Mining, IT and Biomedicine, IT and Clinical Medicine, IT and Laboratory Medicine, IT and Preclinical Medicine, IT and Medical Informatics, Architecture of Educational Information Systems, Building and Sharing Digital Education Resources on the Internet, Collaborative Learning/Training, Computer Aided Teaching and Campus Network Construction, Curriculum Design and Development for Open/Distance Education, Digital Library, e-Learning Pedagogical Strategies, Ethical and Social Issues in Using IT in Education, Innovative Software and Hardware Systems for Education and Training, Issues on University Office Automation and Education Administration Management Systems, Learning Management Information Systems, Managed Learning Environments, Multimedia and Hypermedia Applications and Knowledge Management in Education, Pedagogical Issues on Open/Distance Education, Plagiarism Issues on Open/Distance Education, Security and Privacy issues with e-learning, Software Agents and Applications in Education. Accepted and presented papers highlight new trends and challenges of Medicine and Education. The presenters showed how new research could lead to novel and innovative applications. We hope you will find these results useful and inspiring for your future research.

We would like to express our sincere thanks to Steering Chair: Zongkai Lin (Institute of Computing Technology, Chinese Academy of Sciences, China). Our special thanks go to the Program Chairs: Shaozi Li (Xiamen University, China), Ying Dai (Iwate Prefectural University, Japan), Osamu Takahashi (Future University Hakodate, Japan), Dongqing Xie (Guangzhou University, China), Jianming Yong (University of Southern Queensland, Australia), all program committee members, and all the additional reviewers for their valuable efforts in the review process, which helped us to guarantee the highest quality of the selected papers for the conference.

We cordially thank all the authors for their valuable contributions and the other participants of this conference. The conference would not have been possible without their support. Thanks are also due to the many experts who contributed to making the event a success.

June 2013

Yongnian Liu
Xiaohong Jiang
James J. (Jong Hyuk) Park
Qun Jin
Hong Liu

Message from the ITME 2013 Program Chairs

Welcome to the 5th International Symposium on IT in Medicine and Education (ITME 2013), which will be held on July 19–21, 2013, in Xining, China. ITME 2013 will be the most comprehensive conference focused on the IT in Medicine and Education. ITME 2013 will provide an opportunity for academic and industry professionals to discuss the recent progress in the area of Medicine and Education. In addition, the conference will publish high-quality papers which are closely related to the various theories and practical applications on IT in Medicine and Education. Furthermore, we expect that the conference and its publications will be a trigger for further related research and technology improvements in these important subjects.

For ITME 2013, we received many paper submissions, after a rigorous peer review process; only very outstanding papers will be accepted for the ITME 2013 proceedings, published by Springer. All submitted papers have undergone blind reviews by at least two reviewers from the technical program committee, which consists of leading researchers around the globe. Without their hard work, achieving such a high-quality proceeding would not have been possible. We take this opportunity to thank them for their great support and cooperation. We would like to sincerely thank the following keynote speakers who kindly accepted our invitations, and, in this way, helped to meet the objectives of the conference: Prof. Qun Jin, Department of Human Informatics and Cognitive Sciences, Waseda University, Japan, Prof. Yun Yang, Swinburne University of Technology, Melbourne, Australia, Prof. Qinghua Zheng, Department of Computer Science and Technology, Xi'an Jiaotong University, China. We also would like to thank all of you for your participation in our conference, and also thank all the authors, reviewers, and organizing committee members.

Thank you and enjoy the conference!

Shaozi Li, China
Ying Dai, Japan
Osamu Takahashi, Japan
Dongqing Xie, China
Jianming Yong, Australia

Organization

General Conference Chairs

Prof. Yongnian Liu (QHU, China)
Prof. Xiaohong Jiang (FUN, Hakodate, Japan)
Prof. James J. (Jong Hyuk) Park, Seoul National University of Science and Technology, Korea
Prof. Qun Jin (Waseda, Japan)
Prof. Hong Liu (SDNU, China)

General Conference Co-Chairs

Prof. Yu Jianshe (GZHU, China)
Prof. Ramana Reddy (WVU, USA)
Dr. Bin Hu (UCE Birmingham, UK)
Prof. Dingfang Chen (WHUT, China)
Prof. Junzhong Gu (ECNU, China)

Program Committee Chairs

Prof. Shaozi Li (XMU, China)
Prof. Ying Dai (Iwate Prefecture University, Japan)
Prof. Osamu Takahashi (FUN, Hakodate, Japan)
Prof. Dongqing Xie (GZHU, China)
Dr. Jianming Yong (USQ, Australia)

Organizing Committee Chairs

Prof. Mengrong Xie (QHU, China)
Prof. Gaoping Wang (HAUT, China)

Dr. Jiatuo Xu (SHUTCM, Shanghai, China)
Prof. Zhimin Yang (Shandong University)

Local Arrangement Co-Chairs

Prof. Jing Zhao (QHU, China)
Prof. Peng Chen (QHU, China)

Publication Chairs

Prof. Hwa Young Jeong, Kyung Hee University, Korea
Dr. Min Jiang (XMU, Xiamen, China)

Program Committee

Ahmed Meddahi, Institute Mines-Telecom/TELECOM Lille1, France
Ahmed Shawish, Ain Shams University, Egypt
Alexander Pasko, Bournemouth University, UK
Angela Guercio, Kent State University
Bob Apduhan, Kyushu Sangyo University, Japan
Cai Guorong, Jimei University, China
Cao Donglin, Xiamen University, China
Changqin Huang, Southern China Normal University, China
Chaozhen Guo, Fuzhou University, China
Chensheng Wang, Beijing University of Posts and Telecommunications, China
Chuanqun Jiang, Shanghai Second Polytechnic University, China
Cui Lizhen, Shandong University, China
Cuixia Ma, Institute of Software Chinese Academy of Sciences, China
Feng Li, Jiangsu University, China
Fuhua Oscar Lin, Athabasca University, Canada
Hiroyuki Mituhara, Tokushima University, Japan
Hongji Yang, De Montfort University, UK
Hsin-Chang Yang, National University of Kaohsiung, Taiwan
Hsin-Chang Yang, National University of Kaohsiung, Taiwan
I-Hsien Ting, National University of Kaohsiung, Taiwan
Jens Herder, University of Applied Sciences, Germany
Jian Chen, Waseda University, Japan
Jianhua Zhao, Southern China Normal University, China
Jianming Yong, University of Southern Queensland, Australia
Jiehan Zhou, University of Oulu, Finland

Jungang Han, Xi'an University of Posts and Telecommunications, China
Junqing Yu, Huazhong University of Science and Technology, China
Kamen Kanev, Shizuoka University, Japan
Kiss Gabor, Obuda University, Hungary
Lei Yu, The PLA Information Engineering University, China
Li Xueqing, Shandong University, China
Luhong Diao, Beijing University of Technology, China
Masaaki Shirase, Future University Hakodate, Japan
Masashi Toda, Future University, Japan
Mohamed Mostafa Zayed, Taibah University, KSA
Mohammad Tariqul Islam, Multimedia University, Malaysia
Mohd Nazri Ismail, Universiti Kuala Lumpur, Malaysia
Neil Y. Yen, University of Aizu, Japan
Osamu Takahashi, Future University Hakodate, Japan
Paolo Maresca, University Federico II, Italy
Pierpaolo Di Bitonto, University of Bari, Italy
Ping Jiang, University of Hull, UK
Qiang Gao, Beihang University, China
Qianping Wang, China University of Mining and Technology, China
Qingguo Zhou, Lanzhou University, China
Qinghua Zheng, Xi'an Jiao Tong University, China
Rita Francese, University of Salerno, Italy
Roman Y. Shtykh, Waseda University, Japan
Rongrong Ji, Columbia University, USA
Shaohua Teng, Guangdong University of Technology, China
Shufen Liu, Jilin University, China
Su Songzhi, Xiamen University, China
Tianhong Luo, Chongqing Jiaotong University, China
Tim Arndt, Cleveland State University, USA
Tongsheng Chen, Comprehensive Information Corporation, Taiwan
Wei Song, Minzu University of China, Tsinghua University, China
Wenan Tan, Shanghai Second Polytechnic University, China
Wenhua Huang, Southern Medical University, China
Xiaokang Zhou, Waseda University, Japan
Xiaopeng Sun, Liaoning Normal University, China
Xiaosu Zhan, Beijing University of Posts and Telecommunications, China
Xinheng Wang, Swansea University, UK
Xiufen Fu, Guangdong University of Technology, China
Yaowei Bai, Shanghai Second Polytechnic University, China
Yingguang Li, Nanjing University of Aeronautics and Astronautics, China
Yinglong Wang, Shandong Academy of Sciences, China
Yinsheng Li, Fudan University, China
Yiwei Cao, IMC AG, Germany
Yong Tang, South China Normal University, China
Yoshitaka Nakamura, Future University Hakodate, Japan

Yuichi Fujino, Future University, Japan
Yujie Liu, China University of Petroleum, China
Zhang Zili, Southwestern University, China
Zhao Junlan, Inner Mongolia Finance and Economics College, China
Zhaoliang Jiang, Shandong University, China
Zhendong Niu, Beijing Institute of Technology, China
Zhenhua Duan, Xidian University, China
Zhongwei Xu, Shandong University at Weihai, China
Zonghua Zhang, Institute Mines-Telecom/TELECOM Lille1, France
Zongmin Li, China University of Petroleum, China
Zongpu Jia, Henan Polytechnic University, China

Contents

Volume 1

1. The Anti-Apoptotic Effect of Transgenic Akt1 Gene on Cultured New-Born Rats Cardiomyocytes Mediated by Ultrasound/Microbubbles Destruction 1
   Dongye Li, Xueyou Jiang, Tongda Xu, Jiantao Song, Hong Zhu and Yuanyuan Luo

2. Logic Operation in Spiking Neural P System with Chain Structure 11
   Jing Luan and Xi-yu Liu

3. A Mathematical Model of the Knee Joint for Estimation of Forces and Torques During Standing-up 21
   Zhi-qiang Wang, Yu-kun Ren and Hong-yuan Jiang

4. Adaptive Online Learning Environment for Life-Long Learning 29
   Zhao Du, Lantao Hu and Yongqi Liu

5. A Membrane Bin-Packing Technique for Heart Disease Cluster Analysis 39
   Xiyu Liu, Jie Xue and Laisheng Xiang

6. Teaching Chinese as a Foreign Language Based on Tone Labeling in the Corpus and Multi-Model Corpus 51
   Zhu Lin

7. A Systematically Statistical Analysis of Effects of Chinese Traditional Setting-up Exercise on Healthy Undergraduate Students 61
   Tiangang Li, Yongming Li and Xiaohong Gu

8	**Sample-Independent Expression Stability Analysis of Human Housekeeping Genes Using the GeNORM Algorithm**........ Li Li, Xiaofang Mao, Qiang Gao and Yicheng Cao	73
9	**Development of a One-Step Immunochromatographic Strip Test for Rapid Detection of Antibodies Against Classic Swine Fever** .... Huiying Ren, Shun Zhou, Jianxin Wen, Xinmei Zhan, Wenhua Liu and Shangin Cui	81
10	**Cramer-Von Mises Statistics for Testing the Equality of Two Distributions**.............................. Qun Huang and Ping Jing	93
11	**Establishment of Craniomaxillofacial Model Including Temporomandibular Joint by Means of Three-Dimensional Finite Element Method**............................. Zhang Jun, Zhang Wen-juan, Zhao Shu-ya, Li Na, Li Tao and Wang Xu-xia	103
12	**The Teaching and Practice for Neutral Network Control Course of Intelligence Science and Technology Specialty**..... Lingli Yu	113
13	**A New ACM/ICPC-Based Teaching Reform and Exploration of "Design and Analysis of Algorithms"** .... Yunping Zheng and Mudar Sarem	123
14	**Application Studies of Bayes Discriminant and Cluster in TCM Acupuncture Clinical Data Analysis**.............. Xiangyang Feng, Youqun Shi, Qinfeng Huang, Wenli Cheng, Houqin Su and Jie Liu	133
15	**Implanting Two Fiducials into the Liver with Single Needle Insertion Under CT Guidance for CyberKnife® SBRT**....... Li Yu, Xu Hui-jun and Zhang Su-jing	145
16	**On the Statistics and Risks of Fiducial Migration in the CyberKnife Treatment of Liver Cancer Tumors** ...... Li Yu, Hui-jun Xu and Su-jing Zhang	157

17	The Comparative Analysis with Finite Element for Cemented Long- and Short-Stem Prosthetic Replacement in Elderly Patients with a Partial Marrow Type I Intertrochanteric Fracture .... Wang Shao-lin, Tan Zu-jian and Zhou Ming-quan	165
18	The Exploration of Higher Undergraduate Education Mode Based on University-Enterprise Cooperation .... Yunna Wu, Jianping Yuan and Qing Wang	185
19	Higher Education Quality Supervision System Research ..... Yunna Wu, Jinying Zhang, Zhen Wang, Jianping Yuan and Yili Han	195
20	Micro-blog Marketing of University Library Based on 4C Marketing Mix............................... Feng Qing, Shang Wei and Chen Huilan	205
21	On Ethics and Values with Online Education .... Jiayun Wang and Jianian Zhang	213
22	What? How? Where? A Survey of Crowdsourcing.......... Xu Yin, Wenjie Liu, Yafang Wang, Chenglei Yang and Lin Lu	221
23	Hierarchical Clustering by a P System with Chained Rules ... Jie Sun and Xiyu Liu	233
24	Design and Implementation of Key Techniques in TCM Clinical Decision Support System................ Mingfeng Zhu, Bin Nie, Jianqiang Du, Chenghua Ding and Qinglin Zha	243
25	The Effect of a Simulation-Based Training on the Performance of ACLS and Trauma Team of 5-Year Medical Students ..... Jie Zhao, Shuming Pan, Yan Dong, Qinmin Ge, Jie Chen and Lihua Dai	253
26	A Novel Enhancement Algorithm for Non-Uniform Illumination Particle Image........................... Liu Weihua	265
27	Research on Predicting the Number of Outpatient Visits ..... Hang Lu, Yi Feng, Zhaoxia Zhu, Liu Yang, Yuezhong Xu and Yingjia Jiang	273

28 Acute Inflammations Analysis by P System with Floor Membrane Structure 281
Jie Xue and Xiyu Liu

29 Different Expression of P_{53} and Rb Gene in the Experimental Neuronal Aging with the Interference of Cholecystokinin 293
Feng Wang, Xing-Wang Chen, Kang-Yong Liu, Jia-Jun Yang and Xiao-Jiang Sun

30 Attitudes Toward and Involvement in Medical Research: A Survey of 8-year-Program Undergraduates in China 307
Jie-Hua Li, Bin Yang, Jing-Xia Li, Yan-Bo Liu, Hui-Yong Chen, Kun-Lu Wu, Min Zhu, Jing Liu, Xiao-Juan Xiao and Qing-Nan He

31 Study the Effect of Different Traditional Chinese Medicine Treatment which to the Elasticity Modulus of Asthma Rats' Lung 321
Zhao-xia Xu, Xue-liang Li, Na Li, Peng Qian, Jin Xu, Yi-qin Wang and Jun-qi Wang

32 Cloning and Characterization of Two cDNA Sequences Coding Squalene Synthase Involved in Glycyrrhizic Acid Biosynthesis in *Glycyrrhiza uralensis* 329
Ying Liu, Ning Zhang, Honghao Chen, Ya Gao, Hao Wen, Yong Liu and Chunsheng Liu

33 Ontology-Based Multi-Agent Cooperation EHR Semantic Interoperability Pattern Research 343
Jian Yang and Jiancheng Dong

34 Visual Analysis on Management of Postgraduate Degrees 353
Chen Ling and Xue-qing Li

35 An Energy-Saving Load Balancing Method in Cloud Data Centers 365
Xiao Li and Mingchun Zheng

36 Application of a New Association Rules Mining Algorithm in the Chinese Medical Coronary Disease 375
Feng Yuan, Hong Liu and ShouQiang Chen

37 Design and Development of a Clinical Data Exchange System Based on Ensemble Integration Platform 385
Wang Yu, Guo Long, Tian Yu and Jing-Song Li

38	The Management and Application of a Radio Frequency Identification System in Operating Rooms Jun-Der Leu, Yu-Hui Chiu and Hsueh-Ling Ku	393
39	Exploiting Innovative Computer Education Through Student Associations Wei Hu, Daikun Zou, Wenfei Li, Hong Guo and Ning Li	403
40	Traditional Chinese Medicine Literature Metadata: A Draft Technical Specification Developed by the International Organization for Standardization Tong Yu, Meng Cui, Haiyan Li, Shuo Yang, Yang Zhao and Zhang Zhulu	413
41	A Visualization Method in Virtual Educational System Guijuan Zhang, Dianjie Lu and Hong Liu	421
42	Moral Education with the Background of Information Globalization Liying Xiang	431
43	A Bayes Network Model to Determine MiRNA Gene Silence Mechanism Hao-yue Fu, Xiao-jun Lu and Xiang-de Zhang	441
44	The Novle Strategy for the Recognition and Classification of the Red Blood Cell in Low Quality Form Images Qiyou Cao, Xueqing Li and Qi Zhang	449
45	Scalable and Explainable Friend Recommendation in Campus Social Network System Zhao Du, Lantao Hu, Xiaolong Fu and Yongqi Liu	457
46	Application of Virtual Reality Technology in Medical Education Yan-Li Shi	467
47	An Improved Outlier Detection Algorithm Based on Reverse K-Nearest Neighbors of Adaptive Parameters Xie Fangfang, Xu Liancheng, Chi Xuezhi and Zhu Zhenfang	477
48	A Practical Study on the Construction of Diversified Network Monitoring System for Teaching Quality Jia Bing, Jiang Fengyan and Li Di	489

49	Reformation and Application of "Project-Tutor System" in Experimental Course Teaching of Fundamental Medicine Li-fa Xu and Jian Wang	501
50	A Knowledge-Based Teaching Resources Recommend Model for Primary and Secondary School Oriented Distance-Education Teaching Platform Meijing Zhao, Wancheng Ni, Haidong Zhang, Ziqi Lin and Yiping Yang	511
51	A Fast and Simple HPLC–UV Method for Simultaneous Determination of Emodin and Quinalizarin from Fermentation Broth of *Aspergillus. ochraceus* lp_0429 ShaoMei Yu and Ping Lv	523
52	Alteration of Liver MMP-9/TIMP-1 and Plasma Type IV Collagen in the Development of Rat Insulin Resistance Jun-feng Hou, Xiao-di Zhang, Xiao-guang Wang, Jing Wei and Kai Jiao	531
53	Evaluation Method for Software System Reliability Han Lu, Shufen Liu, Zhao Jin and Xue Fan	545
54	P System Based Particle Swarm Optimization Algorithm Qiang Du, Laisheng Xiang and Xiyu Liu	553
55	Specifying Usage of Social Media as a Formative Construct: Theory and Implications for Higher Education Tao Hu, Ping Zhang, Gongbu Gao, Shengli Jiao, Jun Ke and Yuanqiang Lian	565
56	Unsupervised Brain Tissue Segmentation by Using Bias Correction Fuzzy C-Means and Class-Adaptive Hidden Markov Random Field Modelling Ziming Zeng, Chunlei Han, Liping Wang and Reyer Zwiggelaar	579
57	An Adaptive Cultural Algorithm Based on Dynamic Particle Swarm Optimization Liu Peiyu, Ren Yuanyuan, Xue Suzhi and Zhu Zhenfang	589
58	A Modified Approach of Hot Topics Found on Micro-blog Lu Ran, Xue Suzhi, Ren Yuanyuan and Zhu Zhenfang	603

59	Computational Fluid Dynamics Simulation of Air Flow in the Human Symmetrical Six-Generation Bifurcation Bronchial Tree Model..................... Shouliang Qi, Zhenghua Li and Yong Yue	615
60	Discrimination of Solitary Pulmonary Nodules on CT Images Based on a Novel Automatic Weighted FCM.............. Zhang Xin, Jiaxing Li, Wang Bing, Ming Jun, Yang Ying and Zhang Jinxing	625
61	Investigation of Demands on On-Campus Health Information Education Services....................... Zhao-feng Li, Xuan Li, Xi-peng Han, Xing Tu, Tong Li and Wen-bin Fu	635
62	Suicidality in Medication-Native Patients with Single-Episode Depression: MRSI of Deep White Matter in Frontal Lobe and Parietal Lobe.................................... Xizhen Wang, Hongwei Sun, Shuai Wang, Guohua Xie, Shanshan Gao, Xihe Sun, Yanyu Wang and Nengzhi Jiang	647
63	Relating Research on ADC Value and Serum GGT, TBil of Lesions in Neonatal Hypoxic Ischemic Encephalopathy.... Yue Guan, Anhui Yan, Yanming Ge, Yanqi Xu, Xihe Sun and Peng Dong	659
64	Design and Implementation of the Regional Health Information Collaborative Platform .... Kong Hua-Ming, Qin Yao, Peng-Fei Li and Jing-Song Li	669
65	A Multi-objective Biogeography-Based Optimization with Mean Value Migration Operator.................... Xiang-wei Zheng, Kai-ge Gao, Xiao-guang Wang and Chi-zhu Ma	679
66	Observation of Curative Effect on 200 Cases of Myasthenia Gravis Treated with Traditional Chinese Medicine .... Wang Di and Wang Zhenqiu	687
67	Integrating Social Question–Answer Sites in Learning Management System................................. Yongqi Liu, Zhao Du, Lantao Hu and Qiuli Tong	695
68	The Study of Dynamic Threshold Strategy Based-On Error Correction .... Zhimin Yang, Jie Li, Gaofeng Han, Yue Wang and Songnan Zhao	705

69	Identification of Evaluation Collocation Based on Maximum Entropy Model LingYun Zhao, FangAi Liu and Zhenfang Zhu	713
70	Comparison of Beta Variable Gene Usage of T Cell Receptor in Peripheral Blood and Synovial Fluid of Rheumatoid Arthritis Patients Jianwei Zhou, Cui Kong, Xiukui Wang, Zhaocai Zhang, Chengqiang Jin and Qin Song	723
71	New Impossible Differential Cryptanalysis on Improved LBlock Xuan Liu, Feng Liu and Shuai Meng	737
72	Speckle Noise Reduction in Breast Ultrasound Images for Segmentation of Region Of Interest (ROI) Using Discrete Wavelets S. Amutha, D. R. Ramesh Babu, M. Ravi Shankar, R. Mamatha and S. Vidhya Suman	747
73	Sonic Hedgehog Signaling Molecules Expression in TGF-β1-Induced Chondrogenic Differentiation of Rat Mesenchymal Stem Cells In Vitro Yingchao Shi, Ying Jia, Shanshan Zu, Yanfei Jia, Xueping Zhang, Haiji Sun and Xiaoli Ma	755
74	A FCA-Based Approach to Data Integration in the University Information System Yong Liu and Xueqing Li	763
75	Research and Design on Agent-Based Collaborative Learning Model for Sports Students Zhaoxia Lu, Lei Zhang and Dongming Liu	773
76	Toxicology Evaluation and Properties of a New Biodegradable Computer Made Medical Biomaterial Jinshu Ma, Chao Zhang, Jingying Sai, Guangyu Xu, Xiaotian Zhang, Chao Feng, Fan Li and Fang Wang	783
77	Investigation and Analysis on Ear Diameter and Ear Axis Diameter in Maize RIL Population Daowen He, Hongmei Zhang, Changmin Liao, Qi Luo, Guoqiang Hui, Zhirun Nan, Yi Sun and Yongsi Zhang	795

78	Descriptive Statistics and Correlation Analysis of Three Kernel Morphology Traits in a Maize Recombinant Inbred Line Population........................ Changmin Liao, Daowen He and Xiaohong Liu	803
79	Study on Two Agronomic Traits Associated with Kernel Weight in a Maize RIL Segregation Population............ Changmin Liao	811
80	Improved Single-Key Attack on Reduced-Round LED....... Feng Liu, Pei-li Wen, Xuan Liu and Shuai Meng	819
81	Automatic Screening of Sleep Apnea-Hypopnea Syndrome by ECG Derived Respiration....................... Qing Qiao, Guangming Tong and Rui Chen	829
82	Research on the Informatization Top-level Design Methods... Zhang Huilin, Tong Qiuli and Xie Suping	837
83	Research on Optimization of Resources Allocation in Cloud Computing Based on Structure Supportiveness..... Wei-hua Yuan, Hong Wang and Zhong-yong Fan	849
84	Ambidextrous Development Model of University Continuing Education in Yunnan Province Based on CRM............ Hong-wu Zuo, Ze-jian Li and Ming Pan	859
85	Bibliometric Analysis on the Study of Education Informatization................................ Qiaoyun Chen	869
86	A Method for Integrating Interfaces Based on Cluster Ensemble in Digital Library Federation................ Peng Pan, Qingzhong Li and XiaoNan Fang	879
87	Long Term Web Service Oriented Transaction Handling Improvement of BTP Protocol .... Zhi-Lin Yao, Lu Han, Jin-Ting Zhang and Shu-Fen Liu	889
88	The Verification of a Newly Discovered Hepatitis B Virus Subtype Based on Sequence Analysis.............. Qingqing Yi, Lei Ma, Qinan Jia and Jianfeng He	899
89	A Primary Study for Cancer Prognosis based on Classification and Regression Using Support Vector Machine............ Jia Qinan, Ma Lei, He Jianfeng, Yi QingQing and Zhang Jun	909

Volume 2

90 Feature Extraction and Support Vector Machine Based Classification for False Positive Reduction in Mammographic Images 921
Q. D. Truong, M. P. Nguyen, V. T. Hoang, H. T. Nguyen, D. T. Nguyen, T. D. Nguyen and V. D. Nguyen

91 Research on Distributed Synchronous CAD Collaborative Design System 931
Chen Li

92 Enterprise Evolution with Molecular Computation 941
Xiuting Li, Laisheng Xiang and Xiyu Liu

93 Research and Implementation of Auxiliary System for Waken-up Craniotomy 951
Liu Yu, Feng Wu, Hongmin Bai and Weimin Wang

94 Investigation Performance on Electrocardiogram Signal Processing based on an Advanced Algorithm Combining Wavelet Packet Transform (WPT) and Hilbert-Huang Transform (HHT)* 959
Jin Bo, Xuewen Cao, Yuqing Wan, Yuanyu Yu, Pun Sio Hang, Peng Un Mak and Mang I Vai

95 Study on Self-Adaptive Clinical Pathway Decision Support System Based on Case-Based Reasoning 969
Gang Qu, Zhe Liu, Shengnan Cui and Jiafu Tang

96 Wireless Body Sensor Networks with Cloud Computing Capability for Pervasive Healthcare: Research Directions and Possible Solutions 979
Xiaoya Xu and Miao Zhong

97 Robust Predictive Control of Singular Systems with Structured Feedback Uncertainty 989
Xiaohua Liu and Rong Gao

98 Image Enhancement Methods for a Customized Videokeratography System Designed for Animals with Small Eyes 1001
Bin Chen, Shan Ling, Hongfei Cen, Wenfu Xu, Kee Chea-su, Yongjin Zhou and Lei Wang

99	Cloning and Expression of Catechol 2,3-dioxygenase from *Achromobacter Xylosoxidans* LHB21 .... Shuang Yu, Naiyu Chi and QingFang Zhang	1011
100	Design of Trust Model Based on Behavior in Cloud Computing Environment .... Yong Sheng Zhang, Ming Tian, Shen Juan Lv and Yan Dong Zhang	1021
101	The Study of Community–Family Remote Health Supervisory System Based on IOT .... Dongxin Lu and Wei Li	1029
102	Consistent Metric Learning for Outcomes of Different Measurement Tools of Cervical Spondylosis: Towards Better Therapeutic Effectiveness Evaluation .... Gang Zhang, Ying Huang, Yingchun Zhong and Wuwei Wang	1039
103	Design and Creation of a Universal Model of Educational Process with the Support of Petri Nets .... Zoltán Balogh, Milan Turčáni and Martin Magdin	1049
104	The Application of MPC-GEP in Classification Rule Mining .... Min Yao, Zhepeng Xu and Zenhong Wu	1061
105	Effects of Informationization on Strategic Plan of Regional Universities .... Guilin Chen, Shenghui Zhao and Chunyan Yu	1073
106	A Survey on Wireless Camera Sensor Networks .... Xiaolan Liu	1085
107	A Modified Hexagon-Based Search Algorithm for Fast Block Matching Motion Estimation .... Yun Cheng, Tiebin Wu and Minlei Xiao	1095
108	Protection of Xi Lei Powder to Intestinal Mucosa in Enema-Microstructure Observation by TEM and Light Microscope .... Feng Zhang, DuanYing Cai and Juan Xu	1105
109	Study on the Theory Building of Relationship Between National Culture Benefit and Language Education Policy ..... Jingying Ma	1113

110	Study on the Defect and Research About Discipline Speech Act Theory of Educator. Li Ying	1119
111	Study on the Nature of Education Information: The Education of Digital Virtual World Zhang Junmei	1125
112	Study on the Construction of General Framework of Educational Cost Management Mode in Colleges and Universities Xiu Hongbo	1131
113	Study on the Risk Identification and Warning of Tax Administration. Liu Weidong	1137
114	Study on the System Design of Sports Public Service Performance Evaluation Weidong Liu	1143
115	Research on the Construction of Teaching Resources Platform in Universities Qian Meng	1149
116	Applications of Virtualization Technology to Digital Library. Yu Xiaoyi, Wang Zhengjun, Yu Zhenguo, Jin Yuling, Wang Hong, Liang Yufang, Wang Quanhong, Gao Jian and Wang Haiyin	1155
117	The Health Status Among College Teachers: Taking Jiangxi Local Colleges as Example. Kaiqiang Guo, Weisong Bu and Fangping Li	1163
118	Research on Students' Perception and Expectations of Printed Materials in Online Education Jin Yiqiang	1175
119	Task Driven is an Effective Teaching Model of Discrete Mathematics in High Education Liu Shuai, Fu Weina, Li Qiang, Zhao Yulan and Duan Chanlun	1183

120	Evaluation on Application of Scene-Simulation Teaching Method in Oral Medicine Teaching .... Xiaoli An, Qianqian Lin, Wu Fanbieke, YuLin Zhang, Bin Liu and Wang Jizeng	1189
121	Research on Three Convolutions Related Issues in Signal Processing .... Wei Song	1195
122	Evaluation of College Students' Self-Regulated Learning Based on the IT Technology .... X. Wang, B. Qu and Ch. Y. Jia	1201
123	The Association Analysis of P16 in Transitional Cell .... Yu Hui	1207
124	Problem-Based Learning (PBL) in Eight-Year Program of Clinical Medicine in Xiangya School of Medicine: New Mode Needs Exploration .... Jieyu He, Qingnan He, Xiaoqun Qin, Yongquan Tian, Donna Ambrozy and Aihua Pan	1213
125	Design of Virtual Reality Guide Training Room Based on the Modern Education Technology .... Zhang Pengshun	1221
126	Exploration and Practice of Teaching Mode of Mechanical Engineering Control Foundation Based on Project Driving ... Tao Wu and Xiao-Bin Duan	1229
127	Wireless Sensor Network Distributed Data Collection Strategy Based on the Regional Correlated Variability of Perceptive Area......................... Yongjun Zhang and Enxiu Chen	1235
128	The System Design of the Network Teaching Platform of Learning Based on the Concept of Development Evaluation .... Liu Yong	1241
129	3-Dimensional Finite Element Analysis on Periodontal Stress Distribution of Impacted Teeth During Orthodontic Treatment .... Xu-xia Wang, Na Li, Jian-guang Xu, Xu-sheng Ren, Shi-liang Ma and Jun Zhang	1247

130	A Score-Analysis Method Based on ID3 of NCRE Zeng Xu	1253
131	Education Cloud: New Development of Informationization Education in China Liangtao Yang	1259
132	CRH5 EMU Fault Diagnosis Simulation Training System Development Jian Wang, Zhiming Liu, Fengchuan Jiao and Xinhua Zhang	1267
133	A Study on Recruitment Requirements of Small and Medium-Sized Enterprises and the Talent Training of Local Colleges Zhang Weiwei	1277
134	Simultaneous Determination of Atractylenolide II and III in *Rhizoma Atractylodes Macrocephalae* and Chinese Medicinal Preparation by Reverse-Phase High-Performance Liquid Chromatography Xiao-hong Sun and Jian Ge	1283
135	Research on the Pharmacokinetics and Elimination of Epigallocatechin Gallate (EGCG) in Mice Yang Liu, Jian Ge, Meng-xin Wang, Lin Cui and Bao-yu Han	1291
136	Simultaneous Determination of Five Phthalic Acid Esters (PAEs) in Soil and Air Tian-yu Hu, Yang Liu, Hua-jun Hu, Meng-xin Wang, Bao-yu Han and Jian Ge	1299
137	The Relationship Between Employability Self-Efficacy and Growth: The Mediator Role of e-Recruiting Perceived Chun-Mei Chou, Chien-Hua Shen, Hsi-Chi Hsiao, Hui-Tzu Chang, Su-Chang Chen, Chin-Pin Chen, Jen-Chia Chang, Jing-Yi Chen, Kuan-Fu Shen and Hsiang-Li Shen	1307
138	A Study to Analyze the Effectiveness of Video-Feedback for Teaching Nursing Etiquette Xiaoling Zhu, Mulan Wei, Ruoyan Chen, Daolin Jian and Xiaofei Chen	1315

139	A Biomedical Microdevice for Quantal Exocytosis Measurement with Microelectrodes Arrays .... Liguo Sun, Zhimeng Zou, Haifei Li, Peizheng Liu, Keping Tan and Jun Li	1321
140	The Construction of Comprehensive Financial Evaluation System in Higher Vocational Colleges Based on Connotation Construction........................ Zhongsheng Zhu and Fei Gao	1325
141	Spatial Covariance Modeling Analysis of Hypertension on Cognitive Aging............................... Lan Lin, Wei-wei Wu, Shui-cai Wu and Guang-yu Bin	1331
142	A New Practice Mode and Platform Based on Network Cooperation for Software Engineering Specialty .... Ling He	1337
143	Post-newborn: A New Concept of Period in Early Life ...... Long Chen, Jie Li, Nan Wang and Yuan Shi	1343
144	Analysis of the Characteristics of Papillary Thyroid Carcinoma and Discussion on the Surgery (Experience of 392 Cases).......................... Jia Liu, Guimin Wang, Guang Chen, Shuai Xue and Su Dong	1351
145	Skills of Minimally Invasive Endoscopic Thyroidectomy via Small Incision of Neck (Experience of 1,226 Cases) ...... Jia Liu, Su Dong, Xianying Meng, Shuai Xue and Guang Chen	1359
146	Research on the Contemporary College Students' Information Literacy .... Zhong Wenjuan, Wang Jing, Wang Mei and Guan Yanwen	1365
147	The CEMS Research Based on Web Service .... Wenke Zang and Xiyu Liu	1373
148	Enterprise Development with P Systems .... Xiuting Li, Laisheng Xiang and Xiyu Liu	1383
149	Application of Microblog in Educational Technology Practice Teaching................................. Jiugen Yuan and Ruonan Xing	1389

150 Ultrasound Image Segmentation Using Graph Cuts
with Deformable Prior 1395
Lin Li, Yue Wu and Mao Ye

151 Classifying and Diagnosing 199 Impacted Permanent
Using Cone Beam Computed Tomography 1401
Xu-xia Wang, Jian-guang Xu, Yun Chen, Chao Liu,
Jun Zheng, Wan-xin Liu, Rui Dong and Jun Zhang

152 Research Status and Development Tendency of Multi-campus
and Two Level Teaching Quality Monitoring
and Security System 1407
Mu Lei, Liu Xilin, Wang Keqin and Sun Ye

153 Analysis of the Research and Trend
for Electronic Whiteboard 1413
Guiying Guo and Baishuang Qiu

154 Study on Multi-faceted Teaching Model of Common Courses
in Stomatology: Taking Curriculums of "The Oral
Prevention and Health Care" as an Example.............. 1419
Yanyang Xu, Qian Zheng, Yuting Du, XueLi Gou, Guilong Gu,
Jianhua Huang and Bin Liu

155 Teaching Discussion on Pattern Matching Algorithm
in the Course of Data Structure 1425
Yang An and Bo Zhao

156 The Optimal Medical Device Order Strategy: An Improved
EOQ Model in Hospital 1431
Wei Yan, Yong Jiang and Huimin Duan

157 Improve Effectiveness and Quality of Course Practices
by Opening, Reusing and Sharing 1437
Rao Lan and Xinjun Mao

158 Application of PBL Teaching Method in the Experimental
Teaching of Hematologic Examination.................... 1443
Min Sun, Ya Li Zhang, LiJun Gao and XinYu Cui

159 Study on Bilingual Teaching of Heat Transfer Curriculum
Assisted by Distance Education 1449
Shunyu Su, Chuanhui Zhou and Xiongbing Ruan

160	Nonlinear Analysis of Bioprosthetic Heart Valve on Suture Densities.................................... Quan Yuan, Xia Zhang, Xu Huang and Hua Cong	1455
161	Reflections on Primary PostCapacity-Oriented Integrated Practice Teaching of Oral Courses in Higher Vocational Colleges................................... Chun-feng Wang, Jin Ling, Jian-guo Yi, Min-jiang Huang and Guang-ye Zhao	1463
162	Excellent Man Marathon Runners and Plateau, Plateau Training Period Portion of the Blood in the Index Comparison Analysis .... Zhang Sheng-lin	1473
163	The Implication of Collaborative Learning in College English................................... Yan Sufeng and Song Runjuan	1481
164	Bilingual Teaching Efficiency of Prosthodontics in Different Teaching Methods .... Liangjiao Chen, Ting Sun, Hua Fan, Yaokun Zhang, Ruoyu Liu and Longquan Shao	1487
165	Practice of Paradigm Teaching on Circuit Theory........... Yumin Ge and Baoshu Li	1493
166	The Study of Relationship Between the Nature and Other Properties of Traditional Chinese Medicines Based on Association Rules................................... Wang Zhe and Yu Hong-Yan	1501
167	Usage of Turbine Airflow Sensor in Ventilator.............. Yaoyu Wu, Feng Chang and Dongmin Liu	1507
168	Study on the Model of Double Tutors System in Postgraduate Education .... Jian Wang and Zhongyan Han	1515
169	Research on the Mobile Learning Resources Based on Cellphone .... Huang Lehui and Xing Ruonan	1521

170	Data Structure Teaching Practice: Discussion on Non-recursive Algorithms for the Depth-First Traversal of a Binary Tree. . . . . Zhong-wei Xu	1527
171	Contrast Analysis of Standardized Patients and Real Patients in Clinical Medical Teaching . . . . Zhang Yali, Xi Bo, Zhou Rui, Chunli Wu, Feng Jie, Jiping Sun, Jing Lv, Qingzhi Long and Bingyin Shi	1533
172	Effect of Jiangtang Fonglong Capsule on Expressions of Insulin of Deaf Animal Models of Diabetes . . . . Ruiyu Li, Kaoshan Guo, Lizhen Tang, Yanzhuo Zhang, Meng Li and Bin Li	1539
173	The Discussion for the Existence of Nontrivial Solutions About a Kind of Quasi-Linear Elliptic Equations. . . . . Bingyu Kou, Lei Mao, Xinghu Teng, Huaren Zhou and Chun Zhang	1547
174	A Team-Learning of Strategies to Increase Students' Physical Activity and Motivation in Sports Community. . . . . Hongyv Wu, Xiabing Fan and Dinghong Mou	1555
175	Research on Feet Health of College Students . . . . Pan Meili	1561
176	Uncertain Life . . . . Shao-lin Wang and Dian-ming Jiang	1569
177	Large-Scale Clinical Data Management and Analysis System Based on Cloud Computing. . . . . Ye Wang, Lin Wang, Hong Liu and Changhai Lei	1575
178	Satisfaction Changes Over Time Among Dentists with Outpatient Electronic Medical Record . . . . Hong-wei Cai, Yu Cao, Hong-bo Peng, Bo Zhao and Wan-hui Ye	1585
179	Discussion on English Collaborative Learning Mode in Vocational Schools Under the IT-Based Network Environment. . . . . X. Yang and H. H. Tan	1591

180	The Design of Learner-Centered College Teaching Resource Libraries Cui Wei, Liang Lijing and Hua Wei	1597
181	Research on Practice Teaching of Software Engineering Lianying Sun, Chang Liu, Baosen Zhang, Tao Peng and Yuting Chen	1603
182	Construction of Transportation Professional Virtual Internship Platform Zhao Jianguang and Lui Ruijun	1609
183	Chronic Suppurative Otitis Media Bacteriology Culturing and Drug Sensitive Experiment of Er Yannig Wu Liping, Hu Xiaoqian, Li Meng, Hou Jinjie and Li Ruiyu	1615
184	Research Hotspots Analysis of Hypertension Receptor by PubMed Chaopeng Li, Qinting Zhang, Yang Liu, Shuangping Wei, Jungai Li, Jinjie Hou, Ruijuan Zhang, Weiya Guo, Lijun Wang, Yuhong Liu and Ruiyu Li	1619
185	Creative Approaches Combined with Computer Simulation Technology in Teaching Pharmacology Chuang Wang and Jiejie Guo	1625
186	Problems and Counterplans of College English Independent Study Under Network Environment Zhai Fengjie	1633
187	Integrity Verification of Cloud Data Fan-xin Kong and Li Liu	1639
188	Establishing Automotive Engineering School-Enterprise Practice Training Model Based on Excellent Engineer Plan Geng Guo-qing, Zhu Mao-tao and Xu Xing	1645
189	Mechanical Finite Element Analysis to Two Years Old Children's Orbital-Bone Based on CT Jing liu, He Jin, Tingting Ning, Beilei Yang, Juying Huang and Weiyuan Lu	1651
190	Study on Digitalized 3D Specimen Making of Pathologic Gross Specimen Basing on Object Panorama Ran Hua-quan, Jiang Jun and Zeng Zhao-fang	1659

191	Ontology-Based Medical Data Integration for Regional Healthcare Application .... Yu-Xin Wen, Hua-Qiong Wang, Yi-Fan Zhang and Jing-Song Li	1667
192	The Application of Positive Psychology in Effective Teaching .... Yu Lin, Yu Jing, He Zhifang and Li Wuiguo	1673
193	The Exploration of Paramilitary Students Management in Vocational Colleges................................. Wang Haohui	1683
194	Research on a New DNA-GA Algorithm Based on P System .... Shuguo Zhao and Xiyu Liu	1691
195	Study on the Assistance of Microblogging in English Literature Teaching .... Haixia Fang	1699
196	Problem-Based Learning of Food Hygiene in Higher University of Traditional Chinese Medicine .... Daozong Xia	1707
197	Education Security of Bridgehead Strategic in Southwest China: Concept, Problems and Solutions .... Jing Tian and Ling Wang	1713
198	Applications of Network-Based Education in Lifelong Medical Education .... Liyuan Sun, Mingcheng Li and Yundong Zhao	1719
199	The Application of Informatics Technology in Foreign Medical Undergraduates Teaching .... Limei Liu, Taiguang Piao and Wei Li	1725
200	Discussion on the Reform of Teaching Software Development Training Curriculum Based on Application Store .... Yan-jun Zhu, Wen-liang Cao and Jian-xin Li	1731
201	Research on Construction of Bilingual-Teaching Model Course for Bioinformatics................................. Dong Hu, Jiansheng Wu, Han Wei, Meng Cui and Qiuming Zhang	1737

202	Research on Endpoint Information Extraction for Chemical Molecular Structure Images Zhao-man Zhong and Yan Guan	1747
203	Using Video Recording System to Improve Student Performance in High-Fidelity Simulation Wangqin Shen	1753
204	Exploration of Vocational Talents Culture Model of "Promote Learning with Competition, Combine Competition with Teaching" Wen-liang Cao and Xuan-zi Hu	1759
205	Research of Training Professionals in Computer Application Major from the Perspective of the Connection Between Middle and Higher Vocational Education Xuan-zi Hu and Wen-liang Cao	1765
206	Meta Analysis of Teachers' Job Burnout in China Jian-ping Liu, Zhi-fang He and Lin Yu	1771
207	Similar Theory in Material Mechanics Problem Luo Mao and Song Shaoyun	1779
208	Some Reflections on the Course Teaching of Physical Oceanography Hao Liu and Song Hu	1785
209	A Neural Tree Network Ensemble Mode for Disease Classification Feng Qi, Xiyu Liu and Yinghong Ma	1791
210	Application of PBL Model in the Teaching of Foreign Graduate Student Songzhu Xia, Xiaoyong Cao, Guisheng Yin, Haibo Liu and Jianguo Sun	1797
211	The Influence in Bone Mineral Density of Diabetes with Deafness in Different Syndrome Types by Prescriptions of Hypoglycemic Preventing Deafness Ruiyu Li, Kaoshan Guo, Meng Li, Jianqiao Li, Junli Yan, Liping Wu, Weihua Han, Qing Gu, Shuangping Wei and Yanfu Sun	1803

Volume 3

212 Application of Data Mining in the Assessment
of Teaching Quality 1813
Huabin Qu and Xueqing Li

213 A Data Mining System for Herbal Formula
Compatibility Analysis 1821
Li Jinghua, Feng Yi, Yu Tong, Liu Jing, Zhu Ling, Dong Yan,
Shuo Yang, Lirong Jia, Bo Gao and Gao Hongjie

214 The Analysis of the Chronic Patients' Demand of the Hospital
Health Information Service 1829
Guiling Li, Liqun Yang, Lin Ding, Runbin Wu,
Chundi Zhang, Limei Guo and Xiumei Ma

215 Learning from Errors and Learning from Failures:
A Study on the Model of Organizational Learning
from Errors 1833
Yangqun Xie, Jianian Zhang and Xiangzhi Zhuo

216 Employment-Oriented Web Application Development
Course Design Reform 1841
Chong-jie Dong

217 A Process Model of User Reactions to IT System Features 1847
Yan Yu and Zou Jin

218 Application of Modified PBL Mode on Pathophysiology
Courses 1855
Tang Hua, Chen Rong, Zhang Chun-Mei,
Li Zhu-Hua and Zou Ping

219 Meditations on the Semantic Net: Oriented Library
Information Service in Cloud Computing Era 1863
Yumei Liu

220 Synthesis and Antibacterial Activity
of Resveratrol Derivatives 1871
Yuanmou Chen, Fei Hu, Yinghao Gao, Na Ji and Shaolong Jia

221	Comparison of Intravenous Propofol Using Target-Controlled Infusion and Inhalational Sevoflurane Anesthesia in Pediatric Patients Dong Su, Haichun Ma, Wei Han, Limin Jin and Jia Liu	1883
222	Effect of Different Fluids on Blood Volume Expansion in Epidural Anesthesia of Elderly Patients Dong Su, Lei Pang, Haichun Ma, Wei Han and Jia Liu	1891
223	The Application of Association Rule Mining in the Diagnosis of Pancreatic Cancer Song Shaoyun	1899
224	Meta-Analysis of Chinese Herbs in the Treatment of Nephropathy: Huangqi and Danggui Type Formulations Ming-gang wei and Xiao-feng Cai	1905
225	Establishment and Significance of Digital Embryo Library for Enhancing Embryology Teaching Effect Bai Sheng-Bin, Chen Hong-Xiang, Tang Li, Liao Li-Bin, Li Tian, Feng Shu-Mei, Qin Wen, Zhong Jin-Jie and Luo Xue-Gang	1913
226	3D Reverse Modeling and Rapid Prototyping of Complete Denture Dantong Li, Xiaobao Feng, Ping Liao, Hongjun Ni, Yidan Zhou, Mingyu Huang, Zhiyang Li and Yu Zhu	1919
227	Simulation Training on Improving Basic Laparoscopic Skills of Medical Students Ni Hong, Song Ge and Junfang Qin	1929
228	Research on Reforming of Vocational Colleges for Music Majors in Education Liu Li	1935
229	Research on Badminton Sports in National Fitness Activities Yanling Dong and Qiang Ji	1941
230	University Students' Humanity Quality Education of Tai Ji Quan to Cultivate Influence Ji Qiang and Dong YanLing	1947

231	Study Progress of Traditional Chinese Massage Treatment of Lumbar Disc Herniation .... Qing Lan and Weihong Deng	1953
232	Chinese Anti-Inflammatory Herb May Postpone the Forming and Exacerbating of Diabetic Nephropathy (DN)* .... Hongjie Gao, Huamin Zhang, Haiyan Li, Jinghua Li, Junwen Wang, Meng Cui and Renfang Yin	1961
233	Analysis of Electromagnetic Radiation Effect on Layered Human Head Model .... Lanlan Ping, Dongsheng Wu, Hong Lv and Jinhua Peng	1971
234	A Study on Potential Legal Risks of Electronic Medical Records and Preventing Measures .... Hu Shengli, Feng Jun and Chi Jinqing	1979
235	Fostering the Autonomous Learning Ability of the Students Under the Multimedia Teaching Environment .... Zhao-ying Chen and Xiu-qing Wang	1987
236	Pattern Matching with Flexible Wildcard Gaps .... Zhang Junyan and Yang Chenhui	1993
237	Establishment and Practice of the New Teaching Model of Maxillofacial Gunshot Injuries .... Zhen Tang, Xiaogang Xu, Zhizhong Cao and Dalin Wang	1999
238	Research of Database Full-Text Retrieval Based on Related Words Recognition .... Gao Pei-zhi and Li Xue-qing	2007
239	Construction and Application of High Quality Medical Video Teaching Resources .... Chu Wanjiang, Zhuang Engui, Wang Honghai, Xu Zhuping, Bai Canming, Wang Jian and Li Lianhong	2013
240	Research and Construction of Mobile Development Engineer Course System .... Xiufeng Shao and Xuemei Liu	2023
241	Backward Direction Link Prediction in Multi-relation Systems .... Wang Hong, Yuan Wei Hua and Zhou Qian	2031

242	The Innovation of Information Service in University Library Based on Educational Informationization Liu Fang	2037
243	Speculate the Teaching of Medical Microbiology Network Resource Wang Hongying, Zhang Tao, Zhang Chuntao, Ma Haimei, Ding Jianbing and Ma Xiumin	2043
244	Clinical Significance of the Detection of Serum Procalcitonin in Patients with Lung Infection After Liver Transplantation Juan Guo, Wei Cao, Xiao Yang and Hui Xie	2049
245	Exploration of Teaching Strategies in Medical Network Teaching Bing Li, Jian Tan, Zhi Dong, Chen Xu, Zhaohui Zhong and Xiaoli He	2055
246	The Application of Information Technology Means During Clinical Medical Education in China Ying Xing, Shu-lai Zhu and Chun-di Chang	2061
247	Research Hotspots Analysis of Hypertension Treatment by PubMed Hou Jinjie, Chen Lianqun and Li Ruiyu	2067
248	Research Hotspots Analysis of Hepatitis Receptor by PubMed Hou Jinjie and Li Ruiyu	2073
249	The Application of Information Technology in Modern Sports Teaching Xiao Hong Li and Tuan Ting Zhang	2079
250	How to Use Multimedia Technology for Improvement of the Teaching Effect of Medical Immunology Ding Jianbing, Wang Song, Zhou Xiao Tao, Fulati Rexiti, Dilinar Bolati, Wei Xiaoli and Xu Qian	2085
251	Application of Mind Map in Teaching and Learning of Medical Immunology Song Wang, Jianbing Ding, Qi Xu, Xiaoli Wei, Qi Xu and Bolati Dilinar	2091

| 252 | Electron Microscopy Technology and It's Application in the Morphology | 2095 |

Caili Sun, Xiaohong Li, Zhou Li and Tuanting Zhang

| 253 | Empirical Study on the Relationship Between Financial Structure and Economic Growth: An Example of Zhejiang Province | 2103 |

Songyan Zhang

| 254 | The Teaching Design of Digital Signal Processing Based on MATLAB and FPGA | 2109 |

Xiaoyan Tian, Lei Chen and Jiao Pang

| 255 | The Design of an Management Software for High Value Medical Consumables | 2115 |

Zhou Longfu, Hu Yonghe, Fan Quanshui, Zhao Ming, Zhang Chaoqun and Li Zheng

| 256 | Libraries Follow-Up Services in the Era of Fragmentation Reading | 2123 |

Lu Yanxiang

| 257 | Research on Construction of Green Agriculture Products Supply Chain Based on the Model Differentiation | 2129 |

Bo Zhao

| 258 | Visualization Analysis and Research of Scientific Papers and Thesis in University | 2135 |

Jiangning Xie, Xueqing Li, Lei Wang and Ye Tao

| 259 | Multimedia Assisted Case-Based Teaching Application in Intercultural Communication | 2143 |

Huang Fang and Zhao Chen

| 260 | The Informatization Reform and Practice of the Humanities Courses in Nursing Profession | 2149 |

Ying Wang

| 261 | A Modified Minimum Risk Bayes and It's Application in Spam Filtering | 2155 |

Zhenfang Zhu, Peipei Wang, Zhiping Jia, Hairong Xiao, Guangyuan Zhang and Hao Liang

262	Research of CRYPTO1 Algorithm Based on FPGA .... Zhang Haifeng, Yang Zhu and Zhang Pei	2161
263	Change of Plasma Adrenomedullin and Expression of Adrenomedullin and its Receptor in Villus of Normal Early Pregnancy .... Lihong Ruan, Zhenghui Fang, Jingxia Tian, Yan Dou, Wenyu Zhong, Xiue Song, Wei Shi, Aiying Lu, Lizhi Sun, Guihua Jia, Haifeng Yu, Shuyi Han and Hongqiao Wu	2169
264	A Summary of Role of Alveolar Epithelial Type II Cells in Respiratory Diseases........................ Xueliang Li, Yiqin Wang and Zhaoxia Xu	2177
265	Application of Inquiry Teaching in Econometrics Course..... Songyan Zhang	2183
266	Extract Examining Data Using Medical Field Association Knowledge Base .... Li Wang, Yuanpeng Zhang, Danmin Qian, Min Yao, Jiancheng Dong and Dengfu Yao	2189
267	The Analysis and Research on Digital Campus Construct Model................................ Liu Xiaoming and Jiang Changyun	2195
268	Emotional Deficiency in Web-Based Learning Environment and Suggested Solutions .... Cai Li-hua	2201
269	Mapping Knowledge Domain Analysis of Medical Informatics Education............................. Danmin Qian, Yuanpeng Zhang, Jiancheng Dong and Li Wang	2209
270	Negation Detection in Chinese Electronic Medical Record Based on Rules and Word Co-occurrence .... Yuanpeng Zhang, Kui Jiang, Jiancheng Dong, Danmin Qian, Huiqun Wu, Xinyun Geng and Li Wang	2215
271	Design and Implementation of Information Management System for Multimedia Classroom Based on B/S Structure.... Xian Zhu, Yansong Ling and Yongle Yang	2221

272	The Application of E-Learning in English Teaching of Non-English Major Postgraduate Education Qu Daqing	2233
273	The Construction of Semantic Network for Traditional Acupuncture Knowledge Ling Zhu, Feng Yang, Shuo Yang, Jinghua Li, Lirong Jia, Tong Yu, Bo Gao and Yan Dong	2239
274	The New Training System for Laboratory Physician Rong Wang, Xue Li, Yunde Liu, Yan Wu, Xin Qi, Weizhen Gao and Lihong Yang	2247
275	The Investigation on Effect of Tele-Care Combined Dietary Reminds in Overweight Cases Y.-P. Chen, C.-K. Liu, C.-H. Chen, T.-F. Huang, S.-T. Tu and M.-C. Hsieh	2253
276	A Training System for Operating Medical Equipment Ren Kanehira, Hirohisa Narita, Kazinori Kawaguchi, Hideo Hori and Hideo Fujimoto	2259
277	The Essential of Hierarchy of E-Continuing Medical Education in China Tienan Feng, Xiwen Sun, Hengjing Wu and Chenghua Jiang	2267
278	The Reverse Effects of Saikoside on Multidrug Resistance Huiying Bai, Jing Li, Kun Jiang, Xuexin Liu, Chun Li and Xiaodong Gai	2273
279	Research and Practice on "Three Steps of Bilingual Teaching" for Acupuncture and Moxibustion Science in Universities of TCM Xiang Wen Meng, Dan Dan Li, Hua Peng Liu, Sheng Ai Piao, Cheng Hui Zhu and Karna Lokesh Kumar	2281
280	Current Status of Traditional Chinese Medicine Language System Meng Cui, Lirong Jia, Tong Yu, Shuo Yang, Lihong liu. Ling Zhu, Jinghua Li, Bo Gao and Yan Dong	2287
281	The Selection Research of Security Elliptic Curve Cryptography in Packet Network Communication Yuzhong Zhang	2293

282	Improvement of Medical Imaging Course by Modeling of Positron Emission Tomography................... *Huiting Qiao, Libin Wang, Wenyong Liu, Yu Wang, Shuyu Li, Fang Pu and Deyu Li*	2301
283	The Research of Management System in Sports Anatomy Based on the Network Technology................... *Hong Liu, Dao-lin Zhang, Xiao-mei Zhan, Xiao-mei Zeng and Fei Yu*	2307
284	Innovation of Compiler Theory Course for CDIO......... *Wang Na and Wu YuePing*	2315
285	The Design and Implementation of Web-Based E-Learning System................... *Chunjie Hou and Chuanmu Li*	2321
286	Complex System Ensuring Outstanding Student Research Training in Private Universities................ *YueYu Xu*	2325
287	The Influence of Short Chain Fatty Acids on Biosynthesis of Emodin by *Aspergillus ochraceus* LP-316............. *Xia Li and Lv Ping*	2331
288	Relationship Between Reactive Oxygen Species and Emodin Production in *Aspergillus ochraceus*.................. *Ping Lv*	2337
289	A Studies of the Early Intervention to the Diabetic Patients with Hearing Loss by Hypoglycemic Anti-deaf Party........ *Kaoshan Guo, Ruiyu Li, Meng Li, Jianqiao Li, Liping Wu, Junli Yan, Jianmei Jing, Weiya Guo, Yang Liu, Weihua Han, Yanfu Sun and Qing Gu*	2345
290	Effect of T Lymphocytes PD-1/B7-H1 Path Expression in Patients with Severe Hepatitis Depression from Promoting Liver Cell Growth Hormone Combinations from Gongying Yinchen Soup.................. *Zhang Junhui, Gao Junfeng, Zhao Xinguo, Li Meng, Ma Limin, Hou Jinjie, Sun Yanfu, Gu Qing and Li Ruiyu*	2353

291 The Influence of Hepatocyte Growth-Promoting Factors
    Combined with Gongying Yinchen Soup for Depression
    in Patients with Fulminant Hepatitis Peripheral Blood
    T Lymphocyte Subsets and Liver Function 2361
    Liping Wu, Junfeng Gao, Xinguo Zhao, Huilong Li, Jianqiao Li,
    Limin Ma, Meng Li, Weihua Han, Qing Gu and Ruiyu Li

292 The Impact of Hepatocyte Growth-Promoting Factors
    Combined with Gongying Yinchen Soup on Peripheral
    Blood SIL-2R of Depression in Fulminant
    Hepatitis Patients 2367
    Guo Kaoshan, Gao Junfeng, Li Jianqiao, Zhao Xinguo,
    Li Huilong, Ma Limin, Li Meng, Sun Yanfu, Gu Qing,
    Han Weihua and Li Ruiyu

293 Design and Development of Learning-Based Game
    for Acupuncture Education 2375
    Youliang Huang, Renquan Liu, Mingquan Zhou
    and Xingguang Ma

294 Clinical Research on Using Hepatocyte Growth-Promoting
    Factors Combined with Gongying Yinchen Soup to Cure
    Depression in Patients with Fulminant Hepatitis 2381
    Guo Kaoshan, Hou Shuying, Gao Junfeng, Zhao Xinguo,
    Li Jianqiao, Li Huilong, Hou Jinjie, Ma Limin, Li Meng,
    Sun Yanfu, Gu Qing and Li Ruiyu

295 The Development of Information System in General Hospitals:
    A Case Study of Peking University Third Hospital 2389
    Jiang Xue and Jin Changxiao

296 Several Reflections on the Design of Educational
    Computer Games in China 2397
    Nie Yun and L. V. Ping

297 A Rural Medical and Health Collaborative
    Working Platform 2403
    Jiang Yanfeng, Yin Ling, Wang Siyang, Lei Mingtao,
    Zheng Shuo and Wang Cong

298 Application of Internet in Pharmacological Teaching 2413
    Chen Jianguang, Li He, Wang Chunmei, Sun Jinghui,
    Sun Hongxia, Zhang Chengyi and Fan Xintian

299	Assessing Information Literacy Development of Undergraduates .... Fei Li, Bao Xi and Hua Jiang	2419
300	Improved Access Control Model Under Cloud Computing Environment............................. Yongsheng Zhang, Jiashun Zou, Yan Gao and Bo Li	2425
301	Research on Regional Health Information Platform Construction Based on Cloud Computing .... Zhimei Zhang, Xinping Hu, Jiancheng Dong, Jian Yang and Tianmin Jiang	2431
302	Detection of Fasciculation Potentials in Amyotrophic Lateral Sclerosis Using Surface EMG .... Boling Chen and Ping Zhou	2437
303	Biological Performance Evaluation of the PRP/nHA/CoI Composite Material .... Ning Ma, Li Zhang, Di Ying, Pan He, Ming-guang Jin, He Liu and Chun-yu Chen	2443
304	An Integrated Service Model: Linking Digital Libraries with VLEs .... Deng Xiaozhao and Ruan Jianhai	2453
305	The Research and Application of Process Evaluation Method on Prosthodontics Web-Based Course Learning ..... Min Tian, Zhao-hua Ji, Guo-feng WU, Ming Fang and Shao-feng Zhang	2461
306	Application of Multimedia in the Teaching of Pharmacological Experiment Course.................. Wang Chunmei, Li He, Sun Jinghui, Sun Hongxia, Zhang Chengyi, Fan Xintian and Chen Jianguang	2469
307	THz Imaging Technology and its Medical Usage .... Yao Yao, Guanghong Pei, Houzhao Sun, Rennan Yao, Xiaoqin Zeng, Ling Chen, Genlin Zhu, Weian Fu, Bin Cong, Aijun Li, Fang Wang, Xiangshan Meng, Qiang Wu, Lingbo Pei, Yiwu Geng, Jun Meng, Juan Zhang, Yang Gao, Qun Wang, Min Yang, Xiaoli Chong, Yongxia Duan, Bei Liu, Shujing Wang, Bo Chen and Yubin Wang	2475

308	Effects of Project-Based Learning in Improving Scientific Research and Practice Capacity of Nursing Undergraduates Ruiling Li, Dongmei Dou and Yuanyuan Wang	2481
309	Research on an Individualized Pathology Instructional System Kai Hu and Zhiqian Ye	2487
310	Security Problems and Strategies of Digital Education Resource Management in Cloud Computing Environment Li Bo	2495
311	Vocabulary Learning Strategies in Computer-Assisted Language Learning Environment Liming Sun and Ni Wang	2501
312	Bioinformatics Prediction of the Tertiary Structure for the Emy162 Antigen of *Echinococcus multilocularis* Yanhua Li, Xianfei Liu, Yuejie Zhu, Xiaoan Hu, Song Wang, Xiumin Ma and Jianbing Ding	2507
313	IT in Education Application of Computer in Teaching Flavor and Fragrance Technology Guangyong Zhu, Zuobing Xiao, Rujun Zhou, Yalun Zhu and Yunwei Niu	2513
314	Building an Effective Blog-Based Teaching Platform in Higher Medical Education Bailiu Ya, Qun Ma and Chuanping Si	2519
315	Design and Implementation of Educational Administration Information Access System Based on Android Platform Yifeng Yan, Shuming Xiong, Xiujun Lou, Hui Xiong and Qishi Miao	2525
316	The Application of Information Technology and CBS Teaching Method in Medical Genetics Yang Sun, Fang Xu, Yanjie Wang, Mingzhu Li, Ying Liang and Boyan Wu	2535
317	Research on Practice Teaching of Law in the Provincial Institutions of Higher Learning Haiying Zheng	2541

318	Path Selection for Practice Teaching of Law in Institutions of Higher Learning............................ Rongxia Zhang	2547
319	Inhibition Effects of Celery Seed Extract on Human Stomach Cancer Cell Lines Hs746T.................... Lin-Lin Gao, Chang-Xiang Zhou, Xiu-Feng Song, Ke-Wei Fan and Fu-Rong Li	2553
320	Research on the Practice of Teaching Auto Selective Course While China Stepping into Automobile Society....... Zhang Tiejun and Guan Ying	2561
321	An Integrated Research Study of Information Technology (IT) Education and Experimental Design and Execution (EDE) Courses......................... Guoying Wang and Yunsheng Zhang	2567
322	Empirical Study of Job Burnout Among Higher Vocational College Teachers........................... Cheng Wang	2575
323	Appeals on College Moral Education: Based on Open Environment of Laboratories Under Campus Network....... Jun-Yan Zhang	2581
324	Intercultural Pragmatics Research on Written Emails in an Academic Environment .... Su Zhang	2589
325	Construction of a Differentiated Embryo Chondrocyte 1 Lentiviral Expression Vector and Establishment of its Stably Transfected HGC27 Cell Line .... Rui Hu, Yun-Shan Wang, Yi Kong, Pin Li, Yan Zheng, Xiao-Li Ma and Yan-Fei Jia	2599
326	Construction of Expression Vector of miRNA Specific for FUT3 and Identification of Its Efficiency in KATO-III Gastric Cancer Cell Line .... Yong-Hong Xin, Yan-Fei Jia, Qiang Liu, Hong Zhang, Hai-ning Zhu, Xiao-li Ma, Yong-Jun Cai and Yun-Shan Wang	2607

327 Molecular Cloning, Sequence Analysis of Thioesterases
from Wintersweet (*Chimonanthus Praecox*) 2615
Li-Hong Zhang, Qiong Wu, Xian-Feng Zou, Li-Na Chen,
Shu-Yan Yu, Chang-Cheng Gao and Xing Chen

328 Effects of Bodymass on the SDA of the Taimen 2623
Guiqiang Yang, Liying Zhang and Shaogang Xu

329 Effects of Temperature on the SDA of the Taimen 2631
Guiqiang Yang, Ding Yuan and Shaogang Xu

330 Wireless Heart Rate Monitoring System of RSS-Based
Positioning in GSM 2637
Hongfang Shao, Jingling Han, Jianhua Mao and Zhigang Xuan

331 Research of Separable Polygraph Based
on Bluetooth Transmission 2643
Zhan-ao Wu, Tingting Cheng, Jianhun Mao and Feifei Wang

332 The Design of Intelligent Medicine Box 2649
Jianhua Mao, Xiubin Yuan and Hongfang Shao

333 The Questionnaire Survey about the Video Feedback Teaching
Method for the Training of Abdominal Examination
in the Medical Students 2655
Liu Juju, Ma Huihao, Xie Yuanlong, Qin Lu and Jian Daolin

334 Correlation Analysis on the Nature of Traditional
Chinese Medicine 2663
Zhang Pei-Jiang

335 The Classification of Meningioma Subtypes Based
on the Color Segmentation and Shape Features 2669
Ziming Zeng, Zeng Tong, Zhonghua Han,
Yinlong Zhang and Reyer Zwiggelaar

336 An Extraction Method of Cerebral Vessels Based
on Multi-Threshold Otsu Classification and Hessian
Matrix Enhancement Filtering 2675
Xiangang Jiang and Yunli Qiu

337 Architecture of a Knowledge-Based Education System
for Logistics 2683
Dianjun Fang and Xiaodu Hu

Volume 4

338	Research and Practice of University Statistics Sharing Scheme .... Suping Xie, Huaichu Chen, Shixue Yin and Zou Xiangrong	2693
339	A Formal Framework for Domain Software Analysis Based on Raise Specification Language .... Yuanzheng Zhao, Tie Bao, Lu Han, Shufen Liu and Qu Chen	2699
340	Video Feedback Teaching Method in Teaching of Abdominal Physical Examination .... Huihao Ma, Wang Bo, Juju Liu, Daoling Jian and Yuanlong Xie	2707
341	Evaluation of EHR in Health Care in China: Utilizing Fuzzy AHP in SWOT Analysis .... Ying Xiang and Jinchang Li	2715
342	A Method of Computing the Hot Topics' Popularity on the Internet Combined with the Features of the Microblogs .... Yongqing Wei, Zhen Zhang, Shaodong Fei and Wentao Du	2721
343	The Value of CBL Autonomous Learning Style for the Postgraduate of Medical Imageology: Promoting Professional Knowledge Learning Based on the PACS .... Peng Dong, Ding Wei-yi, Wang Bin, Wang Xi-zhen, Long Jin-feng, Zhu Hong and Sun Ye-quan	2729
344	Web-Based Information System Construction of Medical Tourism in South Korea .... Yinghua Chen and Jaekwang Lee	2735
345	Quantitative Modeling and Verification of VANET .... Jing Liu, Xiaoyan Wang, Shufen Liu, Han Lu and Jing Tong	2743
346	Study on the Financial Change of the Primary Health Care Institutions After the Implementation of Essential Drug System .... Changchun Zhan and Yasai Ge	2749

347 Construction of a Recombinant Plasmid for Petal-Specific Expression of HQT, a Key Enzyme in Chlorogenic Acid Biosynthesis 2755
Yuting Bi, Wei Tian, Wen Zeng, Yushan Kong, Yanhong Xue and Shiping Liu

348 Explorations on Strengthening of Students' Programming Capabilities in Data Structure Teaching 2765
Song Yucheng, Jin Shaoli and Xu Fasheng

349 A Study of the Effect of Long-Term Aerobic Exercise and Environmental Tobacco Smoke (ETS) on Both Growth Performance and Serum T-AOC, Ca^{2+}, BUN in Rat 2771
Xiao Xiao-ling, Huang Wen-ying, Wu Tao, Yu Chun-lian and Xu Chun-ling

350 Research on Multimedia Teaching and Cultivation of Capacity for Computational Thinking 2779
Yongsheng Zhang, Yan Gao, Jiashun Zou and Aiqin Bao

351 The Algorithm of DBSCAN Based on Probability Distribution 2785
Ma Yu, Gao Yuling and Song Shaoyun

352 Exploration and Practice on Signal Curriculum Group Construction of Instrument Science 2793
Wang Rui, Liang Yu, Li Hui and Zhou Hao-min

353 On Improving the E-Learning Adaptability of the Postgraduate Freshmen 2799
Ruan Jianhai and Deng Xiaozhao

354 Construction of a Network-Based Open Experimental Teaching Management System 2807
Yan-Rong Tong and Peng-Bo Song

355 Prediction of Three-Dimensional Structure of PPARγ Transcript Variant 1 Protein 2813
Cong Sun, Qiang Wu, Ye-chao Han, Ting-ting Tang and Li-li Wang

356	Interactive Visualization of Scholar Text .... Ming Jing and Xueqing Li	2821
357	Date-driven Based Image Enhancement for Segmenting of MS Lesions in T2-w and Flair MRI. .... Ziming Zeng, Zhonghua Han, Yitian Zhao and Reyer Zwiggelaar	2827
358	On Aims and Contents of Intercultural Communicative English Teaching .... Diao Lijing and Wang Huanyun	2833
359	Research on the Cultivation of Applied Innovative Mechanical Talents in Cangzhou. .... Wang Huanyun	2839
360	On Feasibility of Experiential English Teaching in Higher Vocational Institutes .... Diao Lijing	2845
361	Vi-RTM: Visualization of Wireless Sensor Networks for Remote Telemedicine Monitoring System. .... Dianjie Lu, Guijuan Zhang, Yanwei Guo and Jue Hong	2851
362	The Effect of T-2 Toxin on the Apoptosis of Ameloblasts in Rat's Incisor. .... Sha-fei Zhai, Zhu Yong, Ma Zheng and Yaochao Zhang	2857
363	A Preliminary Study of the Influence of T-2 Toxin on the Expressions of Bcl-2 and Bax of Ameloblasts in Rat's Incisor. .... Sha-fei Zhai, Zhu Yong, Ma Zheng and Yaochao Zhang	2865
364	PET Image Processing in the Early Diagnosis of PD .... Kai Ma, Zhi-an Liu, Ya-ping Nie and Dian-shuai Gao	2871
365	"4 Steps" in Problem Based Teaching in the Medical Internship: Experiences from China .... Huasheng Liu, Mei Zhang, Richard Bae, Muxing Li, Xiaoping Xi, Qin Gao, Yan Li, Di Wu and Bingyin Shi	2879

366	**Applications of Pitch Pattern in Chinese Tone Learning System**.. Song Liu and Peng Liu	2887
367	**Detection of Onset and Offset of QRS Complex Based a Modified Triangle Morphology**........................ Xiao Hu, Jingjing Liu, Jiaqing Wang and Zhong Xiao	2893
368	**Ecological Characters of Truffles**........................ Hai-feng Wang, Yan-ling Zhao and Yong-jun Fan	2903
369	**A Study on Mobile Phone-Based Practice Teaching System**... Tiejun Zhang	2909
370	**Study on Application of Online Education Based on Interactive Platform**................................ Li Fengyun	2919
371	**Analysis on Curative Effect of Exercise Therapy Combined with Joint Mobilization in the Treatment of Knee Osteoarthritis**................................ Wang Hongliang	2927
372	**Predictions with Intuitionistic Fuzzy Soft Sets**............ Sylvia Encheva	2935
373	**Eliciting the Most Desirable Information with Residuated Lattices**............................ Sylvia Encheva	2941
374	**Research on Data Exchange Platform Based on IPSec and XML**................................ Li Bo	2947
375	**Integration and Utilization of Digital Learning Resources in Community Education**..................... Liangtao Yang	2953
376	**Correlation of Aberrant Methylation of APC Gene to MTHFR C677T Genetic Polymorphisms in Hepatic Carcinoma**................................ Lian-Hua Cui, Meng Liu, Hong-Zong Si, Min-Ho Shin, Hee Nam Kim and Jin-Su Choi	2961

377	The Application of Humane Care in Clinical Medical Treatment Chunhua Su	2969
378	Chinese EFL Learners' Metacognitive Knowledge in Listening: A Survey Study Zeng Yajun and Zeng Yi	2975
379	Research on Mobile Learning Games in Engineering Graphics Education Huang Chen, Liang Chen, Jinchang Chen and Jin Xu	2981
380	Design and Implementation of a New Generation of Service-Oriented Graduate Enrollment System Shao Zhenglong, Li Yanxia and Zhong Wenfeng	2987
381	Research on the Quality of Life of Cancer Patients Based on Music Therapy He Wei	2995
382	Design, Synthesis and Biological Evaluation of the Novel Antitumor Agent 2H-benzo[b][1, 4]oxazin-3(4H)-one and Its Derivatives Huanhuan Li, Kailin Han, Qiannan Guo, Fengxi Liu, Peng Yu and Yuou Teng	3003
383	On Structural Model of Knowledge Points in View of Intelligent Teaching Jun Li	3013
384	Evaluation Model of Medical English Teaching Effect Based on Item Response Theory Lanfen Ji, Dianjun Lu and Dianxiang Lu	3019
385	Discussion on Intervention of Chinese Culture in Chinese College Students' English Writing and Dealing Strategies Ruxiang Ye	3025
386	Investigation and Analysis of Undergraduate Students' Critical Thinking Ability in College of Stomatology Lanzhou University Li ZhiGe, Wang Xuefeng, Zhang Yulin, Weng Wulian, WuFan Bieke, Na Li and Liu Bin	3033

387	Surgeons' Experience in Reviewing Computer Tomography Influence the Diagnosis Accuracy of Blunt Abdominal Trauma 3039
	Sun Libo, Xu Meng, Chen Lin, Su Yanzhuo, Li Chang and Shu Zhenbo

388	Analysis of Face Recognition Methods in Linear Subspace.... 3045
	Hongmei Li, Dongming Zhou and Rencan Nie

389	Energy Dispersive X-Ray Spectroscopy of HMG-CoA Synthetase During Essential Oil Biosynthesis Pathway in *Citrus grandis* 3053
	She-Jian Liang, Ping Zheng, Han Gao and Ke-Ke Li

390	The Method Research on *Tuber* spp. DNA in Soil 3059
	Yong-jun Fan, Fa-Hu Li, Yan-Lin Zhao and Wei Yan

391	The Impact of Modern Information Technology on Medical Education 3065
	Zifen Guo, Yong Feng and Honglin Huang

392	In the Platform of the Practice Teaching Link, Study on Environmental Elite Education 3071
	Yu Caihong, Huang Ying, Xu Dongyao, He Xuwen, Wang Jianbing and Yu Yan

393	The Application of a Highly Available and Scalable Operational Architecture in Course Selection System 3077
	Yanxia Li, Zhang Yu, Peng Yu, Chun Yu and Zhenglong Shao

394	Network Assisted Teaching Model on Animal Histology and Embryology 3083
	Xin Ma, Yunjiao Zhao, Limin Wang, Aidong Qian and Winmin Luan

395	Research on Application of Artificial Immune System in 3G Mobile Network Security 3089
	Dongming Zhao

396	Neuromorphology: A Case Study Based on Data Mining and Statistical Techniques in an Educational Setting 3095
	F. Maiorana

397	Construction and Practice of P.E. Network Course Based on Module Theory in University .... Xin-Ping Zhang and Dong-Hai Wu	3103
398	Application and Practice of LAMS-Based Intercultural Communication Teaching .... Bin Long and Jinxi Li	3111
399	A Study on Using Authentic Video in Listening Course ...... Yan Dou	3117
400	Comparison of Two Radio Systems for Health Remote Monitoring Systems in Rural Areas.................... Manuel García Sánchez, Rubén Nocelo López and José Antonio Gay-Fernández	3125
401	3D Ear Shape Feature Optimal Matching Using Bipartite Graph .... Xiaopeng Sun, Wang Xingyue, Guan Wang, Feng Han and Lu Wang	3133
402	Research on Anti-Metastasis Effect of Emodin on Pancreatic Cancer .... Haishuai Yu	3139
403	Research on Chronic Alcoholic Patients with Nerve Electrophysiology .... He Wei	3145
404	Genetic Dissection of *Pax6* Through GeneNetwork.......... Hong Lu and Lu Lu	3151
405	Impact of Scan Duration on PET/CT Maximum Standardized Uptake Value Measurement .... Qiuping Fan, Minggang Su and Luyi Zhou	3157
406	16-Slice Spiral Computer Tomography and Digital Radiography: Diagnosis of Ankle and Foot Fractures .... Hanqing Zhang, Liangzhou Xu, Peng Wang, Huang Bo, Jian Liu, Xiaojun Dong, Nianzu Ye, Wang Fei and Peng Gu	3163

407 Structural SIMilarity and Spatial Frequency Motivated Atlas Database Reduction for Multi-atlas Segmentation 3169
Yaqian Zhao and Aimin Hao

408 Some Reflections on Undergraduate Computer Graphics Teaching 3175
Shanshan Gao and Caiming Zhang

409 The Application of the Morris Water Maze System to the Effect of Ginsenoside Re on the Learning and Memory Disorders and Alzheimer's Disease 3181
Tie Hong, Shunan Liu, Liangjiao Di, Ning Zhang and Xiangfeng Wang

410 The Application of HYGEYA in Hospital's Antimicrobial Drugs Management...................... 3191
Xiangfeng Wang, Xiujuan Fu, Dasheng Zhu, Yadan Chen, Tie Hong, Shunan Liu, Liangjiao Di and Ning Zhang

411 The Analysis of Wavelet De-Noising on ECG............... 3197
Dongxin Lu, Qi Teng and Da Chen

412 Research of Education Training Model by Stages for College Students' Information Literacy 3205
Jinyuan Zhou and Tianling Zhou

413 Effect of Bufei Granules on the Levels of Serum Inflammatory Markers in Rats with Chronic Obstructive Pulmonary Disease Stable Phase................................. 3213
Sijia Guo, Zengtao Sun, Enshun Liu, Jihong Feng, Wei Liu, Peng Guan and Jingshen Su

414 Design of Remote Medical Monitoring System.............. 3221
Dongxin Lu and Yuanbo Qin

415 Development of University Information Service 3227
Chun Yu, Fang Yuan and JunYang Feng

416 Adaptive Tracking Servo Control for Optical Data Storage Systems 3235
Zhizheng Wu, Yang Li, Fei Peng and Mei Liu

417	Optimal Focus Servo Control for Optical Data Storage Systems .... Zhizheng Wu, Qingxi Jia, Lu Wang and Mei Liu	3241
418	Curriculum Design of Algorithms and Data Structures Based on Creative Thinking .... Chen Weiwei, Li Zhigang, Chen Weidong, Li Qing, Tang Yanqin, Wu Yongfen and Shi Lei	3247
419	Questionnaire Design and Analysis of Online Teaching and Learning: A Case Study of the Questionnaire of "Education Online" Platform of Beijing University of Technology............................ Shidong Xu, Shuyi Zhou, Qian Cao, Jin Lei, Xiaoyong Li and Yuhu He	3253
420	The Application of Telemedicine Technology.............. Ming-gang Wang, Ying-jun Mao and Wei Li	3261
421	A Method of Data Flow Diagram Drawing Based on Word Segmentation Technique...................... Shuli Yuwen and Kaifei Wang	3269
422	Chemical Reaction Optimization for Nurse Rostering Problem .... Ziran Zheng and Xiaoju Gong	3275
423	Survey of Network Security Situation Awareness and Key Technologies.............................. Zhang Xuan	3281
424	Mining ESP Teaching Research Data Using Statistical Analysis Method: Using One-Sample t Test as an Example ... Yicheng Wang and Mingli Chen	3287
425	Research on the Impact of Experiential Teaching Mode on the Cultivation of Marketing Talents .... Jia Cai and Hui Guan	3293
426	Lung Segmentation for CT Images Based on Mean Shift and Region Growing................................ Huang Zhanpeng, Yi Faling and Zhao Jie	3301

427	The Application of Psychological Teaching Combined with Daily Life: The Role of the Internet. Chuanhua Gu	3307
428	Developing a Pilot Online Learning and Mentorship Website for Nurses. Sue Coffey and Charles Anyinam	3313
429	Estrogenic and Antiestrogenic Activities of Protocatechic Acid. Fang Hu, Junzhi Wang, Huajun Luo, Ling Zhang, Youcheng Luo, Wenjun Sun, Fan Cheng, Weiqiao Deng, Zhangshuang Deng and Kun Zou	3319
430	A Study on Learning Style Preferences of Chinese Medical Students. Yuemin Ding, Jianxiang Liu and Xiong Zhang	3329
431	Design and Implementation of the Virtual Experiment System. Liyan Chen, Qingqi Hong, Beizhan Wang and Qingqiang Wu	3335
432	Application of Simulation Software in Mobile Communication Course. Fangni Chen and Zhongpeng Wang	3341
433	Study on the Effect of Astragalus Polysaccharide on Function of Erythrocyte in Tumor Model Mice. Chen-Feng Ji, Yu-bin Ji and Zheng Xiang	3347
434	Anti-Diabetes Components in Leaves of Yacon. Zheng Xiang, Chen-Feng Ji, De-Qiang Dou and Kuo Gai	3353
435	Nitric Oxide Donor Regulated mRNA Expressions of LTC4 Synthesis Enzymes in Hepatic Ischemia Reperfusion Injury Rats. FF Hong, CS He, GL Tu, FX Guo, XB Chen and SL Yang	3359
436	An Optimal In Vitro Model for Evaluating Anaphylactoid Mediator Release Induced by Herbal Medicine Injection. Zheng Xiang, Chen-Feng Ji, De-Qiang Dou and Hang Xiao	3367

437	Change Towards Creative Society: A Developed Knowledge Model for IT in Learning M. Yu, C. Zhou and W. Xing	3373
438	TCM Standard Composition and Component Library: Sample Management System Erwei Liu, Yan Huo, Zhongxin Liu, Lifeng Han, Tao Wang and Xiumei Gao	3379
439	The Teaching Method of Interrogation in Traditional Chinese Diagnostics Jingjing Fu, Haixia Yan and He Jiancheng Ding Jie	3389
440	Designing on system of Quality Monitoring on Instruction Actualizing Zhang Yan	3395
441	Comparisons of Diagnosis for Occult Fractures with Nuclear Magnetic Resonance Imaging and Computerized Tomography Ying Li, Huo-Yan Wu, Zhi-Qiang Jiang and Zhang-Song Ou	3401
442	Identifying Questions Written in Thai from Social Media Group Communication Chadchadaporn Pukkaew and Kanchana Kanchanasut	3409
443	A Programming Related Courses' E-learning Platform Based on Online Judge Xiaonan Fang, Huaxiang Zhang and Yunchen Sun	3419
444	Leading and Guiding Role of Supervisors in Graduate Education Administration Huaqiang Zhang, Xinsheng Wang and Hannan Fang	3425
445	Development of Dental Materials Network Course Based on Student-Centered Learning Shibao Li, Xinyi Zhao, Lihui Tang and Xu Gong	3429
446	Research and Practice of Practical Teaching Model Based on the Learning Interest Tao Gao, Bo Long, Pingan Du and Yefei Li	3435

447	Developing and Applying Video Clip and Computer Simulation to Improve Student Performance in Medical Imaging Technologist Education............ Lisha Jiang, Houfu Deng and Luyi Zhou	3441
448	Research on the Quality of Life of Patients with Depression Based on Psychotherapy................................ Zhou Xiaoqiu	3447
449	On Systematic Tracking of Common Problems Experienced by Students.. Sylvia Encheva	3453
450	Research on Nerve Electrophysiology of Chronic Pharyngitis Based on Automobile Exhaust Pollution......... Chunxin Dong	3457
451	The Status and Challenge of Information Technology in Medical Education.................................... Jun Li, Ming Zhao and Guang Zhao	3463
452	The Comparison of Fetal ECG Extraction Methods......... Zhongliang Luo, Jingguo Dai and Zhuohua Duan	3469
453	Study on Evaluation Index System of Hotel Practice Base Based on Bias Analysis and Reliability and Validity Test..... Changfeng Yin	3475
454	Improvement on Emergency Medical Service System Based on Class Analysis on Global Four Cases............ Zhe Li and Feng Hai	3483
455	Educational Data Mining for Problem Identification........ Sylvia Encheva	3491
456	Statistics Experiment Base on Excel in Statistics Education: Taking Zhejiang Shuren University as Example............ Wenjie Li, Yitao Wang and Guowei Wan	3495
457	Simulating the Space Deep Brain Stimulations Using a Biophysical Model................................ Yingyuan Chen, Fei Su, Jiang Wang, Xile Wei and Bin Deng	3501

458	Strategy and Analysis of Emotional Education into the Cooperative Learning in Microcomputers Teaching .... Dongxing Wang	3507
459	Construction and Practice of Network Platform for Training of GPs .... Gang Liu, Guochun Xiang, Heqing Huang, Junsheng Ji, Hong Chen, Haitao Guo, Biyuan Li, You Li, Guangqiong Liu, Zegui Li and Kehou Wang	3513
460	Research on the Construction of Regional Medical Information Service Platform .... Qun Wang, Chuang Ma, Yong Yu and Gen Zhu	3519
461	Study on the Application of Simulation Technology in the Medical Teaching .... Yong Yu, Xiaolin Chen, Qun Wang and Gen Zhu	3525
462	Desynchronization of Morris: Lecar Network via Robust Adaptive Artificial Neural Network .... Yingyuan Chen, Jiang Wang, Xile Wei, Bin Deng, Haitao Yu, Fei Su and Ge Li	3531
463	Building and Sharing of Information Resources in Radio and TV Universities Libraries Under Network Environment .... Liu Juan and Wang Jing-na	3537
464	Research on Network Information Resources Integration Services in Medicine Library .... Zhang Li-min	3543
465	Applied Research of Ultrasound Microbubble in Tumor-Transferred Lymph Node Imaging and Treatment .... Xin Zhao and Guijie Li	3549
466	The Examination of Landau-Lifshitz Pseudo-Tensor Under Physical Decomposition of Gravitational Field .... Peng-Cheng Zhang, Jia Guo, Jun Zhao and Ben-Chao Zhu	3555

467 Exploring of the Integration Design Method of Rectal Prolapse TCM Clinical Pathway System 3561
Zhihui Huang

Author Index 3567

Chapter 212
Application of Data Mining in the Assessment of Teaching Quality

Huabin Qu and Xueqing Li

Abstract More and more attention paid to the teaching quality of college, the assessment of the teaching quality is of great importance. Traditional teaching evaluation methods have a lot of deficiencies, not identifying what factors are really bound up with the quality of teaching. This paper applies the improved Apriori algorithm QApriori based on data mining technology to teaching evaluation model. On the foundation of data mining definition, mining processes, common data mining methods-Apriori and its improved algorithm-QApriori, this thesis emphasizes study on QApriori in the teaching evaluation model. Through the analysis of data mining, we have come to what factors are mainly related with the teaching quality, which will be very important to teaching and education policy-makers.

Keywords Teaching quality evaluation · Data mining · Association rules · Qapriori

212.1 Introduction

Large-scale enrollment in higher education, on the one hand has provided people with more access to higher education, while on the other hand, students' quality is bound to decline due to the relative reduction of educational resources. Therefore, strengthening the building of faculty, and strengthening the quality of teaching evaluation is of great significance. However, teaching evaluation methods are almost used to just evaluate the level of teaching quality bad or good, which is difficult to explain what factors are related with the teaching level really, that is, it

H. Qu (✉) · X. Li
Shandong University, Jinan, China
e-mail: qhbsky@126.com

is difficult to indicate our teachers in which features, quality of teaching will be relatively high. Especially with the rapid development of computer technology, and the widely used database management system, more and more data is accumulated, but it is not easy to discover hidden relationships in the large data and rules.

Data mining is a decision support process, extracting implicit but potentially useful information and knowledge from a large number of incomplete, noisy, fuzzy and random data. Data mining is the process to find useful information in large data repository automatically [1]. Data mining as a analysis method of deep level applied in the evaluation of the teaching is undoubtedly very useful, analyzing the hidden intrinsic link between the standard of teaching with a variety of factors comprehensively, for example, after the analysis of the data in the database system of teaching evaluation, similar problems can be answered, such as "What are the factors that may affect the level of teacher's teaching", which traditional evaluation methods can not have.

212.2 Data Mining

212.2.1 Concept of Data Mining

Data Mining as an indispensible step of knowledge discovery in databases [2] generally refers to a process that automatically searches hidden information which has a special relationship from the large amount of data process. In other words, that is a process extracting implied, unknown in advance but potentially useful information and knowledge from a large number of incomplete, noisy, fuzzy and random data.

212.2.2 The Process of Data Mining

Data mining process includes the definition of the problem, data preparation, data mining, results analysis and the use of knowledge as shown in Fig. 212.1.

212.2.3 The improvement of Apriori algorithm: QApriori

There are many methods of data mining, including association rules, clustering analysis, decision tree method, and neural grid method and so on. However, the most common is association rules. Apriori algorithm is one of the most influential algorithms of frequent item sets mining Boolean association rules [3]. QApriori

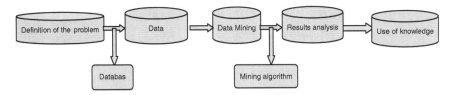

Fig. 212.1 Data mining process

Unlike classic Apriori algorithm data structure uses linked list. There are three nodes, respectively; the itemsets head node, entry node and transaction node. One-level brother node of a linked list ascend order from left to right in accordance with the support count of subset and the benefits of doing so is that even if 1-itemsets is great, it will only produce few candidate 2-itemsets and then generate fewer candidate 3-itemsets, and much fewer go on, the candidate sets will be greatly reduced, thereby system performance is greatly improved. The basic idea of Algorithm QApriori: The improved algorithm QApriori using the data structure of linked list, the head node of k-itemsets K-itemSetHead1 has two pointers, one points the first node K-itemSetNode1 of k-itemsets, and the other points the head nodes of (k + 1)-itemsets. Each item Node also has two pointers, one pointer to the first transaction of the transaction set, and the other to the next node. Transaction node AKN has a pointer which points to the next transaction node. The building process of the linked list is as follows:

(1) The entry node K-itemSetNode1 points ascend order from left to right in accordance with the 1-subset support that will produce fewer candidate sets.
(2) Scan and connect all the 1-itemset nodes according to the order of increasing support, and at the same time merge the same affairs AKN to generate 2-itemset nodes.
(3) Scan and connect all the 2-itemset nodes according to the order of increasing support, and at the same time merge the same affairs AKN to generate 3-itemset nodes.
(4) And so on until new item nodes are not generated.

212.3 Teaching Quality Assessment Model

The quality of teaching has associated with many factors, and we selected eleven major impact indicators, including compliance disciplined, strict management; prepare lessons fully teachers; clear point of view, clear concept; featured content, update knowledge; practice, appropriate illustration; focused, coherent; individualized focus on inspiration; vivid language, easy to understand; various means, blackboard writing orderly; knowledge to grasp, capacity-building; thinking

Table 212.1 Teaching quality evaluation index and weighting coefficient

Index code	Evaluation indicator	Weighting coefficient
1	Compliance disciplined strict management	0.06
2	Prepare lessons fully teachers	0.04
3	Clear point of view clear concept	0.15
4	Featured content update knowledge	0.15
5	Practice appropriate illustration	0.08
6	Focused, coherent	0.07
7	Individualized focus on inspiration	0.12
8	Vivid language, easy to understand	0.08
9	Various means blackboard writing orderly	0.10
10	Knowledge to grasp capacity-building	0.08
11	Thinking pioneering interested inspire	0.07

pioneering interested inspire [4]. Different factors given different weights, we use $R = \Sigma Q_i P_i$ to calculate the evaluation scores for each teacher; Q is the Quantitative Evaluation index Point; W is the weighting coefficient. Weights of various impact indicators are shown in the Table 212.1.

212.4 The Application of Data Mining in Teaching Quality Assessment

212.4.1 Data Selection

We select ten teacher's evaluation data from a large number of teaching quality assessment data stored in the school's information management system. In accordance with the calculation method of teaching quality scores in III, we have come to ten teachers' fraction of the eleven evaluation indicators shown in Table 212.2. 1, 2, 3,..... 11 represent the eleven impact indicators in Table 212.1, 200799017514, 200799017970..... 200893000001 are randomly selected ten teachers.

Table 212.2 Teaching quality assessment information data

编号	1	2	3	4	5	6	7	8	9	10	11
200799017514	5.3	3.55	13.4	13.2	7.1	6.2	10.4	7	8.7	7.1	6
200799017970	5.4	3.8	13.7	13.4	7.4	6.2	10.7	7.3	7.2	7.5	6.3
200893000001	5.6	3.8	13.9	13.4	7.1	6.4	10.6	7.1	9	7.1	6.3
………..	…….	…….	…..	…….	….	…..	…….	…….	…….	…….	…….
201090000012	5.6	3.8	13.9	13.6	7.4	6.5	10.9	7.3	8.9	7.5	6.3

Table 212.3 The binary relation of the teaching quality data

AKN	a	b	c1	c2	c3	c4	d1	d2	d3	e	f	g1	g2	g3	g4	h	i	j	k
1	0	0	0	0	0	1	0	0	1	0	0	0	0	0	1	0	0	0	0
2	0	1	0	1	0	0	0	1	0	1	0	0	1	0	0	1	0	1	1
3	1	1	1	0	0	0	0	1	0	0	1	0	0	1	0	0	1	0	1
...	...	...	...	...	...	...	...	...	...	...	...	...	...	...	...	...	...	...	...
10	0	0	0	0	1	0	0	0	1	0	0	0	0	1	0	0	0	0	0
support	0.5	0.8	0.3	0.2	0.3	0.2	0.3	0.5	0.2	0.4	0.4	0.3	0.2	0.3	0.2	0.4	0.5	0.4	0.5

212.4.2 Data Processing

The evaluation Data in the Table 212.2 is all quantitative attribute. In order to make discretization, we transform it into Boolean type. The following is the transformation rule, 1——>a, segmentation a1>5.55, a2<5.55;2——>b, segmentation b1>3.65, b2<3.65;3——>c, segmentation c1>13.75,13.65<c2< 13.75,13.55<c3<13.65,c4<13.55;4——>d,segmentation d1>13.55,13.35<d2< 13.55,d3<13.35;5——>e segmentation e1>7.25,e2<7.25;6——>f segmentation f1>6.35,f2<6.35;7——>g segmentation g1>10.75,10.65<g2<10.75,10.55<g3 <10.65,g4<10.55;8——>h segmentation h1>7.15,h2<7.15;9——>i segmentation i1>8.85,i2<8.85;10——>j segmentation j1>7.25,j2<7.25;11——>k segmentation k1>6.15,k2<6.15

In order to facilitate the use of the improved algorithm QApriori,we convert the data changed above into a binary relation table. Assuming the support was 40 %, Table 212.3 shows the conversion,

Ascending the order according to the support count, we get the item set {E, F, H, J A, D2, I, K, B}, and frequent itemset 1-itemset is produced. Generating item set and so on according to the improved algorithm QApriori, frequent item set 4-itemset is emerged at last as shown in Fig. 212.2.

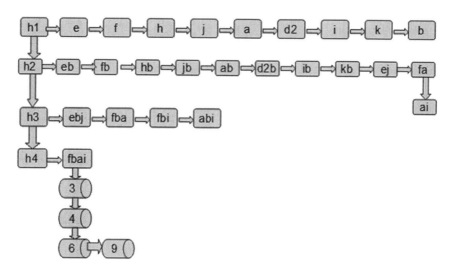

Fig. 212.2 Frequent item set 4-itemset

212.5 Conclusion

This paper describes the importance of teaching quality assessment as well as the assessment of teaching quality defects at the present, showing the advantages and concernment of data mining techniques applied to teaching quality evaluation. Analyzing the classic association rules algorithm Apriori [5] and its shortcomings, put forward an improved algorithm QApriori, and this algorithm is applied to the evaluation of teaching. Exploring several major factors influencing teaching evaluation, we have come to the conclusion that teachers who prepare lessons fully; focus, coherent; various means, blackboard writing orderly generally demand themselves and managing students strictly and the classroom atmosphere is also better. Data Mining applied to the teaching evaluation can not only make the teaching quality get a better rise, but also be more conducive to the work of the education makers.

References

1. Fayya UM, Piatetsky-ShaPiro G et al (1996) Advances in knowledge discovery and datamining. AAAI/MITPress, California
2. Wan A, Wang M, Mao W (2004) Theory and application of data mining technology. Univ Math 06:111–114
3. Agganval CC, Yu PS (1998) Mining large itemsets for association rules. Data Eng Bull 21(1):23–31
4. Yan H, Chen W (2008) Application of association rules in the analysis of student achievement. J Fujian Med Univ (Soc Sci Edn) 9(1):46–48
5. Han J, Kamber M Fan X, Meng M Concepts and techniques of data mining

Chapter 213
A Data Mining System for Herbal Formula Compatibility Analysis

Li Jinghua, Feng Yi, Yu Tong, Liu Jing, Zhu Ling, Dong Yan, Shuo Yang, Lirong Jia, Bo Gao and Gao Hongjie

Abstract In this paper, to mine herb compatibility and especially how formula emerges by some herb combination, we propose a improved association rule algorithm based on herbs frequency and combination, so all the compatibility relationship is displayed in a tree structure, based on which a new data mining system is introduced to analyze the compatibility of herbal formulae in traditional Chinese medicine. This system is mainly based on a tree-based method, and incorporates functions of data cleaning, data selection, data formatting, formula tree generating and result outputting. Experimental results on datasets of viral myocarditis treatment literature in the past 10 years show that this system could serve as a useful tool for data mining of herbal formula compatibility. By which we can infer clearly the relationship of formulas and their derivation, and also shows that the core of TCM treatment of viral myocarditis are forsythia, honeysuckle and licorice root, as the core drug of treatments., to which more attentions should be paid in future pharmacology research.

Keywords Herb · Traditional Chinese medicine · Formula compatibility · Data mining

213.1 Introduction

Traditional Chinese medicine (TCM) has a history of over 2,000 years protecting Chinese people healthcare, in which herb treatments is one of most useful methods. Up to now there has been almost ten thousand herbs applied to patients for

L. Jinghua · F. Yi (✉) · Y. Tong · L. Jing · Z. Ling · D. Yan · S. Yang · L. Jia · B. Gao · G. Hongjie
School of Computer Science and Information Engineering, Zhejiang Gongshang University, Hangzhou 310018, People's Republic of China
e-mail: yfeng@mail.zjgsu.edu.cn

cure all kinds illness. Some herbal combinations with great curative effect are preserved by doctors as formula. Formula, for some extent, is main format for herbal treatment, but we can't accurately explain how multiple herbs form as various kind of formulae.

In this paper, a new data mining system is introduced to analyze the compatibility of herbal formulae in traditional Chinese medicine. This system is mainly based on a tree-based method, and incorporates functions of data cleaning, data selection, data formatting, formula tree generating and result outputting. Experimental results on datasets of viral myocarditis treatment literature in the past 10 years show that this system could serve as a useful tool for data mining of herbal formula compatibility.

213.2 How Formula is Formed

As early as 2,000 years ago, TCM began using herbs to treat disease, and progressed from single herbs to several herbs, from simple combination to complex combination. Over the course of more than 2,000 years, Formulae were constantly tested and continuously applied and improved in the clinical activities, resulting in the creation of the more than ten thousand standard Formulae known today.

Despite there are too many Formulae, we can reckon by mind that the fundamental method forming Formulae: first, an appropriate "base prescription" is chosen according to the given disease syndrome, and then modifications (additions and subtractions) are made depending upon specific signs and symptoms that often vary from individual to individual or change over the course of the disease.

For instance, to the formula Sì Jūn Zǐ Tāng (Four Gentlemen Decoction), bàn xià (Rhizoma Pinelliae) and chén pí (Pericarpium Citri Reticulatae) can be added and form Liù Jūn Zǐ Tāng (Six Gentlemen Decoction), and mù xiāng (Radix Aucklandiae) and shā rén (Fructus Amomi) can be added to Liù Jūn Zǐ Tāng to form Xiāng Shā Liù Jūn Zǐ Tāng (Costusroot and Amomum Six Gentlemen Decoction); and Sì Jūn Zǐ Tāng (Four Gentlemen Decoction) plus Sì Wù Tāng (Four Substances Decoction) constitutes Bā Zhēn Tāng (Eight-Gem Decoction), and so on.

213.3 Why Study on Formula Compatibility

The compatibility, explaining herbal relations in Formulae using TCM theory, is the core of why herbal treatment is effective. In a series of Formulae, some herbs always exist and act as important role, which usually defined as core herb combinations. The effectiveness of core combinations of herbs has been deeply recognized in practice, and their applications are continuously expanding, thus yielding more and more target-specific treatment protocols; therefore, basic formula may have some certain associations with corresponding disease or syndrome in essential. If a basic prescription is found within a series of Formulae that treat similar disease or syndrome, it may indicate that the basic formula has a strong correlation to the nature of the disease or syndrome, and also suggests that the basic formula may be effective in the treatment of the disease in most cases [1].

213.4 Algorithm for Formula Compatibility

In this research we designed an algorithm to mine the compatibility of Formulae cluster by graphical way. In Formulae cluster on one same illness, there are many herbs, most of which are repeated. Herbs combining into Formulae exist in their own rules: first, several important herbs are chosen as base formula according to the essence of the disease; then, modifications (additions and subtractions) are made depending upon specific signs and symptoms that often vary from individual to individual or from the different course of the disease.

To mine herb compatibility and especially how formula emerges by some herb combination, we propose a improved association rule algorithm, which is designed mainly on herbs appearing frequency and their combinations, repeated herbs and their combination is forming a matrix of herbs, most frequency one is calculated out as a tree root and its combination ones continuously calculate the same way to select the next root, until no repeated herb exits the calculation ends. So all the compatibility relationship is displayed in a tree structure, by which we can infer clearly the relationship of formulae and their derivation [2].

213.5 System Design and Implementation

Based on the formula tree analysis algorithm, we design and develop a system including the function of data cleaning, data selection, data format, formula tree generating, and the results output with interactive processing. See as Fig. 213.1.

The front-end development of this system has used Java technology, through JDBC to logic control and database connection, and the back-end database is SQL Server 2000. Detail specifications are as followed.

213.5.1 Formula Data Cleaning

Data cleaning is to process the source data which is not standard, such as the standardization of inconsistent attributes values in formula data, filling the missing values in the formula data, so as to ensure the correctness of results.

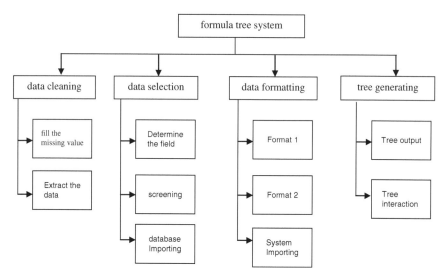

Fig. 213.1 System structure

213.5.2 Formula Data Selecting

We extract a large amount of formula data from traditional Chinese medicine literature, but these data attribute relationships are different, such as the different clinical effect, different quality grades, different composed drugs. In order to make the system output is a clinical reference value, it has the common prescription selection of some aspects, such as effect similar, similar or similar disorders treatment prescriptions and so on, which requires screening from a large number of prescription data, as the input of the system. This system can be used for data selection according to each field source data in the table, such as syndrome, quality grade, pharmaceutical composition, with accurate screening model and fuzzy screening model, and stored screening data in the database in the form of table.

213.5.3 Formula Data Formatting

The processing of formula data formatting mainly includes two aspects: extraction of drugs data as well as the data format conversion. Extraction of drugs data refers to taking the drug data extracted respectively which was originally written in the same field, such as from the field [drugs composition: drugs 1, drugs 2, drugs 3, drugs 4,…drugs n] drugs were extracted respectively. Data format transformation is to turn the formula data into the table form, and stored into the database in the table form.

213.5.4 Formula Tree Generating

This part of System includs the functions of formula tree generation and formula interaction. Formula tree generation function is the core function of this system, to process data according to certain rules format and output to display formula tree model. Formula trees interaction refers to interacting with the source data after formula trees output, when the user select leaf node prescriptions in the tree formula, system can display the ID, name, evidence level, syndrome, drug information of the prescription, which is convenient for user analyzing the formula tree.

213.6 Experimental Results

213.6.1 Viral Myocarditis Formula Data Collecting

To verify the applicability of the system, this paper selects formulae from literatures of viral myocarditis which is of relatively curative effect and of simple pathogenesis, as analysis object. After data acquisition, evidence level evaluation has been finished. See as Fig. 213.2.

213.6.2 Viral Myocarditis Formula Data Processing

System firstly determine whether the chosen data table type need conversion, if need to convert, then system will carries on the data processing, fill the missing

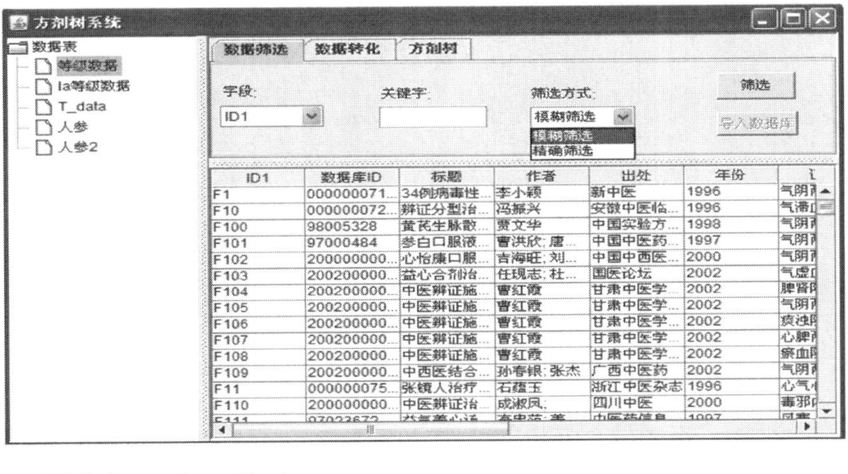

Fig. 213.2 System data collecting

value, extract contains formula drugs, and transform data type, finally data is stored into the database with table form; If not need to transform, the prompt will be given. See as Fig. 213.3.

213.6.3 Viral Myocarditis Formula Tree Generating

System will firstly detect on the selected data sheet format, if the format is correct, according to formula compatibility algorithm, system will calculate and output the formula tree, otherwise will give the that format is not correct. Formula tree output can interact with the data in the data table, displaying proprietary information. See as Fig. 213.4.

213.6.4 Result Analysis

Through system calculation, from 11 high quality treatment of viral myocarditis we achieve the core compatibility relation, six nodes including forsythia, honeysuckle, liquorice, mint, reed rhizome and bamboo leaves, make all Formulae showed as a tree structure, making the clinician got clear of key information of all the treatment, that the nodes nearer the root its' effect is larger. In this sense, forsythia, honeysuckle and licorice root are the core drug of treatments.

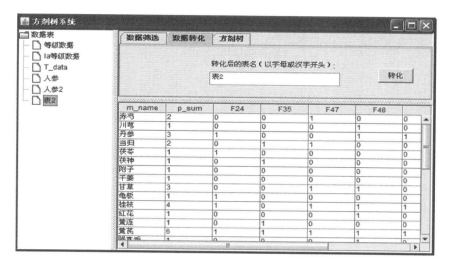

Fig. 213.3 System data processing

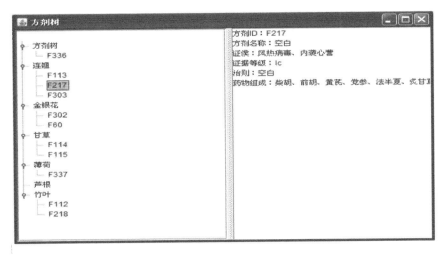

Fig. 213.4 System formula tree generating

213.7 Conclusion

This paper mainly introduces a new data mining system to analyze the compatibility of herbal formulae in traditional Chinese medicine. A new method based on formula tree is proposed and used as the core analysis method of the system. The system incorporates functions of data cleaning, data selection, data formatting, formula tree generating and result outputting. Experimental results on datasets of viral myocarditis treatment literature in the past 10 years show that this system could serve as a useful tool for data mining of herbal formula compatibility.

As a powerful tool, data mining could be applied to acquire knowledge from huge amounts of data, which could as a result improve the academic level of TCM and promote modern research progress. However, at present the application of data mining technology in the field of traditional Chinese medicine is still in its infancy, and is faced with many problems and challenges. This paper is an attempt to use data mining in herbal formula compatibility. In the future we will continue to study for more effective and in-depth mining methods to analyze the massive amounts of formula data in TCM.

Acknowledgments This work is supported by National Natural Science Fund of China (NO. 60905026, NO. 81001560), Zhejiang Science and Technology Plan Project (NO. 2010C33016).

We also thank Dr. Li Jinghua design the framework for the study, Dr. Feng Yi made the improvement of the algorithm, Dr. Yu Tong and Du Xiaolong for developing the software, Dr. Dong Yan, Dr. Zhu Ling and Mrs. Gao Hongjie for polishing this article.

References

1. Li JH, Cui M (2010) Study on algorithm and application of prescription compatibility relation. China Digital Med 5:42–44
2. Cui M, Li JH, Li HY et al (2010) Herbal compatibility of traditional Chinese medical formulas for acquired immunodeficiency syndrome. J Tradit Chinese Med 32(3):329–334

Chapter 214
The Analysis of the Chronic Patients' Demand of the Hospital Health Information Service

Guiling Li, Liqun Yang, Lin Ding, Runbin Wu, Chundi Zhang, Limei Guo and Xiumei Ma

Abstract Information service is the imperative problem that department of health need to resolve,how To provide better services to patients and make harmonious relationship of each other is an issue that we have been studying for a long time. Taking an example of the Chronic patients to research the impact factors of the communication between doctor and patient based on de information communication theory to resolve the problem reasonably.

Keywords The chronic patients information · Requirements Information · Communication information services

Chronic disease is a kind of disease that does not constitute a spread and has accumulated for a long period form damage, mainly caused by the bad behavior habits, lifestyle, environmental pollutants exposure, the long-term neglect of psychological health and balance accumulating occurring in the course of disease. The disease causes large risk of disability and death. Without timely treatment, it will pose a threat to life and property [1].

Health information service is an activity that health department provide needed information using different ways. A task of health information service is providing information to patients. At the same time, it can help patients understand their illness and make doctors know how to treat the disease. A task of medical service is providing high quality medical information service to the patients to make them take participate in treatment actively. In the meantime, it's personnel's duty to provide safe and convenient information services for patients. Taking an example of the Chronic patients to research the impact factors of the communication between doctor and patient based on de information communication theory to realize patient satisfaction.

G. Li (✉) · L. Yang · L. Ding · R. Wu · C. Zhang ·
LimeiGuo · X. Ma
Nursing Institute of Qiqihaer Medical University, Heilongjiang 161006, China
e-mail: wnllgl@sohu.com

Once the information need to be aware of as information demand. Information need is the feeling of dissatisfaction and necessary when people want to solve various practical problems in the practice. Information requirements are divided into potential information needs and information needs of reality. Most of the patients with chronic diseases, especially cancer patients want to know their condition [2]. There are many ways for people to get the source of information, but in hospital, patients want to get information of their disease in doctors and nurses, so it's particularly important to enhance the Information communication between doctor and patient.

1. Theoretical basis and communication mode of the Information communication between doctor and patient.

Information exchange is a symbol system which can be used by people for Information transmission and feedback in some special channels and ways. A pronounced feature of information communication is biphasic. It's a media to realize information exchange and communication between subject and object through the communication which different from the essence of information transfer and information transmission properties. The other feature of information communication is purposeful. Information realize the value of it when people obtain information through communication. Meanwhile, it can promote the use of information and regeneration. The third feature of information communication is targeted. Information exchange is according to the needs and interests of both sides to communicate. The fourth feature of information communication is timeliness. In the process of information communication the timely information feedback is very important. If the information feedback time is too long not only lose communication practical significance and easily lead to interruption of communication.

The fifth feature of information communication is solid righteousness. Information exchange needed a certain symbol, but the connotation of the essence of communication is indicated by the symbol. In order to better reveal the basic rule of communication and guide the practice of information exchange. American politician Lasswell put forward the five basic elements of communication called 5 W mode [3].

But this model is flawed, It doesn't pay attention to the feedback from the elements and ignore the influence of environment on information exchange.

2. Patients with access to medical information and their requirements Patients need to get some information like checking, diagnosis, treatment, rehabilitation care and daily life supplies. The main way to provide information is by medical personnel and medical personnel have a responsibility to do it by the way they can accept it easily. Patients need sincerely listen to the doctor and doctors need to timely feedback problems raised on the patients. Doctors should be able to explain in detail everything that is associated with disease and give suggestions which are beneficial to the treatment and rehabilitation of patients in order to increase the satisfaction of patients [4].

3. The factors that affect the doctor-patient information exchange what the patient needs.

3.1 The aspect of the medical staff. The medical staff has low-income, heavy workload and high risk. The doctor receives a large number of patients per day, making the time that the doctor communicates with the patient is greatly shortened, combined with a strong position by the traditional medical side and work mentality, and improve their own quality ability to pressure, emotional impact, making the weakening of the information on the patient's behavior; thinking of the traditional doctor-patient relationship management model potential patients are sick, need help, incapacity groups, the patients can only passively accept the arrangements of the hospital, management alike, no differences in patient population targeted communication and management, so that the decline in patient satisfaction;

3.2 The aspect of the patient. Different aspects of patients suffering from the disease in patients with and knowledge of the behavior of the ability to understand there is a great difference, and most of the mutual information in information asymmetry, some doctors use jargon in the information exchange, due to the patient's individual big difference, the ability to receive information, resulting in poor information exchange; likely to cause frequent doctor-patient conflicts upgrade and medical malpractice, to establish and maintain the harmonious relationship between doctors and patients seriously affected.

3.3 The neglect of timely feedback to patient information. Patients in the hospital during treatment need to get good medical services, establish harmony between doctors and patients, so that the disease as soon as possible is cured, therefore, it requires mutual understanding and communication between doctors and patients, and more consideration from the other point of view, patients after consumption of medical services are satisfied or dissatisfied with the two results, if being satisfied with medical services, the patient may be to other patients with publicity and repeat consumption, if being not satisfied, the patient may choose to leave or complain and so on. The traditional management model, hospitals will focus in the process of providing services for patients, is an active–passive doctor-patient relationship, the hospital unilaterally makes feedback and evaluation, and neglects patients for medical services feedback. Third, the discussion

Chronic disease has become a major public health problem what is harmful to the health of our people, because of its morbidity and mortality what has been a clear upward trend, including malignant tumors, cardiovascular disease, cerebrovascular disease, respiratory disease had been listed the top four cause of death of the Chinese residents [5].

Facing the grim situation of chronic disease, Health Minister Chen Zhu in the 2011 towel countries chronic disease prevention and control Forum cum Chinese health Union at the inaugural meeting, considered that China had presented a chronic disease "blowout" situation. The main results of the Fourth National Health Services Survey released by the Ministry of Health showed clear diagnosis of the number of cases of chronic diseases reached 260 million in 2008, circulatory system disease cases from 037 million in 1993 to 114 million over two hypertensive patients billion, and increased to 7,000,000 annually; By the year of 2009, chronic disease accounts for the death of the Chinese population constitutes up to

85 %, the World Bank in 2011 considered that the chronic disease has become the number one health threat in China, if not timely take effective strategy By 2030, the number of Chinese people over the age of 40, suffering from diabetes, cardiovascular disease, cancer and chronic respiratory diseases will increase 2–3 times [6].

As WHO Director-General Margaret Chan said, today's chronic diseases are no longer just a medical issue, it is no longer just a public problem. Chronic diseases are a development issue, a political issue, can be seen in chronic non-communicable diseases has been a serious threat to people's health, positive prevention is very important.

We focused on hospitalized chronic disease health information what needs to be analysed, the theoretical basis of the above chart information exchange model point of view, in the hospital, both patients and health care workers need to dissemination of information to each other and produce good results, provide timely feedback, overcome the unfavorable factors in the exchange of medical personnel, the health care must communicate with patients according to the patient's needs in a timely manner, because of the chronic patients contains cancer patients, therefore, the health care should be based on the patient's different, providing patients with appropriate medical solutions, and establish a good doctor-patient communication, so that patients recover as soon as possible.

Management of patients with differentiated classification must depend on the individual patient so that the differentiated management is closer to the patient's needs. Timely processing of patient complaints and timely feedback to the needs of patients, at the same time, and understanding the changes in the condition in communication with patients can make the medical staff to give the active treatment. As a result, the patients recovered earlier.

References

1. Ren J (2011) Research on community health service: based on perspective from NCD patients demand. Master's thesis, p 5
2. Huang X, Butow PN, Meiser B et al (1999) Attitudes and information needs of Chinese migrant cancer patients and their relatives. Aust NZ J Med 29:207–213
3. Luo A (2012) Health information management. People's Medical Publishing House, Beijing, p 8
4. Zhang X (2008) Doctor-patient communication skills in clinical application. China's Practical Med 3(19):163–165
5. In 2008 China health statistics [R], The web site of the ministry of health
6. Chen R (2012) The study of behavioral intervention noncommunicable disease risk factors control based on health promotion. Doctoral dissertation, Shandong University, 5.26

Chapter 215
Learning from Errors and Learning from Failures: A Study on the Model of Organizational Learning from Errors

Yangqun Xie, Jianian Zhang and Xiangzhi Zhuo

Abstract Errors is ubiquitous and unavoidable in the process of organizational production, serving and management. Once the exterior trigger conditions are met, they could lead to organizational failure. Up to now, though there are a few studies about learning from failures, there are few studies of learning from errors in the area of organizational learning. Firstly, this paper clarifies the relations among learning from errors, learning from failures and organization learning, with emphasis on learning from errors a very important resource of organization learning. Secondly, this paper also puts forward the learning models and processes of learning from errors in organization. Its aim arises more attention to be paid to them.

Keywords Learning from errors · Learning from failure · Organizational learning

215.1 Introduction

Organization consists of pluralistic individuals with diversity of cultural background, knowledge base, mental state, and communication skills, etc. Everyone can make errors because of lacking of relevant knowledge, shortcoming of training, working pressure, and so on. As a Chinese proverb says: nobody is perfect, and everybody may make mistake. There is the same meaning of "to err is human" in the Latin language. These words illuminate that errors is ubiquitous. Therefore, errors is unavoidable in the process of production, management and services, furthermore, it is impossible to be fully eradicated in organization.

Y. Xie (✉) · X. Zhuo
Management School of Huaibei Normal University, No. 100, Dongshan St, Huaibei 235000, China
e-mail: xieyangqun1980@163.com

J. Zhang
Educational School of Huaibei Normal University, Huaibei 235000, Anhui, China

The results of errors can be much different from one another. Some errors' emergence do not lead to any ill consequences. For example, a builder without a safety helmet entered construction site and worked a day. Though there was not emergence of injuring his or her safety, the error behavior was taken place. Some errors give birth to slips. For example, a nurse gave a more tablet to patient who took them and did not unfold serious consequence. Though some errors have the tendency of grievous aftermaths, they are detected timely and adopted recovery measures i.e., near-miss. For example, when nurse gave medicines to patient, she found the dosage of a kind of medication increased 1,000 times than usual. After communicated with physician and pharmaceutists of pharmacy, they confirmed that pharmaceutists misread the dosage and a possible critical incident was avoided. Some errors can result in disasters which called failures. For example, The Space Shuttle Challenger disaster occurred on January 28, 1986. Disintegration of the entire vehicle began after an O-ring seal in its right solid rocket booster (SRB) failed at lift-off. The Rogers Commission found NASA's organizational culture and decision-making processes had been key contributing factors to the accident (Wikipedia). The Chernobyl disaster was a catastrophic nuclear accident that occurred on 26 April 1986 at the Chernobyl Nuclear Power Plant in Ukraine, which was under the direct jurisdiction of the central authorities of the Soviet Union. There were two official explanations of the accident: the first, later acknowledged to be erroneous, the catastrophic accident was caused by gross violations of operating rules and regulations. The second is operating instructions and design deficiencies found (Wikipedia).

Failures are the serious results of a few erroneous behaviours which caused of less cognitive effort. In studies of organizational learning, there are many studies focusing on learning from failures [1–3]. These studies showed that the organization should learn from failures of themselves or others and draw lessons in order to avert the similar failures occurrence. By comparison, studies of learning from errors are infrequent. Although errors resulted in failures should be attached to more attention, there are massive errors that are concealed or not uncovered just as the iceberg below sea level. This chapter tries to integrate learning from failures and learning from errors into organizational learning from organizational learning, and construct the model of learning from errors in organization for advancing the performance levels of production, management and services.

215.2 Relations Among Learning from Errors, Learning from Failures and Organizational

215.2.1 Learning from Errors

From the perspective of problem-solving, Zhao [4] proposed advanced learning from errors as the process through which individuals (a) reflect on errors that they have made, (b) locate the root causes of the errors, (c) develop knowledge about action–outcome relationships and the effects of these relationships on the work environment, and (d) use this knowledge to modify or improve their behavior or decision making. From this perspective, learning from errors is an effortful activity—it involves purposeful reflection on, and analysis of, errors and application of new knowledge into decisions or actions [4], p. 436).[1] The content of learning from errors includes contextual information of errors emergence, status information of the operator, information of operative environment, detecting information, reporting information, corrected information of errors, and so on.

Through information accessing, arranging, analyzing and attributing, the deficiency of knowledge could be found in organization system. For example, is instruction of production perfect? Is the organizational structure adaptive to new technology application? Is there unreasonable part in organizational management? Are there any problems in the training system of employees' knowledge and skills in organization? Just as Deming pointed out that the managers should bear the 85 % responsibility of the quality problem, and the operator should only bear the 15 % responsibility [5]. From this point of view, once errors are found in organization, organization should bear more responsibilities, and prompt organizational learning and transformation in knowledge management, organizational structure, organizational system, organizational production mode, etc.

215.2.2 Organizational Learning

The definition of learning is accessing knowledge by self-regulation learning and self experiences, an art of pertaining and applying knowledge, skills, abilities, attitudes and standpoint, a transformation of experience-based behavior [6]. The true learning arises in the obvious behavior, and expresses through behavior changing. Learning also embodies in reflecting on individual experience and drawing lessons from the results.

What is organizational learning? [7] suggested organizational learning "as any modification of an organization's knowledge occurring as a result of its experience" (p. 453). Goal of organizational learning is to facilitate organization accommodating the change of internal and external environment, and constantly renew and improve its performance level and abilities, thereby realizing the organizational goal. According to Marquardt's viewpoint: adaptive learning will happen, when individual and organization learn from the experience and reflection [8]. The content of organizational learning is mainly from their experience [9], Organizations constantly seek new ways to improve their processes and outcomes. Their success depends largely on their capacity to learn from their experiences [10, 11]. The experiences include successes, failures and errors.

---

[1] B. Zhao [5]. Learning from errors: The role of context, emotion, and personality. Journal of Organizational Behavior. 32, 436.

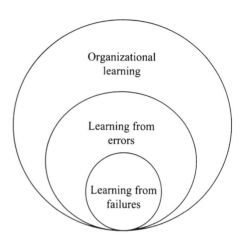

Fig. 215.1 Relations of learning from failures, learning from errors and organizational learning

215.2.3 Learning from Failure

Learning from failure is the process that organization analyses, summarizes and finds out the failure during their production, service and management, thus putting forward the countermeasure to avoid the same failure in the future. For example, the organization can do things like increasing efforts of knowledge learning and training, modifying the operational rules of organization to fit new technology and equipment, reforming system of organizational structure and strengthening the enterprise culture construction. Recent work has explored organizational learning from prior failure experience, disaggregated from total prior experience [12, 13].

However, the researches are not richer than those of learning from success. Baumard and Starbuck [2] bemoaned the scarcity of empirical studies in this domain, stating that "there have been so few studies of learning from failures" (p. 282).[2]

215.2.4 Relations of Learning from Failures, Learning from Errors and Organizational Learning

In order to clarify the relations of three areas, this paper depicts a figure (see Fig. 215.1). It contains different relations among them, hereinto. Learning from failures is a subset of learning from errors. Learning from errors is also a subset of organizational learning. Organizational learning are serious results of part of errors. Errors are those behaviors that deviate the standards, goals or rules in

---

[2] Baumard, P., & Starbuck, W. H. [2]. Learning from failures: Why it may not happen. Long Range Planning, 38, 282.

organization and some of them maybe lead to failures. The range of organizational learning is widest. In order to boost performance level and development of organization, there are two ways. On the one hand, it should constantly introduce new knowledge system, including new technology, fangles, new operational rules, new management system, etc. The aim is to update the dated knowledge On the other hand, reformation offers the opportunity for organizations to find problems and support innovation from errors and failures of themselves or others. Consequently, organization realizes disruptive innovation [14].

215.3 Model Constructing of Organizational Learning from Errors

215.3.1 Information Flow and Knowledge Flow of Organizational Learning

Before constructing the model of organizational learning from errors, we should defecate and understand the model of information flow and knowledge flow in organizational learning. Organizational learning, learning from errors and learning from failures are based on the interaction, sharing and utilizing of information. Without information flow, there is no learning. The results of organizational learning, learning from errors and learning from failures thus facilitate renewal and evolution of knowledge. Then organizational learning, learning from errors and learning from failures are also the kind of knowledge flowing, interacting in organization, transforming and sharing. Therefore, their final goals are to advance the levels of performance and abilities of organization (see Fig. 215.2).

215.3.2 Constructing the Model of Learning from Errors in Organization

From the analysis above, failures are results of error behaviors. Learning from failures thus is a subset of learning from errors. This paper only involves how to integrate learning from errors into organizational learning (see Fig. 215.3).

The nature of learning from errors is a process of problem-solving. It can be divided into four parts: detecting and identifying errors, analyzing and attributing errors, developing and implementing program, evaluating and giving feedback. According [15], organizational learning includes five parts: learning preparation, learning and communication, knowledge acquisition and practice, knowledge integration and transformation, evaluation and giving feedback. In order to correspond to the process of learning from errors, this chapter combines phases of the knowledge acquisition and integration and transformation.

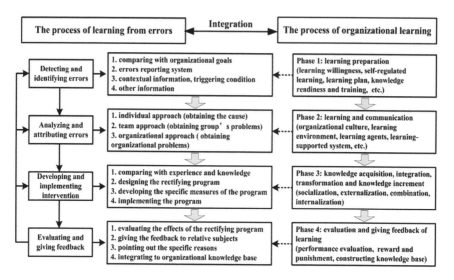

Fig. 215.2 Information flow and knowledge flow among the three learning

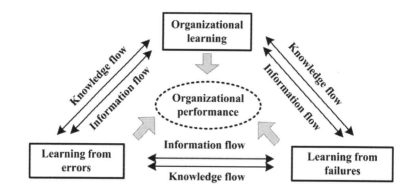

Fig. 215.3 Process of integrating learning from errors to organizational learning

- **Phase 1 detecting and identifying errors:** In this phase, there are several measures to adopt. For example, through comparing current states with normal states, it can be identified if current states deviate from organizational goals. Through error reporting system, subjects of organization can hold the contextual information, trigger conditions and other information of errors' occurring. Correspondingly, phase 1 is the process of learning preparation during organizational learning. Subjects must have the thirst for learning, acquiring knowledge, planning learning, error training, etc. Its aim is to advance their skills and knowledge of detecting and identifying errors through learning from experience (including errors and failures).

- **Phase 2 analyzing and attributing errors:** The measures of this phase include three types. Firstly, through individual approach organization can analyze the cause of errors' emergence, such as which knowledge and skills he or she is lack of? Secondly, through team approach can locate the group's problems, such as which barriers and problems exist in cooperating, communicating and understanding among team members? Finally, through organizational approach can obtain the organizational problems. It is a macroscopical and systemic approach. Organization can find the problems of organizational system, structure, operational flow and knowledge system. Correspondently, organizational learning emphasizes information change and communication. During this phase, organizational culture exerts a major influence on information or knowledge communicating and sharing. Especially, organization should promote no blame culture for active reporting of errors and handling timely. Otherwise, there are some factors including knowledge and skills of learning agents, training methods and guidance, and learning supportive system.
- **Phase 3 developing and implementing intervenes:** In the light of the context of errors and comparing with existing experience and knowledge, subjects design the correcting program and develop countermeasures and implement it in order to avoid adverse effect. In organizational learning process, subjects acquire, integrate, transform and increment knowledge through correcting errors. On the one hand, through explicit knowledge internalized, they integrate the prior knowledge and skills into their operational procedures. On the other hand, through tacit knowledge transformed into explicit knowledge and the experience of correcting errors sublimed, they communicate with others in order to sharing the experience and the experience is socialized.
- **Phase 4 evaluation and giving feedback:** According to evaluating the effects of measures to rectify errors, organization should give feedback to the subjects. If it is not achieve previous goals, the errors give birth to failure. Then, organization should help the subject to analyze and find specific causes. Organization also can collect and classify and pack up the information of errors in order to become an example of organizational knowledge base. In the process of organizational learning, it is the similar to learning from errors.

215.4 Conclusion

Overall, theoretical framework and results of this study display an intriguing picture of integrating learning from errors into organizational learning in organization. From this angle, we regard errors as learning resources, that is a type of knowledge in organization and very important to avoid adverse effects and find opportunity of innovation to improve organizational performance.

References

1. Muehlfeld K, Rao SP, Van WA (2012) A contextual theory of organizational learning from failures and successes: a study of acquisition completion in the global newspaper industry. Strateg Manag J 1981–2008 33(8):938–964
2. Baumard P, Starbuck WH (2005) Learning from failures: why it may not happen. Long Range Plan 38(3):281–298
3. Edmondson AC (2004) Learning from mistakes is easier said than done: group and organizational influences on the detection and correction of human error. J Appl Behav Sci 40(1):66–90
4. Zhao B (2011) Learning from errors: the role of context, emotion, and personality. J Organ Behav 32:435–463
5. Zhao S (2012) Cultivating the manager with responsibility. http://news.china.com.cn/rollnews/2012-03/13/content_13241383.htm. Accessed 20 Oct 2012
6. Gilley JW, Eggland SA (1989). Principles of human resource development. Perseus Books, MA, pp 120–121
7. Madsen PM, Desai Vinit (2010) Failing to learn? the effects of failure and success on organizational learning in the global orbital launch vehicle industry. Acad Manag J 53(3):451–476
8. Marquardt M (1996) Building the learning organization. McGraw-Hill, New York, p 38
9. Darr E, Argote L, Epple D (1995) The acquisition, transfer, and depreciation of knowledge in service organizations: productivity in franchises. Manage Sci 31:1750–1762
10. McGrath RG (2001) Exploratory learning, innovative capacity, and managerial oversight. Acad Manag J 44:118–131
11. Reagans R, Argote L, Brooks D (2005) Individual experience and experience working together: predicting learning rates from knowing who knows what and knowing how to work together. Manage Sci 51:869–881
12. Baum JA, Ingram P (1998) Survival-enhancing learning in the manhattan hotel industry. Manage Sci 44:996–1016, 1898–1980
13. Haunschild PR, Sullivan BN (2002) Learning from complexity: effects of prior accidents and incidents on airlines' learning. Adm Sci Q 47:609–643
14. Cannon MD, Edmondson AC (2005) Failing to learn and learning to fail (intelligently): how great organizations put failure to work to innovate and improve. Long Range Plan 38:299–319
15. Gilley JW, Maycunich A (2000) Organizational learning, performance, and change: an introduction to strategic HRD. Perseus, MA
16. Wikipedia. Chernobyl disaster. http://en.wikipedia.org/wiki/Chernobyl_disaster. Accessed 8 Jan 2013
17. Wikipedia. Space Shuttle Challenger disaster. http://en.wikipedia.org/wiki/Space_Shuttle_Challenger_disaster. Accessed 8 Jan 2013

Chapter 216
Employment-Oriented Web Application Development Course Design Reform

Chong-jie Dong

Abstract For the current grim IT employment situation and goals to train computer professionals of vocational colleges, the reform ideas of employment-oriented and the core of competency training is used in the teaching process of the web application development course design, and through a variety of teaching methods to stimulate students' motivation to learn and enthusiasm, helping student to bring up the ability of analyzing problems and solving problems, improving the quality of teaching, laying a good foundation for student employment.

Keywords Web application development course design · Employment-oriented · Capacity-building · The quality of teaching

216.1 Introduction

Along with rapid development of computer technology and the widespread application of computer technology in each industry, the social demand for IT talents is more and more obvious, especially software development related to talent demand is more and more big. Higher vocational colleges to cultivate out high skills, hands-on ability of graduates received more social favor. Our hospital as a new higher occupation colleges, since building a courtyard always adhere to the "employment-oriented" principle, based in Dongguan, facing the Pearl River Delta' market research to optimize the specialty structure, additional social need professional. By actively conducting market research, confirm industry talent demand. The contents of investigation include relevant industry market demand, development trend, technology requirements, post setting and personnel needs; moreover seriously organize the internal and external experts and scholars are

C. Dong (✉)
Department of Computer Engineering, Dongguan, China
e-mail: dchj2008@163.com

analyzed and proved the results, so as to determine the professional settings. Web application development technology as core course of computer application specialty, closely around the "employment-oriented, competency-based training as the core" teaching philosophy, in various of teaching means and method have carried out a series of reforms.

216.2 Analysis of Teaching Situation About Design of Web Application Development Curriculum

Web application development technology is a practical application of the theory and practice are highly oriented professional core curriculum, mainly introducing basic principle and development method of Web application development technology. In the process of software development, the Web application development technology has become an important technology for software development. Design of Web application development curriculum as the practice of Web application development technology after studying speculative knowledge, pay more attention to improve the ability of students to use the knowledge to analyze and solve problems. However, in the traditional teaching process, teachers often give about five subjects for students to choose, each student according to the selected topic through the analysis of demands, the design of logical structure, the design of physical structure, the implementation of system to achieve.

Mainly has the following problems of this kind of teaching mode:

1. Subjects are so much little, the inevitable existence of copying phenomenon among students, so not only can not improve the practical ability of students, but help to develop students 'bad habits of getting without any labor, which is not conducive to the students can adapt to the fierce competition in the society after graduation.
2. The initiative of students is poor. Each of the students faces the subject of their choice, feeling very difficult to complete the questions, often feeling no place to start, so the quality of completing the curriculum design can imagine.
3. The shortage of resources exist among teachers, so many teachers can not update the knowledge structure and teaching methods according to the practical need of society, and follow the beaten track.

216.3 Take the Employment as the Guidance to Reform Design of Web Application Development Curriculum

Higher vocational education should start from the needs to graduates of the society and the enterprise, the employment as the guidance, focus on training students' occupation ability and practical skills, Adhere to the theory of teaching as principle for servicing the occupation skill training, building and strengthening occupation skill training, focus on training and improving students' basic skills and the overall quality required for working in the future, to meet the demands of employing for society and enterprises, in order to adapt to the change of economic social and industrial structure. At present, whether the jobs of website construction and software development in the IT industry, Web application development technology is an important technical support. In the process of taking the employment as the guidance to reform design of Web application development curriculum, we formulate the teaching objective, teaching methods, teaching process, teaching effect and reflection, this four aspects are as follows.

216.3.1 The Development of Teaching Objective

The main goal of design of Web application development curriculum is to make the students fully understand the basic theory of Web application development, comprehensively grasping the basic concept and basic method of Web application development technology, having the ability of using Web application development technology to solve a variety of problems in the process of software project. The teaching goal of Web application development curriculum can be embodied in three aspects in quality education, knowledge teaching and occupation ability:

The goal of quality education: Training students' ability in project cooperation, team spirit and team communication; Training students' ability in the logical thinking and problem analysis; training the students' ability in using Web application technology development to solve the practical problems in the process of developing management information system.

The goal of knowledge teaching: Mastering the basic principle, basic concepts and methods of the Web technology application; with design and development ability of developing management information system in Microsoft platform.

Training occupation ability: Having ability to apply related knowledge to the design and development of a simple Web system; Cultivating ability to apply Web application technology to development of management information system.

216.3.2 Choosing the Teaching Method

In the process of teaching, Choosing proper teaching method directly affect the teaching effects. Therefore, according to the nature and goals of design of Web application development curriculum, we choose project and experiment teaching method. The project and experiment teaching method carry out experimental teaching activities through the implementation of a complete project, emphasis of "student-centered" teaching method in the experimental teaching, theory combining with practice teaching, fully exploring the independent innovation ability of students, improving student's comprehensive ability to apply the knowledge to solve practical problems. The project and experiment teaching method, by teachers put forward the target of system developing, the students choose project topics in groups, complete development project under the guidance of teachers, students experience the practice by themselves, apply what we have learned in class, effective exploring and learning new knowledge, so as to improve the professional skills, and feel pleasure of experience and the spirit of collaboration.

216.3.3 The Implementation Teaching's Process

Teaching process is a most important part of Web application development curriculum, according to the actual situation of the IT industry first-line talents job requirements and our college students majoring in computer science, our college has a good hardware and software environment for the development of teaching process of Web application development curriculum. The implementation of the teaching process as shown in Fig. 216.1.

The specific content of the seven links of the implementation of the teaching process:

1. Arrangement of project tasks. First of all, teachers give the goal, requirement and content based on the aim of design of Web application development curriculum. Then, show a complete software project, and introduce the corresponding requirements associated with the project to students in the process of demonstration, let the students have a good understanding of curriculum design.
2. Project identification. First of all, teachers issued the grouping task in accordance with the "free combination,a group of three or four" principle, divide students into several groups under the guidance of teachers. Then, the tutor gives about 15 project topics for students to choose, students can also determine the project topic, and allows the students group chose the project topic not more than two repeated. Finally, teachers distribute report template of design of Web application development curriculum to students, and tell mission requirements of each paper to students.
3. Requirements analysis. Requirements analysis is a very important section, the student group needs to determine the task must be completed according to the

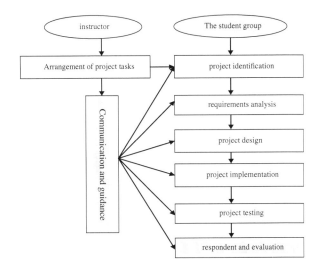

Fig. 216.1 The implementation of the teaching process

project what they have chosen, is also put forward complete, accurate, clear, specific requirements on the system. Students can consult background information related to the project through the network, reference books and so on, and make the summary of the work, complete the requirement analysis report combined with the experience of life. The teachers give comments and suggestions to report in time, students make appropriate modifications to the report.

4. Project design. The main work of project design is to complete database design of the project, including database concept structure design, logic structure design, physical structure design and E-R design.
5. Project implementation. The main work of project implementation is project programming, students can choose JSP, ASP.NET or the other development tools. When the student group have difficulty in solving technical problems, teachers can give proper guidance. Of course, for the common problems of the student group in the process of project development. Teachers give demonstration and discussion to students, and give ideas and solutions, inspire students' logical thinking and innovative ability.
6. Project testing. The main work of the project testing including unit testing, integration testing and system testing. The purpose of project testing is to find problems in each function module, in order to correct the problems in time. Project testing can improve the students' understand ability, above all it can improve the students' understanding of the importance of teamwork spirit.
7. Respondent and evaluation. The main work of the respondent and evaluation is project demonstration. The materials of project demonstration include PPT introducing the project, source files and the electronic version report of curriculum design. Each team choose two representatives to demonstrate project, teachers and students as the judges give project evaluation for each team and

puts forward the existing problems, guide students to reflect and review the project, sum up gain and loss, which is good for the training of ideation and innovation.

216.4 Assessment Methods

The reform of employment-oriented Web application development curriculum carries out teaching through the project, it's aim is to improve the students' professional skills, cultivate talents for IT industry in line. Therefore, it demands reformation to traditional appraisal way. Assessment mainly includes two aspects of usual assessment and project appraisal content. The usual assessment mainly includes attendance, classroom performance, counts as 20 % of the course grade; Project appraisal mainly includes needs analysis report, database design, design and implementation of software interface and function, result of demonstration and reply about the project, report of curriculum design, counts as 80 % of the course grade.

216.5 Conclusion

Employment-oriented IT vocational education take on importance mission of training applied technological talents for the IT industry. As IT professional teachers in higher vocational colleges, we should according to the industrial structure to adjust structure of specialties, and take professional construction as an opportunity, focus on the construction of curriculum system, especially the practice of professional core courses, taking raises students' employability skills as the master line, taking improves students' skills as the core of the reform of curriculum design, strengthen students' social practice ability and job skills, and achieved certain teaching effect and social benefit.

References

1. Pan D (2006) Employment-oriented vocational talents training mode of IT. Vocat Educ Res (12):123–124
2. Yaqi G, Jie S (2011) Discussion on employment-oriented curriculum reform in higher vocational education. Educ Vocat 27:125–126
3. Zhifeng Z, Wenbing W (2010) The research of teaching reform of cultivating the overall abilities of the students with employment orientation. Comput Educ 21:99–101

Chapter 217
A Process Model of User Reactions to IT System Features

Yan Yu and Zou Jin

Abstract It is critical to understand more about the processes contributing to user reactions of these initiatives. We develop a process model based on theories related to organizational sense making to help understand user reactions to IT systems. This paper suggests that IT system features can also send signals to users, user extract cues from their environment and interpret them based on situational characteristics and personality, these cognitive interpretation can influence subsequent emotional reactions and behavior.

Keywords Users reaction · IT system · Feature · Cognitive · Emotional

217.1 Introduction

In today's fast-paced and competitive business environment, many consultants, academics, and futurists view human capital as the principal corporate asset that must be effectively managed. The use of information technology (IT) to perform all kinds of work has been steadily increasing over the last decade. As

---

The research was supported part by a grant from overseas humanities and social sciences dynamic tracking plan of Wuhan University. The research was also supported part by a grant from high-level international journals nurture project of Wuhan University.

Y. Yu
Department of Psychology, School of Philosophy, Wuhan University, Wuhan 430072, Hubei, China
e-mail: yanyu@whu.edu.cn

Z. Jin (✉)
School of Information Management, Central China Normal University, Wuhan 430072, Hubei, China
e-mail: bertha_zj@yahoo.com.cn

organizational functions become increasingly reliant on IT systems, it is important to fully examine the effects of such systems on the numerous stakeholders. IT systems promise stakeholders many advantages, such as more effective distribution of work activities, increases in productivity and efficiency, and better tracking and sharing of information [4, 6].

Klein (1996) have consistently found that stakeholders react psychologically and emotionally to new IT systems during the implementation phase, making assumptions about how the new system will change their role in the organization, how they are supposed to act, and what management values. These assumptions are based on a variety of signals available in the organizational environment, including statements made by organizational leaders, training sessions offered, and rewards for learning and using new technologies.

The current focus from an IT perspective appears to be on user reactions such as ease of use and frustration that are linked to actual system usage [3]. This paper suggests that IT system features can also send signals to users, and considering user reactions to system features early in the design process will help alleviate problems experienced later in implementation. Few existing research has attempted to examine the effects of system features on users. Thus, this study hopes to demonstrate that system design issues can affect user reactions. However, it focuses on macroscopic system characteristics rather than the microscopic characteristics, or system-design features, which we believe may also send important signals to users that affect their reactions to the IT system.

217.2 The Study of User Reactions

Existing literature on several models and theories have been used in recent years to examine user reactions, including the Technology Acceptance Model (TAM), Social Cognitive Theory (SCT), and the Theory of Planned Behavior (TPB). Research utilizing these theories and models is reviewed below.

217.2.1 Technology Acceptance Model

One central model used in the IT literature to examine user reactions to new systems is the Technology Acceptance Model. In TAM, user acceptance of a new system is based on perceived ease of use and usefulness. In other words, if users feel that the system is easy to use and will help them get their jobs done, they are more likely to accept and use it. TAM includes self-efficacy in the prediction of user acceptance in that individuals with high self-efficacy are expected to perceive that a system is easier to use. Researchers have replicated the basic findings of TAM in many situations and have extended the model to consider concepts such as social exchange and even gender [10].

217.2.2 Social Cognitive Theory

More psychologically oriented theories such as Social Cognitive Theory has also been used to examine usage of new computer systems. SCT focuses on the effect of self-efficacy on performance, considering the fact that performance can also impact future self-efficacy. Compeau, Higgins, and Huff (1999) used SCT to examine the relationships among self-efficacy, outcome expectations, user affect, anxiety, and computer use. They found that self-efficacy and outcome expectations predicted affect and computer use, with affect also demonstrating a direct effect on use.

217.2.3 Theory of Planned Behavior

TPB suggests that computer usage is a function of individuals' behavioral intentions, which are influenced by attitudes, norms, and behavioral control. Chau and Hu [2] used TPB to examine implementation of new medical technology for physicians. They found that perceived usefulness and individual attitudes were important predictors of physicians' intention to use the technology.

217.3 The Feature of Information Technology System

In addition to looking at the impact of the IT system as a whole, certain design elements can reflect important attributes about organizations. Four key system characteristics can demonstrate the link between design decisions and organizational attributes: the purpose of the system, user control, accessibility, and perceived innovativeness.

217.3.1 Purpose

The purpose of the system includes both the stated purpose and the implied purpose. The purpose of the system may not be directly related to the functionality of the system, but it should be given the same consideration as any other design-related feature. It is a more general or high-level design factor that can influence functionality-oriented IT systems.

217.3.2 Operate

Another feature relevant to organizational attributes is the amount of operate available to the user. Operate refers to the amount of self-direction granted to the user. This is similar to the concept of learner control, which occurs when learners can make choices about how to proceed with a training course. These choices include the behavior of the learner and how engaged to become with the learning [5].

217.3.3 Accessibility

Accessibility is an important design factor that has two components. One component is having access to data kept in the system. Systems vary in how much data users can access. The other component of accessibility considers whether the system provides access to required information, help, and support. Cappelli [1] describes how technology can improve the recruiting function, using hiring management systems (HMSs) to improve recruiters' responsiveness to applicants.

217.3.4 Perceived Innovativeness

Perceived innovativeness refers to the timing and sophistication of the system as perceived by the users. The level of innovativeness of the technology reflects upon the organization. It can make an organization look progressive, current, or outdated. This connection has been noted in the recruiting literature. Some evidence indicates that test takers view the use of multimedia testing as more modern [7], which could be attractive to applicants.

217.4 A Process Mode of User Reactions

Research in HR, OB, and I/O psychology has determined that individuals interpret and make sense of the environment in different ways. Consequently, different people may interpret the same objective event, process, or system very differently. As discussed above, feature of IT systems such as purpose, operate, accessibility, and perceived innovativeness can send messages to users. Users interpret and respond to these messages and influence the success of system implementation. Unfortunately, organizations often make design decisions based solely on money, time, and technology, and fail to explicitly consider the potential impact on user reactions. Based on the key concepts of this paper, we developed a process model (see Fig. 217.1) that allows us to examine employee reactions to IT systems.

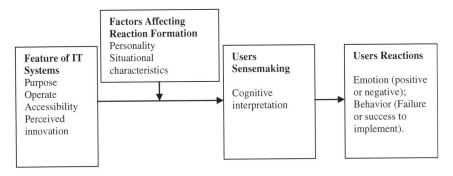

Fig. 217.1 A process mode of user reactions to it system features

This model is based on psychological reaction-formation processes such as sensemaking. Sensemaking theories examine how people interpret new and ambiguous events. People need to make sense of the change and determine how it will affect them. In this sensemaking process, people extract cues from their environment and interpret them based on situational characteristics and personality. These cognitive interpretations can influence emotional reactions and behavior.

This model begins with the organization's system-design decisions around purpose, control, accessibility, and perceived innovation. Based on the sensemaking and socialization literatures reviewed above, we suggest that employees will observe and interpret these design decisions, making inferences about organizational priorities, values, and intentions. These inferences will lead to a variety of possible reactions.

Proposition 1 System-design decisions will indirectly affect user emotional and behavior reactions. Individual's cognition plays a mediator role between the Features of IT systems and user reactions.

The literature reviewed above strongly suggests that sense making processes, therefore, user cognitive interpretation to a particular event, will be affected by both individual personality and situational characteristics. Thus, the model portrays a block of constructs that may moderate the relationship between system-design features and user cognitive interpretation. These constructs include individual personality characteristics, strategic fit and levels of trust in the organization, and could affect the relationship between design factors and user cognitive interpretation in several ways. We review a subset of potential moderators below.

Proposition 2a User characteristics such as personality will moderate the relationship between system feature and user cognitive interpretation.

Proposition 2b Situational characteristics such as strategic alignment, trust, and employee involvement will moderate the relationship between system design and user cognitive interpretation.

Finally, the last step in the model suggests that user cognitive interpretation will impact their subsequent emotional and behavioral outcomes. Lazarus' cognitive motivational relational (CMR) theory (2000) has been the model of choice for researchers investigating relations between cognition and emotion (e.g. [9]). Smith and Kirby [8] also explained how cognitive interpretation lead to emotions and subsequent behavior. Based on these theories, we anticipate that positive cognition will be associated with positive emotion and successful implementation and vice versa. Clearly, more research needs to be done on this aspect of the model.

Proposition 3a Positive user cognition will lead to positive emotion and more favorable implementation outcomes.

Proposition 3b Negative user cognition will lead to negative emotion and less favorable implementation outcomes.

217.5 Future Research Directions

The ideas developed in this paper suggest several directions for future research. Certainly, empirical testing of the propositions described above is critical. Do feature of IT system indirectly affect user reactions? Or will reactions be more dependent on individual and situational characteristics such as locus of values and trust?

What other characteristics will impact the reaction-formation processes described in the model? Further research should also be conducted to investigate the extent to which there are design factors that must be considered beyond the four presented in the model. For example, similar to the TAM concept of "ease of use" is the notion of "ease of learning." Alternatively, variation in cognitive load or mental workload may be best conceptualized as an individual difference that impacts the relationship between design factors and user reactions.

From a more practical perspective, research is needed on methods for obtaining user input across the full range of reactions, including affective, behavioral, and cognitive. It will likely take users more than an hour of interacting with the system to fully develop reactions. What kind of testing process will allow us to elicit and measure reactions effectively?

Experimental work looking at different IT design processes would also be useful, integrating the user into the design and testing process at different stages with different responsibilities and looking at how these variables affect the range of user reactions. One potentially interesting multidisciplinary direction for future research is to expand the breadth of outcomes studied in the more traditional models used in research related to IT systems. We have suggested several other cognitive, affective, and behavioral reactions to consider, such as dissatisfaction, interpretation of corporate values and goals, and sabotage.

References

1. Cappelli P (2001) Making the most of on-line recruiting. Har Bus Rev 79(3):139–146
2. Chau PYK, Hu PJ (2001) Information technology acceptance by individual professionals: a model comparison approach [Electronic version]. Decis Sci 32(4):1–13
3. Fisher SL, Howell AW (2004) Beyond user acceptance: an examination of employee reactions to information technology systems. Hum Resour Manage 43(2/3):243–258
4. Greengard S (2000) Technology finally advances HR. Workforce 79:38–41
5. Howell AW (2000) A process model of learner behavior and engagement during web-based training. Unpublished dissertation, Michigan State University, East Lansing
6. Jossi F (2001) Taking the e-HR plunge. HR Mag September:96–103
7. Richman-Hirsch WL, Olson-Buchanan JB, Drasgow F (2000) Examining the impact of administration medium on examine perceptions and attitudes. J Appl Psychol 85:880–887
8. Smith CA, Kirby LD (2009) Putting appraisal in context: toward a relational model of appraisal and emotion. Cogn Emot 23(7):1352–1372
9. Uphill MA, Dray K (2009) Giving yourself a good beating: appraisal, attribution, rumination, and counterfactual thinking. J Sports Sci Med 8:5–12
10. Venkatesh V, Morris MG (2000) Why don't men ever stop to ask for directions? Gender, social influence, and their role in technology acceptance and usage behavior. MIS Quart 24:115–139

Chapter 218
Application of Modified PBL Mode on Pathophysiology Courses

Tang Hua, Chen Rong, Zhang Chun-Mei, Li Zhu-Hua and Zou Ping

Abstract The aim of this research was to evaluate the effectiveness and feasibility of modified Problem-based learning (PBL) mode in Pathophysiology courses. 294 students were divided into two groups: the study group comprising 148 students was exposed to the modified PBL method, whereas the control group comprising 146 students was given the lecture-based traditional teaching. The teaching effectiveness of both groups was compared by a questionnaire and a formative assessment. Of the study group, above 71.6 % were in favor of the modified mode of PBL, which could motivate them to learn, enhance their ability of problem-solving, self-expressing and team-cooperating, foster their critical and clinical thinking, and contribute to the construction of systemic and comprehensive knowledge system; while only below 53.5 % of the control group took the traditional teaching that way. According to the results of formative assessment, students from study group scored higher in the final exam than those from control group, especially in the subjective questions, which is closely related to the self-study records and teacher's evaluation ($r = 0.568$, $r = 0.692$, $P < 0.05$). Our findings suggest that the modified PBL could improve the students' comprehensive quality, and might be a better teaching mode fitting in with the situations of our college and country.

Keywords Problem-based learning · Educational reform · Pathophysiology

The Problem-based learning (PBL) mode has been generally carried out in China these years. Based on clinical cases, conventional PBL induces students to proceed from self-study and discussion, which is good for improving students' ability of independent learning and problem solving as well as clinical thinking [1]. The conventional PBL, however, has its own limitations such as ignoring the systematicness and integrity of basic knowledge, overlooking the effect of teaching experiences of teachers from different subjects on students, great demand for

T. Hua · C. Rong · Z. Chun-Mei · L. Zhu-Hua · Z. Ping (✉)
Department of Pathophysiology, Luzhou Medical College, Luzhou 646000, China
e-mail: lyzouping@163.com

teaching resources, and so on [2]. And furthermore, the widespread using of PBL in china is challenged by variety of problems including the large number of students, the irregularity of students' ability, the influence of traditional education mode, the lack of unified teaching materials and scientific assessment system and many others [3]. Based on the above problems, we conducted a modified PBL mode in the curriculum of Pathophysiology in our college with the specific process as follows.

218.1 Materials and Methods

218.1.1 Study Group

The research was conducted within 294 second-year undergraduate students in Luzhou medical college during the 2011 and 2012 spring terms. The study group (n = 148) was exposed to the modified PBL throughout the Pathophysiology courses, which was based on study-guiding questions and cases and subsequently guided students into self-study, team discussion and classroom presentation. While the control group (n = 146) was given the lecture-based traditional teaching.

218.1.2 The Implementation Process of Modified PBL Mode

218.1.2.1 Compilation of the Specific PBL Textbook

The PBL textbook we used was compiled by the teachers from department of Pathophysiology, in which the key points, study-guiding questions and clinical cases were included in every chapter. Most important of all, unlike the traditional PBL textbook, this one integrated the key points into the form of study-guiding questions supplemented by clinical cases.

For instance, in the chapter of respiratory insufficiency, the study-guiding questions were mainly as follows: (1) What is respiratory insufficiency? What are the diagnostic criteria of it? (2) By what factors inspiratory dyspnea can be caused? What is the mechanism of it? (3) What is chronic obstructive pulmonary disease (COPD)? Can you state the relation between COPD and respiratory insufficiency? (4) What are the common causes of diffusion disorder? Why does not increase of $PaCO_2$ accompany diffusion disorder? (5) Describe the mechanism of respiratory failure. (6) What are the forms of ventilation/perfusion imbalance and the pathophysiological meaning of each form? (7) What is pulmonary heart disease? How does it happen? (8) What is acute respiratory distress syndrome(ARDS)? Please describe its mechanism. (9) What are the common types of acid–base imbalance in patients with respiratory failure and how do they happen? (10) What are the cautions in the oxygen therapy—the treatment of respiratory failure? And why?

218.1.2.2 Self-Study and Team Discussion

The students were presented with the study-guiding questions and the cases a week in advance, and then worked out their individual answers through consulting related textbooks, professional literatures or network resources. Subsequently, all the members of each team discussed and exchanged their opinions and finally formed the team answers. The record of team discussion was set up as one of the basis of formative assessment.

218.1.2.3 Classroom Presentation and Teachers' Summary

The presentation and discussion in class were hosted by the tutor, which were conducted by the team representatives with the auxiliary of board writing or PowerPoint and with the supplement or different opinions proposed by other students. Finally, a summary was made by the tutor based on the knowledge students had mastered. In the class, there was another teacher—the teaching secretary, who mainly participated in team discussion, checked up the discussion record, took notes of class presentation, and made evaluation of students' performance during PBL.

218.1.2.4 Evaluation of Teaching Effectiveness

A questionnaire coupled with a formative assessment was used to evaluate the teaching effect. The formative assessment system was composed of the following aspects: (1) record of self-study and team discussion, which accounts for 10 % of the total score; (2) classroom test, accounting for 10 %; (3) stage examination, accounting for 20 %; (4) self and peer evaluation, accounting for 20 %, the criteria of which include the ability of analyzing and problem-solving, consulting related information, and cooperating, etc.; (5) teacher's evaluation, accounting for 20 %, which covers expression ability, question answers, production level of PowerPoint, and team collaboration, etc.; (6) final examination, accounting for 30 %, which is in the form of writing exams with case analysis added.

218.1.3 Statistics Analysis

All the data were analyzed in the SPSS statistical software. The measurement data were presented as mean ±SD, and the differences were analyzed by t test; the enumeration data were presented as frequency, and the differences were analyzed by Chi square test. P values of <0.05 were considered statistically significant.

218.2 Results

218.2.1 Results of the Questionnaire

A total of 294 students in both groups completed the questionnaire effectively. Over 71.6 % of the study group approved of the modified PBL mode, and considered that it could motivate them to learn, improve the ability of self-study and learning efficiency, help them to learn more systemically and comprehensively, enhance the ability of analyzing, problem-solving, self-expressing and cooperating, and also foster the clinical thinking. The corresponding proportion of control group, however, was significantly lower, all below 53.5 %. The difference between the two groups had statistical significance by Chi square analysis ($P < 0.01$, Table 218.1).

218.2.2 Results of the Formative Assessment

Table 218.2 compares the average scores obtained by students from two groups in the final examination. The average scores of the study group overweighed those of the control group, especially in the subjective questions, such as essay questions and case analysis ($P < 0.05$), while the average scores in the objective questions such as true-false, multiple-choices and blank questions showed no significant difference in the two groups ($P > 0.05$, Table 218.2). The results indicate that our modified PBL mode benefits students in improving the ability of analyzing and solving practical problems, but without benefits in memory training.

Among all the aspects of formative assessment, the self-study records and teacher's evaluation were found to be closely related to the students' performance

Table 218.1 Comparison of evaluation of teaching effect between control and study group

	Control group		Study group	
	n	%	n	%
Arouse interest in learning	68	46.6	123	83.6*
Motivate the initiative to learn	47	32.2	128	86.5*
Improve the ability of self-study	54	37.0	134	90.5*
Increase learning efficiency	72	49.3	114	77.0*
Enhance the systematicness and integrity of knowledge	78	53.5	106	71.6*
Cultivate the clinical thinking	74	50.7	138	93.2*
Improve the ability of analyzing and problem-solving	42	28.8	140	94.6*
Improve the expression ability	35	24.0	141	95.3*
Improve the cooperative ability	52	35.6	137	92.6*
Improve staff-student communication	70	47.9	143	96.6*

* $P < 0.01$

Table 218.2 Comparison of average scores in the final examination between two groups

	Control group (n = 146)	Study group (n = 148)
Scores in objective questions	48.59 ± 4.21	50.11 ± 2.37
Scores in subjective questions	22.05 ± 5.14	31.12 ± 3.68*
Average scores	72.18 ± 7.49	79.82 ± 8.02*

* $P < 0.05$

in the final examination (r = 0.568, r = 0.692, P < 0.05), which shows that the more initiatives the students have in their usual study, the better performance they will give in the final examination, and that this formative assessment system can really reflect the students' learning effect, fully mobilize their initiatives and urge them to plunge into the usual study.

218.3 Discussion

The lecture-based teaching is proved to benefit students in constructing systemic and comprehensive knowledge system, but usually fail to improve the independent learning ability. The conventional PBL mode, comparatively, is one could motivate students to learn and increase the ability of self-study but at the cost of systematicness and integrity of basic knowledge. Accordingly, the modified PBL mode we carried out in Pathophysiology courses was a reform due to the situations of our college, which was different from the traditional PBL in compilation of textbook and study-guiding questions, executing process as well as evaluation system of teaching effect. It has been confirmed that most of students exposed to the modified mode of PBL had higher satisfaction with teaching activity, and considered that it not only improved the comprehensive quality of students, but also contributed to the construction of systemic and comprehensive knowledge system, as shown in Table 218.1. The students could integrate new information with current knowledge structures in their mind meaningfully and transfer it into long-term memory to use when needed. Furthermore, they could fully understand the studied material with underlying concepts, principles, or mechanisms and use higher cognitive skills, such as the application of the knowledge, analysis, critical thinking, or synthesis. Consequently, high-quality learning and the associated potential for better academic achievement occurred.

The formative assessment made in this research demonstrates that students from the study group obtained higher scores in final examination than those from the control group, which was closely related to two aspects of formative assessment—the self-study records and teacher's evaluation. Such close relation reveals that the higher score could be a result of better student engagement, active learning and peer interactions due to the exposure to the specific PBL exercises.

Based on the above advantages, the modified PBL mode we are trying out is one suiting the situations of our college and country and is worth carrying out further. The followings are some experiences in the implementation process for your reference.

(1) The crucial part of our modified PBL was design and compilation of the study-guiding questions and clinical cases. As the traditional PBL mode tries to lead students into independent learning by means of clinical cases which is short of reflection of the integrity and systematicness of basic knowledge, the weakness of basic knowledge has an inevitable influence on students' learning and understanding of clinical problems, which consequently makes it difficult for students to abstract the knowledge points required in the cases from variety of resources [4]. Therefore, we integrated the key points into the study-guiding questions with the complement of clinical cases so that students could not only master the knowledge fully and systematically, but also use a combination of knowledge they have learned to resolve clinical practical problems.

(2) In order to facilitate students' self-study, we established a PBL learning room for Pathophysiology courses providing all sorts of resources like books, magazines, computers, network, and teacher consultation etc., which narrowed the range of resources students had to consult, and thus increased their efficiency of obtaining useful information.

(3) We set up an interactive platform on the Pathophysiology teaching website of our college, through which students from different teams could share information resources they had gained, and exchange the questions and disagreements generated in discussion; and meanwhile, based on the feedback on line, teachers could offer necessary study instruction in time, and regulate the schedule and style of classroom presentation and discussion.

(4) The tutor should always serve as a guider to keep the classroom presentation and discussion moving along smoothly, and try not to make conclusive opinions on the various viewpoints proposed by students, but point out the mistakes in principles and understanding, so as to encourage students' critical and creative thinking. Within the relaxed discussion environment, students got increasingly autonomous and active.

(5) The study activities were evaluated fully and objectively from more than one angle. Self and peer evaluation made the students act as the real subjects of assessment system; the teaching secretary participating in team discussion and taking notes of every students' classroom presentation made us focus on the evaluation of the whole learning process, through which we could evaluate students' performance truly and reasonably, and moreover students could be urged to learn more autonomously.

Undoubtedly, there are still problems in our practice of modified PBL mode, for example, some students had been used to lecture-based teaching for a long time and were not active enough in the classroom discussion; students could not find the clues and highlights of some more complicated pathogenesis through team discussion, and still need teachers to summarize the depth of knowledge and the interrelation of each main points; limited to the textbooks and some common search engines, the students' approaches of looking up information outside of class were not wide enough with less utilization of professional literatures; insufficient atmosphere of team discussion and incomplete discussion record made the formative assessment difficult to practice, and so on. Therefore, in the future implementation, we will improve it further, and search for a better teaching mode suiting the situations of our country.

References

1. Bosse HM, Huwendiek S, Skelin S et al (2010) Interactive film scenes for tutor training in problem-based learning (PBL): dealing with difficult situations. BMC Med Edu 10:52
2. Nouns Z, Schauber S, Witt C et al (2012) Development of knowledge in basic sciences: A comparison of two medical curricula. Med Edu 46:1206–1214
3. Frambach JM, Driessen EW, Chan LC et al (2012) Rethinking the globalisation of problem-based learning: how culture challenges self-directed learning. Med Educ 46:738–747
4. Cheng-ren Li, Hong-li Li, Yun-lai Liu et al (2010) Practice of improved problem-based learning (PBL) in histology and embryology teaching. China High Med Edu 10:86–101

Chapter 219
Meditations on the Semantic Net: Oriented Library Information Service in Cloud Computing Era

Yumei Liu

Abstract Semantic Net and Cloud Computing, standing out as the epitome of immense influence of IT upon the library information service, have found their way into processing the expanding digital products. Intellectualization and humanization have been projected upon the cloud cyber source platform with the application of RDF and RSS, which is constantly changing the traditional library as well as the mode of digital service.

Keywords Digital library · Semantic net · Cloud computing · Web 3.0 · Resources push

219.1 Introduction

Now total global data has been exceeded one trillion GB, such large amount of data has been insufficient to describe with a broad array. As the active of personal digital creation, its size is series-style rising. The data size of the expansion in the digital library is to increase the difficulty for the users to obtain the required information. Released "Statistical Report about status of the 30th China Internet Development" in July 2012, the China Internet Network Information Center (CNNIC) in Beijing, the users of Chinese Internet has reached 538 million as of the end of June 2012, in which the users of Internet using the platform of mobile phone has reached to 388 million, the mobile phone gone beyond the computer become the first major Internet terminal. The field of using mobile phone in the future of digital library services is a new direction. At the same time, mobile video and microblogging continue the momentum of rapid growth in 2011. In the end of

Y. Liu (✉)
Library of Huaihai Institute of Technology, Lianyungang, China
e-mail: Lymlyg110@sina.com

June 2012, the utilization rate of Microblogging in using mobile phone increased by 5.3 % points to 43.8 %, as the main application of the web 2.0, microblogging application on mobile platforms increases sharply. Due to the applications of Web 2.0 in the Internet has already matured, and recognized by the majority of Internet users. With upgrading the ability of the 3G network and the development of Web 2.0, it will greatly enhance the interactivity of various value-added services for the mobile Internet. The platform of Mobile Internet provided technical possibility for carrying out this great cell phone service in libraries and laid a solid foundation for the launch of the cell phone service in libraries [1].

We are witnessing a great era of Internet innovation from web 1.0 to web 2.0 as well as the upcoming web 3.0, Information resources from the mode of the simple release—Browse (web 1.0) to participate in the interactive (web 2.0) mode as well as the initiative to push (web 3.0) mode is gradually changing the way of searching resources, accessing to the platform and its habits, improving the efficiency in the use of our network greatly, thus promoting the transformation of the service model of digital library resources. All this bases on the development of Internet bandwidth, the hardware and software-based. Especially the rise and development of cloud computing, it makes possibility for multi-source consolidation and virtualization of heterogeneous platforms, the efficiency in the use of hardware resources, deployment of degrees of freedom has improved greatly. The costs of resource application are significantly reduced.

Integrating the interlibrary integration into a distributed network library, digital library on the Internet, like a giant network server through the network service of the "Cloud" it provides services for the readers. In this mode, it will be the behavior of the users for the information as a starting point and foothold and track the behavior of the users for the information, dynamic adaptability aggregate information resources, the systems of information services help users solve the problem through the services. This innovative ideas on the service model and technique of cloud computing, expand the new development space for the integration of information resources and the services of innovation towards the cloud era [2].

219.2 Intelligent Internet: Semantic Net

The Web 3.0 first proposed by Jeffrey Zeldman in 2006 [3], so far, its concept has been raised when it varied different, with a more appropriate way: Semantic Net or Pragmatic Web. By semantic technology, the computer improving the ability to understand the data, has a special significance for the integration of large data sets. By using the semantic technology, it can improve the extent of the intelligent identification for search engine, the computer speculated relational meaning of the words in keywords with multiple meanings in search engine and did semantic identify. All the digital library in the future will become more humanized and intelligent.

Now, through the RDF (Resource Description Framework), OWL (Web Ontology Language), Sparql (Simple Protocol and RDF Query Language), the technology of data organization XML the page information in web via RSS (Really Simple Syndication) Semantic Net aggregated together to form a structured data,the structured data like a database is conveniently inquired and used for the users.

In addition, for the hardware, with the development of hardware technology, the bandwidth of network continuously improving the long-distance transmission of large amounts of data has become more convenient. For the software, peak-based multi-source heterogeneous platform integration and virtualization enter the applications continuously. Making data storage, and the costs of application are further reduced. It seems to be able to hear the web 3.0 footsteps getting closer and closer to us, to promote the development of hardware and software technology service model of digital library resources into a new phase. The main features of this model are:

219.2.1 Initiative

Basing on the platform of digital library resources under the web 3.0 environment, we can take the initiative to understand the needs of users, with the characteristics of precise push digital resources for the users. And analyze the user's preferences of searching engine personalized as the basis of users preference about information processing and a variety of operations performed and various requirements proposed by the users under the Web 3.0 environment. It concluded by preference system and grouped together again, form a content aggregation through the interface in a particular content themes and then take the initiative push [4].The data accuracy is an important indicator for evaluating the web 3.0 features. This indicator produced through the system push resources by the readers.

219.2.2 Personalized

Allow readers to customize a personalized service based on the the web 3.0 environment of digital library resources platform, while allowing cross-platform embedded module. Web 3.0 is designed as the main considerations for the user preferences. In introduced for the screening filtering based on the UGC (user generated content) the preference information processing and personalization engine technology, at the same time to preference information processing personalize the behavioral characteristics of users, as well as the analysis of various requirements for user, and its search used to organize, mining, and then look for the release of high credibility of UGC source is to help Internet users search for information quickly and accurately to their own interest [5]. Such as product information, multimedia information and user information, Internet data, books and serial novels, etc., on this basis, analyzed the depth of the information intelligent, and handled to achieve user-personalized, dynamic needs. It can be said, with Web 3.0 arrival it changed the way of users accessing to the information and user behavior. The degree of personalization is another important indicator for evaluating platform of web 3.0 characteristics.

219.3 The Following Issues in Service Model of Library Should be Handled Under Semantic Net Environment

219.3.1 The Depth Analysis of Readers' Virtual-Behavior

The service model of digital library resources under the Web 3.0 mode will bid farewell to this way of the resource described, obtained, distinguished, then converted into a digital library resources platform to track users, analyze, push, and fix this service model. Readers no longer care about how to obtain resources, and evaluate the digital resources of platform push simply. Digital library not only play the role of provider of digital resources for the users, and track the habits of readers using resources, but analyze the resources evaluated by readers, in order to assess the tendency of the reader data resources, it constantly push the users' personalized to make correction. Improve the precision of push for resources of digital library.

The analysis needed by individuality is firstly based on the readers individual, different from the simple single platform with different professional readers classification can be cross-platform to individual readers all behavior described in the virtual digital world and into the digital library system and become part of the digital library system platforms readers a description of the individual data analysis through the program. Second, analysis of the strategy is the key. The readers' behavior in the virtual world is more fully, this description fits the higher real needs for individuals with the readers. The platform push the reader to get more accurate data. To achieve above objectives requires a reader virtual behavior description language, and evolving analysis strategies to improve the description of the behavior for readers fit. The technology of Semantic Grid is that you can make use of ontology formalization grid information, it has high intelligence, can automatically carry out information processing, and use "service" to shield the heterogeneity of resources to achieve distributed, share the resources under the heterogeneous environment fully and use effectively, therefore, semantic grid which is distributed, heterogeneous, implements ideal platform of large-scale, strong timeliness, accuracy, intelligent, personalized recommended by automated digital libraries under massive information environment [6].

219.3.2 The Capabilities of Customizing Cross-Platform by Readers

Readers realize the content of library resource and the form of customization through cross-platform. Including the colors in interface, layout, appearance, function of platform, operating, module settings, the tendencies of readers' resources digital and the features of deep customization. The platform of Digital Library provides users with a custom data service that can be achieved by providing an open API. Readers can use it through these APIs public data interface. This open API has the following features:

(1) The way of using is a simple and intuitive. It is conveniently available to readers of different levels in different areas of the non-computer professional to use.
(2) It must follow certain data standards of Input and Output data (I/O). It can be easily embedded in the corresponding modules of different data platforms.
(3) The open API can provide the information to the system platform described by the readers and tracking the habits used by readers.

The behavior of the customization of digital library platform for the users will also become part of the description of the virtual world, included in the tendency of readership figures.

219.3.3 Readership Tracking, Identified and Unified

Under a different system platforms and different terminal platform the identity of readers identified and unified will be able to largely rich individual virtual behavioral data for the readers, to improve the fit of the description. The rapid development of the mobile phone platform actually promote the realization of this goal. With the advancement of technology in the future, the Internet of Things and the development of could computing, the identity of readers identified and unified supported by hardware, in the digital library you would be like in real life of flesh and blood, lifelike.

Currently part of the network platforms already have some features of web 3.0, RSS has become the most common basic applications based on semantic net technology. Now many large portals support RSS applications such as Sohu, Sina, Netease, Tencent and so on. Moreover, it will also bring some new depth reflection about the problem for the Web 3.0 era.

219.4 Some New Issues Form Web 3.0 Era are Also Worth Thinking Deeply

219.4.1 Authentication for Security and Legitimacy of the Cross-Platform Module

Now the copyright identification of Creative Commons (CC) based on Semantic Net technology has entered the field of network applications. It can provide flexible copyright licensing agreement for the copyright works. In March 2006, CC mainland China forum city. RDF based on CC search engine can automatically extract, identify and understand the information of copyright and provide a great convenience for the legitimate use of different levels of IP network works. Online photo site Baba (bababian.com) has been integrated CC Chinese mainland version of the license agreement, the user of "Baba," can select the knowledge-sharing projects provided the License Agreement by mainland China and to authorize the use of pictures to enjoy copyright works.

219.4.2 The Contradictions Between the Tracking Analysis of Readers Virtual Behavior and the Protection of the Readers' Privacy on the Network

With the development of science and technology, privacy online in the virtual world lost and theft more easily, logicaly digital tendency of human being is from the real needs, privacy online and realistic privacy overlap. The contradictions between tracking analysis about virtual behavior and network privacy significantly highlight. As said by Zhao Shuizhong "Who Peeping Your Privacy Online" in the sentence: "You browse the network also the network views you" [7]. Currently, the first well-known American online privacy protection organizations TRUSTe, an independent nonprofit organization was established in June 1997 by the American Business Network Group and co-founded the Electronic Frontier Foundation, its main task is to formulate strategies and protection of personal information and issue certification mark, currently it provides certification services for 3500 many websites, including the leading portals such as Microsoft, Yahoo, IBM, Apple, Oracle etc. and other famous companies.

219.4.3 High Precision Resource Initiative to Push Lower Readers Virtual Acts of Initiative and the Contradiction Between the Needs and Evolution

When Network intelligence allows the reader to get the precise nature of resources to achieve a certain ceiling, the platform push to achieve resource evaluation more than their expectations by readers, the digital behavior of readers' active will significantly reduce, or even stagnate. The tendencies of readership figures stop evaluating. How to balance the relationship between the two become a topic of program research and analysis of digital tendency for the readers.

219.5 Conclusion

In short, the future of Libraries would be likely to become one of the physical premises for the readers to use digital resources, generalized library should be a standing in the cloud, to shared services, shared resources based on the vast resources of the network service platform. The emergence of cloud computing model, has provided an infinite number of possibilities for us to use the network, and has brought opportunities to play a central role in information resources by digital library under the Internet environment, and provided a guarantee for the sharing of inter-library information resources.

The library in regions, universities, research institute and information technology departments will become a member of this huge cloud services, it not only provides resources for cloud services while readers can enjoy the services of cloud resources. The users anywhere in the cloud service can adopt and use a simple terminal to access equipment (computers, cell phones, etc.) to obtain the cloud computing services conveniently, quickly and safely, the users can perform the inquiry of book Information, browse or obtain the information anytime, anywhere through the mobile devices, it has greatly changed the depth and breadth of library information service, and really achieve the goals pursued information services everywhere, omnipotently by libraries [8]. With the library community's concern for cloud computing technology and the wide application of security technology, we believe that Semantic Net Information service of library in China will enter a new era.

References

1. Zang L (2010) On the status and countermeasures of mobile phone-based service of public library. Libr Work Study 10
2. Wang C, Ai F (2011) Study on information resources integration and service mode innovation of digital library under the cloud computing environment. Libr Work Study 1:48–51

3. Jeffrey Z (2006) Web 3.0: a list apart (Blog) Jan 16
4. Zangnai Z (2009) Web 3.0 and personalized information services. New Century Library, vol 2
5. Wu Y (2011) Research and application of the Lib3.0's new service pattern based on web3.0. Library
6. Sunyusheng D (2009) Based on semantic grid digital library personalized recommendations studies: architecture and general framework. Inf Theor Pract 6
7. Zhao S (2004) Who peeping your privacy online. Electronics Industry Press, Beijing, p 49
8. Li S,Li Q (2011) Study on the application of cloud computing in the library union. libr Work Study 5

Chapter 220
Synthesis and Antibacterial Activity of Resveratrol Derivatives

Yuanmou Chen, Fei Hu, Yinghao Gao, Na Ji and Shaolong Jia

Abstract Resveratrol (3,5,4′-trihydroxy-trans-stilbene), which is a naturally occurring phytoalexin produced by a wide range of plants in response to environmental stress or pathogenic attack, is found in various medical plants. It has attracted increasing attention over the past decade because of its multiple beneficial bioactivity. In this paper, a set of 12 methoxylated trans-stilbene resveratrol analogues were prepared from methoxybenzoic acids. In addition, all compounds have been evaluated for their antibacterial activity against both types of Gram negative and Gram positive bacteria compared to resveratrol. Pharmacological data indicated that several derivatives showed a marked antibacterial activity, especially the most promising compound 2c, which has the low MIC 60 ~ 90 μg/mL value compared to the resveratrol. Both minimal inhibitory concentration (MIC) and inhibition zones were determined in order to monitor the efficacy of the synthesized compounds. Certain compounds inhibit bacterial growth with low MIC (μg/mL) value. The substitution pattern of the resveratrol derivatives at electronegative groups such as Cl was most important for the activity. Overall, identification of the potential efficacy of these compounds could serve as the bases for the development of novel antibacterial agents.

Keywords Resveratrol derivatives · Synthesis · Antibacterial activity · Structure–activity-relationship

Y. Chen (✉) · F. Hu · Y. Gao · N. Ji · S. Jia
Key Laboratory of Industrial Microbiology of Ministry of Education College of Biotechnology, Tianjin University of Science and Technology, No. 29, 13th Avenue 300457 Tianjin, China
e-mail: chenyuanmou400@126.com

220.1 Introduction

Resveratrol (3,5,4'-trihydroxystilbene) was identified as one ingredient of red wine, which could cause the so-called "French paradox" [1]. This compound, was first isolated from the roots of the white hellebore lily *Veratrum grandiflorum* by O.Loes in 1940 [2]. Since the discovery of its cardioprotective activity in 1992, resveratrol research has steadily accelerated. In past years, there have been a large of reports about resveratrol exert a variety of biological activities. Among the most significant activities of resveratrol are its cancer chemo-preventive properties [3, 4], antioxidant [5], antibacterial and anti-inflammatory activities [6–8]. Some of these has been reported to inhibit LDL oxidation in human [9], in addition to its blocking of platelet aggregation[10] and vasorelaxing activities [11]. In yeast assays, resveratrol was also found to significantly mimic calorie restriction by stimulating Sir2 [12] which is the most homologic homologue of Sirt1 of mammalian and extended lifespan by 70 % [13].

In recent years, a large number of papers have been published on resveratrol, which report a wide range of novel discoveries, such as new extraction methods, new applications [14–16] and resveratrol analogs [17–19]. This intrigued us to prepare its analoges and their derivatives. In this work, analogs with different substituents such as methoxy or halogens was designed and evaluated the antibacterial activity. The compounds were tested for their potency against *Escherichia coli*, *Staphylococcus aureus* and *Bacillus licheniformis* bacterial strains. In the light of the data obtained from the in vitro assays, the antibacterial of a few analogs were superior availability than resveratrol. The electronegative groups such as Br and Cl of the stilbenic backbone has been identified as crucial for the antibacterial effect of 1, 2, 7 and 8c. In addition, a better understanding of the structure—activity provide the basis for the development of resveratrol derivatives with more potent antibacterial activity.

220.2 Results and Discussion

220.2.1 Chemistry

The derivatives were prepared according to Scheme 220.1. Only for the construction of the trans-olefins was obtained, Wittig-Horner reaction is considered as the key route to prepare a series of resveratrol analogues. In this work, methoxylated analogues of resveratrol were started from methoxybenzoic acid, the compounds 1a were prepared in good yield, followed by reduction with $LiAlH_4$. Subsequent treatment of 2a with tribromophosphine afforded 3a in about 91.2 %. The compounds 4a were obtained by refluxing 3a with $P(OEt)_3$ using Wittig-Horner reaction, which was condensed with aromatic aldehydes in NaH/THF to offer compounds 1–12c, only the trans isomer was obtained. These synthesized compounds were characterized by elemental and spectral (^{1}H-NMR and MS) analysis.

220.2.2 Biological Activities

In the present study we evaluated the antibacterial activity of the resveratrol and the synthesized compounds (1c−12c) that were carried out against both types of Gram negative bacteria (*Escherichia coli*) and Gram positive bacteria (*S. aureus* and *B. lincheniformis*) in vitro. Diameter of zone of inhibition (in mm) and MIC (μg/mL) of all the compounds were demonstrated in order to monitor the antibacterial efficacy, the biological activity data were given in Table 220.1. Dimethyl sulfoxide treated group served as a control.

According to the test results, the compounds 1–12c exhibited various antibacterial response against different types of bacterial strains, but the compounds having electronegative groups such as halogens, showed better results than the other compounds. From Table 220.1, the compounds 3c, 9c and 5c, 11c (having none and 2-Methoxyl, respectively) were short of antibacterial activity against Gram positive bacteria *B. lincheniformis* and Gram negative bacteria *E. coli* respectively. These compounds 3c, 9c showed moderate activity against Gram negative bacteria E. coli and Gram positive bacteria *S. aureus* with MIC 180 and 240 μg/mL respectively, but compound 5c, 11c exhibited activity against Gram positive bacteria *S. aureus* and *B. lincheniformis* with MIC 240 and 270 μg/mL respectively. Among the compounds 1–12c, the compound 4c, 10c, and 6c, 12c (having 4-Methoxyl and 2,3-Methoxyl, respectively) exhibited antibacterial activity against Gram negative bacteria *E. coli* and Gram positive bacteria *S. aureus* and *B. lincheniformis* with MIC 180 ∼ 270 μg/mL for each. Out of these compounds, 1, 2, 7 and 8c exhibited significant antibacterial activity against different types of bacterial strains. Furthermore, the compound 2c (having chlorine group) has shown most potent antibacterial activity against Gram negative bacteria *E. coli* (MIC 90 μg/mL) Gram positive bacteria *S. aureus* with lowest MIC 60 μg/mL as compared to the standard resveratrol (MIC 120 and 90 μg/mL, respectively).

The preliminary structure–activity-relationships (SARs) suggested that substituted electronegative groups such as Br and Cl are essential for the antibacterial activity. The compound 2 and 8c having chlorine group exhibited good antibacterial activity against Gram negative bacteria *E. coli* and Gram positive bacteria *S. aureus*, *B. licheniformis* with MIC 60 and 90 μg/mL for each. Moreover,

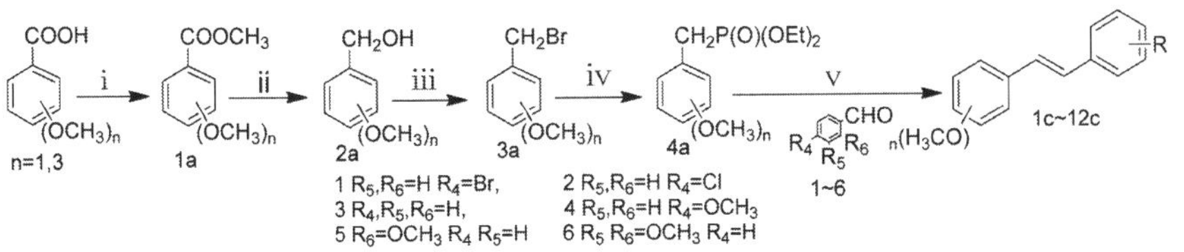

Scheme 220.1 Synthetic pathway for stilbenes 9–18a. Reagents and conditions: (**i**) H_2SO_4, CH_3OH, reflux; (**ii**) $LiAlH_4$, THF, 0 °C; (**iii**) PBr_3, CH_2Cl_2, rt; (**iv**) $P(O)(OEt)_3$, reflux; (**v**) NaH, ArCHO, THF, 0 °C

Table 220.1 Inhibitory-zone diameter (in mm) and MIC (μg/ml) of synthesized compounds 1–12c against the tested bacterial strains

Comp.	R	Antibacterial activity						
		Diameter of the inhibition zone (in mm)			Minimal inhibitor concentration (MIC μg/mL)			
		Escherichia coli	*Staphylococcus aureus*	*Bacillus licheniformis*		*Escherichia coli*	*Staphylococcus aureus*	*Bacillus licheniformis*
1c	4-bromo	20	14	12		90	120	120
2c	4-chloro	23	23	21		90	60	60
3c	–	7	12	–		180	240	–
4c	4-methoxy	10	10	10		240	180	180
5c	2-methoxy	–	10	–		–	240	270
6c	2,3-dimethoxy	10	11	12		270	240	270
7c	4-bromo	18	12	12		90	120	120
8c	4-chloro	16	20	21		90	60	90
9c	–	10	–	–		180	240	–
10c	4-methoxy	12	10	13		180	180	150

(continued)

Table 220.1 (continued)

Comp.	R	Antibacterial activity					
		Diameter of the inhibition zone (in mm)			Minimal inhibitor concentration (MIC μg/mL)		
		Escherichia coli	Staphylococcus aureus	Bacillus licheniformis	Escherichia coli	Staphylococcus aureus	Bacillus licheniformis
11c	2-methoxy	–	12	11	–	240	270
12c	2,3-dimethoxy	14	13	10	210	180	240
Resveratrol	–	21	23	20	120	90	60

compounds 1 and 7c having bromo group showed good activity against Gram negative bacteria E. coli with MIC 90 μg/mL and mild antibacterial activity against S. aureus and B. licheniformis with MIC 120 μg/mL. This study may provide valuable information for further design of resveratrol derivatives as potential antibacterial agents.

220.3 Conclusion

In summary, a series of resveratrol analogues was designed and synthesized by Wittig-Horner reaction and have been screened for their antibacterial activity against E. coli, S. aureus and B. licheniformis. The SAR analysis demonstrated that the substituted electronegative groups such as Br and Cl promotes antibacterial activity. The structural components studies revealed that responsible for the potency of compound 2c have been identified as chlorine group substitutions. Consequently, the bioactive research on 2c indicated its potential inhibitory effect against E. coli, S. aureus and B. licheniformis bacterial strains, with MIC value of 90, 60 and 60 μg/mL, comparable with that of resveratrol (120, 90 and 60 μg/mL, respectively).

220.4 Experimental

220.4.1 Chemistry

220.4.1.1 Materials and Measurements

^{1}H NMR spectra was obtained at Bruker AM-400 NMR spectrometer using CDCl$_3$ as the solvent except where otherwise specified, the chemical shifts are reported in δ values (ppm) relative to Me$_4$Si line as internal standard and J values are reported in Hertz. Mass spectra were determined on a Jeol SX 102 (FAB) spectrometer. Unless otherwise stated, reagents and solvents were of reagent grade and used as obtained from commercial sources without further purification. Dichloromethane was distilled from CaH$_2$, THF from sodium prior to use and DMF were dried over anhydrous sodium sulfate. Thin layer chromatography (TLC) was performed using E. Merck silica gel 60 GF$_{254}$ precoated plates (0.25 mm). Silica gel (particle size 200–400 mesh) was used for flash chromatography.

220.4.1.2 General Procedures

General Procedure 1 (GP1) for the Preparation of Aromatic Esters from Methoxybenzoic Acids

In a round-bottomed flask, to a well-stirred suspension of a mixture of methoxybenzoic acids (1 eq.) in CH_3OH (35 ml) was added a few drops of concentrated sulphuric acid at room temperature. After the mixture was stirred at 80 °C for 8 h, the solution was poured into 100 mL ice-water and stirred for 10 min. Neutralized with $NaHCO_3$, the resulted mixture was extracted with ethyl acetate and the organic layer was washed with water and brine, dried over anhydrous sodium sulfate. The solvent was concentrated in vacuo to yield the pure product as a white solid in good yield aromatic esters (1a).

General Procedure 2 (GP2) for the Preparation of Aromatic Alcohol from Aromatic Esters

$LiAlH_4$ (0.5 eq.) was added slowly to a solution of aromatic esters (1 eq.) in THF (50 mL) at 0 °C for 1 h. The reaction mixture was stirred for 10 h at room temperature. Ice-water (10 mL) was added slowly to the reaction mixture and stirred for 10 min, followed by concentrated 2 M HCl to neutralize the base. The reaction mixture was extracted with ethyl acetate, and the ethyl acetate layer was washed with water and brine, dried anhydrous sodium sulfate. The solvent was removed in vacuo to yield the pure product in good yield aromatic alcohol (2a).

General Procedure 3 (GP3) for the Preparation of Benzyl Bromine from Aromatic Alcohol

A solution of tribromophosphine (3 eq.) in CH_2Cl_2 (15 mL) was added dropwise to a solution of aromatic alcohol (1 eq.) in CH_2Cl_2 (30 mL) at 0 °C. The reaction mixture was stirred for 2 h and then warmed up to room temperature. After 4 h, the solution was poured into 50 mL ice-water and stirred for 10 min. Then the organic layer was washed with water and aq $NaHCO_3$ (3 × 20 mL), dried over anhydrous sodium sulfate and evaporated to yield the pure product as a solid benzyl bromine (3a).

General Procedure 4 (GP4) for the Preparation of Methoxylated Diethyl Benzylphosphonates from Benzyl Bromine (Arbuzov Rearrangement)

A mixture of bromide (1 eq.) and triethyl phosphite (2 mL 5 eq.) was stirred at 135 °C for 3 h. Triethyl phosphate (2 mL 5 eq.) was added again and stirred another 4 h. After the reaction was completely finished, the mixture was cooled to room temperature and purified by distillation at 4×10^{-3} bar and 120 °C to yield yellow oils methoxylated diethyl benzylphosphonates (4a). The crude product was used directly for the next step without further purification.

General Procedure 5 (GP5) for Synthesis of Compounds 1c–6c and 1d~6d (Wittig-Hornor Condensation) [20]

Methoxylated diethyl benzylphosphonates (1 eq.) in the round-bottomed flask was added dropwise to a suspension of NaH (4 eq.) in THF (20 mL) at 0 °C and stirred for 1 h. Then the mixture was treated with aromatic carboxaldehyde (1–6a) (1 eq.) at 0 °C for 2 h. The reaction mixture was warmed up to room temperature and further stirred for 15 h. The solution was poured into 150 mL ice-water, neutralized with 2 M HCl, and extracted with ethyl acetate. The ethyl acetate layer was washed with water and brine, dried over anhydrous sodium sulfate, and concentrated. The crude product purified by crystallization or flash column chromatography to afford compounds 1c~6c and 1d~6d.

220.4.1.3 Syntheses

3,4,5-Trimethoxyl-4′-bromo-trans-stilbene (1c)

This compound was prepared in 51.6 % yield by following GP 4 and 5. White solid: ^{1}H NMR (400 MHz CDCl$_3$): δ/ppm 7.48 (d, J = 8.8 Hz, 2H), 7.37 (d, J = 8.4 Hz, 2H), 7.02 (d, J = 16.4 Hz, 1H), 6.93 (d, J = 16.4 Hz, 1H), 6.73 (s, 2H), 3.92 (s, 6H), 3.87 (s, 3H). MS (m/z): 349.04 [M$^+$].

3,4,5-Trimethoxyl-4′-chloro-trans-stilbene (2c)

This compound was prepared in 55.5 % yield by following GP 4 and 5. White solid: ^{1}H NMR (400 MHz CDCl$_3$): δ/ppm 7.43 (d, J = 8.4 Hz, 2H), 7.01 (d, J = 8.8 Hz, 2H), 7.01 (d, J = 16.4 Hz, 1H), 6.94 (d, J = 16.4 Hz, 1H), 6.73 (s, 2H), 3.92 (s, 6H), 3.87 (s, 3H). MS (m/z): 305.08 [M$^+$].

3,4,5-Trimethoxyl-trans-stilbene (3c)

This compound was prepared in 38.4 % yield by following GP 4 and 5. White solid: ^{1}H NMR (400 MHz CDCl$_3$): δ/ppm 7.51 (d, J = 7.2 Hz, 2H), 7.36 (t, J = 7.6 Hz, 2H), 7.26 (t, J = 7.4 Hz, 1H), 7.05 (d, J = 16.4 Hz, 1H), 7.00 (d, J = 16.4 Hz, 1H), 6.74 (s, 2H), 3.92 (s, 6H), 3.87 (s, 3H). MS (m/z): 271.33 [M$^+$].

3,4,5,4′-Tetramethoxyl-trans-stilbene (4c)

This compound was prepared in 34.2 % yield by following GP 4 and 5. White solid: ^{1}H NMR (400 MHz CDCl$_3$): δ/ppm 7.44 (d, J = 8.4 Hz, 2H), 6.97 (d, J = 16.4 Hz, 1H), 6.89 (d, J = 16.4 Hz, 1H), 6.89 (d, J = 8.8 Hz, 2H), 6.71 (s, 2H), 3.91 (s, 6H) 3.86 (s, 3H), 3.82 (s, 3H). MS (m/z): 301.14 [M$^+$].

3,4,5,2′-Tetramethoxyl-trans-stilbene (5c)

This compound was prepared in 45.2 % yield by following GP 4 and 5. White solid: ^{1}H NMR (400 MHz CDCl$_3$): δ/ppm 7.57 (d, J = 8.8 Hz, 1H), 7.36 (t, J = 16.4 Hz, 1H), 7.24 (q, J = 8.8 Hz, 1H), 7.04 (d, J = 16.4 Hz, 1H), 6.97 (t, J = 7.6 Hz, 1H), 6.91 (d, J = 8.4 Hz, 1H), 6.76 (s, 2H), 3.92 (s, 6H), 3.90 (s, 3H), 3.87 (s, 3H). MS (m/z): 301.24 [M$^+$].

3,4,5,2′,3′-Pentamethoxyl-trans-stilbene (6c)

This compound was prepared in 49.4 % yield by following GP 4 and 5. White solid: ^{1}H NMR (400 MHz CDCl$_3$): δ/ppm 7.34 (d, J = 16.4 Hz, 1H), 7.22 (d, J = 9.2 Hz, 1H), 7.06 (t, J = 8 Hz, 1H), 7.05 (d, J = 16.4 Hz, 1H), 6.84 (d, J = 9.2 Hz, 1H), 6.77 (s, 2H), 3.93 (s, 6H), 3.89 (s, 3H), 3.87 (s, 3H), 3.86 (s, 3H). MS (m/z): 331.15 [M$^+$].

4-Methoxyl-4′-bromo-trans-stilbene (1d)

This compound was prepared in 24.9 % yield by following GP 4 and 5. White solid: ^{1}H NMR (400 MHz CDCl$_3$): δ/ppm 7.45 (d, J = 6.4 Hz, 2H), 7.43 (d,

J = 6 Hz, 2H), 7.34 (d, J = 8.4 Hz, 2H), 7.04 (d, J = 16.4 Hz, 1H), 6.89 (d, J = 8.8 Hz, 2H), 6.89 (d, J = 16.4 Hz, 1H), 3.83 (s, 3H). MS (m/z): 290.02 [M$^+$].

4-Methoxyl-4'-chloro-trans-stilbene (2d)

This compound was prepared in 31.8 % yield by following GP 4 and 5. White solid: ^{1}H NMR (400 MHz CDCl$_3$): δ/ppm 7.43 (d, J = 8.8 Hz, 2H), 7.40 (d, J = 8.4 Hz, 2H), 7.30 (d, J = 8.4 Hz, 2H), 7.02 (d, J = 16.4 Hz, 1H), 6.90 (d, J = 16.4 Hz, 1H), 6.89 (d, J = 8.8 Hz, 2H), 3.83 (s, 3H). MS (m/z): 246.16 [M$^+$].

4-Methoxyl-trans-stilbene (3d)

This compound was prepared in 23.4 % yield by following GP 4 and 5. White solid: ^{1}H NMR (400 MHz CDCl$_3$): δ/ppm 7.49 (d, J = 7.6 Hz, 2H), 7.45 (d, J = 8.8 Hz, 2H), 7.40 (t, J = 7.6 Hz, 2H), 7.21 (t, J = 7.6 Hz, 1H), 7.06 (d, J = 16 Hz, 1H), 6.97 (d, J = 16 Hz, 1H), 6.90 (d, J = 8.4 Hz, 2H), 3.83 (s, 3H). MS (m/z): 211.11 [M$^+$].

4,4'-Dimethoxyl-trans-stilbene (4d)

This compound was prepared in 40.2 % yield by following GP 4 and 5. White solid: ^{1}H NMR (400 MHz CDCl$_3$): δ/ppm 7.40-7.44 (m, 4H), 6.93 (s, 2H), 6.87-6.90 (m, 4H), 3.82 (s, 6H). MS (m/z): 241.01 [M$^+$].

2,4'-Dimethoxyl-trans-stilbene (5d)

This compound was prepared in 20.2 % yield by following GP 4 and 5. White solid: ^{1}H NMR (400 MHz CDCl$_3$): δ/ppm 7.55 (d, J = 8 Hz, 1H), 7.45 (d, J = 8.4 Hz, 2H), 7.34 (d, J = 16.4 Hz, 1H), 7.20 (t, J = 7.2 Hz, 1H), 7.05 (d, J = 16.4 Hz, 1H), 6.94 (t, J = 7.6 Hz, 1H), 6.87 (d, J = 8.4 Hz, 3H), 3.85 (s, 3H), 3.79 (s, 3H). MS (m/z): 241.31 [M$^+$].

2,3,4'-Trimethoxyl-trans-stilbene (6d)

This compound was prepared in 25.3 % yield by following GP 4 and 5. White solid: ^{1}H NMR (400 MHz CDCl$_3$): δ/ppm 7.49 (d, J = 8 Hz, 1H), 7.32 (t, J = 16.4 Hz, 1H), 7.22 (d, J = 8 Hz, 1H), 7.08 (d, J = 16.4 Hz, 1H), 7.04 (t, J = 8 Hz, 1H), 6.90 (d, J = 8.8 Hz, 2H), 6.81 (d, J = 8.4 Hz, 1H), 3.89 (s, 6H), 3.84 (s, 3H), 3.83 (s, 3H). MS (m/z): 271.21 [M$^+$].

220.4.2 Biological Studies

220.4.2.1 Antibacterial Activity

The antibacterial activities of the synthesized compounds 1–12c with *E. coli*, *S. aureus* and *B. licheniformis* bacterial strains at a concentration of 300 μg/mL in vitro were screened by the filter paper disc-method, and resveratrol at the same concentrations was introduced as positive control. DMSO served as control and there was no visible change in bacterial growth due to this. Solution is put into each bottle which are kept in the hot-air oven at 150 °C before and the discs are transferred to the inoculated plates with a pair of fine pointedtweezers. Before using the test organisms, grown on nutrient agar, they were subcultured on nutrient broth at 37 °C for 18–20 h. Each disc was applied to the surface of the agar without lateral movement once the surface had been touched. Then the plates incubated were incubated for 24 h at 37 °C.

220.4.2.2 Minimal Inhibitory Concentration (MIC)

The antibacterial activity was assayed in vitro by Two-fold broth dilution against the bacterial strains. The MICs (μg/mL) were defined as the lowest concentrations of compound that completely inhibited the growth of each strain. The synthesized compounds and resveratrol dissolved indimethylsulphoxide solution were diluted to the culture media. Mueller–Hinton Broth for bacteria was used to obtain the final concentrations ranging from 300 to 3 μg/mL. Inocula consisted of approximately 5×10^4 bacteria/mL. The MICs were read after incubation at 37 °C for 24 h.

References

1. Richard JL (1987) Coronary risk factors the french paradox. Arch Mal Coeur Vaiss 80:17–21
2. Takaoka MJ (1940) Of the phenolic substances of white hellebore. J Faculty Sci 3:1–16
3. Kopp P (1998) Resveratrol, a phytoestrogen found in red wine. A possible explanation for the conundrum of the 'French paradox'? Eur J Endocrinol 138:619–620
4. Jang M, Pezzuto JM (1999) Cancer chemopreventive activity of resveratrol. Drugs Exp Clin Res 25:65–771
5. Stivala LA, Savio M, Carafoli F, Perucca P, Bianchi L, Maga G, Forti L, Pagnoni UM, Albini A, Prosperi E, Vannini V (2001) Specific structural determinants are responsible for the antioxidant activity and the cell cycle effects of resveratrol. J Biol Chem 276:22586–22594
6. Daroch F, Hoeneisen M, Gonzalez CL, Kawaguchi F, Salgado F, Solar H, Garcia A (2001) In vitro antibacterial activity of chilean red wines against helicobacter pylori. Microbios 104:79–85
7. Wang WB, Lai HC, Hsueh PR, Chiou RY, Lin SB, Liaw SJ (2006) Inhibition of swarming and virulence factor expression in proteus mirabilis by resveratrol. J Med Microbiol 55:1313–1321
8. Zaidi SF, Ahmed K, Yamamoto T, Kondo T, Usmanghani K et al (2009) Effect of resveratrol on helicobacter pylori-induced interleukin-8 secretion, reactive oxygen species generation and morphological changes in human gastric epithelial cells. Biol Pharm Bull 32:1931–1935
9. Arichi H, Kimura Y, Okuda H, Baba K et al (1982) Effects of stilbene components of the roots of polygonum cuspidatum on lipid metabolism. Chem Pharm Bull (Tokyo) 30:1766–1770
10. Pace-Asciak CR, Hahn S, Diamandis EP, Soleas G, Goldberg DM (1996) The red wine phenolics trans-resveratrol and quercetin block human platelet aggregation and eicosanoid synthesis: implications for protection against coronary heart disease. Clin Chim Acta 235:207–219
11. Chen CK, Pace-Asciak CR (1996) Vasorelaxing activity of resveratrol and quercetin in isolated rat aorta. Gen Pharmacol 27:363–366
12. Wood JG et al (2004) Sirtuin activators mimic caloric restriction and delay ageing in metazoans. Nature 430:686–689
13. Howitz KT, Bitterman KJ, Cohen HY, Lamming DW et al (2003) Small molecule activators of sirtuins extend *Saccharomyces cerevisiae* lifespan. Nature 425:191–196

14. Wang RH, Sengupta K, Li C, Kim HS, Cao L et al (2008) Impaired DNA damage response, genome instability, and tumorigenesis in SIRT1 mutant mice. Cancer Cell 14:312–323
15. Rocha-Gonzalez HI, Ambriz-Tututi M, Granados-Soto V (2008) Resveratrol:A natural compound with pharmacological potential in neurodegenerative diseases. CNS Neurosci Ther 14:234–247
16. Vieira de Almeida LM, Pineiro CC, Leite Marina MC, Brolese G, Leal RB, Gottfried C, Goncalves CA (2008) Protective effects of resveratrol on hydrogen peroxide induced toxicity in primary cortical astrocyte cultures. Neurochem Res 33:8–15
17. Ali HA, Kondo K, Tsuda Y (1992) Synthesis and nematocidal activity of hydroxystilbenes. Chem Pharm Bull 40:1130–1136
18. Thakkar K, Geahlen RL, Gushman M (1993) Synthesis and protein-tyrosine kinase inhibitory activity of polyhydroxylated stilbene analogs of piceatannol. J Med Chem 36:2950–2955
19. Murias M, Handler N, Erker T et al (2004) Resveratrol analogues as selectivecyclooxygenase-2 inhibitors: synthesis and structure–activityrelationship. Bioorg Med Chem 12:5571–5578
20. Cristau HJ, Darviche F, Torreilles E (1998) Mechanistic investigations of the formation of TTF derivatives via the phosphonate way. Tetrahedron Lett 39:2103–2106

Chapter 221
Comparison of Intravenous Propofol Using Target-Controlled Infusion and Inhalational Sevoflurane Anesthesia in Pediatric Patients

Dong Su, Haichun Ma, Wei Han, Limin Jin and Jia Liu

Abstract Propofol is used for the hypnotic effect and is characterized by a short onset of action and a prompt recovery from anesthesia. The target-controlled infusion system can administer drugs to patients more precisely and consistently. Sevoflurane is a popular inhalational anesthetic for general anesthesia in children. We conducted this study to compare the intravenous propofol using TCI system and inhalational sevoflurane anesthesia in pediatric patients. We collected clinical data of 128 pediatric patients who were underwent surgery from February, 2011 to February 2013 in the First Hospital of Jilin University. Patients were randomly assigned into two groups of either propofol TCI (group P, n = 64) and sevoflurane (group S, n = 64) using a computer generated randomization list. All patients were monitored with an electrocardiogram (ECG), non-invasive blood pressure (BP) and pulse oxygen saturation (SPO2). Patients in group P received an intravenous propofol infusion using a TCI system. Patients in group S received inhalational sevoflurane anesthesia. There was a significant difference between the two groups in hemodynamic variables after anesthesia and intubation and the group P decreased greater than group S ($P < 0.05$). There was significant difference in the time of loss of consciousness, intubation, recovery of spontaneous respiration, and the cases of respiration depression between two groups ($P < 0.05$). The time of loss of consciousness and intubation was longer in the group S than the group P ($P < 0.05$). But the time of recovery of spontaneous respiration and consciousness was shorter in group S ($P < 0.05$). There was less cases of respiration depression in group S ($P < 0.05$). Both of the groups can provide satisfied anesthesia and have their own advantages and disadvantages. We should make good use of the doses of the infusion or inhalation of anesthetic drugs.

D. Su · H. Ma · W. Han · L. Jin
Department of Anesthesia, The First Hospital of Jilin University, Changchun 130021, China

J. Liu (✉)
Department of Thyroid Surgery, The First Hospital of Jilin University, Changchun 130021, China
e-mail: sosea@sina.com

Keywords Anesthesia · Propofol · Sevoflurane · Pediatric

221.1 Introduction

Every anesthetic, even a routine superficial procedure in pediatric patients, can result in a challenge: communication can be impossible; everything can happen from lowest weight or unexplained depression, hypoxia and pulmonary aspiration to anesthetic reaction. Main of our duties as anesthesiologists is anticipation: to be prepared. But the key point of all is how to make good use of the anesthetic agents. Propofol is used for the hypnotic effect and is characterized by a short onset of action and a prompt recovery from anesthesia. Additionally, in maintaining an appropriate level of sedation, it is necessary to maintain the serum level of drugs through a continuous administration of drugs rather than an intermittent one. The target-controlled infusion (TCI, Ochestra Base Primea, Fresenius Kabi Company, Brezins, France) system can administer drugs to patients more precisely and consistently [2]. Sevoflurane is a popular inhalational anesthetic for general anesthesia in children. It is especially characterized by a lower blood/gas partition coefficient, less irritation to the airway, less cardiac depressive effect, and less toxicity to the liver or kidney as compared with other volatile anesthetics. Anesthesiologists prefer those characteristics for pediatric use. We conducted this study to compare the intravenous propofol using TCI system and inhalational sevoflurane anesthesia in pediatric patients and assess which one is an effective and safer method of anesthesia for children.

221.2 Materials and Methods

221.2.1 Patients Selection

The protocol was approved by the Hospital Ethics Committee and informed consent was obtained by the patients' parents. We collected clinical data of 128 pediatric patients who were underwent surgery (include appendectomy 52 cases, hernia repair 46 cases, cryptorchidism surgery 30 cases) from February, 2011 to February 2013 in the First Hospital of Jilin University. There were 97 boys and 31 girls whose age range was 3–8 years, weight was 11–42 kg. The operation time was 0.5–1.5 h. Patients were randomly assigned into two groups of either propofol TCI (group P, n = 64) and sevoflurane (group S, n = 64) using a computer generated randomization list.

221.2.2 Methods

All pediatric patients were restricted from oral intake of clear fluid for 2–3 h. Thirty min before transferring children to the operation room, an intramuscular atropine (0.02 mg/kg) was performed in the ward. In the operation room, an intravenous access on the dorsum of a hand was established immediately and infusion of 5 % Glucose solution was commenced slowly. All patients were monitored with an electrocardiogram (ECG), non-invasive blood pressure (BP) and pulse oxygen saturation (SPO2). Patients in group P received an intravenous propofol (1 % Fresenius Kabi, Deutschland GmbH) infusion using a TCI system. The initial effectsite target concentration of propofol was set at 2.0 μg/ml. Patients in group S received sevoflurane anesthesia for concentration of 8 % with mask at first. After 2–3 min, we will down-regulate the concentration according to the patients' situation. After the concentration of propofol or sevoflurane reached the target level and the patients lost the consciousness, laryngeal mask airway would be established to keep the spontaneous respiration. Then epidural or caudal anesthesia was performed in lateral position. Local anesthesia was performed using 0.33 % ropivacaine, which was the mixture of 1 % ropivacaine (AstraZeneca AB), 2 % lidocaine and 0.9 % saline solution (1:1:1). We regulated the target concentration of propofol and sevoflurane according to the clinical effects and vital signs. During the surgery, we kept the spontaneous respiration and before the operation was over, we stopped anesthetic agents infusing or inhaling, and removed the laryngeal mask when the children could not endure it any more.

During the anesthesia, ECG, BP and SPO2 were monitored and recorded continuously. We also recorded the time of consciousness loss, laryngeal mask intubation, and the cases of cough, respiration depression. We defined the time of looking for food as the consciousness recovery and evaluate the waken status within two hours (perfect: crying time $\leq$ 10 min, well: 11–20 min, bad: > 20 min).

Data are expressed as mean $\pm$ standard deviation (SD). The level of statistical significance was set at $P < 0.05$. Statistical analysis was performed with SPSS version 12.0 (SPSS Inc., Chicago, IL, USA).

221.3 Results

There was no significant difference in demographic variables between the two groups ($P > 0.05$) (Table 221.1). There was no significant difference in hemodynamic data before anesthesia between the two groups ($P > 0.05$). There was significant difference in the mean value of measured time in each group ($P < 0.05$) (Fig. 221.1, 221.2, 221.3). There was a significant difference between the two groups in hemodynamic variables after anesthesia and intubation and the group P decreased greater than group S ($P < 0.05$) (Table 221.2).

Table 221.1 Demographic Variables

	Group propofol (n = 64)	Group sevoflurane (n = 64)
Age (year)	5.2 ± 0.6	5.0 ± 0.8
Weight (kg)	22.1 ± 1.6	21.9 ± 0.9
Height (cm)	108.6 ± 16.3	111.9 ± 15.2
Duration of operation (min)	56.6 ± 10.2	57.8 ± 6.3
Duration of anesthesia (min)	73.1 ± 14.6	72.8 ± 15.3

Data are expressed as mean ± SD. There is no significant difference between groups

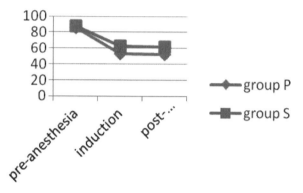

Fig. 221.1 Systolic blood pressure at measured time

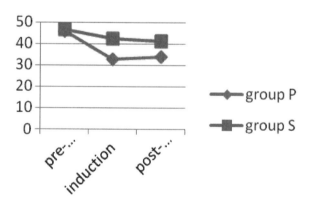

Fig. 221.2 Diastolic blood pressure at measured time

There was significant difference in the time of loss of consciousness, intubation, recovery of spontaneous respiration, and the cases of respiration depression between two groups ($P < 0.05$). The time of loss of consciousness and intubation was longer in the group S than the group P ($P < 0.05$). But the time of recovery of spontaneous respiration and consciousness was shorter in group S ($P < 0.05$). There was less cases of respiration depression in group S ($P < 0.05$). There was no significant difference in the cases of cough and movement during the process of intubation and status of recovery between the two groups ($P > 0.05$) (Table 221.3).

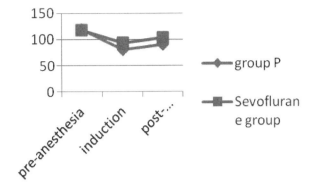

Fig. 221.3 Heart rate at measured time

Table 221.2 Pre-anesthesia, induction and post-intubation records of systolic and diastolic blood pressure and heart rate

	Group propofol (n = 64)	Group sevoflurane (n = 64)
Pre-anesthesia		
Systolic pressure	85.8 ± 4.6	88.0 ± 3.2
Diastolic pressure	45.7 ± 1.1	46.7 ± 2.9
Heart rate	118.7 ± 3.4	117.8 ± 3.9
Anesthesia induction		
Systolic pressure	52.9 ± 4.0*#	62.2 ± 0.9*
Diastolic pressure	32.6 ± 1.4*#	42.3 ± 1.1*
Heart rate	80.9 ± 6.9*#	93.7 ± 4.8*
Post-intubation		
Systolic pressure	52.2 ± 0.9*#	62.0 ± 1.1*
Diastolic pressure	33.8 ± 1.4*#	41.3 ± 1.8*
Heart rate	90.2 ± 6.3*#	103.7 ± 4.2*

Data are expressed as mean ± SD
*$P < 0.05$ vs Pre-anesthesia
# $P < 0.05$ vs group propofol

221.4 Discussion

With the development of surgery and anesthesia, many pediatric selective or emergent operations are chosen to be performed in the childhood. The young patients have their own character and specificity of physiology and pathology. The stability of respiration and circulation is very important to them. It is great challenge to the anesthesiologists. In addition to the carefully monitoring, sedation and anesthesia drug is the key point of all [8].

Inhalational anesthesia has been the mainstay in pediatric anesthesia till recent times [10]. Sevoflurane is a popular inhalational anesthetic for general anesthesia in children. It is especially characterized by a lower blood/gas partition coefficient, less irritation to the airway, less cardiodepressive effect, and less toxicity to the liver or kidney as compared with other volatile anesthetics. Anesthesiologists

Table 221.3 Data during the process of anesthesia

	Group propofol (n = 64)	Group sevoflurane (n = 64)
Time of loss of consciousness (s)	30 ± 13	49 ± 12*
Time of intubation (s)	130 ± 18	189 ± 19*
Time of recovery of spontaneous respiration (s)	420 ± 32	300 ± 22*
Time of recovery of consciousness (min)	27.5 ± 2.1	18.2 ± 2.6*
Status of recovery (%)		
Perfect	22 (34.4)	23 (35.9)
Well	31 (48.4)	29 (45.3)
Bad	11 (17.2)	12 (18.8)
Cases of cough and movement (%)	9 (14.1)	8 (12.5)
Cases of respiration depression (%)	8 (12.5)	2 * (3.1)

Data are expressed as mean ± SD
*P < 0.05 versus group propofol

prefer those characteristics for pediatric use. But with the advances in understanding of pharmacology and availability of new fast-acting drugs and the modern infusion pumps, the target-controlled infusion (TCI) system can administer drugs to patients more precisely and consistently and has become an attractive option in the administration of general anesthesia in children. Additionally, in maintaining an appropriate level of sedation, it is able to maintain the serum level of drugs through a continuous administration of drugs rather than an intermittent one. In this article, we compared the intravenous propofol using target-controlled Infusion and inhalational sevoflurane anesthesia in pediatric patients during the anesthesia induction, maintaining, recovery and hemodynamic influence. It showed that propofol and sevoflurane were all safe to the pediatric patients, but the hemodynamics was more stable in the group sevoflurane. The propofol could provide quicker anesthesia and the sevoflurane could provide quicker recovery.

However, concern has been raised over its propensity to result in significant excitatory emergence in the immediate recovery phase of anesthesia. Emergence agitation is a major source of dissatisfaction for parents, nurses, and others taking care of these children [3]. The irritable, uncooperative, incoherent child who is inconsolably crying, moaning, kicking, or thrashing is at risk for injury and requires extra nursing care and supplemental sedative and/or analgesic medications, which may delay patient discharge from hospital. Pediatric anesthesiologists mostly agree that anesthetic agent causes a higher incidence of emergence agitation [7]. Various methods, including treatments against surgical pain and prescriptions of sedative premedication, have been tried to prevent emergence agitation after anesthesia, but their validities have not been well clarified [12]. In the study, we paid attention to this serious problem though the status of perfect and well weighted the bad. The etiology of emergence agitation derives from multiple factors, including pain, preoperative anxiety, type of surgical procedures, personal character of the patient, too rapid awakening, and type of anesthetics. No sole factor can explain the etiology of emergence agitation. Although pain is definitely a major reason for emergence agitation, screaming as a result of pain should be distinguished from emergence agitation. However, especially in younger children, it is sometimes not possible to distinguish between them. It is widely believed that reducing or eliminating pain decreases the incidence of emergence agitation after anesthesia. Several studies demonstrated that regional block, opioids, and non-steroidal antiinflammatory drugs decrease the incidence of emergence agitation. However, emergence agitation often occurs even after adequate pain treatment or after procedures that are not associated with pain.

Target-controlled infusion (TCI) pumps currently do not satisfactorily cater for the pediatric population [6], particularly for those under 5 years. Growth and development are two major aspects of children not readily apparent in adults, and these two aspects influence clearance (CL) and volume of distribution (V). In simple terms, V determines initial dose, and CL determines infusion rate at steady state [1]. Three major covariates (size, age, and organ function) contribute to parameter variability in children [4]. Although pharmacokinetics (PK) in children is receiving increasing attention and is eminently programmable into a TCI device, pharmacodynamic (PD) measures in children remain poorly defined, partly because the depth of anesthesia monitoring are inadequate. Both PK and PD are necessary for safe use of TCI pumps [9]. Propofol PK in children has been investigated in numerous publications [5] with different estimates in each study. Both the administration method (intravenous bolus or infusion) and the collection of venous blood for assay rather than arterial blood will have influence on PK parameter estimates. Schuttler [11] pooled data from adults and children to investigate covariate effects using allometry. The allometric exponent for clearance was estimated as 0.75.

In summary, the both groups can provide satisfied anesthesia and have their own advantages and disadvantages. We should make good use of the doses of the infusion or inhalation of anesthetic drugs. Pay more attention to the pharmacodynamics of propofol and emergence agitation after anesthesia is necessary and important in the pediatric population.

References

1. Allegaert K, de Hoon J, Verbesselt R (2007) Maturational pharmacokinetics of single intravenous bolus of propofol. J Paediatr Anaesth 17:1028–1034
2. Anderson BJ (2010) Pediatric models for adult target-controlled infusion pumps. J Pediatric Anesthesia 20:223–232
3. Cohen IT, Finkel JC, Hannallah RS, Hummer KA, Patel KM (2003) Rapid emergence does not explain agitation following sevoflurane anaesthesia in infants and children: a comparison with propofol. J Paediatr Anaesth 13:63–67
4. Hu C, Horstman DJ, Shafer SL (2005) Variability of target-controlled infusion is less than the variability afterbolus injection. J Anaesthesiology 102:639–645

5. Jeleazcov C, Ihmsen H, Schmidt J (2008) Pharmacodynamic modelling of the bispectral index response to propofol-based anaesthesia during general surgery in children. J Anaesth 100(4):509–516
6. Munoz HR, Cortinez LI, Ibacache ME (2006) Effect site concentrations of propofol producing hypnosis in children and adults: comparison using the bispectral index. J Acta Anaesthesiol Scand 50:882–887
7. Kuratani Norifumi, Oi Yumiko (2008) Greater incidence of emergence agitation in children after sevoflurane anesthesia as compared with halothane. J Anesthesiology 109:225–232
8. Daniel Mellon R, Simone Arthur F, Rappaport Bob A (2007) Use of anesthetic agents in neonates and young children. J Pediatric Anesthesia 104:509–520
9. Saint-Maurice C, Cockshott ID, Douglas EJ (1989) Pharmacokinetics of propofol in young children after a single dose. Br J Anaesth 63:667–670
10. Schultheis LW, Mathis LL, Roca RA (2006) Pediatric drug development in anesthesiology: an FDA perspective. J Anesth Analg 103:49–51
11. Schuttler J, Ihmsen H (2000) Population pharmacokinetics of propofol: a multicenter study. J Anesthesiology 92:727–738
12. Voepel-Lewis T, Malviya S, Tait AR (2003) A prospective cohort study of emergence agitation in the pediatric postanesthesia care unit. J Anesth Analg 96:1625–1630

Chapter 222
Effect of Different Fluids on Blood Volume Expansion in Epidural Anesthesia of Elderly Patients

Dong Su, Lei Pang, Haichun Ma, Wei Han and Jia Liu

Abstract Relative hypovolemia is generally considered to be the cause of the reduction of the blood pressure during epidural anesthesia, especially in the elderly groups. In this study, we compared the effect of 6 % hydroxyethyl starch 130/0.3, succinyl gelatin and lactated Ringer's solution on blood volume expansion in epidural anesthesia of aging. Sixty ASA I-II elderly patients scheduled for elective radical mastectomy requiring epidural anesthesia were recruited. Patients were randomly assigned into three groups of infusing different fluid. An intravenous fluid load of 1,000 ml of 6 % hydroxyethyl starch 130/0 (group A), succinyl gelatin (group B) or lactated Ringer's solution (group C) was given at a constant rate over 60 min via an infusion pump. Intravenous ^{125}I-HSA1 ml (5–10 μCi) was injected into the cubital vein of infusing fluid. The plasma volume, basis of blood volume, blood volume of different time, blood volume change and fluid remained were calculated from the equation. The incidence of hypotension was higher in group C than other two groups ($P < 0.01$). During the surgery, the systolic and diastolic blood pressure declined in all groups and the difference was significant in group A, B ($P < 0.05$) and group C ($P < 0.01$). The BV increased significantly 30 min after anesthesia to 60 min after completing infusing in all groups ($P < 0.05$). Compared with group C, △BV, FR increased significantly in group A and B from completing infusing to 60 min later ($P < 0.05$). 6 % hydroxyethyl starch 130/0.3 and succinyl gelatin are better to keep the hemodynamic stability in elder patients after performing epidural anesthesia and can last longer in the circulation.

Keywords Elderly · Epidural anesthesia · Plasma volume

D. Su · L. Pang · H. Ma · W. Han
Department of Anesthesia, The First Hospital of Jilin University, Changchun 130021, China

J. Liu (✉)
Department of Thyroid Surgery, The First Hospital of Jilin University, Changchun 130021, China
e-mail: sosea@sina.com

222.1 Introduction

With an increasing number of elderly people (individuals 65 years of age and older), the demand for surgery will continue to increase. Regional anesthetic techniques are frequently used in elderly patients undergoing surgery. Aging influences the pharmacokinetics and pharmacodynamics of local anesthetics after perineural administration. Relative hypovolemia [2] is generally considered to be the cause of the reduction of the blood pressure during epidural anesthesia, especially in the elderly groups. Although the mechanisms accounting for any arterial hypotension are probably different, hemodilution is frequently induced by volume loading with different solutions before induction of anesthesia to prevent decrease in arterial pressure. The purpose of using volume expanders before and during surgery is to maintain stable hemodynamics. Applying an appropriate fluid with enough volume at this stage may prevent systemic hypoperfusion and cellular hypoxia, which lead to systemic lactic acidosis. Furthermore, after surgery, patients experience systemic inflammatory responses, which lead to fluid extravasations. Therefore correct volume administration is recommended in this stage. There is controversy regarding the different types of solutions used during anesthesia, and various researchers have used materials such as crystalloid solutions or colloids, including gelatin, and hydroxyl ethyl starch solutions. Volume expansion is an important aspect of these solutions, however, side effects, such as inflammatory responses, and effects on organs such as the kidney should also be considered during their administration. This article is to compare the effect of three different fluids (6 % hydroxyethyl starch 130/0.3, succinyl gelatin, lactated Ringer's solution) on blood volume expansion in epidural anesthesia of aging.

222.2 Materials and Methods

222.2.1 Patients Selection

Sixty ASA I-II elderly patients whose age range was 65–75 years scheduled for elective radical mastectomy requiring epidural anesthesia were recruited in the first hospital of Jilin University from February, 2010 to February, 2011. The study was approved by the Hospital Research Ethics Committee and written informed consent was obtained from all patients before the start of the study. Excluded criteria included the diseases of cardiovascular and hematological systems. Patients were randomly assigned into three groups of either 6 % hydroxyethyl starch 130/0.3 (group A, n = 20), succinyl gelatin (group B, n = 20) and lactated Ringer's solution (group C, n = 20) using a computer generated randomization list.

222.2.2 Procedures

After fasting overnight, all patients underwent surgery. When entering the operating room, a cannula was placed in the cubital vein of one arm for purpose of infusing fluid and a radial artery catheter was inserted for sampling and continuous measurement of arterial blood pressure. Then all patients were monitored with an electrocardiogram (ECG), invasive blood pressure (BP) and pulse oxygen saturation (SPO2). Patients were placed in the right lateral decubitus position, an epidural catheter was inserted through a 17-gauge Tuohy needle at T2–3 and advanced 3 ~ 4 cm, and a catheter was aspirated to excluded intrathecal or i.v. placement and then secured. The patient was then returned to the supine position. At first, 4 ml of 2 % lidocaine was injected through epidural catheter as a test dose. Five min later, the patient was given an anesthetic solution of mixture of 1 % ropivacaine (AstraZeneca, Sweden) and 2 % lidocaine (1:1) without epinephrine in increments of 8 ml. According to the surgery, the mixture solution was given 4 ml internal 90–120 min and the level of anesthesia was controlled between T2–T7. All the patients inhaled 100 % oxygen with mask. An intravenous fluid load of 1000 ml of 6 % hydroxyethyl starch 130/0.3 (Fresenius Kabi, Germany), succinyl gelatin (Changyuan Company, Changchun, China) or lactated Ringer's solution (Pharmacia, Baxter, Shanghai, China) was given at a constant rate over 60 min via an infusion pump (IEC 601-1, Class 1, Abbott Laboratories, North Chicago, IL) respectively in different groups.

222.2.3 Measurement

Heart rate, arterial blood pressure and pulse oxygen saturation were monitored and recorded every three minutes. Hypotension was defined as a decrease in systolic blood pressure by more than 30 % of the pre-anesthetic value, or a systolic blood pressure <90 mm Hg. Hypotension was treated by injecting intravenous dopamine 2 mg.

Intravenous ^{125}I-HSA1 ml (5–10 μCi, Radiation immunity analysis technology co., Shanghai) was injected into the cubital vein of infusing fluid. At the same time, we kept 1 ml of the same concentration sample as control to analysis radiometric (A) with ria counter. Opposite cubital venous blood (5 ml) was collected in 10, 15 and 20 min after infusing different fluid. Analysis and calculate the radiometric of plasma of time 0 (S) with logarithm transformation. Arterial blood (2 ml) was collected 30 min after anesthesia, 30 and 60 min after infusing to measure the Hb concentration, hematocrit (Hct).

222.2.4 Calculation

The plasma volume (PV), basis of blood volume (BV0), blood volume of different time (BVn), blood volume change ($\triangle$BVn) and fluid remained (FR) were calculated from the following equation (V was the vascular albumin volume; D is the times of dilution (500); A and S were the radio-metric of plasma; f was the ratio of hematocrit value and was 0.864 usually):

$$PV = A \times V \times D/S \quad (222.1)$$

$$BV = PV/(1 - f \times HCT) \quad (222.2)$$

$$BV_n = BV_0 \times Hb_0/Hb_n \quad (222.3)$$

$$\triangle BV_n = BV_n - BV_0 \quad (222.4)$$

$$FR = \triangle BV_n/1000 \times 100\% \quad (222.5)$$

Data are expressed as mean ± standard deviation (SD). The methods of statistical evaluation were simple and multiple linear regression analysis, Fisher's exact test, one-way ANOVA, two-way ANOVA, and the group t test. $P < 0.05$ was considered statistically significant.

222.3 Results

There was no significant difference in demographic variables of the groups ($P > 0.05$) (Table 222.1). There were no significant differences in systolic and diastolic blood pressure of the three groups before infusing ($P > 0.05$). Ten minutes after anesthesia, the systolic and diastolic blood pressure declined in all groups but the difference in group C was significant ($P < 0.05$). After twenty minutes, there were 1 case of hypotension in group A, 1 case in group B and 5 cases in group C. Totally there were 26 cases of hypotension in the study and 3 cases in group A, 4 cases in group B and 19 cases in group C. The incidence of hypotension was higher in group C than other two groups ($P < 0.01$). During the surgery, the systolic and diastolic blood pressure declined in all groups and the difference was significant in group A, B ($P < 0.05$) and group C ($P < 0.01$) (Table 222.2). The BV increased significantly 30 min after anesthesia to 60 min after completing infusing in all groups ($P < 0.05$). Compared with group C, $\triangle$BV, FR increased significantly in group A and B from completing infusing to 60 min later ($P < 0.05$) (Table 222.3).

Table 222.1 Demographic Variables

	Group A (n = 20)	Group B (n = 20)	Group C (n = 20)
Age (year)	66.4 ± 1.2	65.9 ± 1.0	66.1 ± 1.3
Weight (kg)	63.4 ± 5.8	62.5 ± 6.9	64.4 ± 6.0
Height (cm)	157.6 ± 8.3	155.0 ± 8.2	157 ± 7.7
Duration of operation (min)	109 ± 37	106 ± 29	106 ± 34
Duration of anesthesia (min)	120 ± 11	123 ± 16	119 ± 19

Data are expressed as mean ± SD. There is no significant difference between groups

Table 222.2 Systolic and diastolic blood pressure in pre-infusing, 10 min after anesthesia and mean in surgery

	Group A (n = 20)	Group B (n = 20)	Group C (n = 20)
Pre-infusing			
Systolic blood pressure (mm Hg)	115.5 ± 5.0	114.5 ± 4.5	110.3 ± 5.8
Diastolic blood pressure (mm Hg)	69.3 ± 5.9	70.2 ± 6.5	70.0 ± 6.7
10 min after anesthesia			
Systolic blood pressure (mm Hg)	110.7 ± 5.5	108.7 ± 3.8	99.6 ± 1.2*
Diastolic blood pressure (mm Hg)	63.6 ± 3.2	65.1 ± 2.2	60.0 ± 1.7*
Mean in surgery			
Systolic blood pressure (mm Hg)	105.3 ± 1.7*	106.5 ± 3.3*	89.5 ± 5.4#
Diastolic blood pressure (mm Hg)	67.6 ± 1.2*	64.1 ± 5.1*	60.4 ± 1.7#

Data are expressed as mean ± SD. *$P < 0.05$, #$P < 0.01$ versus Pre-anesthesia

Table 222.3 BV, △BVn and FR at measured time

	Group	Pre-infusing	30 min after anesthesia	Infusing-completed		
				0	30 min	60 min
BV (ml)	A	4507 ± 423	4584 ± 422*	4905 ± 458*	4840 ± 482*	4612 ± 448*
	B	4938 ± 503	5043 ± 473*	5438 ± 488*	5358 ± 516*	5084 ± 468*
	C	4486 ± 475	4556 ± 510*	4598 ± 510*	4602 ± 502*	4556 ± 510*
△BVn (ml)	A		77 ± 58	398 ± 85*#	333 ± 97*#	105 ± 73*#
	B		105 ± 90	500 ± 107*#	420 ± 94*#	146 ± 113*#
	C		70 ± 55	112 ± 94	116 ± 89	70 ± 38
FR (%)	A		7.7 ± 5.8	39.8 ± 8.5*#	33.3 ± 9.7*#	10.5 ± 7.3*#
	B		10.5 ± 9.0	50.0 ± 10.7*#	42.0 ± 9.4*#	14.6 ± 11.3*#
	C		7.0 ± 5.5	11.2 ± 9.4*#	11.6 ± 8.9*#	7.0 ± 3.8*#

Data are expressed as mean ± SD. *$P < 0.0501$ vs Pre-infusing, #$P < 0.05$ versus group C

222.4 Discussion

The elderly population is steadily increasing in both absolute and relative terms as a result of the aging of the baby boomers, healthier lifestyles, and advances in health care [9]. Physical function and cognitive dysfunction are reported to predict 5-year mortality in this population. Cognitive declines that may result from surgery and anesthesia are of particular concern in older adults. The advantages of any anesthetic technique need to be balanced against the associated risks. For example, with hypotensive anesthesia, the advantages of reduced blood loss need to be balanced with the possibility of decreased cerebral perfusion and subsequent cognitive impairment. Several studies [5, 10] suggest a connection between low blood pressure and increased mortality in people older than 75 year. In addition, blood pressure levels show a complicated relationship with cognitive impairment [12, 14]. Elevated rates of cognitive decline have been associated with both low and high blood pressures, with the pattern of decline depending on the nature of the blood pressure change with age. Among the elderly, orthostatic hypotension has been shown to be a risk factor for cognitive decline. The lack of any short- or long-term cognitive impairment in the study by Williams-Russo et al. [15] with the use of hypotensive epidural anesthesia is encouraging, suggesting the safety of these transient episodes of low blood pressure.

In this study, we measured the plasma volume with ^{125}I marked albumin. It was simply, safe and accurate method to value the blood volume [3, 13]. The dose in this study was safe to human and even three times was harmless. Albumin is a kind of small protein and can pass the wall of blood vessel with certain rate of 5.4 % in the 1st h. So after 10 min after injecting, the corrected radio-metric was 1 % higher than the calculated. So we evaluated with logarithm transformation to reduce the error.

Previous studies showed that relatively inadequate circulating blood volume resulting from sympathetic block is one of the main mechanisms responsible for hypotension during the onset of epidural anesthesia (Mark and Steele 1989). Blood is pooled in the capillary vessels of legs at the expense of cardiac filling (Arndt et al. 1985). With the regimen described, our results showed that at 10 min after infusion, the blood pressure decreased, more rapidly in the group of lactated Ringer's solution. At the same time, the hemodilution, volume expansion and volume expansion efficiency become greater accordingly in group 6 % hydroxyethyl starch 130/0.3 and group succinyl gelatin in elderly patients undergoing epidural anesthesia probably indicates an altered relationship in compliance with the volume expansion between the intravascular fluid compartment and the interstitial fluid, to the advantage of the dilated intravascular fluid compartment [6]. In the present study we also found that the fluid retained in circulation was increased after infusing different fluid and the remained time were all over 120 min. But the increased extent was higher and the remained time was longer after infusing 6 % hydroxyethyl starch 130/0.3 and succinyl gelatin than lactated Ringer's solution. They could keep the hemodynamic more stable in elder patients after performing epidural anesthesia. Some researchers [1, 7, 8], and [11] have shown that hydroxyethyl starch reduced inflammation and endothelial damage. It also maintained the cell's integrity and function. Lower-molecular weight hydroxyethyl starch molecules had an effect on the arteriolar integrity and could reduce arterioleinduced oedema in clinical and experimental models. Reported effects of hydroxyethyl starch usage were improvement in the microcirculation and the oxygenation of organs and the oxygenation of organs. Hydroxyethyl starch also had an effect on inflammation. Reduction of macrophage inflammatory protein (MIP-2), IL-1β and TNF-α level was found to be a mechanism for reduction of inflammation after the use of hydroxyethyl starch, also had an effect on inflammation. Reduction of macrophage inflammatory protein (MIP-2), IL-1β and TNF-α level was found to be a mechanism for reduction of inflammation after the use of hydroxyethyl starch.

In summary, 6 % hydroxyethyl starch 130/0.3 and succinyl gelatin are better to keep the hemodynamic stability in elder patients after performing epidural anesthesia and can last longer in the circulation.

References

1. Boldt J, Brosch CH, Rohm K, Papsdorf M, Mengistu A (2008) Comparison of the effects of gelatin and modern hydroxyethyl starch solution on renal function and inflamnatory response in elderly cardiac surgery patients. J Br Anaesth 1–8
2. Charlson ME, MacKenzie CR, Gold JP, Ales KL, Topkins M (1990) Intraoperative blood pressure. Ann Surg 212:567–580
3. Fairbanks VF, Klee GG, Wiseman GA et al (1996) Measutement of blood volume and red cell mass: re-examination of ^{51}Cr and ^{125}I methods. J Blood Cells Mol Dis 22:169–186
4. Fried LP, Kronmal RA, Newman AB, Bild DE, Mittelmark MB, Polak JF, Robbins JA, Gardin JM (1998) Risk factors for 5-year mortality in older adults: the cardiovascular health study. JAMA 279:585–592
5. Gold JP, Charlson ME, Williams-Russo P, Szatrowski TP, Peterson JC, Pirraglia PA, Hartman GS, Yao FSF, Hollenberg JP, Barbut D, Hayes JG, Thomas SJ, Purcell MH, Mattis S, Gorkin L, Post M, Krieger KH (1995) Improvement of outcomes after coronary artery bypass: A randomized trial comparing intraoperative high versus low mean arterial pressure. J Thorac Cardiovasc Surg 110:1302–1314
6. Halmaja K, Bishop G, Bristow P (1997) The crystalloid versus colloid controversy: present status. J Balleres Clin Anaesth 11:1–13
7. Hahn RC, Drobin D, Stahle L (1997) Volume kinetics of Ringer's solution in female volunteers. J Br Anaesth 78:144–148
8. Lang K, Boldt J, Suttner S, Haisch G (2001) Colloids versus crystalloids and tissue oxygen tension in patients undergoing major abdominal surgery. J Anesth Analg 93:405–409
9. Muravchick S (1998) The aging process: Anesthetic implications. Acta Anaesth Belg 49:85–90
10. Williams-Russo P, Sharrock NE, Mattis S (1999) Randomized trial of hypotensive epidural anesthesia in older adults. J Anesthesiology 91:926–935
11. Alavi SM, Baharvand B, Baharestani B, Babaei T (2012) Comparison of the effects of gelatin, Ringer's solution and a modern hydroxyl ethyl starch solution after coronary artery bypass graft surgery. J Cardiovasc J Africa 23:428–431

12. Swan GE, Carmelli D, Larue A (1998) Systolic blood pressure tracking over 25 to 30 years and cognitive performance in older adults. J Stroke 29:2334–2340
13. Thosmsen JK, Fogh-Andersen N, Bulow K et al (1991) Blood and plasma volumes determined by carbon monoxide gas, 99mTc-labelled erythrocytes, ^{125}I-albumin and the T 1824 technique. J Scand J Clin Lab Invest 51:185–190
14. Williams-Russo P, Sharrock NE, Mattis S, Szatrowski TP, Charlson ME (1995) Cognitive effects after epidural vs. general anesthesia in older adults: a randomized trial. JAMA 274:44–50
15. Williams-Russo P, Sharrock NE, Mattis S, Liguori GA, Mancuso C, Peterson MG, Hollenberg J, Ranawat C, Salvati E, Sculco T (1999) Randomized trial of hypotensive epidural anesthesia in older adults. J Anesthesiology 91:926–935

Chapter 223
The Application of Association Rule Mining in the Diagnosis of Pancreatic Cancer

Song Shaoyun

Abstract The method of association rule mining used in cases of diagnostic work, you can find out the relationship between the etiology level factors from a large number of cases recorded, from mining association rules in the diagnosis of pancreatic cancer database to discover the relationship pancreatic cancer and blood group age, gender, environment, diet, genetic predisposition, mood state factors, which found that the factors of pancreatic disease it may rule, diagnosis and prevention of pancreatic cancer cases are important guiding significance.

Keywords Data mining · Association rules · Diagnosis of pancreatic cancer

223.1 Introduction

(1) Data sets: a collection of all affairs (i.e. database), each transaction T(task) is a collection of some of the projects.
(2) Association rules: Assume X, Y are itemsets and $X \cap Y = \phi$, Implication formula $X \Rightarrow Y$ called association rules.
(3) Support: The number of transactions is called support. Data set D contains itemset X number of itemsets X support. Denoted R_X, Itemsets X support is $s(X) = \frac{R_X}{|D|} \times 100\%$, where $|D|$ is all items in database D.
(4) Confidence: The confidence of Association rules $X \Rightarrow Y$ is $c(X \Rightarrow Y) = \frac{s(X \cup Y)}{s(X)} \times 100\%$, it is the credibility of the association rules.

S. Shaoyun (✉)
Information Technology Engineering Institute, Yuxi Normal University, Yuxi, Yunnan, China
e-mail: mathsong@126.com

(5) Frequent itemsets: Itemsets X support s(X) is not less than the minimum support and confidence of user settings called frequent set.
(6) Strong rules: support and confidence greater than the minimum support and minimum confidence association rules given by the user.

223.2 Improved Apriori Algorithm

The frequency of occurrence of all projects with an element of the first step in simple statistics, and find out which is greater than or equal to the minimum support itemsets to generate a one-dimensional frequent itemsetsLt. Starting from the second step loop handle frequent itemsets until unable to re-produce a higher dimension. Cycle: k-1 step generated k-dimensional frequent item sets in the k-th step, k-dimensional candidate itemsets k-1 dimensional frequent item sets, we can achieve the centralized the event of a number of elements in the counting process, and therefore a certain element, if it is the number of counts is less than k-1, then, can advance to remove the elements, so as to exclude all combinations caused by the element of large size. This is because of an element to become an element of the set of the K-dimensional item, the element concentration of counts in the k-1 order frequent items must be up to K-1, otherwise it is impossible to generate the K-dimensional set of items. Then Apriori algorithm to test all of the new K-dimensional frequent item sets k-1 dimensional itemsets is already included in the K-1 dimensional frequent item sets have been obtained. If one of which is not included, you can delete the combination, so that a truly useful K-dimensional frequent item sets election itemsets. The candidate itemsets, you can scan the database D, each transaction tid retain the transaction, if the transaction candidate itemsets containing at least one of the C_K, otherwise, the end of the transaction record database no transaction record for delete mark on the exchange, and moved to the database end transaction record delete marked a record finish scanning the entire database for the new.

Transaction database D 'in. As K increases, the decrease in D 'in the transaction record large earth, can be significant savings for the next transaction scan I/O overhead. Customers generally may be time to share buy some merchandise delete this virtual method can achieve a large number of transactions recorded in the excavation kick out for higher dimensional data, in the few remaining record mining can greatly save time.

223.3 Application Examples

It is possible to reduce the morbidity and mortality of the population of pancreatic cancer to explore and discover effective and suitable for China's national conditions pancreatic cancer interventions, raise public awareness and ability of self-care, mining association rules used in the pancreas simple data sets for cancer diagnosis, trying to discover the relationship between the environmental, dietary factors, genetic susceptibility factors of pancreatic cancer diagnosis, to discover rules pancreatic cancer disease and it may, these rules mode important guiding significance for the diagnosis and prevention of pancreatic cancer cases.

Database D is taken as a region of Liaoning Province from 1996 to 1999, the residents have a family history of pancreatic cancer, with a history of pancreatic cancer over the age of 35 and mixed with a small number of 35-year-old rural residents of the obvious symptoms of pancreatic disease the medical records of 3033 [7], in the region of the high incidence of pancreatic cancer illness, many patients 35 to 60 years, medical records representative, the study of pancreatic disease have a certain credibility; relatively concentrated due to the patient's age, disease and gender relationship is not significant, the patient's age, gender information is omitted, the name switch to medical records code on the patient's medical records, blood type, eating habits, family history of pancreatic cancer, a history of chronic pancreatitis, drinking habits, normal life stress, often sulking attributes such as association rule mining more data to the data table is only a

Table 223.1 Medical records database

Medical record code	X	A	B	C	D	E	F	G	H	I	Pancreatic Cancer
1025	B	1	1	1	0	1	1	1	1	1	1
0759	O	0	0	0	1	1	0	0	1	0	0
1108	AB	1	0	1	0	1	1	1	0	0	0
...	...	...	...	...	...	...	...	...	...	...	...

Table 223.2 Frequent 5-itemsets

TID	Itemset	Support (%)
1	B-type blood, pancreatic cancer, family history, history of chronic pancreatitis, often sulking, pancreatic cancer	19
2	No family history of pancreatic cancer, normal life, not nervous, drinking habits, eating fresh fruits and vegetables, no pancreatic cancer.	16
3	Eat preserved foods, history of chronic pancreatitis, life is stressful, eat smoked food, pancreatic cancer.	17.3
4	Type O blood, drinking habits, life is not nervous to eat fresh fruits and vegetables, no pancreatic cancer	18.4
5	B blood type, history of chronic pancreatitis, often sulk, eat smoked food, pancreatic cancer	15.1

Table 223.3 Mining results

Ruler	Cancer	X	A	B	C	D	E	F	G	H	Suppot(%)	Confidence(%)
1	1			B	–	1	1	–	–	1	–	–	19	86
2	1	–	1	–	1	–	1	–	–	1	17.3	77
3	0	0	–	–	–	1	1	–	1	–	18.4	76

partial list of data is easy and intuitive, the property values in the table are boolean, as shown in Table 223.1.

Figures in the Table: 1, 0 no, X is the blood type A to eat preserved foods, B has a family history of pancreatic tumors, C is a history of chronic diseases, D drinking habits, E normal life stress, F often the depressed, G to eat fruits and vegetables, the H eat smoked food I smoking.

Table 223.1 with improved Apriori algorithm, whichever support = 15 % of the database D scan to identify large items are shown in Table 223.2.

By frequent 5-itemset mining step (2), take confidence = 70 %, draw strong rules: pancreatic⇒{pancreatic cancer, family history, history of chronic pancreatitis, often sulking}; no pancreatic⇒{pancreatic cancer family history, everyday life stress, drinking habits},mining results are shown in Table 223.3.

Analysis blood type in Tables 223.2 and 223.3 have B, family history of pancreatic cancer, history of chronic pancreatitis, often sulk, eat marinated smoked food dominant pancreatic cancer cases; drinking habits, life is not nervous to eat fresh fruits and vegetables protective factors for pancreatic cancer. Above focuses on medical history, the results of the association rules of pancreatic cancer, given the minimum support minsup = 0.15 and the minimum credibility minconf = 0.75 mining three association rules, Table 223.3 lists the support and confidence of these meaningful association rules, and these rules, the so-called meaningful association rules that support and confidence of not less than the minimum support rate and minimum credible degree rules, these rules reveal the information contained in the database, and the general law, can be used as reference for the diagnosis of new cases, can explore and discover effective and suitable for China's national conditions, pancreatic cancer interventions, improve the people's awareness of self-care and abilities. Mining association rules, the domestic and international complexity of pancreatic cancer etiology research, can be analyzed as follows.

223.4 Conclusion

Patients with pancreatic cancer family history of cancer and pancreatic cancer history was significantly higher than that in the control group [7], their family members, family members than non-pancreatic cancer patients suffering from 2 to 3 times higher risk of pancreatic cancer, pancreatic cancer family aggregation causes both genetic factors, there are living together environmental factors, including diet, lifestyle, the environment and other people suffering from chronic pancreatitis, especially people suffering from chronic atrophic pancreatitis, are more prone to pancreas cancer the acidic environment of the normal pancreas can kill bacteria decomposing enzyme, chronic atrophic pancreatitis in patients with pyloric glandular mucosa surface environment the most suitable for the bacteria to settle, is chronic atrophic pancreatitis and pancreatic cancer more susceptible to reason. Freshly fruits and vegetables have a protective effect on pancreatic cancer, fresh fruits and vegetables in addition to the low nitrite content, and also contains a lot of vitamin C and carotene and other ingredients, the anti-cancer effects of these substances, has been recognized by the scientific community. Instead, eat pickled manufacturing smoked food, in addition to high nitrite content, but also the lack of a lot of vitamin C and carotene and other ingredients, and promote the formation of pancreatic cancer life advocate to eat more fresh fruits and vegetables, eating pickled and smoked food barrier off the formation of nitrite, amine and ammonium nitrite, blocking the formation mechanism of pancreatic cancer. Similarly, drinking green tea is an effective protective factors of pancreatic cancer. Moreover, in pancreatic cancer risk factors, often sulking, depression, quality and usually life is stressful and significantly associated with pancreatic cancer, these factors normal immune function, reduced ability to resist carcinogenic factors, increased susceptibility to cancer patients.

References

1. Shao F (2003) Principle of data mining algorithms Beijing: China Water Power Press, 93–95
2. Agrawal R, Imieliski T, Swami A (1993) Mining Association Rules Between Sets of Items in Large Database. In: Mproceedings of ACMS IGMOD international 1 conference on management of data (SIGM OD. 93), 207–216
3. Houtsma M, Swami A (1995) Set-oriented Mining for Association Rules in Relational Databases. In: MProceedings of the 11th IEEE international conference on data engineering, Taipei, 25–34
4. Lei C (2001) Data mining and its application in medical research. Inf Syst 24(5):368–370
5. Armed S (2003) Literature association rules in tumor diagnosis. Comput Eng 29(12):8–10
6. Li H (2003) Cai Chinese association rules in medical data analysis. Microcomput Dev 13(6):94–97
7. Guohai J, Bao-Sen Z, Guan P (2001) Pancreatic cancer prevention early epidemiological evaluation of the effect of health statistics in China 18(2):69–73

Chapter 224
Meta-Analysis of Chinese Herbs in the Treatment of Nephropathy: Huangqi and Danggui Type Formulations

Ming-gang wei and Xiao-feng Cai

Abstract *Objective* Numerous Chinese patients with Diabetic nephropathy (DN) have benefited from chinese herbs. However, there is no systematic evaluation about them. *Methods* We conducted a meta-analysis to all eligible randomized clinical trials (RCTs) to assess the effect of Chinese herbs on DN for the first time. *Results* (1) Five eligible RCTs with 356 participants; (2) Chinese herbs brought a favorable increase in total remission (TR) (RR2.60, 95 %CI 1.55 to4.34, $I^2 = 0$ %) compared with non-Chinese herbs treatment; (3) Exploiting subgroup meta-analysis, Chinese herbs led to significantly improvements of DN with ACEI treatment with regard to the decrease of urinary proteinuria excretion (UPE) (MD −23.65 ug/min, 95 % CI −29.37 to −17.92, $I^2 = 0$ %) *Conclusion* Chinese herbs was certainly a valuable and promising treatment remedy for DN.

Keywords Diabetic nephropathy · Chinese herbs · Drug therapy · Meta-analysis

224.1 Introduction

DN is a secondary glomerulonephritis defined histologically by the presence of glomerular accompanied with high level of blood glucose in the absence of systemic disease. DN still represents the majority of secondary glomerular disease, and is the most common cause of end-stage renal disease in the world [1]. The increasing incidence and poor outcome of DN result in a large expenditure of healthcare resources and a significant burden for patients and society. According to the way of immunosuppressive therapy, cyclophosphamide, cyclosporine A and mycophenolate mofetil have been used in DN treatment [2]. Despite the clinical

M. wei (✉) · X. Cai
The First Affiliated Hospital of Soochow University, 215006 Suzhou, China
e-mail: weimg@sina.com

efficacy of these therapies, many patients do not acquire clinically meaningful remission. Furthermore, the relatively high cost of the drugs has hampered the access to these therapies in many patients with DN in poor countries.

Astragalus mongholicus and angelica root (huangqi and dang gui medicinal broth, HDMB) are the member of the Chinese herbs family of medicine plants. In Traditional Chinese Medicine (TCM), they have been widely used to treat the symptoms correlating with the chronic kidney diseases (CKD) such as edema, hypodynamia and waist soreness and so on. Exciting results derived from randomized controlled trials (RCTs) in China, which have already demonstrated the efficacy and safety of Chinese herbs in the treatment of DN [3–7].The significant therapeutic benefit of HDMB in patients with primary glomerulonephritis (GN) and secondary kidney disease has also been widely reported based on findings in clinical trials [3–8]. Recently a meta-analysis of HDMB for DN in adults has been accomplished. It was found that HDMB indeed resulted in a significant increase of (TR) (OR 2.6, 95 % CI 1.55 to 4.34) compared with angiotensin converting enzyme inhibitor (ACEI) or placebo.

During the past ten decades, hundreds of thousands of Chinese patients with DN have been successfully treated with HDMB, just like the primitive situation of HDMB in hemophthisis treatment. In recent years, a few RCTs concerning the effect of HDMB on DN have been designed [3–7]. However, there is no systematic evaluation of this remedy for DN. Thus, we carried out a meta-analysis of RCTs to assess the efficacy and safety of HDMB in the treatment of DN.

224.2 Materials and Methods

Inclusion and exclusion criteria RCTs that evaluated the efficacy and safety of a special preparation of HDMB on DN. The "special preparation" is defined as that astragalus mongholicus and angelica root prescribed as the special proportion is 5 to 1. The preparations of HDMB such as decoction and formula were excluded. Any other forms of Chinese herbals other than astragalus mongholicus and angelica root were excluded. Studies were also excluded if any drugs other than ACEI were investigated or served as comparisons. We also excluded nRCTs, for example controlled clinical trials (CCTs).

224.3 Search Strategy

PubMed/MEDLINE, EMBASE, Cochrane Central Register of Controlled Trials (CENTRAL), Science Citation Index(SCI), Chinese Biomedical Literature Database (CBM), Chinese science and technology periodicals databases (CNKI,VIP, and Wan Fang) were searched (February 2013). The following medical subject heading items and free-text words were used: diabetic nephropathy, DN, huangqi, danggui, huangqi danggui mixture, danggui buxue medicinal broth, randomized controlled trial, controlled clinical trial, randomized, randomly, placebo, and trial.

224.4 Study Validity Assessment

The commonly-used Jadad scale for assessing quality of bias for RCTs has been discouraged by the Cochrane Collaboration. We evaluated the validity of studies using a specific tool which has recently been recommended by the Cochrane Collaboration. The tool for assessing risk of bias addresses such specific domains as sequence generation, blinding, incomplete outcome data, and selective outcome reporting. Each domain comprises a description and judgement for each included study. This description provides a succinct summary of which judgement of risk of bias can be made, whereas the judgement involves answering a specific question for each domain. In all cases, the answer "Yes" indicates low risk of bias, "No" indicates high risk of bias, and "Unclear" indicates either lack of information or uncertainty over the potential for bias.

224.5 Data Collection and Analysis

Data were extracted from all included studies in terms of participant characteristics of the study sample, baseline of study, and intervention characteristics for each group. Primary outcomes were remission rates of proteinuria, the total remission (TR) which was defined as proteinuria <0.15–1.0 g/day or the decrease of protein excretion >50 % accompanied by stable serum creatinine (increase of serum creatinine <25 % of baseline). Secondary outcomes included the level of urinary protein excretion (UPE), serum albumin, and serum creatinine.

224.6 Statistics Analysis

All statistics analyses were performed using Review Manager (RevMan) (Version 4.3. Copenhagen:The Nordic Cochrane Centre, The Cochrane Collaboration). The results were expressed as risk ratio (RR) for dichotomous data, and mean difference (MD) for continuous data, with 95 % confidence intervals (95 % CI). Heterogeneity among included trials was analyzed using chisquared (x^2) test.

224.7 Results

The details of characteristics of the five included studies are summarized in Table 224.1. We identified 5 RCTs involving HDMB in the treatment of DN. All five studies have low risk of bias concerning "incomplete outcome data": no missing outcome data existed in the studies, and missing outcome data were balanced in numbers. Main outcomes were all reported in the studies. In a word, the overall level of included studies validity was acceptable. Data for primary outcomes of TR at the end of studies were available in five trials with a total sample size of 356 participants (190 were assigned to the HDMB groups and 166 in non- HDMB groups). HDMB resulted in an increased TR rate and the similar result of fasting blood glucose (FBG) compared with controls (RR2.60, 95 % CI 1.55 to4.34, $I^2 = 0$ % for TR) and (RR-0.27, 95 % CI $-0.59 - 0.04$, $I^2 = 0$ % for FBG) Figs. 224.1, 224.2, 224.3.

Subgroup analysis was also preformed among two RCTs [3, 6] which compared HDMB with non-HDMB in the treatment of DN. There was still a significant increase in TR (RR 4.08, 95 %CI 1.74 to 9.54, $I^2 = 0$ % for TR). These results indicated that the direction of effect of subgroup analysis was the same as that of total analysis, with the effect size being greater than that of total analysis. Secondary outcomes of UPE were reported in three RCTs which compared the effects of HDMB with ACEI for DN [4, 5, 7]. UPE decreased with an overall effect size of MD -23.65 ug/min(95 % CI -29.37 to -17.92, $I^2 = 0$ %) in favor of the HDMB groups at Fig. 224.4.

Table 224.1 Characteristics of the five included studie

Studies	Baseline characteristics of participants	Interventions/controls
2005 Li [3]	N:76; Gender:M44, F32	HDMB/placebo
2007 Zhao [4]	N:46; Gender:M24, F22; UPE: 47–150 μg/min	HDMB/ACEI
2007 Zhao [5]	N:54; Gender:M29, F25; UPE: 57–171 μg/min	HDMB/ACEI
2008 Li [6]	N:60; Gender:M30, F30	HDMB/placebo
2009 Gong [7]	N:52; Gender:M26, F26; UPE: 41–142 μg/min	HDMB/ACEI

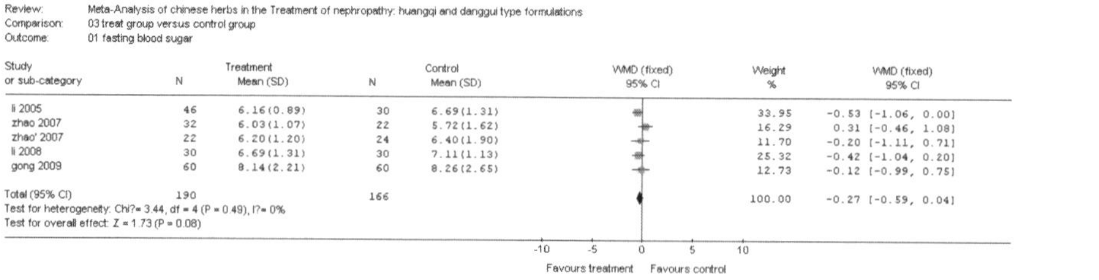

Fig. 224.1 The meta-analysis of FBG

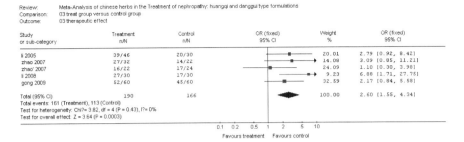

Fig. 224.2 The meta-analysis therapetic effect

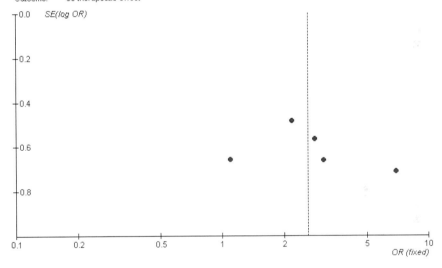

Fig. 224.3 The meta-analysis of funnel plots of therapetic effect

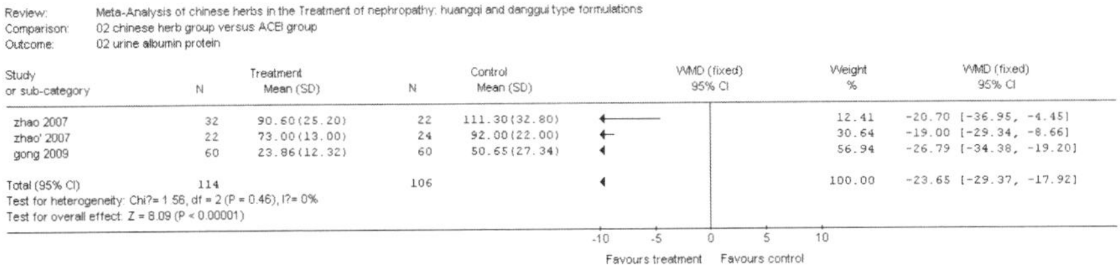

Fig. 224.4 The meta-analysis of UPE

224.8 Discussion

To our best knowledge, this is the first meta-analysis to appraise the efficacy and safety of HDMB in the treatment of DN. All of the nRCTs including CCTs were excluded, and thus the strength of this meta-analysis implicated acceptable standards and methodology. In this analysis, about 84.72 % (161/190) of patients with DN could acquire significant therapeutic benefits (total remission rate of proteinuria) from HDMB. The results of this meta-analysis indicated that patients with DN could benefit from HDMB. In the trial, HDMB with ACEI in the treatment of DN [4, 5, 7], there was significant difference in terms of TR (RR 4.08, 95 % CI 1.74 to 9.54, $I^2 = 0$ % for TR). Although HDMB still contains a variety of components, evidence suggests that tha main components such as astragalus polysaccharides and ferulaic acid, are the most abundant and responsible for the treating DN effects [8, 9]. The mechanisms by which HDMB exert its dramatic antiproteinuric effect on DN is not fully elucidated. Recently, HDMB revealed powerful in vivo anti-proteinuric and podocyte-protected effects, which were accompanied by the suppression of cytoskeleton disruption, and nephrin and podocin abnormal expression [10].

In previous studies, the release of inflammatory and fibrogenic factors in glomerular mesangial cells, such as fibronectin (FN), laminin (LN) and transforming growth factor-beta (TGF-beta), has proved a critical downstream event in the pathogenesis and progression of DN [11, 12]. Recently, the mechanisms of HDMB on the progressive GN have been investigated [13, 14]. HDMB could ameliorate proteinuria, lessen mesangial injury and improve renal function. HDMB significantly attenuated the glomerular expression of TGF-beta of GN. In addition, the mechanisms underlying the effect of HDMB on experimental chronic progressive GN involved suppression of TGF-beta, FN, and LN, as well as inhibition of glomerular infiltration of inflammatory cells. These findings suggested that HDMB was a potential multi-target agent for various injurious factors observed in human DN.

The results of meta-analysis interpreted with caution and warrants further investigation for several reasons. First, the relatively small sample size (356 participants) may influence the extent of the effect of HDMB. Secondly, the follow-up periods (2–3 months) were relatively short and thus inadequately powered to detect the long-term outcomes of renal function deterioration and more serious adverse events. However, this issue was attributed to the fact that all of the included RCTs with high standards and acceptable methodology were conducted within the most recent 10 years. Taken together, HDMB may be efficient and safe for the clinical treatment of DN, and the mechanisms underlying the dramatic antiproteinuric effects of HDMB could be multiple.

Acknowledgments The work is supported by the grant from the Natural Science Foundation of China (No. 81273723).

References

1. Fang C, Jing-tao D (2012) Insulin selections ofdiabetic nephropath. J Drug Evalutation 9:21–25
2. Ling Q (2006) New treatment progress of diabetic nephropathy. Foreign Med Geriatr Med 27:16–19
3. Mei-ru L, Qing-feng G, Xi-jun F (2005) Clinical observation on efficaly of jiawei danggui buxue decoction in treating 46 patients with diabetic nephropathy in clinical stage. Chinese J Pract Chinese Mod Med 28:572–573
4. Xue-lan Zh, Zhao-yun Q, Jin-ling W et al (2007) Clinical observation on efficaly of huangqi danggui decoction compasing with benazepril in treating patients with diabetic nephropathy. Clin Focus 22:131–132
5. Xue-lan Zh, Song-juan L, Lin-lin Zh et al (2007) Huangqi danggui decoction in treating patients with diabetic nephropathy. Chinese Tradit Pat Med 29:641–644
6. Shi-yun L, Dao-kuan L, Su-pu N (2008) Huangqi danggui decoction in treating patients with diabetic nephropathy. J New Chinese Med 40:21–22
7. Cui-fen G, Xiao-li Q, Jing-hua W et al (2009) Danggui buxue decoction and benazepril in treating patients with diabetic nephropathy at erarlier stage. Shanxi Chinese Med 30:974–976
8. Ling-yun Y, Shu-yu Y, Xue-jun L (2012) Research progress of the control mechanisms of astragalus polysaccharides on diabetic nephropathy. Med Recapitulate 18:172–1728
9. Li CR, Cai F, Yang YQ et al (2010) Tetrahydroxystilbene glucoside ameliorates diabetic nephropathy in rats:involvement of S1RT1 and TGF-B_1 pathway. Eur J Pharmacol 649:382–389
10. Ming-gang W, Li N, Ling Zh et al (2012) protecion mechansms of modified danggui buxue decoction for podocytes in adriamycin-induced nephropathy rats. Chin J Integr Med 32:1077–1087
11. Cover-smith A, Hendry BM (2008) The regulation of mesangial cell proliferation. Nephron Exp Nephrol 108:e74–e79
12. Tahara A, Tsukada J, Tomura Y et al(2008) Effect of vasopressin on type IV collagen production in human mesangial cells. Regul Pept 147:60–66
13. Ming-gang W, Wei S, Pei-hua X et al (2012) Antifibrotic effect of the Chinese herbs modified danggui buxue decoction on adriamycin-induced nephropathy in rats. Chin J Integr Med 18:591–598
14. Ming-gang W, Pei-hua X, Ling Zh (2013) Effect of Chinese herbs on immunoglobulin A nephropathy: a randomized controlled trial. J Tradit Chinese Med 33:65–69

Chapter 225
Establishment and Significance of Digital Embryo Library for Enhancing Embryology Teaching Effect

Bai Sheng-Bin, Chen Hong-Xiang, Tang Li, Liao Li-Bin, Li Tian, Feng Shu-Mei, Qin Wen, Zhong Jin-Jie and Luo Xue-Gang

Abstract With the rapid development of the computer and network technology, the digital information provides a good platform for reform of medical teaching mode. The traditional teaching type and teaching mode in the classroom can gradually not adapt to the needs of the development of information society [1, 2]. The increasing popularity of student-centered teaching mode gradually grew up along with the emergence of multimedia and network technology. Digital multimedia network teaching methods of embryology is the core of the multimedia

---

Z. Jin-Jie (✉)
Xinjiang Medical University, Xinyi road 393, 830011 Urumqi, China
e-mail: zhongjinjie@sina.com

B. Sheng-Bin · C. Hong-Xiang · T. Li · L. Li-Bin · L. Tian · F. Shu-Mei · Q. Wen · Z. Jin-Jie · L. Xue-Gang
Department of Histology and Embryology, Preclinical Medicine, Xinjiang Medical Univerity, Urumqi, Xinjiang, China
e-mail: bsbxx@126.com

C. Hong-Xiang
e-mail: chenhongxiang@126.com

T. Li
e-mail: tangli123@126.com

L. Xue-Gang
e-mail: xgluo@xysm.net

B. Sheng-Bin · C. Hong-Xiang · T. Li · L. Li-Bin · L. Tian · F. Shu-Mei · Q. Wen · Z. Jin-Jie · L. Xue-Gang
The People's Hospital in Xinjiang Uyghur Autonomous Region, Urumqi, Xinjiang, China

B. Sheng-Bin · C. Hong-Xiang · T. Li · L. Li-Bin · L. Tian · F. Shu-Mei · Q. Wen · Z. Jin-Jie · L. Xue-Gang
The First Filiated Medical Hospital of Xinjiang Medical Univerity, Urumqi, Xinjiang, China

B. Sheng-Bin · C. Hong-Xiang · T. Li · L. Li-Bin · L. Tian · F. Shu-Mei · Q. Wen · Z. Jin-Jie · L. Xue-Gang
Department of Anatomy and Neurobiology, Xiangya School of Medicine, Central South University, Changsha, Hunan, China

teaching resource construction, also is the key of realization of multimedia network teaching conditions. Therefore it become a network in the field of application of an important topic. Embryology teaching resource construction is very significant for medical teaching resource construction. It not only improves the objective requirement of the teaching efficiency about Embryology, but also improves the quality of teaching and deepen teaching reform needs. Embryology is a basic medical subject, the course characteristic is very abstract, including microstructure, and large amount of information, and perceptual teaching materials. Because of teaching hours reduced about embryology in recent years, a big increase in the number of enrollment, and students level is uneven, so the traditional teaching mode can not meet the twenty-first century medical morphology teaching need. Through the construction of the resource library to promote network multimedia teaching, we can solve this problem in order to improve embryology teaching effect by establishment of digital embryo library.

Keywords Digital library · Computer technology · Embryology

225.1 Introduction

Embryology is a subject which is very difficult to master and understand it. In recent years it is very important for new students and undergraduate to strengthen the embryology teaching and promote teaching effect, especially for medical students. The embryology "as an independent course", need a lot of specimens, model, pictures and the corresponding sections to meet the needs of teaching in the classroom. In addition, with the increase of new research personnel, record of formal schooling levels rise, old teacher's retirement, and many other reasons, new personnel training in the embryology course is not strong enough. Embryonic specimens aging and embryo specimen mark, record almost blanking, the teacher is not able to recognize of the fetus' exact situation, besides the teaching for students, the student is vague, need to solve these problems. According to investigation we found that the majority of colleges and universities in embryonic specimen deficiency, there is a phenomenon that embryology teaching is not enough attention. In view of the present these problems, our teaching group has do a lot of work for future teaching and training, scientific research and the establishment of digital specimens library. We hope that we can provide good resources environment for the vast number of teachers and students the embryology of study through the establishment of the specimens library.

225.2 Construction and Classification of Digital Embryo Library

It can be classified into five parts: the first part, collect and digitalize human embryo specimen: the specimen are derived from department of gynecology, obstetrics and outpatients service of hospital. For fetus about induced abortion, drug abortion and accidental death which are agreed by relatives of patient. We will collect and fix specimen of fetus. We manage and take notes about mother and fetus' general conditions, cases and store these data. After finishing these work, we will take photos for fetus in different direction and deal with photos by three dimensional methods and store them by digital format [3–5]. Because of network-based platform students shared with others in the university local area network in order to study and research at any time for enhancing learning effect.

The second part, construction of digital section library of human fetus. In the teaching process of human embryology, research group will observe and make sections in different growth period of chicken fetus and frog fetus. We will make special staining and scan these sections one by one through digital scanning section system. We will store them by digital methods for long time to avoid the use of the process of loss, fragmentation of unnecessary waste, but also to ensure the long-term resource storage.

The third part, the construction of digital photo library. From the beginning of 2003, research group has made teaching reform project through the network and Library and each teacher make a variety of access and methods collect Embryology related images and digital processing with related embryology. We save the formation of BMP, JPG and other formats in order to greatly enrich the embryology teaching materials and meet students' learning interest in embryology [6]. Digital photo library has shown this case has been organized in our school campus embryology of top-quality courses, students access levels, better feedback information.

The fourth part, making mouse embryonic specimens. In the period changing from teaching university to the teaching and researching university, research group make comparative study between mice and human embryonic specimens. When human embryos were not collected or insufficiency of the embryonic period, we follow the mouse embryo development regularity and space–time. The anatomic study on mice, the different stage embryos were fixed with human embryonic specimens, made of comparison with the human embryo.

The fifth part, making embryology model. The use of existing resources, the embryology teaching three-dimensional structure is more complex, this part is not easy to explain. For example, the occurrence of heart of the embryonic period, namely the obscure and difficult to hear, space imagination is made, then it needs to change the model of heart. Therefore, the use of digital resources construction of embryology at the same time, making many embryo models about some organs. We also make a benefit of computer to handle the models. All of these work will benefit for us, for our teaching.

225.3 Application of Embryonic Digital Resources in the Teaching Process

Through the construction in recent years, embryo library is gradually perfect, and gradually digitized, exerted great influence on the embryology teaching. Firstly, to update teaching ideas, promote the reform of teaching methods. As a teacher, the digital resources of the library building is a process about knowledge accumulation and summary update. Secondly, to add the resources of the library is to collect students' learning resources, for students to learn to actively cooperate with the role, so that students learn to independence. In addition, the construction of embryonic libraries make embryology study more easy to understand, through the observation of embryonic picture library of embryonic development with overall sensory understanding. By digital embryo library learning, recognizing the embryonic structure and internal development, finally through the comparison of specimens and human specimens of mice. We make full use of all resources to reach the purpose of learning from an evolutionary point of understanding process of development and evolution of the embryo. The concrete implementation measures, research group had combined with the department of embryology practical drawing contest and model making competition. These make students in the learning process, based on the actual behavior, learning and practice, dare to imagine, has the courage to practice, give full play to the space imagination of students. It made medical students for later to study embryology to increase the confidence and motivation. Because of achieved remarkable results, students' understanding of the more profound. The construction and improvement of the digital resource library of embryology more from the network and teaching work, it will be reflected more significantly. As a platform for the use of LAN and campus network, the research group will be come true digital resources for cyber source sharing, truly reflects the power of the network, so that more students and learners are able to enjoy the charm of resources. In addition to traditional learning methods, it is a necessary to find a personalized learning method suitable for their own development. This is the digital resources of the library and network sharing power. Of course, we will establish like Howard hughes medical institute biological virtual laboratory that perfect digital section library is to participate in the work of the goal of teachers. Digital section library construction, not only can for teachers improve teaching quality and teaching efficiency, and actively adapt to the contemporary college students' learning teaching reform. For students to create a better environment of independent study, improve their learning interest, and save a lot of national education funds, avoid unnecessary waste, for medical college education teaching launched more broad prospects.

225.4 The Implementation Effect of Embryonic Digital Resources in the Teaching Process

Generally speaking, establishment of digital embryo library enriched teaching resources, widen teachers and students' field of vision, enhanced embryology teaching effect. The most important is to stimulate students' learning ability and learning interest, learning to adapt to the requirements of the learning method. Through the construction of digital embryo resources, further enrich the embryology teaching resources, construction of deepening the embryology course. Because of web-based courses through the network, it promoted the students to make full use of the digital resources of the library, so that students learn more conveniently, stimulate students interest in learning medical course, improve student achievement. Making learning whenever and wherever possible, as long as there is network, capable of autonomous learning, this is the ultimate goal of our education and teaching. Please ensure running headers are no longer than one line. When dealing with particularly long chapter titles please shorten them to an acceptable length in the running header only.

References

1. Katina Z (2013) Using information and communication technologies to engage students in the later years of schooling in learning content and literacy: case studies of three teachers. Educ Inf Technol 18:205–214
2. Yigang W, Shengli F, Jialin C et al (2012) Practical teaching reform for digital image processing based on project-driven. Emerg Comput Inf Technol Educ Adv Intel Soft Comput 146:9–14
3. Arraez-Aybar L-A, Mérida-Velasco J-R, Rodriguez-Vazquez J et al (1994) A computerised technique for morphometry and 3D reconstruction of embryological structures. Surg Radiol Anat 16:419–422
4. Beckwith JB (2012) Congenital malformations: from superstition to understanding. Virchows Arch 461:609–619
5. Jirkovská M, Náprstková I, Janáček J et al (2005) Three-dimensional reconstructions from non-deparaffinized tissue sections. Anat Embryol 210:163–173
6. David P, Brent B, Neil K (2012) USRC: a new strategy for adding digital images to the medical school curriculum. J Digit Imag 25:682–688

Chapter 226
3D Reverse Modeling and Rapid Prototyping of Complete Denture

Dantong Li, Xiaobao Feng, Ping Liao, Hongjun Ni, Yidan Zhou, Mingyu Huang, Zhiyang Li and Yu Zhu

Abstract An integrated method of reverse engineering and rapid prototyping technology to manufacture complete denture was presented in this paper. Firstly, geometrical surfaces of complete denture were measured by three-dimensional scanner and their point clouds were obtained. Then the point clouds de-noising processing was performed, data was filtered and reduced, the missing data was repaired and triangular surfaces splicing was realized in Geomagic software. 3D model of complete denture was reconstructed in Pro/E software, and the STL file was generated. Finally, the entity model was manufactured by rapid prototyping machine. Through this process the entity model of running-in-period complete denture was manufactured, which can reduce denture repairing time and contribute to health and medical research.

Keywords Reverse engineering · Complete denture · 3D model reconstruction · Rapid prototyping

226.1 Introduction

With the progress of science and technology (especially material science and computer aided technology), molding materials and rapid prototyping technology (such as 3D technology) are also constantly improved in the medical application. According to news, recently, a patient was accepted a successful pioneering surgery in the United States. The surgery used 3D-printing skull to replace 75 % of

D. Li · X. Feng · P. Liao · H. Ni · Y. Zhou · M. Huang (✉) · Z. Li · Y. Zhu
School of Mechanical Engineering, Nantong University, 226019 Nantong, Jiang su, China
e-mail: huang.my@ntu.edu.cn

D. Li
e-mail: ldthh@163.com

the patient's own skulls. In the manufacturing process of the skull, the researchers first scanned the head of the patient, then they used 3D-printing technology to print out skulls for transplantation. Traditional cranial molding materials are: organic glass, silicon rubber, steel plates, Medpor (linear high-density polyethylene material), hydroxyapatite, titanium alloy, etc. [1, 2]. They used PEKK (polyetherketoneketone) as the print material. The customized implants for patients could be completed within 2 weeks, which have a significant impact in the field of plastic surgery.

Reverse engineering is to transform the product model or physical model into a design model and conceptual model, then to anatomy and deepen the existing products and to create again [3]. Reverse engineering application range is very wide in the aerospace, automotive, household appliances, computing machines, machinery, mould, entertainment industries and other industries. In addition, there also has a wide application in the replication of archaeological cultural relics and the body organs, bones and joints. Rapid prototyping and manufacturing technology (RPM) has a fundamental different with the traditional material removing method and material forced molding method. It is to use integral methods to create 3D entity, accumulating layer by layer. At present, with the development of computer 3D reconstruction technology and the improvement of related processing software, the RPM technology applications is becoming a research spot in the field of medicine [4–6].

Complete denture, which is to replace the missing maxillary or mandibles full denture and related organizations. It is mucous membrane support type activity denture in order to restore single or double jaw tooth loss, consisting of two parts: kitto and artificial teeth. Because of the abrasion of denture surface, a pair of ordinary denture should be adjusted teeth occlusion after 3 years and be repaired after 7 years [7]. This paper mainly aims at study of a pair of complete denture after the running-in period (not damaged). 3D data of denture surface was collected with a laser scanner. The data was processed in Geomagic software and the model was reconstructed in Pro/E software. The final 3D replica of denture is obtained by rapid prototyping machine. Through this process the entity model of running-in-period complete denture can be manufactured, which provides reference for clinical application.

226.2 Model Reconstruction

226.2.1 The Data Collection of Parts

Data collection is the foundation of subsequent processing in reverse engineering. According to weather the probe is in contact with the surface in the process of data collection, model digitizing method can be divided into two categories: contact method and non-contact method. Common measurement equipments includes

Fig. 226.1 Laser scanning of complete dentures

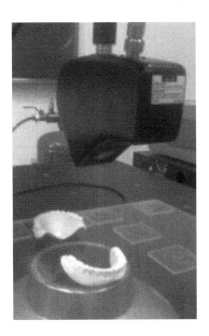

three coordinate measuring machine, laser scanners, grating measuring equipment, numerical control (NC) machine tools, industrial computed tomography (CT) and special digitizer [8]. The surface of complete denture consists of a large number of irregular surfaces; it is suitable to used non-contact laser scanning method to collect data.

This study used the three-coordinate measuring machine (CMM). The machine type is MQ8106, which can not only do contact measurement, can also do non-contact measurement by laser scanning. The HEADER F-Scan laser scanning probe was used to collect data. The main technical indexes are: measuring speed is 9216/s, measuring width is 65 mm, measuring depth of field is 100 mm, and measuring accuracy is 10 μm. The scanning path was planned. Complete denture data collection was shown in Fig. 226.1. Part of the point cloud data collected were opened in Imageware software, as shown in Fig. 226.2.

226.2.2 Data Preprocessing

Point cloud data preprocessing is one of the important part in reverse engineering, which directly affect the quality of later model reconstruction. The main processing including noise point removing, data smoothing and filtering, data compaction, data segmentation, data positioning and alignment [9]. The point cloud data obtained by laser scanning was not only a large amount of data, also have lots of miscellaneous points. This study use observation method to remove noise

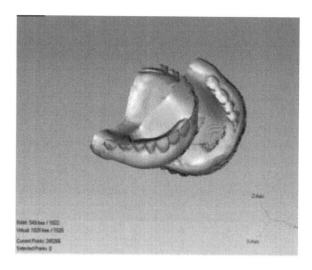

Fig. 226.2 Collected point cloud

points, namely, the user interacts with the CAD system, putting forward clearly the wrong point through visual observation [10]. Point cloud data after removing noise is shown in Fig. 226.3. The two parts of point cloud data were opened in Geomagic software at the same time, the measured point cloud data was regarded as a rigid body, only the coordinates changed when it moved, the shape did not change. Therefore, the alignment of point cloud data of complete denture question boils down to three dimensional rigid body coordinate transformation problem. Through coordinate transformation, the overlapping two parts of the point cloud was joined together as a whole. Three basis points were established in different views. Through the alignment of three basis points, the alignment of the 3D point cloud data could be realized [11, 12]. The point cloud registration was realized through the three matched points we selected as a reference in advance, after that the error was evaluated, as shown in Fig. 226.3.

Point cloud collecting and point cloud split were from the multiple points of view, which provided a large number of redundant data. It was necessary to filter the point cloud. At present, the widely used filtering algorithm is smoothing filter algorithm. Smoothing filter algorithm usually includes average filtering algorithm, Gaussian filtering algorithm, median filtering algorithm, etc. Gaussian filter algorithm was used here. The weight of its sample point is the Gaussian distribution. The average effect is smaller, morphology of the original data was well maintained [13].

The amount of data after filtering was still large, which would affect the efficiency of later manipulation. It was necessary to streamline the data. For scattered point cloud, common streamline methods are: bounding box method, uniform grid method, random sampling method, curvature sampling method, etc. [14]. The shape of denture model is extremely complex, so curvature sampling method was used here. After sampled, the data volume is 59.33 % of the original point cloud data.

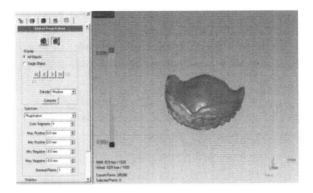

Fig. 226.3 Point cloud collage error

226.2.3 Model Reconstruction and Error Evaluation

There are many methods to reconstruct the model. At present relatively mature surface representation can be divided into two broad categories: (1) The three side surface construction method based on the triangular Bezier surface; (2) quadrilateral surface construction method mainly based on the NURBBS (non-uniform rational B-spline) curve and curved surface [15]. Point cloud data of complete denture model was large and its shape was complex. It was difficult to construct surface by using the method of characteristic curve extraction from model. Direct encapsulation triangular Bezier surface method was more accurate and convenient to use here.

The original point cloud data was seen as a whole. Firstly, the characteristic line was extracted, and on this basis an initial triangle mesh was formed. Then the triangular mesh was subdivided according to the curvature variation. Finally, smooth surface was constructed based on the mesh using the triangular Bezier surface method. The processed point cloud data was encapsulated into triangle surface directly. Triangle surface was edited, holes filled, excess surface removed, wrinkles smoothed, and the triangle number was reduced on the premise of not influencing the precision [16]. The triangular surface was transformed into NURBS surface, as shown in Fig. 226.4.

After the model was reconstructed, it was necessary to evaluate the precision of the model. Precision reflects the size of the gap between products and the reverse model [17]. Every link of reverse engineering can produce error, which resulted in a larger number of cumulative errors. The errors are: prototype error ε_p, measurement error ε_m, data processing error ε_d, processing and manufacturing error ε_c. The total error between reconstructed model and the sample is the transmission cumulative error among each part. The mathematical formula is:

$$\epsilon = \sqrt{\epsilon_p^2 + \epsilon_m^2 + \epsilon_d^2 + \epsilon_c^2} \qquad (226.1)$$

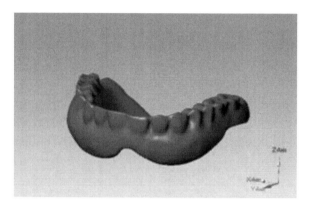

Fig. 226.4 NURBS surface

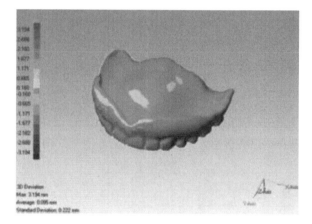

Fig. 226.5 Error between surface and original point cloud

In the formula, it is difficult to determine the weights of all the error. They were treated as equal weight. Due to the size of the various errors was difficult to determine, the accurate value of precision could not be determined. In practice, the distance between measurement point and surface model is usually used as the judgment to determine if model is accurate [18]. Error of reconstructed surface and the original point cloud was evaluated in Geomagic software, shown in Fig. 226.5, the average error is 0.095 mm, it was meet the requirements.

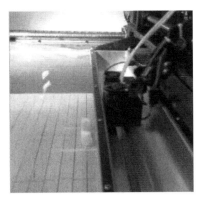

Fig. 226.6 Rapid prototyping process

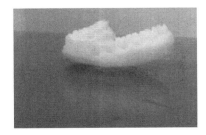

Fig. 226.7 Entity model of complete denture manufactured by rapid prototyping machine

226.3 Rapid Prototyping and Manufacturing of 3D Entity Model

The full name of the manufacturing machine used is Melt extrusion rapid prototyping machine. It is applied to innovative design, product development and rapid prototyping of product or parts. It can quickly manufacture three-dimensional modeling into material object. The machine type is MEM320A, the molding materials is ABS B601, the supporting materials is ABS S301.

The Pro/E CAD model was saved as STL format which is required for rapid prototyping machine, and process parameter was settled. Molding temperature was settled to 260 °C, layering thickness was 0.2 mm. Rapid prototyping process is shown in Fig. 226.6. The forming time was 106 min, and Fig. 226.7 shows complete denture entity manufactured by rapid prototyping.

226.4 Conclusions

Combination of reverse engineering and Rapid prototyping and manufacturing technology provided a good method for repairing of denture model. Reverse measurement of denture model was completed with 3D laser scanner. Then the measured point cloud data was dealt with in reverse engineering software Geomagic. The triangular Bezier surface was used to generate curved surface on the basis of grid structure, the 3D model was reconstructed in Pro/E software. Finally, rapid prototyping machine was used to get reverse products of denture model. The dimension of entity model is consistent with the three-dimensional model. Compared with the machining method, rapid prototyping method does not need a tool and has no influence of cutting force, so it can manufacture thin-walled parts, and the forming time is shorter. The entity model of complete denture can be used for medical analysis. The model can also be used as a reference to make denture mould, and after-running-in-period shaped denture can be made for patients to use,which can shorten the running-in period of complete denture, reduce the pain of patients and provide the basis to improve the level of medical technology and medical research.

Acknowledgments This work was supported by A Project Funded by the Priority Academic Program Development of Jiangsu Higher Education Institutions and A Project Funded by the Graduate Workstation of Jiangsu Enterprises.

References

1. Xiong YF, Qiu JH, Chu SH (2011) Selection and evaluation of different skull moulding materials. Chin J Clin 5(17):5119–5121
2. Anne P, Matthias H, Paul F et al (2012) Bonding of acrylic denture teeth to MMA/PMMA and light-curing denture base materials: the role of conditioning liquids. J Dent 40:210–221
3. Zhang XP (2009) Application of reverse engineering in industry. Mach Manuf Res 8:108–111
4. Chen DM, Liu YR, Liu J (2009) Reconstruction of skull using the rapid prototyping preprocessing technologies. J Biomed Eng Res 28(3):215–218
5. Gittard SD, Roger N, Jason L (2009) Rapid prototyping of scaphoid and lunate bones. Biotechnol J 4(1):129–134
6. Bai ZH, Zhang Y, Yin QS (2010) Bibliometric analysis of rapid prototyping techniques in the field of orthopaedics. 14(48):9046–9050
7. Deng M, Su XH (2010) Application of silicone rubber materials in repair of complete denture. J Clin Rehabil Tissue Eng Res 14(25):4645–4648
8. He YY (2011) Design of link rapid prototyping based on reverse engineering. Small Inter Combust Engine Motorcycle 40(2):69–71
9. Peng YJ, Wang S, Peng XO (2011) Applied research of UG and imageware in 3-D model reconstruction of reverse engineering. Mach Des Manuf 5:85–87
10. Fan HZH, Liu J, Yu N (2007) Data Pre- processing for data from cross section scan in reverse engineering. Mach Des Manuf 9:71–73
11. Akemi G, Andres I, Jaime PP (2012) Iterative two-step genetic-algorithm-based method for efficient polynomial B-spline surface reconstruction. Inf Sci 182:56–76
12. Giordanoa M, Ausiello P, Martorelli M (2012) Accuracy evaluation of surgical guides in implant dentistry by non-contact reverse engineering techniques. Dent Mater 28:178–185
13. Dai J L (2006) A research on preprocessing algorithms of mass point cloud. ZheJiang, China
14. Zhou L, Lin H, Zhong YX et al (2004) The thinning method for measued points cloud in surface reconstruction. Manuf Inf Eng China 33(5):102–104

15. Liu Y, Hu ZHY, Liu YSH (2010) Surface reconstruction about buckle based on imageware. Mach Build Autom 39(5):117–119
16. Wang J, Gu DX, Yu ZY et al (2012) A framework for 3D model reconstruction in reverse engineering. Comput Ind Eng 63:1189–1200
17. Zhu Y, Wu XJ, Lv JJ et al (2011) Three-dimensional reconstruction of dentures based on general CAD technology. J Clin Rehabil Tissue Eng Res 15(13):2345–2348
18. Giordanoa M, Ausiello P, Martorelli M (2012) Accuracy evaluation of surgical guides in implant dentistry by non-contact reverse engineering techniques. Dent Mater 28:178–185

Chapter 227
Simulation Training on Improving Basic Laparoscopic Skills of Medical Students

Ni Hong, Song Ge and Junfang Qin

Abstract *Objective* A Laparoscopic Simulation Training on improving basic skills of endoscopic surgery is evaluated. *Methods* eight test projects are set, include three simple projects, three complex projects, and two comprehensive projects were used to compare the laparoscopic surgical techniques between untrained students (the control group) and students who were trained using above training device 50 h (the experimental group). *Result* Significant difference existed between the two groups in laparoscopic skills. The experimental group had more score than the experimental teams in simple and complex subjects, as the result of comprehensive projects. *Conclusion* A Laparoscopic Simulation Training has significant training effect in using laparoscope surgical instruments and the basic operation technology of laparoscope.

Keywords Laparoscopy · Training · Laparoscopic training instrument

227.1 Introduction

Since twenty first century, endoscopic surgery has been applied in more and more traditional surgical field with revolutionary success, which has been the theme of global surgical development. Due to the remarkable differences between endoscopic surgery and traditional open operation, it is very necessary to carry out endoscopic surgery training [1]. Therefore various medical colleges should greatly introduce laparoscopic Simulation Training system, and then the training based on the system should be conducted to the trainers with various clinical experiences so

N. Hong (✉) · S. Ge · J. Qin
Medical School of Nankai University, Tianjin 300071, China
e-mail: hongni@nankai.edu.cn

as to explore the training result of the laparoscopic simulation training, which can lay a good foundation for the medical students who want to take up the medical work.

227.2 Materials and Method

227.2.1 Laparoscopic Simulation Platform

A set of self-made Laparoscopic simulation platform, the camera and display that are connected with the Laparoscopic simulation platform. Put the camera into the operation box of laparoscopic simulation platform; adjust the lens angle thus the simulation laparoscopic model can be clearly shown on the display. The trainers can carry out the instrument operation training according to the display picture before the display.

227.2.2 Groups

Hundred and two students were selected from medical college. Randomly choose 6 persons as the experimental team (seed team), who will have the complete laparoscopic basic skill training for about 50 h totally. Other 96 persons are grouped into control teams. They will be divided into 16 teams with 6 persons for each team. The students form 07 grade were divided into 4 teams (completing 36 h surgical operation course learning); the students from 09 grade were divided into 5 teams and the students from 10 grade were divided into 7 teams. Before carrying out the test, the experimental teams shall conduct training on the laparoscopic simulation machines for 1.5 h so as to understand the operation instruments and operation method well.

227.2.3 Test Projects

8 test projects are set, include 3 simple projects, namely picking beans, Lead wire threading and tailoring smiling face; 3 complex projects, namely tailoring angle shape, flexible wire threading and skin graft. 9 experimental completed the test; and 2 comprehensive projects, namely, taking the foreign body in the stomach and intestinal suture and cannula. The control team should complete all the test projects; the 16 experimental teams completed the simple projects and 9 teams (three teams from 2007 grade, three teams from 09 grade and three teams from 11 grade) completed the complex project and 5 teams (three teams from 07 grade, two teams from 09 grade) completed the comprehensive projects.

227.2.4 Statistics Methods

All the data was processed with SPSS 17.0, and all the groups of data was expressed with mean ± standard deviation. Matching T test was be used in various grade scores of simple test items and contrast teams. If P value is less than 0.05, it is deemed as that statistical difference between both exists.

227.3 Results

227.3.1 Analysis on the Simple Items Test

In all simple items test, the scores of experimental team are much better than the control teams of various grades. The scores of two items (Picking beans, Lead wire threading) in experimental team are two times much better than that of control teams. In the tailoring smiling face with scissors, the score of experimental team is six times better than that of control teams. Compared to various groups, in the picking beans and tailoring smiling face that can be used to test the ability of using the instruments the teams from 07 grade are much better than the teams from other grade ($P < 0.05$). In the Lead wire threading that can be used to test the manual operation stability, the teams from 09 grade have a better performance (Table 227.1).

227.3.2 Analysis on Complex Items Test

In all complex items test, the test scores of experimental team that have experienced the systematic training are still much better than the control teams from various grades. In the tailoring the angle forms and flexible wire threading, the scores of the experimental team are more than 3 times of the control teams. It can be also known from the analysis on the items that the flexible wire threading items in the experimental team have a remarkable advantage against the control teams (Table 227.2).

Table 227.1 Analysis on the simple item tests

Groups (n)	Picking beans (x ± s)	P value	Lead wire threading (x ± s)	P value	Tailoring smiling face (x ± s)	P value
07 (4)	17.25 ± 3.948	0.058	15.00 ± 5.774	0.009	4.50 ± 1.291	<0.001
09 (5)	10.50 ± 2.646	<0.001	20.00 ± 9.129	0.206	3.75 ± 2.872	<0.001
11 (7)	8.33 ± 4.633	0.001	10.83 ± 11.143	0.059	3.00 ± 2.000	<0.001
Control (1)	23.00 ± 4.000		48.33 ± 18.930		28.33 ± 2.082	

Table 227.2 Analysis on complex items test

Groups (n)	Tailoring the angle (x ± s)	Flexible wire threading (x ± s)	Suture operation (x ± s)	Total score
Experimental (9)	6.00 ± 3.674	22.22 ± 15.635	19.11 ± 11.656	47.33 ± 24.864
Control (1)	21.00 ± 0.000	105.00 ± 0.000	42.00 ± 0.000	168.00 ± 0.000

227.3.3 Analysis on the Comprehensive Items Test

We can know from the test result that just as the same result we get from simple items, the test scores of experimental team are still much better than the control teams from various teams in the comprehensive items. In the item of taking out foreign body in the stomach, the experimental team can complete the item operation nearly 9 min ahead of the best control teams. In the item of intestinal suture and intubation, the score of the experimental team was five times higher than that of the control teams. The total score of the experimental team was 2 times higher than the control teams (Table 227.3).

227.3.4 Comparison of Various Items Between Experimental Teams and Control Team

We compared the average scores of various items between the experimental team and control teams and found that the average scores of various items of the experimental team are remarkably higher than that of the control teams. The improvement degree of eight items can be shown in Fig. 227.1. If the highest difference of 7.19 times and lowest difference of 1.32 are eliminated, we will find that the average score of the experimental team is increased by 3.6 times as that of control teams and that is a remarkable advantage.

The comparison and analysis on the best scores of various items between experimental team and control teams was also compared. It was found that the average scores of various items of the experimental team are remarkably higher than that of the control teams. The improvement degree of eight items can be shown in Fig. 227.2. If the highest difference of 6.30 times and lowest difference of 1.00 are eliminated, we will find that the average score of the control teams is increased by 2.3 times as that of experimental teams and that is a remarkable advantage.

Table 227.3 Analysis on the comprehensive items test

Groups (n)	Taking foreign body	Intestinal suture and intubation	Total score
Experimental (5)	66.40 ± 30.038	16.00 ± 9.849	82.40 ± 33.359
Control (1)	102.00 ± 0.000	86.00 ± 0.000	188.00 ± 0.000

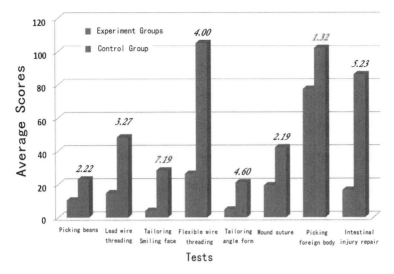

Fig. 227.1 Comparison of average scores between experiment and control group

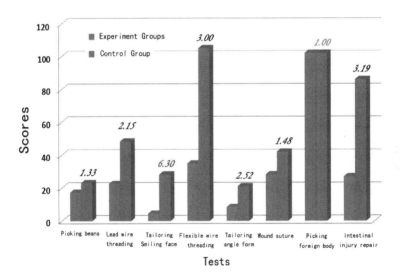

Fig. 227.2 Comparison of the best records between experiment and control group

227.4 Discussion

Laparoscopic surgery, as a new minimally invasive approach, is an evitable trend for the future operation method. With tremendous development of Industrial manufacturing technology, the integration of relevant disciplines can lay a good foundation for developing the new technology and methods. With doctors' operation getting more and more skillful, many operations that were conducted with open operation can take place of the internal urethrotomy, thus increasing the choices for the operation. It is undoubted that mastering the laparoscopic basic technology can play an influential role in improving the medical student surgical operation internship result [2, 3].

In simple item tests (such as picking beans, lead wire threading and tailoring smiling face), according to the control teams, the score of the 07 grade teams are obviously higher than other grade team, it may be related to that they systematically studied the course about operative surgery and got some operation skill training. Just like other control teams, the members of the 07 grade teams didn't receive the complete laparoscopic simulation training, but compared with other grade teams, they obviously have an advantage in mastering the operation of new equipment. Besides 07 grades, the differences of scores of each other grade teams are not conspicuous, but there is a trend that all the scores are increasing with the increase of grade, it shows that the ability of medical students to master the operation of equipment will increase as they spend more time participating in practice courses in medical school. In this study, the score of 08 grade teams are lower, it may be related to that only two teams of it participated in the test, thus their data are too little and the representativeness is poor.

In all the complex item tests (tailoring angle form, flexible wire threading and skin graft suture), the experimental team has obvious advantage, and their score are 3 times more than others in average. In the operation of the integrated item about simulation operation without early training, the performance of the experimental team is still better than other. It shows that enough laparoscopic simulation training has significant training effect and value in having a good command of using laparoscope surgical instruments and the basic operation technology of laparoscope. It is visible that, the necessary laparoscope simulation training can do well to medical students in their future laparoscopic surgery clinical practice. At the same time, the simple laparoscopic equipment and training programs designed in this study have many advantages, such as low cost, good training effect, strong practicability and so on, and they can be used in the future surgery teaching after a further optimization.

References

1. Beyer L, De Troyer J, Mancini J et al (2011) Impact of laparoscopy simulator training on the technical skills of future surgeons in the operating room: a prospective study. American J Surg 202(3):265–272
2. Larsen CR, Oestergaard J, Ottesen S et al (2012) The efficacy of virtual reality simulation training in laparoscopy: a systematic review of randomized trials. Acta Obstet Et Gynecol Scand 91(9):1015–1028
3. Varas J, Mejia R, Riquelme A et al (2012) Significant transfer of surgical skills obtained with an advanced laparoscopic training program to a laparoscopic jejunojejunostomy in a live porcine model: feasibility of learning advanced laparoscopy in a general surgery residency. Surg Endosc Other Intervl Tech 26(12):3486–3494

Chapter 228
Research on Reforming of Vocational Colleges for Music Majors in Education

Liu Li

Abstract Recently years, college students that small number of causes vocational college music education students in specialized courses overall reduction in the level of student learning objectives are not clear, not solid and clear knowledge to grasp the phenomenon. How the status quo student teachers of their ability to training culture by fostering target, learning ability teaching and the ability to organize capacity capability, making them capable of future teaching and other work.

Keywords Teacher training · Student status · Music education · Capacity-building

228.1 Introduction

Emotions is an emotional phenomenon, usually refers to the person's mood, state of mind. Psychology research shows that emotions have impact on many cognitive factors. The emotional state is performance of emotion in the practice of great significance to its people's lives. It may improve the way people work, learning efficiency, and also can reduce people's working and learning efficiency.

Students in grades not go instead to test music in the test into colleges before choosing a vocational music education professional, there is no good study habits are not interested in the professional courses, even those that graduate students can not find a job, not to mention college graduates do not have lofty ideals and aspirations, the goof in school felt that they could get a diploma on the line, late for class absences, do not listen carefully, undisciplined, free class to play phone, exam review, the effort in the examination room.

L. Li (✉)
Teacher's Branch of Beihua University, Jilin, China
e-mail: kingmesh@gmail.com

Vocational music education majors, whether professional courses or cultural studies, knowledge of general knowledge do not know do not understand, such as specialized courses not know what a coloratura, and cultural knowledge do not know the time of the birth of the Communist Party of China a lot of blind students learning music, but in fact they are not low level of cultural studies, and only professional music lovers, go to college, there is no pressure and parental supervision of their studies, the less time spent in learning, the classroom teacher taught knowledge of music story of the students only when listening to the story, the next class to ask questions, what do not remember a lot of teachers in the school at the beginning very few students go to the piano room piano, only before the final exam, in order to feel to the momentum of the students a crash course.

Therefore, studies of computer crime has its special significance, a certain extent, the computer and cyber crimes related to national security, can not be overlooked.

228.2 The Main Ideas of the Domestic and Foreign Scholars and the Criticism

1. A macro-theory is the relationship between the computer and computer research, to define computer crime. So this theory, called the relationship between theory, this theory was also defined as the relevant theory and theory of abuse. The related theory is that: Where the crimes of subjective or objective related to computer crime, known as computer crime. American scholars in the initial study is the concept of computer crime (computer crime). American scholar Don B. Parker (Parker): Computer Crime (Computer Crime) refers to the computer directly involved in the execution of the crime, and further limit the conditions of computer crime.
2. The concern perspective of the micro-computer crime, computer crime, whether the object is a computer system. For example, the Swedish law on computer crime made the following definition: invasion of personal privacy, computer crime, including unauthorized computer and save the private documents and all violations by the data protection acts. German scholar computer crime is characterized as a kind of property vandalism, and this behavior is related to electronic data.

Definition of cyber crime, the microscopic theory of "crimes against computer networks is the use of computer technology on the integrity or normal operation of the computer network information systems to cause damage results constitute a criminal act [2]. The rationale of cyber crime is limited to the object of crime occurred to computer networks and criminal behavior in cyberspace, crime and crime results in the network formation and end. Microscopic theory seems, network implementation, kidnapping, extortion, etc., should be attributed to the traditional crime, does not belong to the scope of cyber crime. As a result, the microscopic theory of cyber crime is only for the criminal acts of the network itself, can be summed up as an object theory. The author believes that too narrow a definition of the microscopic theory of computer and cyber crime, there is no data to defraud and steal computer information and other criminal acts bear came in, nor will use the Internet to include secession act or acts of espionage come. According to China's introduction of the provisions in the draft decision on the maintenance of network and information security, including the use of the Internet to incite ethnic hatred or serious harm to social behavior should be classified as computer crime. Clearly, the definition of the microscopic theory is not comprehensive enough.

3. Intermediate theoretical point of view, instruments of crime of computer crime computer crime computer assets. Referred to in the middle of the theory of instruments of crime refers to computer information systems, including different levels of computer technology. This intermediate theory the definition of computer crime, the macroscopic theory and the microscopic theory of fusion and processing instruments of crime and the criminal purpose of the relationship between the two. Obviously this definition is more comprehensive, more scientific.

228.3 Analysis of Judicial Practice

The legal nature of the generation of a law often is a lag. Because social life is a living, you propose a legislative initiative to research, to make the draft to the discussion through the new social phenomenon came out, that the legal loopholes are inevitable. Lag of the criminal law always seemed more prominent. The existing criminal law, established the principle of "legality". Established the three characteristics of the crime, that is harmful to society, criminal violations, should be subject to criminal penalties. Three are indispensable. The field of computer crime, the reality is that the rapid emergence at present the majority of countries in the world of computer crime law is incomplete, the legal provisions of the lagged far behind that computer crime. This deficiency is not only reflected in the number and scope of application of the law itself, in the proceedings based on the principle of "the law does not sin" before the 1997 Criminal Law by the Court for a lot of computer crime there is no way qualitatively. The situation has been improved, but still a lot of lag, after the enactment of the current Penal Code.

Seen in this light, the term cyber crime is not a statutory concept, but the sense of criminology collectively on a new type of crime. I believe that the meaning of cyber crime is the perpetrator made use of the Internet, the criminal behavior of the devastating attacks in the permit has not been the victim, the injured party's computer or network system. Ministry of Public Security Public Information Network Security Supervision Bureau of Statistics report shows that China's cyber crime since 1986, when the only incidence nine of 2,000 soared to more than 2,700 cases, from 35,000 in 2008. To a District Prosecutor's Office of Shandong Province for the cyber crime cases in the first half of 2006–2010, for example (see figure below):

Information on the Internet and publishing division is not clear. The exchange of multimedia works is attributable to the publication and distribution? The regular publication of a work usually in the form of books, periodicals, newspapers, audiovisual products must have a formal ISBN and publishing license, otherwise you can treat the illegal publication of acts. But on the Internet, and no national boundaries and the police, anyone can feel free to publish their own or others' works. This behavior may not be for commercial purposes, at the same time to see this information free to copy these works and does not require any formalities. Therefore lead to the judicial practice will find some of the issues, the legal principles to determine whether this behavior is illegal, and who will determine whether an offense has become the problem in the judicial practice.

228.4 Computer and Cyber Crime Face New Problems and Reflections

The author believes that many criminal acts on the Penal Code provisions on computer and network crime in the identified lack of Elements, the lack of actual operability facing some new problems.

1. An object of a crime is not clear

For the safe operation of combat cyber crime, the protection of the Internet, our decision on safeguarding Internet security, "issued December 28 2000. Explicitly in the document, to be held criminally responsible Internet behavior which constitutes is a crime. Which the decision first sets out the following acts, including acts of intentionally spreading computer viruses and other destructive programs, attacks on computer systems and communication networks, resulting in computer systems and communication networks suffer damage, in violation of state regulations, unauthorized interruption of computer network or communication service, resulting in the behavior of computer networks or communications systems may not run. In Article IV explicitly refers to the following acts, including the illegal interception, tampering, delete others 'e-mail or other data behavior, violation of the behavior of the citizens' freedom and privacy of correspondence, use the Internet for theft, fraud, extortion behavior.

Seen in this light, the term cyber crime is not a statutory concept, but the sense of criminology collectively on a new type of crime. I believe that the meaning of cyber crime is the perpetrator made use of the Internet, the criminal behavior of the devastating attacks in the permit has not been the victim, the injured party's computer or network system. Ministry of Public Security Public Information Network Security Supervision Bureau of Statistics report shows that China's cyber crime since 1986, when the only incidence 9 of 2,000 soared to more than 2,700 cases, from 35,000 in 2008. To a District Prosecutor's Office of Shandong Province for the cyber crime cases in the first half of 2006–2010, for example (see figure below):

2. The behavior of the objective aspect of crime is unknown

The crime of computer theft, a common Italian sausage surgery this crime is not easy to make the victim aware of the ways in which the victim unconscious to make minor concessions to the interests, add up in order to achieve a criminal purpose. For example, the perpetrator in the victim's computer silently install a Trojan horse program, this Trojan horse programs can be opened in the victim's bank account, password quietly record, while the occasional micro-transfer of money from the victim account, the import of the offender's account. a small amount, is often difficult to immediately find the program to run automatically, so no obvious criminal act. We are usually talking about computer and network "fraud" or "fraud, always the consequences of criminal behavior or taken by the Trojans implantation means to do empirical judgment.

3. The new requirements of the traditional subject of crime

In business, some companies in order to win in the field of commercial competition, or for the protection of their own intellectual property rights of purposes, and to take the network means to limit and even undermine each other's computers and networks, users and competitors piracy. 1997, Beijing has undergone a similar event. An anti-virus software company anti-virus software to its products of a particular model "logic lock" to prevent being pirated, so that the computer installed the software does not work properly. However, the main body of the crime of invasive calculation of the information system in the provisions of section 30, 285, 286 of the Criminal Law, crime and destruction of computer information systems does not contain units. This author believes that it is necessary to the unit main body into the scope of computer crime regulation.

228.5 Conclusion

Principal penalty five and additional punishment of three kinds of penalties prescribed by the Criminal Law of China. From the existing case, the penalty's deterrent and protective enough. Computer and cyber crime body total fascination with this form of crime, punishment after the crime occurred usually to prevent criminal acts from happening again, so the introduction of new types of penalties is particularly important. Eligible for punishment can be included in China's penal system, as new types of penalties. Eligible for punishment including the public authority, parental authority and occupational deprivation of the right. Computer and cyber crime as a high-tech career criminal, set or provide deprived of their professional qualification in computer and networking industry, will play a very prominent role in the containment and prevention of crime.

References

1. Zhe H (2002) The essential characteristics of cyber crime and its criminal jurisdiction. Shandong Public Secur Coll 3:68–71
2. Yao L (2010) The meaning of computer and cybercrime legal perspective Study. BUPT (Social Science Edition) 2:24–28
3. Cyber crime cases continued to increase attention should be paid [EB/OL]. http://news.xinhuanet.com/legal/2010-09/12/c_12542964.htm
4. Jinyuan L Analysis of computer crime challenge the existing criminal law and criminal legislation to improve. http://fjfy.chinacourt.org/public/detail.php?id=10280
5. Barrett N (2008) Digital crime. Liaoning Education Press, Hao marine Translation. p 2–6

Chapter 229
Research on Badminton Sports in National Fitness Activities

Yanling Dong and Qiang Ji

Abstract Particle Swarm Optimization (PSO) is a swarm intelligence algorithm to achieve through competition and collaboration between the particles in the complex search space to find the global optimum. Basic PSO algorithm evolutionary late convergence speed is slow and easy to fall into the shortcomings of local minima, this paper presents a multi-learning particle swarm optimization algorithm, the algorithm particle at the same time to follow their own to find the optimal solution, random optimal solution and the optimal solution for the whole group of other particles with dimensions velocity update discriminate area boundary position optimization updates and small-scale perturbations of the global best position, in order to enhance the algorithm escape from local optima capacity. The test results show that several typical functions: improved particle swarm algorithms significantly improve the global search ability, and can effectively avoid the premature convergence problem. Algorithm so that the relative robustness of the search space position has been significantly improved global optimal solution in high-dimensional optimization problem, suitable for solving similar problems, the calculation results can meet the requirements of practical engineering.

Keywords Badminton movement · National Fitness · Value

229.1 Introduction

Particle Swarm Optimization algorithm proposed in 1995 by Eberhart and Kennedy (particle swarm optimization, PSO) is a global optimization evolutionary algorithm, invented it from the predatory behavior of flocks of birds and schools of

Y. Dong (✉) · Q. Ji
Institute of Physical Education, Beihua University, Jilin, China
e-mail: jlsbhjq@163.com

fish populations and evolutionary computation technology, is a new kind of global optimization evolutionary algorithm, through the sharing of information between the groups and the individual's own lessons learned to fix individual action strategies, and ultimately strike the optimization problem solution. PSO has been widely used in function optimization, neural networks, pattern classification, fuzzy system control in areas such as the core swarm intelligence (Swarm Intelligence), has formed a theoretical system. Particle Swarm individual represents a possible solution of the problem, each particle position and velocity of two describe the amount of particle position coordinates corresponding objective function value as the fitness of the particles, PSO algorithm to measure the particle's fitness pros and cons. This paper proposes a new improved PSO algorithm—multi-adaptive learning PSO (CLSPSO), both the accuracy and convergence speed. The idea of this algorithm is proposed based on a particle populations, a particle on the one hand to develop their own expertise, on the other hand, to learn the best particle populations in the same skills, and also other particles in the stochastic learning same advantages skills. The algorithm is to determine the rate of change during operation, according to the group fitness current optimum particles mutation probability, mutation operation, enhanced particle swarm optimization algorithm's ability to escape from the local optimal solution. Experimental results show that the improved particle swarm algorithm has been significantly enhanced into a local optimum capacity of preventing the same time, the algorithm for high-dimensional optimization problems in global optimal solution with respect to the robustness of the search space position has been significantly improved.

229.2 Improve Optimization of the Particle Swarm Algorithm

First, according to the basic information to initialize to be optimized for a group of random particles, the so-called "particles" is to be a potential solution of the optimization problem, which is a bird of the search space, it is to adjust according to their flying experience flying experience and peer their flight in the D-dimensional target in the search space, by population size for P (pop size), composed of particles communities particle i experienced during the flight the best position for the eq. (229.1) group as a whole experienced the most excellent location for the BS, each particle can remember own search for the best solution to CS, as well as the entire particle swarm optimal position for DE. Kennedy and Eberhart the earliest proposed by PSO algorithm formula is as follows: EF.

$$pb_i = pb_{i1}, pb_{i2}, \ldots, pb_{iD} \qquad (229.1)$$

$$gb_i = gb_1, gb_2, \ldots, gb_D \qquad (229.2)$$

$$v_{id}^{k+1} = v_{id}^k + c_1 r_1 (pb_{id}^k - x_{id}^k) + c_2 r_2 (gb_{id}^k - x_{id}^k)$$
$$x_{id}^{k+1} = x_{id}^k + v_{id}^k \tag{229.3}$$

229.3 GA Description

GA maintains a population of candidate solution regions using a sampling sequence to select the optimal solutions that work well from the problem. Process described as follows. Genetic algorithm (GA) is an evolutionary search strategy based on rules of biological population theories and genetics of evolution

$$\{q^e\} = [T]\{Q^e\}$$

$$\{q^e\} = \{u_1 \ v_1 \ w_1 \ u_2 \ v_2 \ w_2 \ u_3 \ v_3 \ w_3 \ u_4 \ v_4 \ w_4\}^T$$
$$\{Q^e\} = \{U_1 \ V_1 \ W_1 \ U_2 \ V_2 \ W_2 \ U_3 \ V_3 \ W_3 \ U_4 \ V_4 \ W_4\}^T$$

$$\begin{Bmatrix} u \\ v \\ w \end{Bmatrix} = [N]\{q^e\}$$

$$[N] = \begin{bmatrix} N_1 & 0 & 0 & N_2 & 0 & 0 & N_3 & 0 & 0 & N_4 & 0 & 0 \\ 0 & N_1 & 0 & 0 & N_2 & 0 & 0 & N_3 & 0 & 0 & N_4 & 0 \\ 0 & 0 & N_1 & 0 & 0 & N_2 & 0 & 0 & N_3 & 0 & 0 & N_4 \end{bmatrix}$$

where the shape function Ni (i = 1, 2, 3, 4) as follows:

$$N_1 = \tfrac{1}{4}(1-\xi)(1-\eta) \quad N_2 = \tfrac{1}{4}(1+\xi)(1-\eta)$$
$$N_3 = \tfrac{1}{4}(1+\xi)(1+\eta) \quad N_4 = \tfrac{1}{4}(1-\xi)(1+\eta)$$

$$u_{,x} = \sum_{i=1}^{4} \frac{\partial N_i}{\partial x} u_i; \quad u_{,y} = \sum_{i=1}^{4} \frac{\partial N_i}{\partial y} u_i; \quad v_{,x} = \sum_{i=1}^{4} \frac{\partial N_i}{\partial x} v_i$$

$$v_{,y} = \sum_{i=1}^{4} \frac{\partial N_i}{\partial y} v_i; \quad w_{,x} = \sum_{i=1}^{4} \frac{\partial N_i}{\partial x} w_i; \quad w_{,y} = \sum_{i=1}^{4} \frac{\partial N_i}{\partial y} w_i$$

$$\begin{Bmatrix} \partial N_i/\partial \xi \\ \partial N_i/\partial \eta \end{Bmatrix} = \begin{bmatrix} \partial x/\partial \xi & \partial y/\partial \xi \\ \partial x/\partial \eta & \partial y/\partial \eta \end{bmatrix} \begin{Bmatrix} \partial N_i/\partial x \\ \partial N_i/\partial y \end{Bmatrix} = [J] \begin{Bmatrix} \partial N_i/\partial x \\ \partial N_i/\partial y \end{Bmatrix}$$

$$[J] = \begin{bmatrix} \sum_{i=1}^{4} \left(\frac{\partial N_i}{\partial \xi} x_i\right) & \sum_{i=1}^{4} \left(\frac{\partial N_i}{\partial \xi} y_i\right) \\ \sum_{i=1}^{4} \left(\frac{\partial N_i}{\partial \eta} x_i\right) & \sum_{i=1}^{4} \left(\frac{\partial N_i}{\partial \eta} y_i\right) \end{bmatrix} \quad \begin{Bmatrix} \partial N_i/\partial x \\ \partial N_i/\partial y \end{Bmatrix} = [J]^{-1} \begin{Bmatrix} \partial N_i/\partial \xi \\ \partial N_i/\partial \eta \end{Bmatrix}$$

The procedure description of panel drawing direction constraint function maximizes to single objective function. Suppose that:

$$\begin{cases} n_x = N_1 n_x^1 + N_2 n_x^2 + N_3 n_x^3 + N_4 n_x^4 \\ n_y = N_1 n_y^1 + N_2 n_y^2 + N_3 n_y^3 + N_4 n_y^4 \\ n_z = N_1 n_z^1 + N_2 n_z^2 + N_3 n_z^3 + N_4 n_z^4 \end{cases}$$

$$r = -t_1 \cdot \boldsymbol{n}_{,x} = -\sum_{i=1}^{4} \frac{\partial N_i}{\partial x} n_x^i$$

$$t = -t_2 \cdot \boldsymbol{n}_{,y} = -\sum_{i=1}^{4} \frac{\partial N_i}{\partial y} n_y^i$$

$$s = -t_1 \cdot \boldsymbol{n}_{,y} = -\sum_{i=1}^{4} \frac{\partial N_i}{\partial y} n_x^i$$

$$s = -t_2 \cdot \boldsymbol{n}_{,x} = -\sum_{i=1}^{4} \frac{\partial N_i}{\partial x} n_y^i$$

The rules, which ensure the non-negative feasible region of drawing direction, indicate that each cell normal has the corresponding unit vector half spherical surface of feasible region on the unit vector spherical surface. The normal nA of cell A corresponding the unit vector half spherical surface RA as well as the RB. However, the RA ∩ RB corresponding the unit vector spherical surface based on normal nA and nB. Therefore, the feasible region unit vector spherical surface can be obtained by the cell normal of the panel. The intersection R of feasible region unit spherical surfaces is the feasible region of panel drawing direction (Tables 229.1, 229.2, 229.3).

Table 229.1 List of frequent nodes based on confidence limit

	11	12	13	14	15	Support (%)	Confidence (%)
1	1	1	0	0	0	42	55.34
2	1	0	1	0	0	42	55.34
3	0	1	1	0	0	42	27.35
4	1	1	1	0	0	18	44.935
5	1	1	0	0	1	18	44.935

Table 229.2 List of frequent nodes based on confidence limit

	11	12	13	14	15	Support (%)	Confidence (%)
1	1	1	0	0	0	42	55.34
2	1	0	1	0	0	42	55.34
3	0	1	1	0	0	42	27.35
4	1	1	1	0	0	18	44.935
5	1	1	0	0	1	18	44.935

Table 229.3 Mutated cloned for every item sets

1	2	3	4	5
11000	10101	1101	10100	11001
11000	11100			
11000				

229.4 Conclusion

The proposed drawing punch can enter into the cavity without contact. The contact area between the punch and sheet is maximum so that realize the uniform stress during the drawing process. The minimum drawing limit depth and the uniform depth of each drawing direction realize the accurate and comprehensive constraint conditions.

In the feasible region of drawing direction that determined by unit vector spherical surface method, the optimal drawing direction could automotive confirmed by using genetic algorithm. The test indicates that the acquisition of optimal drawing direction can provide basic reference of mould structure design and the sequent technics plan. The optimization algorithm can automotive accomplish without manual operation. The results are accuracy and its operation is efficient and has good robustness.

References

1. Gong K, Hu P (2006) Method for generating additional surface in die face design of automotive panel. J Jilin Univ (Engineering and Technology Edition), 36(1): 63–66
2. Pernot J-P, Moraru G (2006) Filling holes in meshes using a mechanical model to simulate the curvature variation minimization. Comput Graph 30:892–902
3. Rayevskaya V, Larry L (2005) Multi-sided macro-element spaces based on Clough–Tocher triangle splits with applications to hole filling. Comput Aided Geom Des 22:57–79
4. Wang J, Manuel M (2007) Filling holes on locally smooth surfaces reconstructed from point clouds. Image Vis Comput 25:103–113

Chapter 230
University Students' Humanity Quality Education of Tai Ji Quan to Cultivate Influence

Ji Qiang and Dong YanLing

Abstract The right panel drawing direction is an important prerequisite for generating qualified parts, an important step before the panel forming simulation is to determine the reasonable direction of the drawing. Manually adjust parts in order to overcome rely on experience, the drawbacks to the drawing direction, the direction of the drawing punch and forming the contact area of the sheet as the goal of automatic determination algorithm. Objective function of the direction of the drawing for the variable contact area in the drawing direction of the feasible region, the use of heritage algorithms to optimize the objective function of the contact area and, ultimately feasible within the contact area corresponding to the drawing direction, that is the best drawing direction. The measured results show that the direction of the drawing based on genetic algorithm, the automatic algorithm can fast and accurate to obtain the optimal direction of drawing.

Keywords Humanistic quality · Cultivate · Tai Ji Quan education

230.1 Introduction

As an important component of frame car body, the qualified panel is the key factor to guarantee the automobile manufacturing quality. In order to ensure the forming quality and development period of panel, the designed mould should conduct forming simulation before the panel drawing forming. The most important process of forming simulation pretreatment is to determine drawing direction. As the main factor to effect the flow direction and velocity of sheet metal, the unreasonable drawing direction would lead to fold and wrinkle of panel [1–3]. Moreover, the reasonable drawing direction is an important basis of drawing mould structure and

---

J. Qiang · D. YanLing (✉)
Institute of Physical Education, Beihua University, Jilin City, China
e-mail: jlsbhjq@163.com

the subsequent process design. The traditional drawing direction of panel depends on the experience of technician that constantly rotating part, which rely on the experience of technician and would consume more time and labor force, furthermore, it is difficult to stable obtain the optimal direction in the feasible region of the drawing direction. A lot of researches about the automatic panel drawing direction have been studied, which mainly conducted the relevant objective optimization in the feasible region of drawing direction that provided by the 2-D cross-section data of panel model [4]. The application results showed that the simplified 2-D cross-section data replace the 3-D entity process would lead to data loss, which result in a narrow region and finally change the optimal solution. In order to overcome the disadvantages of traditional algorithm for drawing direction, it has proposed that the spatial information of pre-processing grid of panel was utilized and the genetic algorithm was adopted to optimize the normal plane projected area of parameter drawing direction of panel, which was in the feasible region decided by unit sphere. In addition, the corresponding parameters of the maximum projected area were determined as the optimal drawing direction. The measured data indicated that the automatic algorithm of panel drawing direction acquired the optimal drawing direction without manual operation, and it had fast computation speed and good robustness.

230.2 Establish Optimized Model of Drawing Direction

The constraint conditions of drawing direction optimized model include the following aspects:

The drawing punch can enter into the cavity without touch.
For ensuring the drawing punch can enter into the cavity without touch, the angle between the normal of panel cell and the parameter drawing direction should less than 90°, otherwise the punch cannot enter into the cavity.
Maximize the initial contact area between punch and sheet. Large contact area can realize smooth and uniform stress during drawing process.
Minimize the drawing limit depth. Large depth of drawing is the main reason to the defects of break, fold, wrinkle and thin.
Uniform the drawing depth each direction. The uniform drawing depth realizes the same deflection of sheet and feed resistance that is advantage to manufacture qualified panels.

According to the geometry size of the physical model, the geometric center of panel is determined and establishes local coordinate system that use the geometric center as the origin. The arbitrary drawing direction Zi ($i = 0,1,\ldots, n$) is set through the origin of coordinate system as well as the series normal plane of drawing direction. They should isometric intersect with the parts. The section interval is usually 3–6 mm. The height of section Z1 is always the 1/30 of total height. The schematic of the normal plane of drawing direction is shown in Fig. 230.1.

Fig. 230.1 Schematic of the normal plane of panel drawing direction

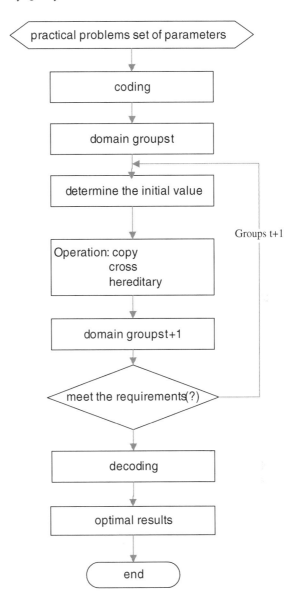

In the feasible region, the objective function of panel drawing direction Z based on constraint conditions is shown as:

The contact area between punch and sheet is maximum in the beginning of drawing. The function is expressed as:

$$F_1(Z) = \max\left\{\sum_{i=1}^{k} s_i\right\} \quad (230.1)$$

where the s_i is projected area of panel finite element mesh in section z_0 according to the drawing direction.

Inform the drawing depth in each direction during the drawing process. The function is expressed as:

$$f_3(Z) = \min(z_n - z_{n-1}) \tag{230.2}$$

Minimize the panel drawing final depth at the end of the drawing. The function is expressed as: $f_2(Z) = \min(z_n - z_0)$.

230.3 Confirm the Feasible Region of Drawing Direction

The angle between drawing direction and cell normal is less than 90°, which is the essential condition to constrain the feasible region of panel drawing direction and is called non-negative angle. It is equal to the angle less than $\pi/2$, and that the mathematics analytic expression is $f(z, n_i) = \cos\alpha_i \geq 0$. Here, n_i is the normal direction of cell i, a_i is the angle between drawing direction Z and cell n_i (i=1,2,…, m).

Establish the unit vector spherical surface of feasible region of drawing direction that uses the local coordinate system origin as globe. The parameter function of unit vector spherical surface expresses as:

$$\begin{cases} x = \cos\theta\cos\phi \\ y = \cos\theta\sin\phi \\ z = \sin\theta \end{cases} \left(-\frac{\pi}{2} \leq \theta \leq \frac{\pi}{2}, -\pi \leq \phi \leq \pi\right) \tag{230.3}$$

The rules, which ensure the non-negative feasible region of drawing direction, indicate that each cell normal has the corresponding unit vector half spherical surface of feasible region on the unit vector spherical surface, as shows in Fig. 230.2. The normal nA of cell A corresponding the unit vector half spherical surface RA as well as the RB. However, the RA ∩ RB corresponding the unit vector spherical surface based on normal nA and nB. Therefore, the feasible region unit vector spherical surface can be obtained by the cell normal of the panel. The intersection R of feasible region unit spherical surfaces is the feasible region of panel drawing direction.

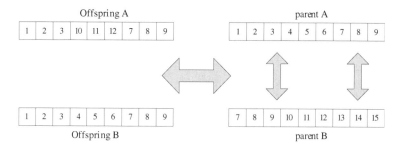

Fig. 230.2 Feasible domain of drawing direction

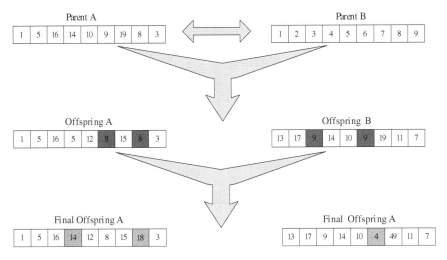

Fig. 230.3 Crossover when duplicated information number produced

230.4 Structure the Genetic Algorithm Function

Genetic algorithm has a very strong adaptability to optimize the single-objective function in disperse feasible region. The mathematical function expresses as:

$$\begin{cases} \max F(x) \\ st.\ x \in R \end{cases}$$

Here, F (x) shows the objective function of expected optimization. The matrix form of independent variable is $x = [x_1, x_2, \cdots, x_n]^T$, R is the gather of constraint conditions, which is also the feasible region of independent variable.

The optimization objective function of panel drawing direction based on genetic algorithm could solve the optimal drawing direction by means of programming. The structure composition of genetic algorithm program is shown in the following (Fig. 230.3).

230.5 Conclusion

The proposed drawing punch can enter into the cavity without contact. The contact area between the punch and sheet is maximum so that realize the uniform stress during the drawing process. The minimum drawing limit depth and the uniform depth of each drawing direction realize the accurate and comprehensive constraint conditions.

In the feasible region of drawing direction that determined by unit vector spherical surface method, the optimal drawing direction could automotive confirmed by using genetic algorithm. The test indicates that the acquisition of optimal drawing direction can provide basic reference of mould structure design and the sequent techniques plan. The optimization algorithm can automotive accomplish without manual operation. The results are accuracy and its operation is efficient and has good robustness.

References

1. Yong tae J (2005) A piecewise hole filling algorithm in reverse engineering. Comput Aided Des 37:263–270
2. Gabrielidesa NC, Ginnisa AI, Kaklisa PD (2007) G1-smooth branching surface construction from cross sections. Comput Aided Des 39:639–651
3. Yang Y-J, Yong J-H, Zhang H (2006) A rational extension of Piegl's method for flling n-sided holes. Comput Aided Des 38:1166–1178
4. Cheng P-F, Yan H-W, Han Z-H (2008) An algorithm for computing the minimum area bounding rectangle of an arbitrary polygon. J Graph 1:122–126

Chapter 231
Study Progress of Traditional Chinese Massage Treatment of Lumbar Disc Herniation

Qing Lan and Weihong Deng

Abstract This paper reviews the literature on the Chinese massage treatment of lumbar disc herniation clinical treatment method, curative effect and mechanism in recent years. This paper thinks Chinese massage has certain curative effect on lumbar disc herniation. This paper can provide ideas and approaches for clinical summary and mechanism of further scientific study.

Keywords Lumbar disc herniation · Massage therapy · The therapeutic mechanism

231.1 Research Survey

Lumbar disc herniation is a degenerative disease of lumbar intervertebral disc, under the action of external force, the annulus fibrosus of intervertebral disc part or all of the nucleus pulposus prolapse of rupture, outward. Due to external forces or pathogenic wind and cold stimulation, spinal internal and external imbalance, prominent nucleus and surrounding tissue injury in inflammatory changes in the formation of mixed projection, irritation or compression of the nerve and spinal cord or cause lumbago and a series of neurological symptoms, referred to as "lumbar disc herniation".

With the development of modern medical technology, understanding the pathogenesis, people on prolapse of lumbar intervertebral disc pathological characteristics of the more in-depth, clinical diagnosis method is more specific and

Q. Lan (✉) · W. Deng
P. E Institute of Yichun University, Xuefu Road 576, Yichun 36000, China
e-mail: jxlanqing@163.com

W. Deng
e-mail: dwh0227@126.com

intuitive, treatment means increasingly diverse. The treatment methods, generally can be divided into operation and non operation therapy in two categories, various methods have advantages and characteristics of its own, such as the effect of operation treatment on some long-term conservative treatment is invalid, and seriously affect daily life and work of prolapse of lumbar intervertebral disc is good, data showed that: Patients 60–90 % treated by operation with satisfactory results, and patients with 6–14 % still exists or recurrence of low back pain, great attention has been caused clinician. If you can't grasp the operation indications, blindly expanding the operation range of use, it may be some drawbacks and side effect of operation therapy emerged, such as dangerous operation itself, surround operation period higher infection rate and complications such as postoperative adhesions, and the data show that: after the operation only short-term curative effect is better than that of conservative therapy with conservative therapy had no significant difference in long-term effect, postoperative vertebral body and joint ligament damage caused by spinal stability decreased, and postoperative lumbar disc herniation and prominent, causing operation therapy of long-term curative effect of uncertainty. Because the operation method of equipment requirements higher, medical expense, to make use of the therapy has great limitations. So, now most physicians have different levels of commitment to conservative treatment, according to the Adam report, only less than 10 % of patients (including central huge disc herniation) had the operation indications. According to the United States Center for public health data show: only a few patients with lumbar disc herniation need operation treatment, most can chiropractic therapy, functional training, wear the back waist circumference or epidural injection of steroid drugs ease. In traditional Chinese medicine conservative treatment of lumbar disc herniation, massage therapy is one of the important aspects, massage therapy with good effect, simple treatment method, less side effects, is not affected by the medical environment, medical conditions such as low—cost advantages, is widely used in the clinical doctors, received the majority of patients are recognized. In this paper, massage therapy for treatment of the disease were reviewed.

231.2 Methods of Treatment and Therapeutic Effect of Massage

A method of manipulation in the treatment of lumbar disc herniation, according to the key techniques of different, generally divided into pulling and rotating side pulling two major classes of techniques.

231.2.1 Pulling and Stretching Manipulation

This kind of technique is similar to the mechanical traction effect, but also with other necessary auxiliary means, avoiding violent pull on muscle, ligament injury. Li Qian used massage method, method of main pressure in order to point, press, elbow, palm and fist shock, passive activities of upper limb and 74 cases of disc herniation of lumbar traction, acupuncture treatment, the total effective rate was 90.5 %. Lei Hao used dorsal extension method combined with physiotherapy in conservative treatment of lumbar intervertebral disc herniation. Partial dorsal extension method combined with physiotherapy treatment (treatment group) and traditional traction manipulation therapy (control group) with 50 cases in each. Dorsal flexion method take the prone position, in preparation for release technique after the end, take the lift the shoulder pressing waist and leg pressing waist methods make the waist back stretch, and then combined with the point pressing, and computer intermediate frequency treatment, one times a day, 10 days are one period of treatment; the control group only use the SD-502 Japan traction treatment machine, patients take supine position, the traction weight from 25 kg began to increase, according to the conditions of patients, continuous traction 25 min, one times a day, 10 days are one treatment course. Results: the total effective rate of treatment group 98 %, control group was 84 %, there was significant difference ($P < 0.05$), the treatment group curative effect surpasses the control group. Hua Cui used massage and traction in 48 cases of lumbar disc herniation treated, method is by pushing, kneading, massage to relax the muscles of waist string, 2 min, after using JQ-3C type multifunctional automatic traction bed against programmed lumbar traction for lumbar muscle spasm tension eased, the traction for patients weighing 1/4 weight, select the intermittent traction, or traction 4 min, intermittent 1 min, before all time is 20 min, one times a day, 10 times for one course of treatment. 48 patients after treatment, the cure was 35 cases, accounting for 72.92 %; effective in 10 cases, accounting for 20.83 %; 3 cases were improved, 6.25 %. From the point of view of action forms of intervertebral disc, stepping lumbus should belong to pull out a method combined with the press, such as Caigui Luo using the toe pressure on the waist method for treatment of this disease, the total effective rate was 91 %; Bingcheng Zhou used traction Caiqiao reduction method in Treating 200 cases of this disease, cure 85 cases (42.5 %), effective in 61 cases (30.5 %), improved in 47 cases (23.5 %), invalid in 7 cases (3.5 %), the total efficiency of 96.5 %.

231.2.2 Rotary Side Pulling Manipulation

Jirong Zhao was observed in 310 cases of patients with lumbar disc herniation, clinical effects of spinal manipulation in the treatment of lumbar disc herniation with different. Divided into two groups, the treatment group of 250 cases with spinal fixed-point spin reduction treatment, control group of 60 patients with mechanical traction treatment, symptoms, signs, imaging changes were observed before and after treatment. The results show that: two groups after treatment of lumbar pain, lower limb pain, numbness of lower limb function, spinal mobility and paravertebral contact radiation pain, straight leg raising and strengthening test were significantly improved ($P < 0.01$); technique improvement in pain, numbness symptoms than the control group ($P < 0.05$). 20 cases were ineffective protrusion and canal area ratio exceeds 40 %. Treatment with rotating side rotatory manipulation of massage for this disease effective rate is higher than that of pure traction therapy. Minghui Ding used simple traction (control group) with rotary manipulation traction (treatment group) in the treatment of lumbar disc herniation, the treatment group in the spinous processes of rotatory reduction manipulation combined with traction, 6 and 12 weeks after treatment to assess the efficacy. The results showed that: in 6 weeks after simple traction group, the total efficiency of 57.14 %, rotary manipulation and traction group, the total effective rate was 85.71 %, there was significant difference between two groups ($P < 0.05$). In 12 weeks after simple traction group total effective rate was 52.38 %, of rotatory reduction manipulation and traction group total effective rate was 80.95 %, with significant difference ($P < 0.05$). In order to get the rotatory reduction manipulation and traction traction therapeutic effect is better than simple conclusion.

231.3 The Mechanism of Manipulation in the Treatment of Lumbar Disc Herniation

At present, generally, massage can make the intervertebral disc nucleus returning, thereby reducing the light of nerve root pressure relief of symptoms, and can play an analgesic effect effectively.

231.3.1 Biomechanical Study of Massage

Biomechanical study of lumbar spine specimens, using various techniques of the simulation. Weizhuang Jiang with micro sensors in determination of lumbar posterior displacement of joint in different poses and stress, the joint adjustment on the same side of the rotary manipulation is bigger, also found that application of this technique after intra-articular pressure wavy, the first half distance is lower, the empress half distance goes up, so in the spinous process the thumb push pressure should appear a little earlier, to match the reduction tendency of joint. Limin Xie through the analysis of 30 cases of patients with lumbar disc herniation treatment before and after quantization, manipulation can longitudinal ligament and fiber ring tension inward thrust force, forcing the nucleus pulposus of intervertebral space also satisfied to. He also found that massage disc in cross section of vertex position and curvature changed obviously, it actually validates what change position between the protrusion and the application techniques of nerve root. Conclusion, this change may achieve decompression and releasing the nerve root adhesion, protrusion of the intervertebral disc also satisfied and deformation is an important mechanism of massage in the treatment of lumbar disc herniation. Da Ma found through experiments the maximum lumbar flexion lateral rotation of lumbar facet joint activities, the vertical rotation method. Confirm the manipulation can make a part of the outer fiber ring is complete, the nucleus pulposus has not yet been degenerated nucleus pulposus also satisfied or partially also satisfied, but because after end of treatment of spinal manipulation and return to their original form, as a result, repetitive activity of facet joint, expansion joint capsule changed the morphology and size of intervertebral foramen, releasing the nerve root adhesion around. Ying Zhang through the change of dynamic measurement technique of nucleus pulposus pressure results show, rotatory reduction manipulation process, does not make the nucleus pulposus pressure decrease, instead will make the nucleus pulposus pressure increased, and in the way successful nucleus pulposus pressure increased, so that the manual process can not make the nucleus pulposus pressure in the negative pressure change, also therefore cannot make the herniation of the nucleus pulposus is satisfied. Sheng Bi simulation lumbar traction rotatory manipulation biomechanical experimental results show that, the normal intervertebral space in flexion, axial rotation traction composite under stress, change does not produce enough nucleus pulposus pressure. Directly observed and can be measured by lumbar flexion, tensile and torsional composite should be displacement distance under the action of the force of the intervertebral disc protrusion from the nerve root. So that the therapeutic mechanism of massage lumbar disc herniation is to reduce or eliminate the stimulation and oppression of nerve root by changing the displacement between the protrusion and the nerve root, so as to improve or eliminate pain, not the nucleus also satisfied.

231.3.2 Analgesic Effect of Manipulation

Massage is very effective in analgesia experiment proves the massage clinical remission has been recognized: massage on pain through several links to achieve, as can improve the content of hypothalamic beta-endorphin, content can be reduced 5-serotonin, bradykinin, prostaglandin, platelet degradation products, substance P inflammatory mediators, can correct or mitigate systemic and local circulation disorder, also can explain the principle of massage analgesia through gate control theory. In recent years, many people made beneficial exploration in this respect. As Yefu Li measured the changes of 5-HT use massage therapy in the treatment of lumbar disc herniation with norepinephrine and other indicators, found that patients recovered and effect of two distinct change, mechanism of massage in the treatment of this disease and prompt adjustment of the two kinds of substances in the body content of. Xi Chen study found that massage therapy can reduce 5-serotonin, norepinephrine, and the increase of β-EP, DA, can improve microcirculation, promote absorption of edema of nerve root and relieve pain, nerve endings of the allergic state, increase the pain threshold, both anti-inflammatory and analgesic role play. Hong Jiang through the study found, low back and leg pain endorphin content in patients with lower than normal, massage can increase the content of endogenous analgesic substance—the patient's body endorphin.

231.4 The Indication, Contraindication and Evaluation of Massage Therapy

Conservative therapy is not reach the acme of perfection, clinical must master the indications and contraindications, in order to obtain a satisfactory effect, in which a lot of people through retrospective summary to explain. Most people think: nucleus pulposus calcification, or associated with spinal stenosis, lateral recess stenosis, should be treated by surgical operation. Lei Wang believe that conservative treatment methods including massage therapy for central type, large rupture type herniation and intervertebral disc calcification and ossification of ligament and prominent with severe stenosis is not applicable; patients age, long course of disease, central type protruding relative age is small, short duration, unilateral and bilateral type, then the long course of treatment, the cure rate is low, poor effect. Dechun Liu observed 786 patients with disc herniation were treated with lumbar, of which 68 were treated by massage therapy is poor or ineffective operation treatment of patients, has obtained the satisfactory curative effect, combined with the analysis of the cases of conservative treatment and operation of treatment satisfaction, indication and contraindication of conclusion, consider the following the situation should not be used or continue treatment: (1) central protrusion in patients with larger, have obvious cauda equina symptoms; (2) calcification of posterior longitudinal ligament or protrusion cause nerve root compression techniques, the conservative treatment of 1–3 treatment and poor effect; (3) giant herniation of the disc, protrusion is greater than 0.7 cm, severe pain, postural special and after dehydration treatment effect is not obvious; (4) intervertebral disc herniation accompanied by severe nerve root canal stenosis and clinical symptoms consistent; (5) lumbar disc herniation has manipulation system for 3 months, and poor efficacy, recurrent; (6) disc and facet joint degeneration is heavy and is accompanied by marked hypertrophy of ligamentum flavum of lumbar spinal canal stenosis; (7) the prominence than 0.5 cm are still in heavy manual labor, patients should be replaced by operation or other treatment.

231.5 Conclusion

From the above situation, the massage treatment for lumbar disc herniation mechanism analysis can be seen, massage on the research focus of this disease in the massage treatment of biomechanical effect on nucleus pulposus, namely the improvement of nerve root compression of the protruded nucleus pulposus, in this regard, many conclusions are made to improve the situation symptoms and signs of manipulation therapy based on speculation, while CT, MRI and so on lack of evidence, may be because such findings cannot reflect the fine anatomic changes, and how to accurately the clinical observation, a lack of strong support. In addition, although the biomechanical study of lumbar intervertebral disc herniation has made great achievements, but because of the big difference between pathological model and character in general use, so the technique effect in the model to simulate the doesn't really in the clinic with repeatability, some experimental results and the actual situation of mechanical treatment is still errors, which can only investigate possible theory. So, how to establish the corresponding research model in vivo has become a pressing matter of the moment.

References

1. Li Q (2008) Traction combined with acupuncture and massage therapy effect of lumbar disc herniation. Mod Medicine Health 24(14):2125–2126
2. Lei H, Limin Z, Wenli X (2000) And 50 cases of conservative treatment of lumbar disc herniation with dorsal extension method. Liaoning J Tradit Chin Med 29(3):158–159
3. Hua C (2009) With massage and traction for the treatment of lumbar disc herniation. Chin Med J 21(10):1154–1155
4. Bingcheng Z, Xihua L, Xiaoming L (2009) Analysis on the effect of massage rocker comprehensive treatment of lumbar disc herniation. Massage Guided 25(5):24–25
5. Minghui D, Zaiwen L, Dongfeng H et al (2000) Of rotatory reduction manipulation combined with traction and simple observation of traction for the treatment of lumbar disc herniation. Chin J Rehabil Med 15(4):212–214
6. Sheng B, Yikai L, Fugen W et al (2001) Mechanism of manipulation in the treatment of lumbar disc herniation. Chin J Rehabil Med 16(1):8–10
7. Hongzhu J (2000) Based massage. Shanghai
8. Li Y, Hu Q, Zhou W et al (2001) Traction in the treatment of central type massage lumbar changes of monoamine neurotransmitters in disc herniation and saliva analysis. Chin Basic Med 8(3):237–238
9. Chen Xi, Li Yan (2000) Discussion on the mechanism of massage therapy for prolapse of lumbar intervertebral disc. Massage Guidance 17(2):37
10. Liu Dechun, Zhu Chen, Yang Yonghui et al (2001) Operation for the treatment of lumbar disc herniation invalid cases. Tradit Chin Med 13(12):27–28
11. Askar AL (2003) Flavum.Preserving approach to the lumbar spinal canal. Spine 28(19):385–390
12. Yorimitsu SL (2001) Term out comes of standard discectomy for lumbar disc herniation: a follow. Up study of more than 10 years, Spine 26(6):652–657

Chapter 232
Chinese Anti-Inflammatory Herb May Postpone the Forming and Exacerbating of Diabetic Nephropathy (DN)*

Hongjie Gao, Huamin Zhang, Haiyan Li, Jinghua Li, Junwen Wang, Meng Cui and Renfang Yin

Abstract Background: Diabetic Nephropathy (DN), a serious microvascular diabetic complication, is one of the main causes of death. Modern medical treatment is still not able to completely prevent the development and deterioration of DN despite the the fact that it has curative effect to some degree,at present. Therefore, how to effectively prevent the occurrence and development of DN has become a problem that should be solved as soon as possible in the medical community. Method: A valuable scientific hypothesis can be achieved by analyzing keywords frequency in open irrelevant literature in the field of Traditional Chinese Medicine to study literature about Diabetic Nephropathy and by discovering the hidden connection among irrelevant literature about DR,. By verifying the obtained hypothesis by experts to guide and realize the discovery of knowledge, we can explore more effective Chinese medicine treatment and methods of DN so that much more references can be provided for scientific researchers and clinical workers. Result: Among the target set C of keywords, the keyword "Anti-inflammatory herb (Traditional Chinese Medicine)" was screened out. Conclusion: Chinese Anti-inflammatory Herb may postpone the forming and exacerbating of Diabetic Nephropathy (DN), and plays an important role in the treatment of DN.

Keywords Chinese anti-inflammatory herb · Diabetic nephropathy (DN) · Swanson's analytical method of irrelevant literature

H. Gao (✉) · H. Zhang · H. Li · J. Li · J. Wang · M. Cui · R. Yin
Institute of Medical Informatics, China Academy of Chinese Medical Sciences, Beijing 100700, China
e-mail: jiehonggao@163.com

232.1 Background

With the rapid development of science and technology, the specialized division of labor is getting more and more detailed. There may be undiscovered valuable connection among various literature on different disciplines which seem to be totally irrelevant on the surface. It may play an important promoting role for the scientific development to discover these implicit associations among these literatures (Fig. 232.1).

In 1985, Don. R Swanson, the medical professor in University of Chicago created a medical method—Irrelevant Literature Knowledge Discovery Method which can reveal the logical connections among knowledge segments that have not been discovered yet in published literature and propose hypothesis for researchers' further confirmation. The process of Swenson's discovery of knowledge can be divided into two steps: the formation of hypothesis and the confirmation of it. The process of the formation of hypothesis is called Open Irrelevant Literature Knowledge Discovery Method (open). Its concrete process is C → B → A, which means that the interesting theme C is considered as an initial point, the middle set B is found out, and the connection between C and A is confirmed through the connection between middle set B and literature set A, as shown in the illustration i, while the process of the confirmation of hypothesis is called Closed Irrelevant Literature Knowledge Discovery Method. Its route is C → B←A, which means that A and C is considered as the initial point and so the middle word B is found out, as shown in illustration 2. The open method of formation of hypothesis can seek for a new method of treatment or a new target for drugs. If researchers have already formed the hypothesis by Open Irrelevant Literature Knowledge Discovery Method, they can detailedly prove the hypothesis on the base of literature. In 2000, American Society of Information Science and Technology (ASIST) awarded D. R. Swanson its highest achievement award (Tables 232.1, 232.2, 232.3).

Diabetic Nephropathy (DN) is the severe microvascular complication of Diabetes Mellitus (DM). According to the statistics by Renal Data System of the United States: Among patients who have diabetes with microalbuminuria over 10 years, about 50 % of them progressed to DN, and after 5–10 years appeared the

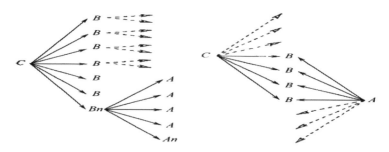

Fig. 232.1 Knowledge discovery process

Table 232.1 Search results

Databases	Literature quantity after initially searching (strip)	Literature quantity after screening (strip)	Literature quantity after excluding repetition (strip)
Traditional Chinese medical literature analysis and retrieval system	2896	2455	
Chinese biomedical literature database	9400	3033	
Total	12295	5488	3718

Table 232.2 Radix salviae miltiorrhizae results

Databases	Literature quantity after initially searching (strip)	Literature quantity after screening (strip)	Literature quantity after excluding repetition (strip)
Traditional Chinese medical literature analysis and retrieval system	27084	351	
Chinese biomedical literature database	17895	128	
Total	44979	479	400

Table 232.3 Astragalus root results

Databases	Literature quantity after initially searching (strip)	Literature quantity after screening (strip)	Literature quantity after excluding (strip)
Traditional Chinese medical literature analysis and retrieval system	35418	556	
Chinese biomedical literature database	13704	122	
Total	49122	678	572

end-stage renal failure, more than 30 % of which is caused by diabetes and the proportion has increased by yeas. It is both a serious threat to human health and a leading cause of death resulted from diabetes. Currently modern medical treatment pay more attention to keeping a diet, controlling blood sugar, lowering blood pressure, adjusting lipid metabolism and so on. And dealysis, renal transplantation are also applied to treatment. However, all of these could not prevent its development and deterioration and bring heavy economic burden to patients despite the fact that they do have some effect. Therefore, how to effectively prevent the occurrence and development of DN is not only a problem that should be urgently solved in the medical community but also a hot issue that physicians pay attention to.

A valuable scientific hypothesis can be achieved by applying the Open Irrelevant Literature Knowledge Discovery Method to the Chinese medical field of treating diabetic nephropathy to study literature about Diabetic Nephropathy and by discovering the hidden connection among irrelevant literature about DR,. By verifying the obtained hypothesis by experts to guide and realize the discovery of knowledge, we can explore more effective Chinese medicine treatment and methods of DN so that much more references can be provided for scientific researchers and clinical workers.

232.2 Methods

232.2.1 Choice of Specific Research Methods

Open Irrelevant Literature Knowledge Discovery Method can be based on either literature headings frequency statistical method or literature keywords frequency statistical method. As keywords can be better response to literature main content because they are standardized words or phrases to express the theme in the indexing and retrieval, Open Irrelevant Literatures Knowledge Discovery Method based on subject words frequency statistics is applied in this study.

232.2.2 Choice of Database

The study applies two Chinese databases, which are Chinese biomedical literature database and Traditional Chinese Medical Literature Analysis and Retrieval System established by the Institute of Medical Informatics of China Academy of Traditional Chinese Medical Sciences. Both of the databases used the Medical Subject Headings Notes Table (MeSH) of American National Library of Medicine and the standard subject words standard by "Chinese Medicine Thesaurus" which are compiled by China Academy of Traditional Chinese Medical Sciences, widely used in academic circles, and can be compatible with the "Medical Subject Headings Notes Table". They can relatively accurately reflect the main content of the literatures.

232.2.3 Specific Research Steps

232.2.3.1 The Collection of Source Subject Words Set C

Download literature whose subject words contain "Diabetic Nephropathy" from both the Traditional Chinese Medical Literature Analysis and Retrieval System and Chinese Biomedical Literature Database, exclude literature which don't belong to the classification of Traditional Chinese Medicine and the repetitive literature, summarize all the subject words in these literature, and form the source subject words set C.

The scope of literature search and retrieval strategy:

(1) Traditional Chinese Medical Literature Analysis and Retrieval System (1984–2008)
(2) Chinese Biomedical Literature Database (1978–2008)
    Search Type Subject words: Diabetic Nephropathy

The criteria of selection and exclusion of literature:

(1) The range of selection: traditional Chinese medicine, traditional Chinese drugs or TCM combined with Western medicine clinical and experimental research literatures related to diabetic nephropathy.
(2) The range of exclusion: literature not related to traditional Chinese medicine research; Chinese basic research literatures; review literatures; repetitive literatures and literatures about Diabetic Nephropathy with other diseases.

Search Results
According to calculation, there are totally 5488 strips of literature in the above two databases. After removing the repetitive literature, the remaining 3718 form the source literature Set C.

232.2.3.2 The Formation of Intermediate Set B of Subject Words

Extract the subject words in Set C, remove the subject words "diabetic nephropathy"; arrange the remaining subject words in descending order of the frequency of occurrence and we get 1730 subject words. According to Chinese medicine classification MeSH tree structure, extract subject words of C Class (TCM disease) and part of the D Class (medicine and prescription) subject words in Thesaurus of Traditional Chinese Medicine from these 1730 subject words, there are 503 remaining subject words.

Ask for advice of Chinese medicine clinical experts and screen five subject words related to traditional Chinese medicine treating diabetic nephropathy out of 503. They are: astragalus root, radix salviae miltiorrhizae, rhubarb, dried rehmannia root, pseudostellaria root, Chinese angelica root and rhizoma of sichuan lovage. Intersecting the word, radix salviae miltiorrhizae and astragalus root are extracted. The intermediate Set B form.

232.2.3.3 The Formation of Intermediate Set A of Subject Words

Download literature whose subject words contain the terminology including the words "astragalus root" and "radix salviae miltiorrhizae" from the Traditional Chinese Medical Literature Analysis and Retrieval System and Chinese Biomedical Literature Database and exclude the literature which don't belong to the field of Traditional Chinese Medicine or the repetitive documents.

The scope of literature search and retrieval strategy:

(1) Traditional Chinese Medical Literature Analysis and Retrieval System (1984–2008)
(2) Chinese Biomedical Literature Database (1978–2008)
    Search Type (1) Subject words: radix salviae miltiorrhizae (2) Subject words:astragalus root

The criteria of election and exclusion of the literature:

(1) The range of selection: Chinese medicine or TMC combined with Western medicine clinical and experimental research literature about either of radix salviae miltiorrhizae or astragalus root; pharmacological literature about either radix salviae miltiorrhizae or astragalus root.
(2) The range of exclusion: research literature about compound pharmaceutics of radix salviae miltiorrhizae and astragalus root and their effective content analysis; literature not related to traditional Chinese medicine; Traditional Chinese medicine basic research literature except Traditional Chinese medicine pharmacology literature; review literature and repetitive literature.

Search Results

According to calculation, there are totally 479 strips of literature. After removing repetitive literature, there are 400 remaining. Extract the subject words from the 400 literature, arrange them in descending order of the frequency of occurrence and we get 692 subject words.

According to calculation, there are totally 678 strips of literature. After removing repetitive literature, there are 572 remaining. Extract the subject words from the 572 literature, arrange them in descending order of the frequency of occurrence and we get 982 subject words.

Extract subject words in sort C and sort D of Traditional Chinese Medicine Thesaurus from the 692 subject words of radix salviae miltiorrhizae. There are 14 subject words remaining. Extract subject words in sort C and sort D of Traditional Chinese Medicine Thesaurus from the 982 subject words of astragalus root, there are 91 subject words remaining. After summarizing those two parts, we get a total subject words of 135. Consult Chinese medicine clinical experts about these 135 subject words terminology, then screen the special experience and methods about Chinese medicine treatment of Diabetic Nephropathy, and reach the following screening words: Cold and Heat Interwoven Syndrome, anti-inflammatory herbs (traditional Chinese medicine), Jade-scree powder, Chinese angelica root herb broth for blood-enriching, ferulenol, earth worm, Shen Xian Decoction. After intersecting experts' opinion, "anti-inflammatory herb (TCM)" is screened.

232.3 Results

In summary, based on Chinese Biomedical Literature Database and Traditional Chinese Medical Literature Analysis and Retrieval System established by the Institute of Medical Informatics of China Academy of Traditional Chinese Medical Sciences, the source subject words Set C formed. Among the subject words in set C, subject words "radix salviae miltiorrhizae" and "astragalus root" are found. That is to say "radix salviae miltiorrhizae" and "astragalus root" have something to do with Diabetic Nephropathy. Through the subject words "radix salviae miltiorrhizae" and "astragalus root", "anti- inflammatory herbs" (TCM) is spotted, which means "anti-inflammatory herb (TCM) " has something to do with "radix salviae miltiorrhizae" and "astragalus root". So according to Doc. Swanson's open analysis method of irrelevant literature, the screened "anti-inflammatory herb (TCM) "may be related to the treatment of Diabetic Nephropathy. The "anti-inflammatory herb "may postpone the development of DN and have some therapeutic effects on it.

232.4 Discussion

In recent years, numerous research studies show that inflammatory factor is a factor that can not be ignored for the occurrence and development of Diabetic Nephropathy. Many scholars proposed "inflammatory pathogenesis" when they explore the etiology of Diabetic Nephropathy.

DM normal proteinuria, microalbuminuria and clinical proteinuria in acute phase proteins such as C-reactive protein (CRP), a-acid glycoprotein, ceruloplasmin and sialic acid are all higher than the normal control group, indicating the body in DM is in the state of chronic inflammation. The inflammatory proteins increasing with the increase of microalbuminuria, indicates that chronic inflammation is closely related to the damage of the kidney [1]. When caused DN, inherent pathophysiological changes such as hyperglycemia in DM, hemodynamic disorders lead to the damage of intrinsic cells of kidney and cause cytokine release and accumulation of inflammatory cells to the intrarenal inflammatory disease. And agent of inflammatory cells result the continuity and development of inflammatory disease by autocrine and paracrine cascade reaction, which makes progress to DN. Pathology data also confirmed in DN kidney, there are infiltration of inflammatory corpuscle such as macrophage. And the expression of cytokines such as MCP —1, IL—6, TNFa, adhesion molecules, TGF-a and PDGF increase. Meanwhile these agents of inflammatory disease and are closely related to the change of urinary protein, renal function, mesangial cell proliferation, ECM accumulation, glomerulosclerosis and interstitial fibrosis, which proves the existence of inflammation in DN kidney and verifies that inflammation is the key to DN progress. Therefore, anti-inflammatory treatment is an important method to hamper the progress of DN.

In recent years, clinical researches and experimental studies have proofed that a lot of Chinese medicine have good anti-inflammatory effects, and less toxic side effect, such as Rhizoma Coptidis, Cortex Phellodendri Amurensis, Radix Scutellariae Baicalensis, Flos Lonicerae, Fructus Forsythiae Suspensae, Folium Isatidis, Herba Houttyniae Cordatae, Herba Andrographitis Paniculatae, Herba Portulacae Oleraceae, Radix Isatidis, Herba Taraxaci Mongolici, Aconitum Carmichaeli Debx, Sinomenium acutum (Thunb.) Rehd.et Wils., Radix Sophorae Flavescentis, Radix Bupleuri Chinensis, Herba Asari Mandshurici, Agkistrodon, Radix Platycodi, Radix et Rhizoma Tripterygii, Radix Gentianae Macrophyllae [2, 3]. Now it is generally considered that the mechanism of Chinese anti-inflammatory herbs have related to pituitary, adrenal cortex (HPA) axis function, inhibition of inflammatory mediators, nitric oxide (NO) inhibition and effects of arachidonic acid metabolism and other factors. Chinese medicine is natural medicine, and one contains many elements. The fact is that not only there are a lot of anti-inflammatory effects in one Chinese herbal ingredient but also many ingredients in one medicine have anti-inflammatory effect. In short, the mechanism of anti-inflammatory of Chinese medicine is very complex. Chinese medicine plays anti-inflammatory role of by various ways through multiple links [4].

232.5 Conclusion

Chinese anti-inflammatory herb may postpone the forming and exacerbating of Diabetic Nephropathy. It plays an important role for the treatment of DN. Although the conclusion has already passed the verification of Chinese medicine literature, it still needs to be verified in Chinese medicine clinical research and basic research. We expect that it can provide much more references and effective treatment for the Chinese medical treatment of Diabetic Nephropathy.

Acknowledgments Thanks the second free topics of China Academy of Traditional Chinese Medical Sciences for supporting the research topic group—Chinese Medicine Diagnosing and Treating Knowledge Discovery Research of Diabetic Nephropathy Based on Irrelative Literature Analysis (Z02050).

References

1. Bing H, Ping H, Xianke L (2003) The relation between acute phase protein in patients with diabetic2 and diabetic nephropathy. J Endocrinol Metab 19(4):260–262
2. Tiebing S, Tao Y (2006) Common anti-cushion Chinese medicine and its function. J Chin Med 4(6):177
3. Delian M, Ling G, Xinhua L, Qin L (2003) Herbal immune function. China J Exp Tradit Med Formulae 9(5):63–65
4. Xiuneng T, Naiping W, Renbin H (2008) Summary of studying anti-inflammatory mechanism of Chinese drugs. Chin Pharmacists 11(5):583–586

Chapter 233
Analysis of Electromagnetic Radiation Effect on Layered Human Head Model

Lanlan Ping, Dongsheng Wu, Hong Lv and Jinhua Peng

Abstract This paper deal with interaction of electromagnetic wave with the human body by using the algorithm of Frequency-Dependent Finite-Difference Time-Domain method ($(FD)^2$ TD method). The detailed algorithms of $(FD)^2$ TD method are presented in this paper when the electromagnetic wave propagates in dispersive medium. Thereby a similar three tiers spherical model of 2-D human head is built which from outside to inside is divided into the skin layer, the bone layer and the brain layer. And more, the distribution of specific absorption rate (SAR) is utilized to analyze the effect of the electromagnetic wave on the human head at 900 MHz job-frequency point. Compared with the usual international safe standards, the simulation results are below the safe standard when human head exposure to electromagnetic radiation in a short time.

Keywords: $(FD)^2TD$ method · Dispersive medium · Human head · SAR · Electromagnetic radiation

233.1 Introduction

With the use of mobile phone widely, electromagnetic radiation of mobile phone antenna on human health has raised national and international attention. It had been reported on this question as early as 1978 [1], and then there were a lot of reports about "phone-induced cancer" [2] immediately. Therefore, the effect of electromagnetic radiation has become an important research subject in Bioelectromagnetics.

L. Ping (✉) · D. Wu · H. Lv · J. Peng
School of E&IE, AnHui JianZhu University, Hefei 230601, China
e-mail: pinglan09@126.com

When the external electromagnetic waves enter into the organisms, the electromagnetic interaction with biological systems directly is the major factor in the biological effects. Therefore it is very important to calculate the distribution of the electromagnetic waves in organisms. The electromagnetic dosimetry is an main analysis method about electromagnetic waves effect on the human body. Through theoretical analysis or experimental test, the SAR distribution in human body has been gotten. The SAR is defined as unit biological mass which is exposed to the electromagnetic field absorbing average power. According to different tissue regions, SAR is divided into local SAR (SAR_L), SAR every 1 g tissue (SAR_{1g}) and average SAR of all tissue model (SAR_{av}) [3].

In order to get more accurate SAR, a human body dispersive medium model is established in this paper. And the electromagnetic fields in human tissues is made by $(FD)^2 TD$ method [4–7]. Firstly, the SAR of homogeneous medium is calculated, the result is agreeable with reference, which demonstrate that the given $(FD)^2 TD$ method is an effcient and accurate method. Then a three tiers spherical model of 2-D human head is calculated, the SAR_L, SAR_{1g} and SAR_{av} are given. The conclusion is got by compared the results with the international mobile communication health standards.

233.2 Theoretical Analysis

The dispersive medium is defined that dielectric coefficient and conductivity vary at different frequencies. For example: plasma, muscle tissue, radar absorbing materials and so on. Commonly there are some frequency domain models of the dispersive medium as follows [5]: (1) Drude model. It is usually used in the description of the dispersive characteristics of plasma, metal and other media description. (2) Debye model. It is usually used to describe the dispersive characteristics of soil, water, human tissue medium. (3) Lorentz model. It is usually applied to the describe the dispersive characteristics of biological tissue, optical material and artificial dielectric medium. The actual dielectric coefficient need to be gained by experiment test and then fit it with the above model. If the interest frequency range is wide, all above models can be used jointly.

There are some methods to analyse the dispersive model commonly by $(FD)^2 TD$ algorithm as follow [5]: Recursive Convolution methods (RC-FDTD), Z transforms methods (Z-FDTD), Auxiliary Differential Equation methods (ADE-FDTD), Shift Operator methods (SO-FDTD) and so on. Z-FDTD is used to analyse electromagnetic field distribution in human tissues in this paper.

Human tissues is a typical dispersive medium, its dielectric coefficient is [4]:

$$\varepsilon(\omega) = \varepsilon_r + \frac{\sigma}{j\omega\varepsilon_0} + \varepsilon_1 \frac{\omega_0}{(\omega_0^2 + \alpha^2) + j2\alpha\omega - \omega^2} \qquad (233.1)$$

Where ε_r is relative dielectric coefficient, σ is conductivity, ω_0 denote resonance frequency. Inserting Eq. (233.1) into $D(z) = \varepsilon(z)E(z)\Delta t$ and taking the Z transforms, we get

$$D(z) = \varepsilon_r E(z) + \frac{\sigma \Delta t/\varepsilon_0}{1-z^{-1}} E(z) + \varepsilon_1 \frac{e^{-\alpha \Delta t} \sin(\omega_0 \Delta t) \Delta t z^{-1}}{1 - 2e^{-\alpha \Delta t}\cos(\omega_0 \Delta t)z^{-1} + e^{-2\alpha \Delta t}z^{-2}} E(z)$$

(233.2)

We will define two auxiliary parameter:

$$I(z) = \frac{\sigma \Delta t/\varepsilon_0}{1-z^{-1}} E(z)$$

(233.3)

$$S(z) = \varepsilon_1 \frac{e^{-\alpha \Delta t}\sin(\omega_0 \Delta t)\Delta t}{1 - 2e^{-\alpha \Delta t}\cos(\omega_0 \Delta t)z^{-1} + e^{-2\alpha \Delta t}z^{-2}} E(z)$$

(233.4)

The electric field of the human tissue can be calculated by

$$E(z) = \frac{D(z) - z^{-1}I(z) - z^{-1}S(z)}{\varepsilon_r + \sigma \Delta t/\varepsilon_0}$$

(233.5)

$$I(z) = z^{-1}I(z) + \frac{\sigma \Delta t}{\varepsilon_0} E(z)$$

(233.6)

$$S(z) = 2e^{-\alpha \Delta t}\cos(\omega_0 \Delta t)z^{-1}S(z) - e^{-2\alpha \Delta t}z^{-2}S(z) + \varepsilon_1 e^{-\alpha \Delta t}\sin(\omega_0 \Delta t)\Delta t E(z)$$

(233.7)

We can calculate (D,I,S) → E by Eq. (233.5), E → I by Eq. (233.6), and E → S by Eq. (233.7), then get cycle formation of E → H → D → E.

233.3 Results and Analysis

To validate the effectiveness of (FD)^2 TD method, the electric field distribution of homogeneous medium is investigated firstly. The calculation region is 150*150, the tissue is a spherical model that its radius is 10 cm, and its electromagnetic parameters are: $\varepsilon_r = 36$, $\varepsilon_1 = 2$, $f_0 = 100\,MHz$, $\delta = 0.25$ $\omega_0 = 2\pi f_0$, $\sigma = 0.6$. The incident field is a harmonic plane wave with incident frequency 900 MHz, input power 0.6 W. The grid size $\delta = 0.33$ cm, and time step 650. Figure 233.1 shows the electric field distribution after it reaches stable field.

After electric field within tissue is calculated at every node, we can use the following formulas to calculate SAR_L of each node and SAR_{av}. The formula for SAR_L is [6]

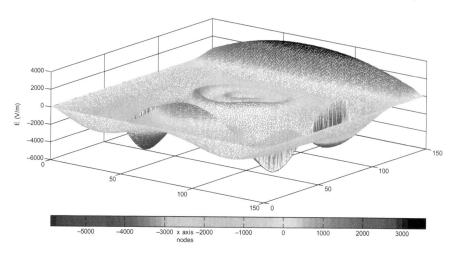

Fig. 233.1 The electric field distribution of homogeneous medium

$$SAR_L = \frac{\sigma(i,j,k)}{2\rho(i,j,k)} |E(i,j,k)|^2 \qquad (233.8)$$

Where ρ is the human tissue density (kg/m^3), because of human tissue density approximately equal, we set to $1.0*10^3$, kg/m^3 E(i,j,k) is the electric field intensity.
The formula for SARav is

$$SAR_{av} = \frac{1}{2\sum_i\sum_j\sum_k \delta^3(i,j,k)\,\rho(i,j,k)} \left[\sum_i\sum_j\sum_k \delta^3(i,j,k)\,\sigma(i,j,k)\,|E(i,j,k)|^2\right]$$

(233.9)

The Fig. 233.2 shows the SAR$_L$ and SAR$_{1g}$ which change with electromagnetic field penetration depth. We can see that the SAR is gradually decreased with increase of the electric field penetration depth. The peak value of SAR$_L$ is more than two times the SAR$_{1g..}$ The conclusion is agreeable with Ref. [6].

The SAR value of three layered spherical human head model is studied, which from outside to inside is divided into the skin layer, the bone layer and the brain layer. The Table 233.1 shows that geometric parameters of layered spherical human head model and corresponding dielectric parameters in 900 MHz [6].

The SAR distributions of human head is given in Fig. 233.3. We can found that the SAR distributions of electromagnetic field in human head are big different. The SAR$_L$ peak value of the skin which is close to the radiation source is the maximum, achieve 0.39 W/Kg. The SAR$_L$ peak value of the bone is 0.057 W/kg and the brain is 0.2 W/Kg. The SAR$_{1g}$ peak value of skin, bone and brain are 0.12 W/Kg, 0.042 W/Kg and 0.07 W/Kg respectively. The SAR$_{av}$ is also calculated, it

Fig. 233.2 The SAR value of homogeneous medium

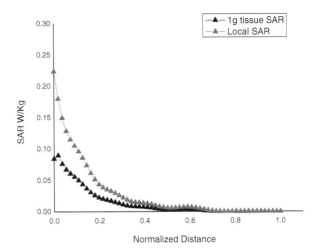

Table 233.1 Geometric parameters of layered spherical human head model and corresponding dielectric parameters in 900 MHz

Parameters	Skin layer	Bone layer	Brain layer
Relative dielectric coefficient ε_r	36	8	55
Conductivity σ (S/m)	0.6	0.11	1.23
Geometric radius/mm	5	10	95

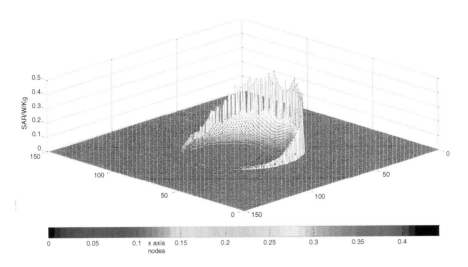

Fig. 233.3 The local SAR peak value of human head model

is 0.97 mW/Kg. Comparing with current universal safety standards (TEEC95.1-1991) [8], the SAR_{1g} peak value of the head model less than the safety standards 1.6 W/Kg, and the SAR_{av} is also lower than Standard limit 0.08 W/Kg.

233.4 Conclusion

The paper apply $(FD)^2 TD$ algorithm to simulate the electric field distribution of homogeneous medium through the establishment of human dispersive model firstly. With the value of electric field, the SAR can be calculated easily. We can found that the SAR is gradually decreased with increase of the electric field penetration depth. Thus it is indicated that the FDTD algorithm is an effective method to study the influence of electromagnetic radiation on he human body. And then three tiers spherical model of human head is studied, the SAR_L, SAR_{1g} and SAR_{av} are calculated. Compared with the international mobile communication health standards, electromagnetic radiation has little influence on the human body in short time communication. Because a 2-D human head model is studied in this paper, also the head model is simplified different form the real prototype, the calculation error is hardly avoided. But there is not affect correctness of the conclusion. Future, the author will make further research, through the establishment of antenna model [9], fine division of 3D human head models [10], more accurate and reasonable SAR value will be provided for the study of the Bio-electromagnetics effect.

Acknowledgments Our work is supported by Anhui Colleges and Universities Natural Scientific Research Project (grant No. KJ2011A060), National Natural Science Foundation of China (grant No. 61071001), Doctor/Master Scientific Research Launch Projects, Special Foundation for Young Scientific Research of Anhui Jianzhu University 2011 (grant No. 2011183-13).

References

1. Balzano Q, Garay O, Steel FR (1978) Heating of biological tissue in the induction field of vhf portable radio transmitters. IEEE Trans Veh Technol 27(2):51–56
2. Toftgard J, Hornsleth SN, Andersen JB (1993) Effects on portable antennas of the presence of person. IEEE Trans AP 41(6):739–746
3. Liu Y (2002) Biological electromagnetic effect. Beijing University of Posts and Telecommunications Press, BeiJing
4. Franek O, Pedersenf GF (2006) Numerical modeling of aspherical array of monopoles using FDTD method. IEEE Trans antennas and propag 54(7):1952–1963
5. Ge D, Yan Y (2011) Finite-difference time-domain method for electromagnetic waves, 3rd edn. XiDian University Press
6. Zhou X, Lai S (2003) Numerical simulation of interaction system between monopole handset and layered human head model. J South China Univ Technol 31(12):5–8

7. Reyhani SMS, Ludwig SA (2006) An implanted spherical head model exposed to electromagnetic fields at a mobile communication frequency. IEEE Trans on Bio Eng 53(10):2092–2101
8. IEEC95.1-1991, IEEE Standard for Safety Levels with Respect to Human Exposure to Radio Frequency Electromagnetic Fields, 3 kHz to 300 GHz
9. Han Y, Lu Y, Zhang J, Zhang H (2008) Specific absorption rate distribution in human body caused by PIFA for bluetooth applications. Chinese J Radio Sci 23(2):360–364
10. Niu Z, Hou J, etc (2006) The bioelectromagnetics dosimetry and numerical analysis of electromagnetic dose absorbed by human body. Chinese J Biomed Eng 25(5):580–589

Chapter 234
A Study on Potential Legal Risks of Electronic Medical Records and Preventing Measures

Hu Shengli, Feng Jun and Chi Jinqing

Abstract *Objectives* This paper aims at ensuring relevant parties' interests of electronic medical records and promoting in-depth application and rapid development of electronic medical records in clinic. *Methods* We probe into the legal risks existing in the actual application of electronic medical records such as the laws and regulations, electronic signatures, electronic certification institutions, time stamp certification institutions, privacy protection, traceability of electronic medical records and legal consciousness. *Results* We put forward the measures to prevent them. *Conclusions* Our study has a very important significance in perfecting the existing laws and regulations, reducing medical accidents, improving medical treatment and promoting the healthy and orderly development of the electronic medical records.

Keywords Electronic medical records · Laws and regulations · Electronic signature

234.1 Introduction

With the development of medical information, electronic medical records are becoming the core of the digital hospital. It improves the quality and normalization of medical records, reduces the workload of doctors and greatly reduces the occurrence of malpraxis. Furthermore, the spread of electronic medical records turns the information sharing of health care system into reality.

Electronic process of medical records is spontaneous, high-speed and out of order, but the legal effect of electronic medical records is the key and premise to

---

H. Shengli (✉) · F. Jun · C. Jinqing
Information Construction Office, Cangzhou City Central Hospital, No. 16, Xinhua Western Road, Hebei Province 061001 Hebei, China
e-mail: hushenglihsl@139.com

decide whether the electronic medical records can be widely used. At present, it is a problem whether the electronic signatures are legal and modifying traces can be retained. Therefore, we have a lot of work to do to make the electronic medical records paperless in the future.

In recent years, with the enhancement of the consciousness of patients' protection, in the medical dispute, the user of electronic medical records is the hospitals and the hardware and software is under the control of the hospital, so the hospital must adduce evidence to prove herself faultless. As a result, the hospital will be very passive. So the study on potential legal risks of electronic medical records and preventing measures has the very vital significance to ensure patients' and medical personnel's legitimate rights and interests and promote the healthy development of electronic medical records.

234.2 Potential Legal Risks of Electronic Medical Records

234.2.1 Lag of Laws and Regulations

At present, due to the rapid development of medical information, health information legislation is relatively backward which, to some extent, restricted the in-depth development of hospital information. Since March 1, 2010, all the medical institutions in China have implemented Article IV of the amended Basic Criteria for Documentation of the Medical Records, that is to say, the medical records should be written in ink and the medical records to be replicated can be written by ballpoint pen, which are the provisions made for the paper medical records. The medical records mentioned in Medical Malpractice Management Regulations performed on September 1, 2002 and its supporting documents refer to the paper records, not electronic medical records. No clear requirements and standards for electronic medical records in the policy and laws have been put forward up to now.

Electronic medical records established its legal status secured law security [1–5] in Electronic Signature Law of the People's Republic of China (hereinafter referred to as Electronic Signature Law) taken into effect on April 1, 2005 and Electronic Medical Records Basic Norms (Trial Edition) (hereinafter referred to as Basic Norms) taken into effect on April 1, 2010. The court has recognized the legal status of such records in trial practice of the medical institutions. The application of any new technologies is likely to face the contradictions of lag of the relevant laws and regulations. Moreover, the legal evidence of electronic medical records are called for in special statutory provisions.

234.2.2 Problem of Electronic Signature

Article 14 of Electronic Signature Law stipulates that a reliable electronic signature with the handwritten signature has the same legal effect as the seal. The signature in the electronic medical records will meet with legal issues if we can't guarantee that the electronic signature is safe and reliable.

However, at present, most hospitals have not use technology of electronic signature and there are many problems in the application of the electronic signature. For example, some hospitals only scan the physician's signature and save on their computer in image form. When used, the signature is copied to the desired location. This signature is not legally recognized by a third party and has no effective encryption and time stamp, therefore, it is not a real electronic signature.

234.2.3 Selection of Electronic Certification Institutions

It is stipulated in Article 16 of Electronic Signature Law that the electronic signature requiring the third-party must be certified by authentication institutions in accordance with the legislation. At present, the authentication institutions of digital certificate are mainly in the field of electronic commerce, there are no specific certification institutions for the health. According to the current situation, although electronic signatures are adopted by some hospitals, they don't choose the authorized and legitimate electronic authentication agencies, which can not guarantee the legal effectiveness of electronic medical records.

234.2.4 Selection of Time Stamp Authentication Institutions

We will face many legal risks, if we only use digital signature. For example, the certificate will be invalid and the content and timing of electronic medical records will be amended when the doctors re-sign them. Besides, each electronic signature of electronic medical records is recorded as the time of the server, the server is placed in the hospital, thus, the time can be easily adapted by the hospital, which is the hidden danger of medical disputes. Then the electronic signature will loss legal effect. In order to ensure the safety and reliability of electronic signatures, and an authoritative third-party is needed to provide reliable time stamp service. In practice, some hospitals do not use reliable time stamp, some use software of time stamp provided by the manufacturers issuing a time stamp, other hospitals adopt the time stamp provided by the non-credible time stamp institutions [2]. The above-mentioned time stamp will put the hospital into law risk when in dispute.

234.2.5 Protection of Privacy

Article 22 of Law on Medical Practitioners of the People's Republic of China taken into effect on May 1, 1999 stipulates that physician has the obligation to protect patient privacy. Article 37 also stipulates if the physician releases the privacy of patients, thereby causing serious consequences, he shall be given a warning light, suspend the practice activities, revoke the practicing certificate and investigate criminal responsibility etc., according to the seriousness of the case. Therefore, the hospital workers should fully respect the privacy of patients, and ensure the interests of patients [6].

234.2.6 Traceability of Electronic Medical Records

It is stipulated in Article 58 of Law of Tort Liability of the People's Republic of China promulgated on December 26, 2009 that the patients are damaged for the medical records are forged, falsified and destroyed, the medical institutions will be presumed to be at fault. In view of the above, you can see that whether Electronic medical records have been tampered with is often the bone of contention. Electronic medical records are a new form of medical records and the data can be modified, once the medical dispute appears, the patients or their families will question the authenticity of the medical records. Therefore, electronic medical records system should have the function of the traces, which can trace the man, the date and the content of modification of electronic medical records to protect the legitimate rights and interests of patients.

234.2.7 Weak Legal Awareness

Some medical personnel have the weak legal awareness and are lack of self-protection awareness. They are not aware that the medical records are not only a comprehensive record of the diagnosis and treatment process, but also the important evidence in dispute between hospitals and patients. Because they pay little attention to the written records, medical records are not standardized. For example, in order to write medical records quickly, some doctors make copy in electronic medical records which leads to the similarity of the medical records of the same disease and can't really reflect the occurrence, development and outcome of the disease. This not only affects the quality of medical records, but also plants a hidden danger for medical disputes.

234.3 Preventing Measures

234.3.1 Speed-up of Health Information Legislation

We should actively learn from the international legal results to perfect laws and regulations of health care as soon as possible. For instance, stipulations covering electronic medical records should be added in Electronic Signature Law. Regulations on the medical record security and privacy protection are called for to establish the legal status of electronic medical records in the form of law, benefit the doctors and patients and embody the seriousness, fairness and justice of the electronic medical records as a valid legal document.

234.3.2 Selection of Appropriate Digital Certification Services

In order to guarantee the legal effect of electronic medical records, we must first select the appropriate digital certification services. So far, Health Ministry has issued four name-lists of qualified digital certification services, these services has been tested and can provide electronic certification service for the health system.

234.3.3 Selection of Credible Time Stamp Agencies

Credible time stamp must be issued by time stamp service center of the authorized third-party. Time Stamp Authority is the only the third party credible time stamp service agencies, the authority time is guaranteed by National Time Service Center. The National Time Service Center is responsible for safeguarding the time of granting and punctuality of monitoring. Time can not be modified by any institutions including time stamp center in order to ensure the authority of the time. The time stamp has legal effectiveness. In addition, in advanced electronic signature format, the reliable time stamp is also put forward to ensure the long-term electronic signatures.

234.3.4 Protection of Patients' Privacy

Various measures are adopted to protect patients' privacy in electronic medical records system. Firstly, in the aspect of technology, we adopt different security classification to manage according to the different patients' identity. At the same time, we assign different permissions to hierarchical management according to the different title and position of the medical workers. Automatic hidden security classification is higher than the user permissions, the user is warned to use the electronic medical records in accordance with the regulations, when the medical workers need to see the non-directly related patient's electronic medical records. Electronic medical records provide anonymized patient treatment, so that it can protect patients' health and privacy. The progress note, discussion of difficult case, suggestion of consultation and so on in electronic medical records do not open directly to the patient and will be hidden. Secondly, in the aspect of management, the privacy of patients should be considered first for scientific research, medical exchange and references, the name, address, telephone number, identification card numbers of the patient and other sensitive personal information should not be provided. Medical workers must strengthen their own quality and culture to protect the privacy of patient. Hospitals and patients should establish a strict privacy protection system, in the whole process of doctor-patient communication, the hospital shall inform patients and their families of the right of privacy, and take measures to adequately protect patients' privacy according to the request.

234.3.5 Retaining Traces

Data in electronic medical records can be easily changed, so the system provides specific identification methods for the system operator such as setting up their corresponding permissions and classifying permissions, the operator is responsible for his own identity. In the log, all the operations by the users will be saved when the electronic medical records are modified or deleted. The corrections, accurate modification time, modified content and the modifier information will be saved when the superior physicians review and amend the junior doctor's medical records.

234.3.6 Security of Patients Information

Validity of data in electronic medical records should be ensured from two aspects of technology and management. First, firewall and anti-virus software should be used to prevent hacker attacks, computer viruses, counterfeit electronic signature damaging system data. Set the appropriate permissions to consult, copy, print electronic medical records for medical workers. Without authorization, any unit or individual can not be allowed to make access to consulting or copying the electronic medical records. Second, the medical institution shall establish the security and confidentiality system of electronic medical records information. If the physician practices when his certificate is not valid, it may cause harm to patients. We should copy or duplicate the electronic medical records for the applicant in strict accordance with the relevant provisions in Basic Norm.

234.3.7 Improving Physicians' Self-Protection Awareness

The hospital should organize the medical workers to study the relative laws and regulations in the field of health care, improve the quality of medical records, enhance the legal awareness, regularly carry out the training on preventing and handling medical dispute and recognize that electronic medical records is important for maintaining the interests of the patients, doctors and hospitals and plays a very important role in the medical dispute.

234.4 Conclusion

With the development of technology of IT and network, the use of electronic medical records is inevitable for the management of modern hospital medical records. However, the lag of related laws and regulations restricts the promotion of electronic medical records to some extent and the rapid development of electronic medical records must exist a lot of potential legal risk, so the study on potential legal risks and preventing measures for the electronic medical records has a very important significance in realizing the real digital hospital management and improving our medical level.

References

1. Guo T, Wang X-D, Wang Q-H, Tang J-P (2010) Three legal issues of electronic medical record. Univ Med Nanjing (Soc Sci) 2(39):112–115
2. Ji J (2010) The legal effect of electronic medical records is the key to electronic medical records pilot. China Inf Times (E-Healthc) 11:18–20
3. Li lei tian jianmei wang xiaodong (2010) On the legal authentication of electronic medical records. Jiangsu Healthc Adm 21(6):102–103
4. Liang M-H, Yu R-L (2010) Discussion on legislation principles of electronic medical record in China. China Digital Med 5(5):5–8
5. Zheng L-C (2010) Electronic medical records, the value of legal evidence of. Zhejiang Arch 9:31–32
6. Wang X-L, Jun Y (2007) Analysis and research on potential legal liability in electronic medical record [J]. Chin J Hosp Adm 23(2):140–142
7. Dai J, Xu Y (2011) A feasibility discussion on electronic medical records and paper medical records function equivalence. Chin Med Rec 12(1):38–40
8. Yang L, Liu J (2010) Digital signature and time-stamp technology is the key to the development of paperless electronic medical records. Chin Med Rec 11(12):38–40
9. Chen Y, Wang G, Liu X (2009) The application of electronic signatures in electronic medical records. Chin J Hosp Adm 25(4):226–228
10. Su S, Cui S, Cheng M (2010) Zhongshan municipal people's hospital electronic medical records paperless storage feasibility study. Med Inf 23(10):3722–3724

Chapter 235
Fostering the Autonomous Learning Ability of the Students Under the Multimedia Teaching Environment

Zhao-ying Chen and Xiu-qing Wang

Abstract This chapter discuss the importance about how to foster the autonomous learning ability of the students under the multimedia teaching environment. Taking example linear algebra and space analytic geometry, it illustrates the multimedia teaching which has brought the convenience such as large amount of information, more lively and visual flash demonstration, intuitive and clear teaching drawing and so on. Meanwhile, due to the objective environment and problem consciousness factors, the multimedia has not reached its full advantages in promoting students to study autonomously. This essay puts forward some of the measures about the autonomous learning ability training of the students, for example, how to strengthen the monitoring of students' autonomous learning, which promotes the cultivation of students' autonomous learning ability, stimulates the students' innovation ability, etc. Moreover, improves academic performance goals, and finally promotes the all-round development of students. In this way, the teaching quality of education will be improved.

Keywords Autonomous learning · Ability training · Multimedia teaching · Linear algebra · Space analytic geometry

235.1 Introduction

Autonomous learning is proposed by the United States and other countries in the 1970s, which is an active and constructive learning. The students themselves

Z. Chen (✉)
School of Mathematical Science, University of Jinan, Jinan 250022, Shandong, China
e-mail: zhaoyingchen@126.com

X. Wang
President Office University of Jinan, Jinan 250022, Shandong, China
e-mail: ujnwxq@163.com

determine the learning objectives, monitor and control the cognition, motivation and behaviour guided by objective and situational characteristics and constraints (1). Since a recent period, autonomous learning attracted more and more attention of the academic research in the field of education (2). Even many countries of the world cultivate the students' autonomous learning ability as an important education goals (3).

235.2 The Existing Problems of the Students' Autonomous Learning Under the Multimedia Teaching Environment

With the development and popularity of information technology, the teaching of linear algebra and space analytic geometry course is now widely used in multimedia auxiliary teaching. This way of teaching has brought not only the convenience such as large amount of information, more lively and visual flash demonstration, intuitive and clear teaching drawing etc., but also the new problems in learning. For instance, the students still play the passive role in class. And this way of teaching is unable to mobilize the enthusiasm and initiative of the students. The students can not participate in the classroom teaching as a master. Particular case is shown as follows:

235.2.1 The Status of Teachers in Teaching is too Conspicuous

The teacher is the core of the whole class who controls the whole process of teaching activities and abides by the teaching routine "concept-theorem-sample-problem" step by step. Sometimes, the content conversion is so fast that the students cannot keep up with teaching progress and they have no space at thinking and understanding, Classroom becomes the teacher's stage of completely.

235.2.2 The Students' Adaptability to the Multimedia Teaching is Poor

This is mainly manifested that few students will take the initiative to preview lesson before class. In this way, it will result in that the students are unable to keep up with teaching progress, let alone make note in class. As time passes, class effect is greatly reduced.

235.2.3 Use of Modern Information Technology is not Comprehensive

The development of information technology has been changing with each passing day (4). A computer network is more necessary to the personal intelligent terminal equipment. But the use of technology still stays in the era of making the multimedia courseware. It is far from satisfying the need for teaching. The integrated use of a variety of technical means should be promoted, such as online counseling, answering questions, changing online assignment, online testing and so on, which helps the students to study from every level of course and improve the effect of learning.

235.2.4 Calculation Software of Teaching and Practice Link Also Needs to be Strengthened

Although the methods involving the use of mathematical computing software are contained in chapters and computer training does not reach the designated position. As is known to all, improving the ability of scientific computing is a very important basic link for modernization of mathematics education in science and engineering, and we should teach the students to lay a solid foundation for the use of mathematical software, to further stimulate students' interest in learning.

235.3 The Measures to Cultivate Students' Autonomous Learning Ability Under the Multimedia Teaching Environment

An important goal of the teaching reform is to strengthen the status of students in teaching and highlight the autonomy of learning. But the comprehensive research on the present situation of teaching indicates that the teachers should understand the students' learning status and class requirements, improve methods classroom teaching, and develop the students' ability of autonomous learning. Therefore, the integrated use of a variety of education information technology should be taken and the use of existing teaching platform in school should be strengthened. Teachers should create autonomous learning platform of multimedia network for students, develop the network database, and build a full range of learning space. The math course practice teaching research need be strengthened, through learning the students can really make use of mathematical software like linear algebra package (LINPACK) to solve some common problems. There are the following several solutions in detail.

235.3.1 The Teacher Should Create Autonomous Learning Platform Supported by Multimedia Network for Students, Develop the Network Database of the Linear Algebra and Space Analytic Geometry, and Build a Full Range of Learning Space, in Particular

Firstly, the teacher can adopt the multimedia teaching system: in class, new knowledge outside the classroom should be introduced to enrich the content and make the classroom teaching orientated and extended. When we teach an abstract concept, it is as far as possible to introduce the background of the application, which lays a good foundation for follow-up professional course, such as using the theory of matrices to determine the single game in the league, and to solve the problem of input and output in economics.

Secondly, the teacher can implement resources sharing of network courseware: to apply computer software adequately to perfect the existing courseware of "linear algebra and space analytic geometry". According to the different professional requirements for this course, the teachers could make the excellent multimedia courseware more convenient which is suitable for all kinds of professional teaching under the network environment. In addition, the teacher can make some vivid and excellent video resources which is suitable for communicating with other students from different universities in the network and achieve resources sharing of network courseware.

Finally, the teacher can accomplish the network tutoring system: after class, the teacher can communicate with the students by setting up an email (Blog or BBS or QQ group). They may know the progress of each student timely, In addition, the teacher tries to upload the process of their teaching video to the Internet, or upload the problem-solving document to the file sharing server, which is convenient for the learners to download. In this way, the teachers have created a convenient, fast and comfortable learning environment for the students who are never restricted by the classroom, and it is enough to help students to take their subjective initiative.

235.3.2 The Teacher Should Help Students Make Clear Their Learning Objectives, Formulate a Set of Reasonable and Effective Study Plan

According to the different learning tasks and goals, the teachers should guide the students to establish their individual learning goals, and provide the students with learning strategies and learning resources independently. Through the network platform, the teachers can help and guide the students timely, and make the independent interactive learning more rational, and promote the students to get independent ability gradually. The students can allocate their study time scientifically, and provide their learning feedback in time.

235.3.3 The Teacher Should Help Students Develop Their Self Monitoring and Self Evaluation Ability

In the process of the multimedia network teaching, the teachers should help students control their learning process. In addition, the teachers can provide the students with online test and check the students' homework through the network platform. Adjusting the learning progress and method according to their actual situation, the teachers guide the students to find the most suitable and efficient, personalized learning methods and learning strategies and reflect their learning effect. Besides, the students still have to learn how to self-assess under teachers' monitoring and achieve the goal of cultivating their autonomous learning ability.

235.4 Conclusions

The teacher should give full play to the advantages of multimedia teaching and the students' subjective initiative, guide the students to learn independently, and highlight the students' learning autonomy so that the students can form individual learning methods and ultimately achieve the goal of their lifelong learning.

Acknowledgments Project supported by the Provincial Teaching Research Foundation of Shandong Province (No. 2012204) and the Teaching Research Fund of University of Jinan (JZC12015).

References

1. Richards JC, Rodgers TS (2000) Approaches and methods in language teaching. Foreign Language Teaching and Research Press, Beijing
2. Smith L (2004) Changes in student motivation over the final year of high school. J Educ Enq 5(2):64–83
3. Zhang X (2008) Thinking about the students' autonomous learning under the network environment. J Soc Sci Hunan Med Univ 10(4):88–90
4. Zhou Y, Sang Q (2007) Summary of the home and overseas research on independent learning. J Anhui Inst Educ 27(1):100–104

Chapter 236
Pattern Matching with Flexible Wildcard Gaps

Zhang Junyan and Yang Chenhui

Abstract Pattern matching is a fundamental application in biomedicine and biological sequence analysis. A wildcard can match any one character in a sequence. Multiple wildcards form a gap. A flexible wildcard gap can match any characters with specific length which is specified by users. Therefore, the effective algorithm performing this kind of matching is in great need. In this paper, we design PMFG algorithm and achieve it by dividing a pattern into multiple sub-patterns with different length based on gap segmentation. After computing the starting positions and ending positions of each subpattern, the effective intervals and effective starting positions can be determined one by one. The number of the elements in the last effective position set equals to the number of the matching. A comparison experiments are done based on three DNA sequences. The results show that PMFG algorithm has better performance in the same fields.

Keywords Pattern matching · Wildcard gap · Sequence

236.1 Introduction

Advances in biomedicine provide a quick reaction to new types of genes. H1N1 was first detected in the middle of April, 2009, and then 40 versions of its DNA sequences are available online on April 27, 2009. Researchers can analyze genes immediately using data mining tools, such as BLAST [1] provided by the same

Z. Junyan (✉) · Y. Chenhui
Information Science and Technology College, Chengdu University, Chengdu, China
e-mail: 67306683@qq.com

Z. Junyan
Key Laboratory of Pattern Recognition and Intelligent Information Processing of Sichuan, Chengdu University, Chengdu, China

website. Pattern matching with wildcards is a key issue to the central of these tools. It is also fundamental in biological sequence analysis, text mining, time series data mining, stream data mining, and computational applications [2].

Usually a DNA sequence is represented by a sequence S with a small alphabet $S = \{A,C,G,T\}$, while a repetitive fragment is represented by a pattern P. A wildcard ϕ is a special symbol in P that matches any character in the alphabet [3] Therefore, pattern $P = CG\phi\phi\phi TAC$ matches any subsequence starting with CG, ending with TAC, and with three "don't care" characters in the middle.

Observations show that repetition of DNA fragments is not error-free, and a phase shift may occur due to the insertion or deletion of a short sequence. Consequently, a more general concept called gap has been coined. A gap $g(N, M)$ is a sequence of wildcards with a minimal size N and a maximal size M.

Often a pattern contains a number of gaps. In many existing works, those gaps should be equal [4].

In order to break this limitation, and enable the user to specify each gap independently, we design PMFG algorithm to obtain more flexibility to control queries in this paper. The pattern matching problem with flexible wildcard gaps is defined in Sect. 236.2. The corresponding algorithm is put forward in Sect. 236.3. Thereinto, the sequential matching is segmented into multiple precise pattern matching. The algorithm analysis shows that our algorithm has better time and space complexity. Finally, the results of experiments based on several DNA sequences prove the algorithm to be correct and effective.

236.2 The Problem

236.2.1 Problem Definition

Definition 1 Let $\sum$ be an alphabet. $S = s_1 s_2 ... s_L \in \sum^*$ is called a string or sequence of $\sum$, where $L = |S|$ is the length of S.

Definition 2 A wildcard ϕ is a special symbol that matches with any character in Σ. A gap $g(N, M)$ is a sequence of wildcards with a minimal size N and a maximal size M. $W = M - N + 1$ is the gap flexibility of $g(N, M)$.
$g(N, M)$ is often represented by $[N, M]$ for brevity. If W is fixed in the given P, the gap is called inflexible. Otherwise, the gap is called flexible.

Definition 3 A pattern is a tuple $P = (p, g)$, where $p = p_1 p_2 ... p_k$ is a sequence of Σ. Each p_i is called a subpattern of P. Let $m_i = |p_i|$ denote the length of each p_i, where $1 \leq i \leq k$. So $l = |P| = \sum_{i=1}^{k} m_i$ is the length of P. And $g = g_1 g_2 ... g_{k-1}$ is a sequence of gaps. $g_j = g(N_j, M_j)$ where $1 \leq j \leq k - 1$ is the gap between p_i and p_{i+1}.

A pattern can also be viewed as a mixture of characters and gaps, and expressed as $P = p_1 g(N_1, M_1) p_2 ... g(N_{k-1}, M_{k-1}) p_k$.

Definition 4 A pattern P with flexible gaps matches a subsequence S' of S iff $S' = P = p_1 g(N_1, M_1) p_2 \ldots g(N_{k-1}, M_{k-1}) p_k$.

Given a sequence S and a pattern P with flexible wildcard gaps, Our purpose is to find the number of subsequences in S that match P, which is denoted by $N(P, S)$.

236.2.2 Problem Analysis

In order to analyze the problem, we consider the problem instance over the DNA alphabet $\sum = \{A, C, G, T\}$ by giving an example.

Example 1 $T =$ ATCGGCTCCAGACCAGTACCCGTTTCCGTGGT.
$P =$ A[6,7]CC[2,6]GT.

In order to find the number of subsequences in S that match P, we decompose the problem into multiple precise pattern matching. For each p_i, we first compute the starting position set. The ending position set of p_i can be calculated easily based on m_i, i.e. the length of p_i.

We adopt *startpos*(p_i) and *endpos*(p_i) to denote the starting position set and ending position set of p_i respectively. Thus, *startpos*$(p_i) = \{S_{i1}, S_{i2}, \ldots\}$, *endpos*$(p_i) = \{E_{i1}, E_{i2}, \ldots\}$. Obviously, $E_{i1} = S_{i1} + m_i - 1$, where $1 \leq i \leq k$.

In Example 1, $p_1 =$ A, *startpos*$(p_1) = \{1, 10, 12, 15, 18\}$. For $m_1 = |p_1| = 1$, we have *endpos*$(p_1) = \{1, 10, 12, 15, 18\}$.

Accordingly, $p_2 =$ CC, *startpos*$(p_2) = \{8, 13, 19, 20, 26\}$, $m_2 = |p_2| = 2$, so *endpos*$(p_2) = \{9, 14, 20, 21, 27\}$. $p_3 =$ GT, *startpos*$(p_3) = \{16, 22, 28, 31\}$, $m_3 = |p_3| = 2$, so *endpos*$(p_3) = \{17, 23, 29, 32\}$.

Therefore, the number of possible matching can be denoted $N'(P,S) = \prod_{i=1}^{k} |startpos(p_i)|$, where $|startpos(p_i)|$ is the number of elements in starting position set of p_i. In this example, $N'(P,S) = 5 \times 5 \times 4 = 100$. Obviously, $N(P,S) \neq N'(P,S)$. That is to say, not all the starting positions are effective. For this purpose, we give the definition of effective interval.

Definition 5 Let *startpos**(p_i) represent effective starting positions set. Each $S_{ij} \in$ *startpos**(p_i) is effective. So the effective interval of S_{ij} is denoted as τ_{ij}. According to the requirement of $g_i = [N_i, M_i]$, we have $\tau_{ij} = [S_{ij} + N_i + 1, S_{ij} + M_i + 1]$, where $1 \leq i \leq k-1$, and $j \geq 0$.

Subsequently, we check each $S_{i+1, j} \in startpos(p_{i+1})$. If $\exists \tau_{ij}, S_{i+1, j} \in \tau_{ij}$, then $S_{i+1, j}$ is effective. Then $E_{i+1, j}$ is added to *startpos**(p_{i+1}).

In order to find $N(P,S)$ and record the effective positions, each $S_{1j} \in startpos(p_1)$ is supposed to be effective, so *startpos**$(p_1) = endpos^*(p_1)$.

Let's review Example 1. In term of Definition 5, for $g_1 = [6, 7]$, so the effective intervals are as follows: $\tau_{11} = [8, 9]$, $\tau_{12} = [17, 18]$, $\tau_{13} = [19, 20]$, $\tau_{14} = [22, 23]$, and $\tau_{15} = [25, 26]$.

In *startpos*(p_2), $8 \in \tau_{11}$, 13 doesn't belong to any effective interval, $19 \in \tau_{13}$, $20 \in \tau_{13}$, $26 \in \tau_{15}$. Therefore, the effective values include 8, 19, 20 and 26. Their corresponding ending positions form new effective intervals, i.e., *startpos**(p_2) = {9,20,21,27}. Similarly, based on *startpos**(p_2) and $g_2 = [2,6]$, the effective intervals of p_2 can be obtained as follows: $\tau_{21} = [12,16]$, $\tau_{22} = [23,27]$, $\tau_{23} = [24,28]$, and $\tau_{24} = [30,34]$. In *startpos*(p_3), $16 \in \tau_{21}$, 22 doesn't belong to any effective interval, $28 \in \tau_{23}$, and $31 \in \tau_{24}$. The effective values are: 16, 28 and 31. Their corresponding ending positions form new effective intervals, i.e., *startpos**(p_3) = {17,29,32}. For the last p_i without g_i, we needn't calculate its effective intervals. The computation process and data are shown in Table 236.1. Obviously, the number of the elements in the last start point set is the value of $N(P,S)$. In Example 1, $N(P,S) = 3$.

236.3 The Algorithm

236.3.1 Algorithm Description

Algorithm 1 is employed to compute starting position set and ending position set for each p_i in S. Here, L is the length of sequence S, and k is the number of subpatterns.

Algorithm 1: Computing starting position set and ending position set.
Input: $S=s_1s_2...s_L$, $p=p_1p_2...p_k$
Output: *startpos*(p_i), *endpos*(p_i)
    for(j=1; j<=k; j++)
        for(i=1; i<=L; i++)
        {if(*S*.regionMatches(i, p_i, 1, p_i.length()))
            {*startpos*(p_i)=i;
            endpos(p_i)=*startpos*(p_i)+m_i–1;}
        }
    }

Table 236.1 Computation process and data for example 1

p_i	$p_1 = A$	$p_2 = CC$	$p_3 = GT$
Startpos(p_i)	{1, 10, 12, 15, 18}	{8, 13, 19, 20, 26}	{16, 22, 28, 31}
m_i	1	2	2
Endpos(p_i)	{1, 10, 12, 15, 18}	{9, 14, 20, 21, 27}	{17, 23, 29, 32}
g_i	[6, 7]	[2, 6]	–
Startpos*(p_i)	{1, 10, 12, 15, 18}	{9, 20, 21, 27}	{17, 29, 32}
τ_{ij}	[8,9],[17,18],[19,20],[22,23],[25,26]	[12,16],[23,27],[24,28],[30,34]	

Algorithm 2 is employed to compute $N(P,S)$. Here, k is the number of p_i, and τ_{ij} is effective interval.

Algorithm 2: Computing $N(P,S)$.
Input: $startpos(p_i)$, $endpos(p_i)$, $g_i(N_i,M_i)$
Output: $N(P,S)$

    $startpos^*(p_1)=endpos(p_1)$;
    for($i=1$; $i<=k$; $i++$)
        {for each $S_{ij} \in startpos^*(p_i)$
            {$\tau_{ij}=[S_{ij}+N_i+1, S_{ij}+M_i+1]$;
            if($S_{i+1,j} \in \tau_{ij}$)
                Add $E_{i+1,j}$ to $startpos^*(p_{i+1})$;}
        }
    $N(P,S)= startpos^*(p_k)$.length;

236.3.2 Algorithm Complexity Analysis

Algorithm 1 is employed to compute starting position set and ending position set. Each position in S should be scanned, and there are k positions need matching each time. So the time complexity is $O(kL)$. Algorithm 2 is employed to compute $N(P,S)$. The times of loop depends on the number of τ_{ij} for each S_{ij} in p_i. No matter how large it is, it is always less than L. So the time complexity is $O(kL)$ approximately. Therefore, the overall time complexity is: $O(kL) + O(kL) = O(kL)$.

Let's compute the space complexity now. In Algorithm 1, we use tow arrays to store S and p, and $L + l$ space are needed. Another 2 two-dimensional arrays are employed to store $startpos(p_i)$ and $endpos(p_i)$. Obviously, the number of starting positions of each p_i is less than L. The number of p_i is k, so the space complexity is $O(L + l + 2kL) = O((2k + 1)L + l)$. In Algorithm 2, we need approximate $2kL$ spaces store effective intervals and approximate kL spaces store $startpos^*(p_i)$. So the space complexity is $O(2kL + kL) = O(3kL)$. Therefore, the overall space complexity is: $O((2k + 1)L + l) + O(3kL) = O((2k + 1)L + l)$.

The results show that the complexity of our algorithm depends on the number of p_i instead of the length of p. So the performance of our algorithms is superior to most others in the same fields.

236.4 Experiments

In this section, we tested our algorithm using the biological sequences downloaded from the National Center for Biotechnology Information website: The first one we used is New York/11/2009(H1N1) No. FJ984346. Its length is 2,151. The second

Table 236.2 Experimental results

Data	P	N(P,S)	Running time of PMFG (ms)	Running time of PAIG (ms)
FJ984346	P1	4.92×10^2	10	10
	P2	6.30×10^3	18	20
	P3	2.96×10^4	25	30
AX829174	P1	2.72×10^4	18	20
	P2	2.29×10^4	18	20
	P3	9.83×10^4	30	40
AB038496	P1	4.28×10^5	150	180
	P2	3.67×10^5	130	170
	P3	1.57×10^6	200	230

one is human DNA sequence AX829174, the length of which is 10,011. The third one is Homo sapiens gene for fukutin AB038490 and its length is 131,892.

Three patterns are chosen for testing: P1 = A[6,7]CC[2,6]GT[0,3]AT, P2 = AT[0,3]AG[1, 5]T, and P3 = GT[2,7]AG[3,6]T. We do some comparison experiments between our algorithm and PAIG[5]. The results are listed in Table 236.2. For brevity, our algorithm is named PMFG.

According to the results in Table 236.2, we can find PMFG has similar running time with PAIG when the values of N(P,S) is smaller. When the values of N(P,S) become larger, the performance of PMFG is better than PAIG.

236.5 Conclusions

In this paper, we have designed PMFG for pattern matching with flexible wildcard gaps. Our algorithm has a polynomial time and space complexity. It can solve pattern matching problem by dividing the long sequence into multiple subpatterns. The comparison experiments are done. And the results show that PMFG has better performance than the similar algorithm in same filed.

References

1. Altschul SF, Gish W, Miller W et al (1990) Basic local alignment search tool. J Mol Biol 215:403–410
2. Crochemore M, Iliopoulos C, Makris C et al (2002) Approximate string matching with gaps. Nordic J Comput 9(1):54–65
3. Kim S, Bhan A, Maryada BK et al. (2007) EGGS: extraction of gene clusters using genome context based sequence matching techniques. In Proceedings of IEEE ICBB, 23–28
4. Haapasalo T, SilvastP I, Sippu S et al. (2011) Online dictionary matching with variable-length gaps. In Proceedings 10th SEA, 76–87
5. Zhang M, Kao B (2011) Mining periodic patterns with gap requirement from sequences. In Proceedings of SIGMOD, 623–633

Chapter 237
Establishment and Practice of the New Teaching Model of Maxillofacial Gunshot Injuries

Zhen Tang, Xiaogang Xu, Zhizhong Cao and Dalin Wang

Abstract Medical education models play an important role in medical education, especially in military medical education. However, there are shortcomings in various existing teaching models of maxillofacial gunshot injuries. To resolve this issue, we integrated a dynamic simulation of image data to create a new, three-dimensional dynamic digital teaching model that was based on our previous completed three-dimensional finite element model of human maxillofacial bone tissue gunshot injuries. This model was applied to teaching practice with good results. The new model has helped us to achieve the teaching objective and improve the teaching efficiency.

Keywords Military medicine · Teaching model · Maxillofacial gunshot injuries

237.1 Introduction

Medicine is a practical science, and students cannot rely solely on theoretical study to fully grasp medical knowledge. In this sense, medical education is difficult to implement. Unlike the teaching methods of other disciplines, which mainly rely on explaining texts, medical education requires more extensive use of non-text methods, such as images, three-dimensional models, and videos, in the teaching process so that students can intuitively comprehend the content explained by the instructor; these non-text methods also make it easier for the instructor to express their intent. Broadly speaking, all non-text media used in the teaching process can be referred to as a teaching model. Due to the specific characteristics of medical education, the quality of a medical teaching model will directly affect the success

Z. Tang · X. Xu · Z. Cao · D. Wang (✉)
Department of Stomatology, Changhai Hospital, The Second Military Medical University, 200433 Shanghai, China
e-mail: tangzhen1999@yahoo.cn

or failure of medical education. This type of education requires medical instructors to continue to improve the teaching model, to explore new areas to establish a teaching model, to constantly improve the medical teaching model, to improve the overall quality of teaching, and to train more qualified medical personnel for the country and society.

Medical teaching models play an important role in medical education, especially in military medical education. Due to the shortcomings in various existing teaching models of maxillofacial gunshot injuries, it has been a challenge to teach military medical school students about maxillofacial gunshot injuries. On the basis of our previously completed three-dimensional finite element dynamic model of human maxillofacial bone tissue gunshot injuries, we converted the dynamic simulation of the image data into a teaching model to better achieve the teaching objective and to improve teaching efficiency.

237.2 Materials and Methods

237.2.1 Establishment of the Finite Element Model of Human Maxillary and Mandible Bone Gunshot Injuries and the Acquisition of Dynamic Simulation Images

In a previous basic research study of maxillofacial gunshot injuries, we used the first digitized female [1] (22 year old, 1620 mm) head and neck computed tomography (CT) scan data in China to obtain a three-dimensional finite element model of human maxillary and mandible bones and completed the dynamic simulation of the three-dimensional finite element model and a biomechanical analysis of human maxillofacial bone tissue gunshot injuries [2, 3]. In the process of performing basic research, we used LS-PREPOST software, which is the postprocessing software of the finite element model, to collate the obtained data and to computer simulate the dynamic process that occurs when bullets and steel balls hit human maxillary and mandible bones from multiple angles and the dynamic distribution of the internal stress of bone tissue during injury. We also recorded the entire changing process by exporting multiple dynamic images, and we obtained a series of dynamic change images in the injury model and images of the dynamic changes of stress distribution under different injury conditions (two projectiles, two sites, and one angle of incidence in the maxillary bone; two projectiles, two sites, and three angles of incidence in the mandible bone).

237.2.2 Image Integration and Teaching Model Establishment

The models were divided into groups based on the injury conditions used in the basic experimental research (projectile, incident site, and incident angle). The maxillary models were divided into four groups, as follows: bullet anterior incident site and posterior incident site models and steel ball anterior incident site and posterior incident site models. The mandible models were divided into 12 groups, as follows: bullet mandibular angle and chin incident site models (three angles: 45, 67.5, and 90°) and steel ball mandibular angle and chin incident site models (three angles: 45, 67.5, and 90°).

According to the grouping criteria, LS-PREPOST software was utilised for the dynamic simulation of the injury process and the stress distribution of each model, and the images of dynamic change were exported in the JPEG format. At least four images of dynamic changes (two angles) were obtained for each model. In total, 64 images of dynamic changes were obtained.

PowerPoint multimedia software was used to create a teaching model, and all levels of subdirectories were established according to the above grouping criteria. Then, the PowerPoint multimedia software was used to create hyperlinks for each directory, which ensured that all subdirectories levels were linked to the corresponding dynamic simulation images of gunshot injuries.

237.3 Results

The dynamic change images were organised into a PowerPoint multimedia slideshow through hyperlinks to establish the three-dimensional dynamic digital teaching model of human maxillofacial bone tissue gunshot injuries. The maxillary and mandible injury processes and the distribution of internal stress when the bone tissue was hit by bullets or steel balls could be dynamically displayed by clicking the hyperlinks, as shown in Figs. 237.1, 237.2, 237.3 and 237.4.

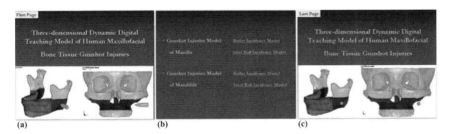

Fig. 237.1 The main body of the three-dimensional dynamic digital teaching model of human maxillofacial bone tissue gunshot injuries. **a, c** The home page and last page of the teaching model. **b** The main page of the teaching model; the font in *yellow* is a hyperlink; click to go to the specific model page

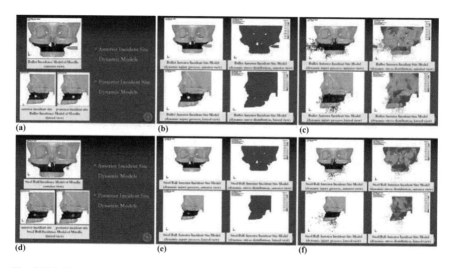

Fig. 237.2 Excerpt diagram of the three-dimensional dynamic digital teaching model of maxillary bone gunshot injuries. **a, d** The main page of the teaching model of maxillary bone bullet and steel ball incidence; the font in *yellow* is a hyperlink, click "Anterior Incident Site Dynamic Models" to go to page (**b**) or (**e**). **b, c** The same page, demo page of the dynamic teaching model of maxillary bone bullet anterior site incidence; demonstrating the initial and end state shown in the teaching model. **e, f** The same page, demo page of the dynamic teaching model of maxillary bone steel ball anterior site incidence; demonstrating the initial and end state shown in the teaching model

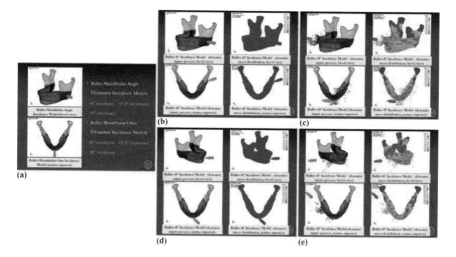

Fig. 237.3 Excerpt diagram of the three-dimensional dynamic digital teaching model of mandible bullet incidence. **a** The main page of the teaching model of mandible bullet incidence, the font in *yellow* is a hyperlink, click "45° incidence" to go to page (**b**) or (**d**). **b, c** The same page, demo page of the dynamic teaching model of bullet 45° incidence at angle of mandible, demonstrating the initial and end state shown in the teaching model. **d, e** The same page, demo page of the dynamic teaching model of bullet 45° incidence at mental region, demonstrating the initial and end state shown in the teaching model

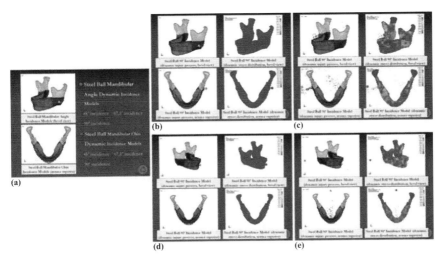

Fig. 237.4 Excerpt diagram of the three-dimensional dynamic digital teaching model of mandible steel ball incidence. **a** The main page of the teaching model of mandible steel ball incidence, the font in *yellow* is a hyperlink, click "90° incidence" to go to page (**b**) or (**d**). **b, c** The same page, demo page of the dynamic teaching model of steel ball 90° incidence at angle of mandible, demonstrating the initial and end state shown in the teaching model. **d, e** The same page, demo page of the dynamic teaching model of steel ball 90° incidence at mental region, demonstrating the initial and end state shown in the teaching model

237.4 Application

Since the establishment of the new teaching model, we have applied it to actual teaching practice. When teaching oral and maxillofacial firearm injuries to military medical school students, we used the three-dimensional dynamic digital teaching model of human maxillofacial bone tissue gunshot injuries instead of the traditional method of explanation, which consists of texts and images. Our practice has proven that the three-dimensional dynamic digital teaching model is intuitive, with a dynamic display of the processes and biomechanical changes of maxillofacial gunshot injuries. The application of this model has quickly attracted the attention of the military medical school students and greatly stimulated the students' interest in learning. At the same time, the model has also made teaching easier. This teaching model demonstrates the abstract and complex process of maxillofacial gunshot injuries and the changes in biomechanical effects through a series of dynamic images, which makes it more convenient for the instructor to explain the characteristics of maxillofacial gunshot injuries, the concept of secondary shrapnel injuries, how to perform emergency treatment, and how to strengthen protection in wartime, thereby achieving the teaching objectives and improving teaching efficiency.

237.5 Discussion

The characteristics that make teaching in military medical schools different from teaching in general medical schools are the distinctive military features of the teaching content. It has been challenging for instructors in military medical schools to help students grasp the characteristics, treatments, and techniques for the protection of war injuries while teaching the medical knowledge.

With the development of modern weapons, the type of war injuries is diverse, but gunshot injuries are still the main war injury type. The maxillofacial area is exposed, and its wartime protection is poor. In addition, the maxillofacial area is also the main target for violence and self-injury. Among all body gunshot injuries, the percentage of maxillofacial gunshot injuries is the highest. Therefore, the treatment of maxillofacial gunshot injuries is the focus of treatments for maxillofacial and even systemic injuries. For the treatment of war injuries, students should be mainly concerned about the mechanisms, injury processes, and biomechanical effects of maxillofacial gunshot injuries, yet these subjects are challenging for military medical schools instructors to teach.

Currently, the teaching of maxillofacial gunshot injuries is mainly based on theoretical knowledge, which is supplemented by images, videos, and three-dimensional models. Among the teaching models of maxillofacial gunshot injuries currently in use, images are commonly used by the instructors, but the images are two-dimensional and cannot provide all the information relevant to maxillofacial gunshot injuries. In addition, a wide variety of images with varying qualities are used in military schools, and some images are even wall charts from decades ago that have also limited the effect of using these images. The introduction of videos showing maxillofacial gunshot injuries is a major change in the development of the military medical teaching model. By using the recorded videos, instructors can present dynamic information on maxillofacial gunshot injuries to the students so that the students will be able to intuitively understand the entire process and the main points relevant to maxillofacial war injuries. However, there are limitations in the video materials. First, certain conditions and equipment are required to obtain a video, making it difficult to acquire a video. Second, a video mainly shows what happens outside the human body, and it is difficult to show the change in stress inside the body. Therefore, the information provided by the video is still not comprehensive enough. There are a wide variety of three-dimensional models of maxillofacial gunshot injuries, including animal models, cadaver models, and models made with artificial materials. These models have been in use for many years. Due to the comprehensive information they provide and their manoeuvrability, they are favoured by military medical school students, which is also the main reason for the enduring appeal of these models. However, it is not easy to obtain these models, and their costs are high. Currently, the use of cadaver models of gunshot injuries is completely prohibited due to ethical considerations. To perform basic research on gunshot injuries, scholars at home and abroad have established experimental animal models of maxillofacial gunshot injuries. In China, the Fourth Military Medical University has completed a great deal of research in this field, and they has converted some basic research results into teaching content and reproduced the results in experimental animal models. However, due to the individual differences in experimental animals, the initial conditions of the experiment are subject to various factors; therefore, it is difficult to maintain consistency. Moreover, the costs of each experiment are high, thus, it is impossible to meet the urgent needs of the students. With the development of engineering techniques and materials science, some scholars have used artificial materials for the research of wound ballistics, but due to the complex anatomical structures of maxillofacial area and the many sinuses and canals, it is still impossible to establish models using artificial materials with an anatomical shape and material characteristics similar to those of the maxillofacial area. Moreover, models made with artificial materials also have the disadvantages of being high cost and time-consuming. Therefore, the development of teaching models of maxillofacial gunshot injuries using experimental animals and artificial materials has faced many problems. The question remains as to how to solve these problems. We believe that when traditional teaching models are facing challenges, we need to seek solutions in new areas.

With the advancements in computer hardware and software, computer-aided modelling and simulation techniques have been applied to various medical fields. The techniques can simplify a biological system into a mathematical model and conduct the computational analysis of these models on a computer, thus replacing complex biomechanical experiments. In this study, the three-dimensional dynamic digital teaching model of human maxillofacial bone tissue gunshot injuries was established based on our previous research, and the three-dimensional dynamic change images of the maxillofacial bone tissue gunshot injuries were integrated to generate a digitised teaching model.

In our teaching practice, we found that the new teaching model can help military medical school students improve their learning of maxillofacial gunshot injuries and grasp the injury conditions, main treatment points, and protective measures of maxillofacial gunshot injuries so that the students can intuitively and dynamically grasp the process and biomechanical effects of maxillofacial gunshot injuries. This teaching model is established based on the most recent results from basic research and has enabled medical school students to have faster access to the frontier of medical research, and it has thus stimulated the students' interest in medical research and cultivated more talents in medical research.

References

1. Zhang SX, Heng PA, Liu ZJ et al (2004) The Chinese visible human (CVH) datasets incorporate technical and imaging advances on earlier digital humans. J Anat 204(3):165–173
2. Tang Z, Tu W, Zhang G et al (2012) Dynamic simulation and preliminary finite element analysis of gunshot wounds to the human mandible. Injury 43(5):660–665
3. Tang Z, Zhou Z, Zhang G et al (2012) Establishment of a three-dimensional finite element model for gunshot wounds to the human mandible. J Med Coll PLA 27:87–100

Chapter 238
Research of Database Full-Text Retrieval Based on Related Words Recognition

Gao Pei-zhi and Li Xue-qing

Abstract With the popularity of application system, there is a growing demand for database full-text retrieval application. Users hope that they can easily find the information they want. This brings more restrict requirement on the Chinese synonyms recognition. At present, the study about Chinese synonym recognition has just begun in the domestic and the application of Chinese synonym recognition in the area is not just as one wish either. In this paper, we build a database full-text retrieval system which supports related words recognition in combination with lucene. The recognition of related words is applied to the full-text retrieval system. The data of related words were extracted from subject and achievement information.

Keywords Recognition of Chinese related words · Chinese word segmentation · Lucene · Database full-text retrieval

238.1 Introduction

With the rapid development of information technology, more and more demands in full-text retrieval systems emerge too. Currently, the implementation of full-text search systems is mostly based on lucene [1].

The current search engines are basically search based on keywords. But it's impossible for us to end the same concept when we input the keyword and users

G. Pei-zhi (✉) · L. Xue-qing (✉)
Department of Computer Science and Technology, Shandong University, Shandong 250101, China
e-mail: lei.ren123@163.com

L. Xue-qing
e-mail: xqli@sdu.edu.cn

cannot get a satisfied result. This promotes the research on synonym recognition. In recent years, foreign researches on the recognition of synonyms mainly adopt three methods: from document set, Internet and dictionary. Domestic researches for the recognition of Chinese synonyms mainly includes: (1) word-form-similarity approach [2] (2) thesaurus based approach [3] (3) the statistics method based on large corpora [4] (4) the method based on dictionary definition [5].

In this paper, the establishment of database full-text retrieval is based on lucene. Based on the thought of lexical co-occurrence analysis, we extract subject-related words from subject information and extracts related words from achievement information with an improved similarity calculation method based on joint probability distribution. In addition, in order to get a reasonable result, we modify the result sort by the term's importance with an improved similarity calculation method based on vector space model.

238.2 Database Full-Text Retrieval Based on Related Words Recognition

238.2.1 The Establishment of Related Words Thesaurus

The establishment of thesaurus is divided into two parts: to extract related words from subject information, and to extract related words from achievement information.

238.2.1.1 Extracting Subject-Related Words and Put it into Thesaurus

The first purpose of this paper is to recognize subject related words. We establish a related words thesaurus with subject information as test data. Subject itself has a containment relationship. Based on the relationship, it is easy to find that the relationship can be expressed by a tree structure.

Based on subject-related tree, we find the related subject and add it into thesaurus. The method of recognizing the related words of vocabulary A: according to the structure of the subject-related tree, the nodes in second layer are different subjects. Starting from the third layer of tree, every node has the same father node, so they are related subjects. When searching, the users wish to search for related subject information. So identification of related words is transformed into the calculations of distance of nodes in the tree. For related words of vocabulary A, the similarity is defined by their distance in subject-related tree. Define the similarity of vocabulary A and B as the following quotation:

$$Sim(A, B) = 0.5^{(level(B)-level(A))} \qquad (238.1)$$

In (238.1), *level (A)* represents the layer of A, *level (B)* represents the layer of B.

238.2.1.2 Extracting Related Words from Achievement Information and Put it into Thesaurus

There are some other terms related to the subject word besides the subject name. For these words, we extract related words from achievement information with the algorithm of similarity calculation based on lexical co-occurrence analysis and put them into subject-related words thesaurus.

In this paper, we take achievement information as test data, and extract achievement name and achievement content from repository with a statistical method based on lexical co-occurrence information. Then we get all participle vocabulary information and make statistics about their co-occurrence frequency from each data record. Set a threshold according to the co-occurrence frequency first, if the similarity of two terms is greater than the threshold, they can be stored in thesaurus as related words. In co-occurrence model, we put co-occurrence distance and co-occurrence window into account to improve the accuracy and reasonableness. We believe that the words appearing in same window is co-occurrence, obviously. Due to the different distance, they have different weight even if they are in a same window. In this paper, we take each record as a window and the words appearing in the same record is considered to co-occurrence. We believe that the closer of the distance, the higher of the similarity. Therefore, in the joint probability formula, we add vocabulary distance limit, transform the formula as follows:

$$Sim(A,B) = \frac{\sum_{i=1}^{P(A,B)} \frac{1}{d_i(A,B)} + \sum_{i=1}^{P(B,A)} \frac{1}{d_i(B,A)}}{P(A) + P(B) - P(A,B) - P(B,A)} \quad (238.2)$$

In (238.2), $d_i(A,B)$ represents the co-occurrence distance of vocabulary A and B in i times. $P(A, B)$ represents the co-occurrence times of vocabulary B follows A, $P(A)$ represents the number of occurrence of vocabulary A.

238.2.2 *Full-Text Retrieval System Based on Subject-Related Words Recognition*

238.2.2.1 Introduction of Full-Text Retrieval Principle Based on Related Words

The principle of full-text retrieval based on related words is combining the keywords and related words of keywords to produce a new keyword and searching it. The specific process is divided into four steps:

1. Word segmentation. For keyword S, it is separated into $S(T1, T2,\ldots, Tn)$ with Paoding analyzer.
2. Get related words $Ti(Ti1, Ti2,\ldots, Tin)$ by query thesaurus for each Ti.
3. Combine Ti and related words into a new keyword $S'(Ti, Ti1, Ti2,\ldots, Tin)$.
4. Search using new keyword S' in index.

238.2.2.2 Problem of Search Results Sort Based on Related Words

When the recognition of related words being applied to full-text retrieval system, we can get a lot of related words from thesaurus, which are different from the keyword, and we cannot search them with the keyword as the same word. So we introduce the concept of relevance to distinguish important-performance between the original words and related words appearing in the result set. This paper presents an improved vector space model (VSM) algorithm: This algorithm uses TF-IDF to transform the handling of the text content simplify into a vector in the vector space, and to transform semantic similarity into space similarity.

Each document is composed of multiple terms, so we can consider each document as D (term1, term2, term3,..., termn). We can consider the index file which contains N term as an n-dimension vector space. Due to the introduction of related words, it is unreasonable that the keyword and the related words as a same word to calculate, so relevance also added to the calculation. We determine rl_k represents the similarity of termk and keyword. If termk and keyword are the same word, then $rl_k = 1$, if termk and keyword are related words, then $rl_k = 0.8*Sim(A, B)$. So the weight of document i: $W_{ik} = tf_{ik} \times idf_{ik} \times rl_k$, for keyword S, we can get new keywords $S'(K1, K2,..., Kn)$. The weight of document i for keyword S is $\sum_{k=1}^{n} W_{ik}$.

238.3 Experiment and Analysis

We take patent data as the test data and the Table 238.1 demonstrates the search results based on Chinese keyword "computer":

The Table 238.1 shows that the keyword-based full-text retrieval can get all data records that exactly match with keywords and return in accordance with the

Table 238.1 Search results

Keywords	Refine search	Related words search sorted by score of lucene	Related words search sorted by relevance
Computer	1 design for computer cases	1 end cutter of flat-end computer aided design system	1 ouma computer information management system for online marking software V2.1.1V2.1.1
	2 end cutter of flat-end computer aided design system	2 end cutter of ball-end computer aided design system	2 design for computer cases
	3 end cutter of ball-end computer aided design system	3 design for computer cases	3 ouma computer election recount system V1.0

lucene scoring rule. For keyword "computer", 128 records will be found, which can meet common search requirement. Full-text retrieval with related words not only can search the records that match the keywords exactly but also can search records that match related words. For keyword "computer" in this system 643 records can be found. The sort result is unsatisfied owing to that it can't distinguish the keyword and related words. Search results that sort based on relevance can find 643 records, Results can reflect the importance of the record. The experiment results suggest that full-text retrieval based on subject-related words can return search results reasonably.

References

1. Lang X, Wang S (2006) Research and development of full text search engine based on lucene. Zhejiang University, Hangzhou
2. Song M (1996) The Chinese vocabulary literal similarity principle after the controlled vocabulary the dynamic maintenance study. Information 04:261–271
3. Wu Z (1999) Economic information retrieval control the vocabulary study. Journal of Nanjing Agricultural University, Nanjing
4. Crouch CJ (1990) An approach to the automatic construction of global thesaurus. Inf Process Manage 26:629–640
5. Lu Y, Hou H (2004) Chinese synonym automatic recognition based on dictionary annotation. In: NCIRCS
6. Cheng T, Shi S, Wang X (2007) Thematic words extracting from Chinese text based on synonym Cilin. J Guangxi Normal Univ: Nat Sci Edn 25(2):145–148
7. Qun Liu, Sujian Li (2002) How net-based lexical semantic similarity calculation. Chin Comput Linguis 7(2):59–76

Chapter 239
Construction and Application of High Quality Medical Video Teaching Resources

Chu Wanjiang, Zhuang Engui, Wang Honghai, Xu Zhuping, Bai Canming, Wang Jian and Li Lianhong

Abstract The construction and application of high quality medical video teaching resource is the important support to higher education teaching reform. Research and development is the key of high-quality medical video teaching resources construction, the key link is teachers' team to determine the topic, attach the traditional teaching resources, modern diagnosis and treatment of digital video resources. Break up the whole into parts in the first class of formal teaching and second class, composite study application of high-quality medical video teaching resources is an important characteristic to modern teaching process and students' Autonomous learning. To strengthen the quality of medical video teaching resource construction and application will be the key to long-term education theme and the process quality of the cultivation of innovative talents and improving the quality of teaching.

Fund Project: Liaoning Province teaching reform in department of higher education research project in 2009 (A119), Chinese Medical Association 2010 medical education research (2010-13-1).Author: Chu, WanJiang (1963-), male, Liaoning, Dalian, master degree, research direction: the integration of modern education technology and higher medical education, the construction and application research and practice of quality video teaching resource.

C. Wanjiang · Z. Engui · W. Jian
Modern education technology department of Dalian Medical University, Dalian 116044, China

W. Honghai
Teaching affair office of Dalian Medical University, Dalian 116044, China

X. Zhuping
Library of Dalian Medical University, Dalian 116044, China

B. Canming
Clinical skills center of Dalian Medical University, Dalian 116044, China

L. Lianhong (✉)
Basic Medical College of Dalian Medical University, Lushun South Road. 9, Dalian 116044, China
e-mail: lilianhong@dlmedu.edu.cn

Keywords High quality medical video teaching resources · Audio-visual teaching · Traditional teaching resources and modern diagnosis · Digital resources · Teacher classroom video · Scientific applications

With the rapid development of modern technology, the reform of higher education promotes to a deeper level. *National Education Reform and Development Medium and Long-term plan* (2010–2020) clearly put forward to strengthen the development and application of high quality educational resources, which fully demonstrates the role and important strategic position of high-quality educational resources in the modern education and teaching [1]. This article describes the construction and application of high quality medical video teaching resources based on many years of teaching practice.

239.1 The Important Role of High Quality Medical Video Teaching Resources in Modern Medical Education

China's higher education has developed into the popularization in recent years which resulted in higher education resources relatively scarce; the growth of knowledge increases exponentially which resulted in the task of higher education is more and more heavy; higher composite and comprehensive quality of talents has being needed gradually in modern society [2]. All of these are calling the new education concepts and new teaching methods, therefore, the modern constructivist teaching mode, PBL teaching mode and double main teaching mode emerge as the times require, changing the traditional teaching mode like Cramming and Indoctrination that profess in the classroom [3]. Nowadays, modern education and teaching is becoming hybrid type, discrete type or compound type, students not only study in classroom [4], but also in home informally extruding the requirement of high quality medical video teaching resources.

Educational psychology research indicates that the video has a unique advantage in showing procedural knowledge [5]. A large part of medical knowledge is procedural knowledge and most medical mechanism, medical process is difficult to describe directly, however the abstract knowledge could transform believable image vividly by video and audio media. For example, how to make people have a clear understanding of one pulse? I'm afraid even the high master of language is difficult to describe it, but if the ECG multiple wave type is recorded by video and heart sound is recorded the pulse could show vividly. For another example, the process of clinical operation is difficult to describe, but we can record the process by video, and then compose a teaching resource by montage, displaying the process of operation beyond the time and the space.

In short, the video can concentrate the objective world, expand the microscopic world, condense time, display space, and also show a world. In the transfer of medical knowledge, it can be widely used. Therefore, it's important to strengthen and improve the construction and application of high quality medical video teaching resources, meeting the demand of higher education increasing.

239.2 The Vital Links of High Quality Medical Video Teaching Resources

239.2.1 The Connotation of Quality Medical Video Teaching Resources

High quality medical video teaching resources should meet two basic characteristics. First, the video could present the teaching content and process very well that meet the needs of teaching design and student self-sufficiency learning, namely scientific, teaching and strong demand. Second the video should have a vivid image of high technical index, namely artistic, edutainment and strong readability. High quality medical video teaching resources should be an audio-visual materials system which is all-round, three-dimensional and multi-level display of teaching contents and teaching process. High quality medical video teaching resources in our school are composed of various disciplines of medical video teaching materials which are useful for the first class and the second class [6]. High quality medical video teaching resources are series with various forms, there are special series, material piece series, classroom teaching series, development of video teaching resource collection series and so on. Special series is composed of many independent and related thematic or module. The material could specifically focus on the display of modular teaching content vividly. Material piece series is the most practical audio-visual fragment lattice which is widely coverage. The material has systematic and flexible knowledge which plays an important role in teaching and autonomous learning. Classroom teaching series is a subject system of classroom teaching live video collection. The material can well demonstrate the teaching process and the atmosphere which is the best auxiliary video teaching resources of autonomous learning and review. Development of video teaching resource collection series is a extracurricular teaching resources which is closely related with the teaching content such as academic lecture, seminar and the new development of the discipline. The material could broaden knowledge and vision which is the best quality education teaching resources [7].

239.2.2 The Vital Links of Development of High Quality Medical Video Teaching Resources

The development of high quality medical video teaching resources is the basis for application of the high quality video teaching construction. There are many links such as topic determination, script and shooting script writing, shooting and post-production, publication and so on in high quality audio-visual production process. In this article we focus on the key steps and strategies.

239.2.2.1 The Abstraction of the Topic

The medical video teaching material has been widely used in modern medical teaching process. That results in the shortage and deterioration of audio-visual material. Therefore, teachers in the process of teaching, often by the audio-visual materials can't satisfy the demand of distress [8]. Therefore, the understanding of what knowledge teachers lack of audio-visual materials, also the most well known point of audio-visual teaching material development, so the research and development of audio-visual materials, to fully rely on the teachers' team of experts in teaching practice topic, this is the key to the development of audio-visual materials [9]. For example, the Dalian Medical University in pathology teaching, teachers team of experts according to the demand of teaching, research and development of the 'Eleventh Five-Year Plan' national key Audiovisual Publishing Planning Ministry of health medical audio-visual material 'Experimental case-based pathology guidance', through ten cases had pathological shown teaching methods and technology of the system, has been widely used in distributed learning first class teaching and second class, has received the good teaching effect.

239.2.2.2 Attach Great Importance to the Traditional Teaching Resources and Modern Diagnosis and Treatment Digital Resources

In the process of quality medical video teaching material construction, digital integration of traditional teaching resources is an important part. Because pass down the traditional teaching pattern, precious slide, mould, anatomical specimens, plasticizing specimens can take pictures through camera, scanning, means of digital acquisition become making audio-visual teaching material. Similarly, the modern medical equipment digitization degree more and more high, many clinical examination process, treatment process can be synchronous digital video recording. These digital video is the conventional video equipment can't be photographed and recorded, but teaching is urgently needed. There are plans to record and organize related material collection, reorganization, is the construction of an important source of audio-visual series materials [10].

For example, in histology and embryology teaching, teachers apply modern teaching methods to organize teaching, various teaching resources scattered, feel inadequate space, time constraints, lack of a system and comprehensive experimental guide series of audio-visual materials. The Dalian Medical University achieved 'Eleventh Five-Year Plan' national key Audiovisual Publishing Project 'the development of human embryo' audio-visual materials. Combining with the teaching practice of traditional teaching resources on a plurality of medical institutions for the digital recombination and modern medical teaching resource optimization, production consists of 5 thematic modules of the human embryo development series of audio-visual materials, in February 2010 by people's medical electronic audio–video publishing house publication, in teaching practice, received a good social effect, according to not complete statistics in the country has issued 358 copies, has been applied widely and sharing. The strategy and method of the same, optimization and reorganization of the traditional and digital teaching resources and modern diagnosis, Dalian Medical University has successfully made the clip series 'chest CT read piece of guidance' the Ministry of health of audio-visual materials.

239.2.2.3 Excavation of the Traditional Teaching Experience

To revitalize the traditional teaching resources, not only reflected in the physical resources can be seen, is applied in order to mouth experience, such as Dalian Medical University in surgical operation in experiment teaching, the accumulation of a large number of mouth of teaching experience, the experience is the experience of several generations of teachers, is the precious wealth of teaching. Now if every teacher in the teaching practice to the mouth again, time is not allowed, audience number is restricted [11]. Therefore, teachers according to the teaching requirements, classification and formed a "surgical operation experimental teaching of common errors" clip series of audio-visual materials manuscript, involving a tsotal of operating procedures common errors and correct 51 basic surgical operation experiment, and won the national "eleven five" focus on the planning of the Ministry of health medical video teaching material making project financial support, produced a clip type series of audio-visual materials, in 2011 February by people's medical electronic and audio-visual publishing house, the national issue copy is 500, applied widely, greatly improves the efficiency of teaching effect, laid a solid foundation for the improvement of teaching quality.

239.2.2.4 Excellent Course Teachers Live Video Teaching

Teacher teaching live video is an important part of the construction of high-quality video teaching resources, the Provincial Education Department of the national Ministry of education, is the focus of attention and the implementation of the work. The classroom video material input of tremendous power, therefore, in the selection of courses and teachers should be under foot, in order to make the classroom video finally formed the authoritative academic, artistic and appeal in form, with demand in the content, the final student love to see and hear, is students' Autonomous learning rare resource is the ultimate goal [12]. Of course, the construction of excellent course videos is a big project, has just started, national and provincial director of teaching department needs, formulate corresponding policies to promote this work to the in-depth development of. If the domestic high school credit can be mutual recognition, courses can be elected, subjects with levels of student textbooks unification into reality, students can independently from the network selection from teachers, school, learning process management and practice is still in the school where the school, so to promote the teaching resource fair, promote teacher resources benefit the majority of students have great benefits, the construction of classroom video will be on the right track [13].

239.3 Application of High-Quality Audio-Visual Teaching Resources to Meet the Teaching Demands Flexible

Nowadays, high-quality audio-visual teaching resources construction in expanding the scale, quality in improving the transmission of audiovisual material, wide application, convenient application, but efficient, and teachers' teaching and students' initiative of learning is inseparable [14]. Dalian Medical University in teaching practice, the use of audio-visual teaching science has achieved remarkable teaching effect. Surgical operation experiment teaching as an example: the series 'surgical operation experiment series (A, B)' and the material piece 'common mistakes in surgical operation' began in 2010 were scientifically applied to surgical operation experiment teaching, the students viewed the materials independently (experiment group), and the students viewed the materials by traditional method (control group). Students in the second classes of independent watch, even in the animal experiment of entity operation, also can at any time to watch the video viewing [15]; teachers in surgical experiment teaching, according to the students' practical situation, can take the small scope of operation guidance, also can use a wide range of video playback instruction, the experimental teaching process. Surgical operation in the process of experimental teaching, scientific application of rich audio-visual materials and its multi-faceted break up the whole into parts, it is its main characteristic; the leading role of the teacher play effectively, the subjectivity of the students are active to reflect [16]. The data were as follows: Table 239.1 statistics average scores of surgical operation between two groups in 4 years of clinical medicine specialty 7 years students of Dalian Medical University, Fig. 239.1 and 239.2 illustrates the scores and growth ratio of two groups. The chart shows the quantification of scientific application of high-quality audio-visual teaching resources to promote the higher grade overall learning performance, and promote the teaching quality of ascension.

Surgical operation experimental teaching is an epitome of reform of Dalian Medical University teaching ideas and methods of the teaching quality of Dalian Medical University, a comprehensive upgrade [17]. Figure 239.3 shows the national clinical skills contest finals score and ranking of Dalian Medical University from 2011 to 2013. The qualification examination in countries in 2012, the rate is higher than the national average of 7 percentage points, the results obtained

Table 239.1 The annual average performance and growth ratio

Grade and school year	2006 2008–2009	2007 2009–2010	2008 2010–2011	2009 2011–2012
Group	Control group	Experiment group I	Experiment group II	Experiment group III
Numer	219	285	271	349
Average performance(score)	80.89	86.50	89.80	84.70
Growth ratio(%)	–	6.93	11.01	4.71

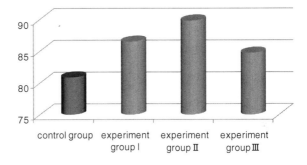

Fig. 239.1 Annual average grade

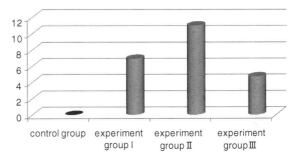

Fig. 239.2 Growth ratio of experiment group

with the Dalian Medical University attaches great importance to the building and Application of video teaching resources, deepening teaching reform, the overall quality of students is inseparable.

239.4 Conclusion

The construction and application of high quality medical video teaching resource is the higher education teaching reform to the important support of the deep development of educational administration; departments at all levels attach great importance to and support of policy, teacher team of experts, in-depth planning

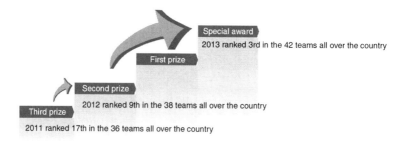

Fig. 239.3 The national clinical skills contest finals score and ranking of Dalian medical university from 2011 to 2013

study design, use modern educational technology professional team roles are important guarantee for the construction and application high quality medical video teaching resources. High quality medical video teaching resource is the design of teaching process, teaching resources and students' Autonomous learning. Practice proves that the quality of medical video sufficient teaching resources, the teaching of the first class and the second class learning would be handy, efficiency and quality will greatly enhance the teaching, students' professional skills and comprehensive quality will have a qualitative leap. To strengthen the quality of medical video teaching resource construction and application will be the long-term education theme.

References

1. Chao H, Jiaming C, Youqun R et al (2013) New trends of research learning under new technology. China Educ Tech 1:1–6
2. Ruqian T (2012) The construction of the community model of teacher internet learning. China Educ Tech 11:82–85
3. Haifeng L, Yonghua M, Yusi K (2013) The recent advances of learning scientific research. China Educ Tech 1:7–15
4. Young J (2002) Hybrid teaching seeks to end the divide between traditional and online instruction. Chron High Educ 48(28):33–34
5. Xu W, Guo G, Wei J (2004) Application of modern education technology. Science and Technology Press, Beijing, pp 173–202
6. Li L, Wang B, Zhang C et al (2011) The practice and experience of medical morphology in the second classroom. Chin Foreign Women Health 19(6):498
7. Bai Q, Li W, Chen B (2011) Research and design of blended learning based on resources. Mod Educ Technol 21(4):42–47
8. Yao P (2012) The construction and development of teaching resources in 'cloud computing era'. Modern Educational Technology 22(12):112–114
9. Chu W, Li L, Hao L et al (2010) The important role of teachers in the medical video teaching material construction. Chin Med Educ Technol 24(3):255–257

10. Chu W, Li L, Xu Z et al (2011) The research and practice of teaching resources reorganization by building a series of medical video teaching material. Exp Technol Manage, 28(6): 89–92
11. Chu W, Bai C, Xu Y et al (2011) The new trend of production and application of medical video teaching material. Res Explor Lab, 30(12):126–129
12. Wang P, Tian J, Jiang Q (2012) Research and countermeasures of open class problems in the construction of college quality video. China Educ Technol 11:86–92
13. Xu DR, Wei ZJ (2012) The construction and thoughts of video open class. Mod Educ Technol 2:54–59
14. Xu X, Zhou F, Wei M et al (2013) Application of constructing support theory teaching in pharmacology. Chin Med Educ Technol 27(1):28–30
15. Wu HJ, Bin TH et al (2012) Research on clinical teaching mode of medical image based on network. Chin Med Educ Technol 26(1):62–64
16. Yan Z (2013) Application of diversified teaching method in gynecology and obstetrics teaching. Chin Med Educ Technol 27(1):113–115
17. Gao S, Gao S, Liu L (2011) Analysis of suitability of constructivism teaching mode in medical education. Chin J Med Educ 31(1):9–11

Chapter 240
Research and Construction of Mobile Development Engineer Course System

Xiufeng Shao and Xuemei Liu

Abstract We begin to deep research aiming at course system about how to train mobile development engineer efficiently based on the mainstream Android platform in this paper, and build a set of comprehensive course modules and solutions. We build different course module and system for the different directions of mobile development engineer, train the design and practice capability based on Android mobile application development course by case and project teaching, provide evidence for training good mobile development engineer.

Keywords Mobile application development · Mobile development engineer · Case teaching · Project teaching

240.1 Foreword

More and more people realize the wide foreground of move internet industry, move application development produces at the same time. As free and open operation system, Android is welcomed by more and more developers. Android is main development platform with open source code, wide application, easy study and master by students and rich study resource. All universities begin Android course building and person train work.

New generation internet is considered as strategic industry based on mobile internet, it will be supported mainly by country policy and investment. We need huge person with ability with rapid development of mobile application industry. The company of communication needs person with practice experience, integrate technology, operation ability and good basis. Because it is rapid development of

---

X. Shao (✉) · X. Liu
Department of Information, Beijing City University, Beijing, 100083 China
e-mail: shaoxiufeng@bcu.edu.cn

the emerging areas of technology, the course system of universities is blank or incomplete and practical experience of teachers is lack. The person with ability exists gap between universities and enterprise.

At present, mobile development engineer includes Android mobile telephone software development engineer, Android mobile telephone game development engineer, Android software test engineer according to market research. We tell how to train mobile development engineer of society need according to ability point aim at above position.

240.2 Ability Point Sum-Up

The ability point of mobile development engineer as follows:

1. The development ability of Android mobile telephone software with JAVA;
2. Master Android system structure or some module, such as UI, Multimedia, OpenGL, network transport and so on;
3. There is a strong Java skills, familiar with Java development environment and libraries;
4. Cooperate work ability with others according to project plan.

The ability point of mobile test engineer as follows:

1. The ability of writing test case and finding design defect;
2. The ability of writing test plan, beginning test and giving analysis report;
3. The ability of tracing mobile telephone software defect;
4. The ability of changing test method and improving test quality;
5. The ability of knowing Android development flow and unitary thinks;
6. The ability of reading code;
7. The ability of writing test case and beginning test under the condition of shorting document.

240.3 Course System's Form

We get necessary course of Android mobile engineer according to above ability point, include base course (software engineering document writing course, JAVA application program course and so on), core course (J2ME system structure and program, Android mobile development course and so on), practice and real train course Android mobile(Android platform project and so on). Then we research period and check standard of all courses, make teaching outline and plan. At last we finish the course system of mobile development engineer (Fig. 240.1).

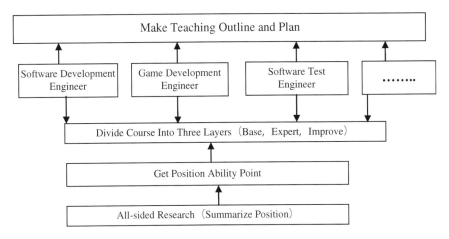

Fig. 240.1 Training process of the mobile engineer

The main course of mobile application development engineer includes three layers:

Base layer: computer basis train, program design (JAVA, C ++) and so on;

Expert layer: web program design (Asp.net, Jsp), Linux operation system, database theory (SQL_Server, Oracle) and so on;

Improve laye: Android mobile application development, mobile telephone test, project management.

We design two or three expert courses aim at mobile development engineer in improve layer. Then we begin expert improve course according to direction. At last, We begin Android advanced application development course aim at mobile telephone software development engineer, begin Android game development course aim at mobile telephone game development engineer, begin mobile telephone test case course aim at mobile telephone test engineer. The concrete period as follows (Table 240.1).

Our students study computer science, math basis knowledge, software engineering basis knowledge according to above flow. All of above include expert basis knowledge of high math, program design, data structure, operation system, computer network, database theory and so on. Our students get expert knowledge of software project management, software document write, mobile application program design and development, mobile telephone game design and development, mobile telephone test and so on. At last we train mobile development engineer that satisfy society need according to real train, practice and get expert competency certificate before graduate.

Table 240.1 Teaching schedule

Course class	Course name	Teaching hours	School time			
			The first year	The second year	The third year	The fourth year
Base	Computer basis train	30	Spring semester			
	C++ program design	60	Spring semester			
	Java program design	60	Autumn semester			
Expert	Asp.net program design	45		Spring semester		
	JSP program design	45		Spring semester		
	Database theory (SQL_server)	60		Spring semester		
	Operation system (Linux)	45		Autumn semester		
	Oracle database	45		Autumn semester		
	Mobile operation system	45		Autumn semester		

(continued)

Table 240.1 (continued)

Course class	Course name	Teaching hours	School time			
			The first year / The second year	The third year	The fourth year
Improve	Android mobile application development	60		Spring semester,	
	Write of mobile software document	45		Spring semester,	
	Project management	45		Spring semester,	
	Android advanced application development (Mobile telephone software development engineer)	45		Autumn semester	
	Android game development (Mobile telephone game development engineer)	45		Autumn semester	
	Design of mobile telephone test case (Mobile telephone software test engineer)	45		Autumn semester	
Practice, real train	Mobile telephone advanced application software development real train (Mobile telephone software development engineer)	45			Spring semester
	Mobile telephone game development real train (Mobile telephone game development engineer)	45			Spring semester
	Mobile telephone software test real train (Mobile telephone software test engineer)	45			Spring semester
Graduate design	Finish development and test works independently in each direction	200			Autumn semester

240.4 Teaching Method and Instrument

We tell teaching method and measure by Android application development course.

We use the combination methods of theory teaching, experiment teaching, case teaching, project teaching in this course. Our aim is to improve student's study ability, solute problem ability and adopt society ability.

Theory teaching is used to train basic concept and theory knowledge, developmental and broody problems are brought forward, and we analysis, discuss and direct students to solute problems by combining some cases, then teachers begin to sum up and demonstrate result or ask students to speak and demonstrate aiming at some knowledge point, then teachers begin to sum up. We change ago teaching modal, add course interest, focus student's energy and improve student's ability of analysis and solute problems.

We arrange relevant experiment after finishing main knowledge point every charter. We give experiment topic according to important knowledge point of every chapter, ask student finish by self, give more touch chance to students. Experiment period over 50 %. Aiming at the students with Android operating system handset, we require them to use real circumstance and deepen understand to experiment. Aiming at student's error, teachers direct after thinking by self. We improve student's think and touch ability by this method. Aiming at original experiment program, teachers invite it's owner to display and exploit student's program design think.

We begin project teaching after finishing every knowledge point of integrated part. At first, we give project topic and project requirement, then students are distributed by group, every group less than three person, mark every person divide the work, then ask students to look up datum after school and begin design work, we check and discuss a project in the middle of period. We arrange reply according to every person divide the work. We improve student's ability of using move application development knowledge point and team collaboration, ground for real project development by project teaching.

We use education investigate method and experiment sum up method during the teaching feedback research, that is investigate during students, know student's satisfaction degree and teaching effect and research exist problems and countermeasure. We regard practice experience conclude, sum and improve and conform all kinds of valuable theory and experience, impenetrate total teaching activity.

We use education investigate and questionnaire method during practice post feedback research and global move application development match research. We conclude the relation between professional skills and obtain employment post, analysis affect and effect of move application development between practice obtain employment post and program design match.

At last, we use the method of sum up experience, that is use this method to sum up successful experiment and solute exist problem in move application development course.

240.5 Conclusion

The user number of China internet gets the scale of a thousand million. There is a rapid increase in the future. The society needs a lot of mobile internet engineers. At present, the research of mobile development engineer course system is blank or incomplete in universities. The form of mobile development engineer course system with huge practicability and innovation, it can accelerate teaching intercommunion in universities, give huge contribution to innovate and train application person with ability, provide proof for training good quality mobile development engineer in our school and other universities.

Acknowledgments This paper is contributed by Beijing City Special Finance Fund (PXM2012_014202_000201).

References

1. Wang X (2010) Android move application development. Tsinghua University Press, p 03
2. Yang F (2010) Android application development unveil. China Machine Press, p 01
3. Zhang L (2010) Android move development case details. Posts & Telecom Press, p 02
4. He X (2009) Practice and research of Java program design elite course build. Mod Educ Sci (1):241-242
5. Zhang hongmei (2010) Think to high Java program design elite course build. Educ Forum, p 14

Chapter 241
Backward Direction Link Prediction in Multi-relation Systems

Wang Hong, Yuan Wei Hua and Zhou Qian

Abstract Recently, many researchers have been attracted in link prediction which is an effective technique to be used in graph based models analysis. To the best of our knowledge, most of previous works in this area have not explored the prediction of links in Multi-relation systems and have not explored the prediction of links which could disappear in the future. We argue that these kinds of links are important. At least they can do complement for current link prediction processes in order to plan better for the future. In this paper, we propose a link prediction model, which is capable of predicting backward direction links that might exist and may disappear in the future in Multi-relation systems. Firstly, we present the definition of multi-relation systems and put forward some algorithms which build Multi-relation systems. Then we give backward direction link prediction algorithms in multi-relation systems. At the end, algorithms above are applied in recommendation systems.

Keywords Multi-relation systems · Backward direction link prediction · Weight similarity · Personalized recommendation

---

W. Hong · Y. Wei Hua · Z. Qian
School of Information Science and Engineering, Shandong Normal University, Jinan 250014 Shandong, China
e-mail: 1456029328@qq.com

Z. Qian
e-mail: 442007728@qq.com

Y. Wei Hua (✉)
School of Computer Science and Technology, Shandong JianZhu University, Jinan 250014 Shandong, China
e-mail: 1456029328@qq.com

241.1 Introduction

More and more scholars have been attracted by the research of how to find unknown relationships from the existing relationships in networks, which helps people to understand and recognize something of the future. Link prediction in networks is a kind of method to solve this problem. Most of previous works in this area lay emphasis on the possibility of generating links between nodes based on information of nodes and structure of networks [1]. This method includes both the unknown links prediction and the future links prediction. However, in this paper, we put forward a kind of link prediction method called backward direction link prediction, which predicts the possibility of links disappearing among nodes in the future. As we know, an enterprise might grow or might decline. If using backward directional link prediction method correctly, the enterprise can take precautions to reduce losses and avoid failure [2].

In reality, complex networks are usually multi-dimensional networks in which relationships among objects are diverse. For instance, behaviors of people on the Internet generally are involved in several network systems such as film and television networks as well as reading networks. If each kind of networks is regarded as a sub-network system, the set of these sub-networks will constitute a multi-dimensional network, which is dynamic changed, or grow up or decay. The generation of new edges in the network indicates the emergence of new relations among nodes [3], and the disappearance of existing edges demonstrates that the mutual relations between nodes in networks no longer exist. It is undoubtedly very important for our future planning if we could accurately forecasted when and where a new edge emerges, an existing one disappears and a disappeared edge appears again between two nodes.

241.2 Dynamic Multi-dimension Networks

Definitions of some related concepts are firstly given as the foundation for the study of link prediction.

Definition 1 (Multi-relation Systems): supposing $V = \{V_1, V_2, \ldots, V_n\}$ is a set which is composed by nodes of n categories, in which $V_i(1 \leq i \leq n)$ is a set of nodes that belong to the same sort. $\forall v_i \in V_i, vj \in Vj \quad j = 1, 2, \ldots i-1, i+1, \ldots n)$, supposing a unordered couples (v_i, vj) indicates the edge between v_i and vj, then $W = \{ (v_i, vj) \mid v_i \in V_i, vj \in Vj, j = 1, 2, \ldots i-1, i+1, \ldots n\}$ is a set of all possible edges between any node v_i in set Vi and any vj in $Vj(1 \leq j \leq n, j \neq i)$, we call a network, which takes V as the node set and takes a subset of W as the edge set, a Multi-relation Systems, described as MS.

Definition 2 (Reduction-relation Systems): in definition 1 of Multi-relation Systems MS, with regard to $\forall p, q \in V_i$, supposing node sets and V_{jq} ($V_{jp} \subseteq V_j, V_{jq} \subseteq V_j$) represent respectively the set of nodes from $V_j(1 \leq j \leq n, j \neq i)$

241 Backward Direction Link Prediction

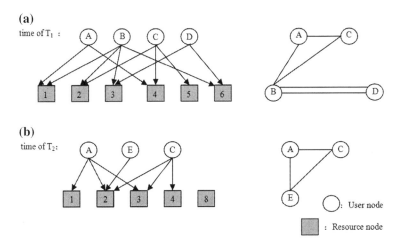

Fig. 241.1 Two-relation system and its reduction relation system

that has connecting edges with p, q. The condition for connecting points p, q is defined as if and only if $V_{jp} \cap V_{jq} \neq \emptyset$. A network is called a Reduction-relation System of MS, which takes Vi as the node set and has connecting edges mentioned above, which is referred to as RS.

Figure 241.1 shows the state of a MS and its corresponding RS at two different time points, in which one kind of nodes is defined as the object node while the other kind is defined as the subject node.

In Fig. 241.1, node A–E are subject nodes, while node 1–6 represent object ones, at time of T_1 the relationship network between subjects and objects and the corresponding reduction dimension networks are shown as (a); counterparts at time of T_2 are shown as (b). Comparing the network state at time of T_2 with that at time of T_1, we find that subject nodes B and D as well as object nodes 5 and 6 left, subject node E and object node 8 joined, and edges of the network changed simultaneously.

241.3 Backward Direction Link Prediction of Multi-relation Systems

In this section, the backward direction link prediction process of this modal will be carried out, which predicts the possibility of existing links disappearing in the future. The main thought is to change weights during the dimension reduction of the system, which means changing the original bigger weight into a smaller one, or vice versa. Then the Forward direction link prediction is conducted, and the outcome is the links that might disappear most likely in the future. The following is the algorithm.

Algorithm 1: Algorithm of the backward direction link prediction in Multi-relation systems.
Input: Multi-relation system and time sequence $T = \{t_1, t_2,...t_n,...\}, t_1 < t_2 <...t_n <...$.
Input: Multi-relation system and time sequence $T = \{t_1, t_2,...t_n,...\}, t_1 < t_2 <...t_n <...$.
Output: Link sequences of subject nodes that might disappear in the future.
BackwardLinkPrediction()
{MultiDimentionModel(); NetworkProjection(); SelectRelation(); DimensionReduction(); Get reduction relation systems called RS = (U, E, W); forEach ($w_{xy} \in W$) {$w_{xy} = 1 - w_{xy}$;}; LinkPrediction();
Put these similarity numbers in a list and sort them descending and get the first L lists}

241.4 Experimental Results and Analysis

There are about 1,496, 1,253 and 1,800 pieces of data in evaluation data sets of movie, TV series and songs respectively. After data processing, each dimension of the experimental data is described in a two-dimensional table, with the following structure as shown in Table 241.1.

In the experiments, each dimension corresponds to a type of project network. As the consistency of the users, the evaluation tables are joined according to userID, a foreign key, to generate the three-dimensional data table for each user.

Table 241.1 Evaluation table structure of users

Identifier	Meaning
UserId	User ID
ItemNum	Project category ID
ItemId	Project ID
Rating	Rating
Timestamp	Timestamp

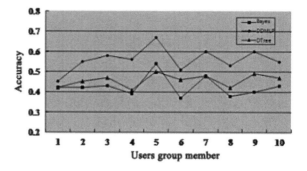

Fig. 241.2 Accuracy comparison

Data sets of users and resources in our experiments are randomly divided into a training set and a test set, with a proportion of 80 and 20 % separately. The training set is used to generate results of predictions and the test set is used to evaluate superior and inferior of recommendation results. Link edges were predicted based on the training set, sorting all the possible links in descending order by the value of similarities, and then extracting the first L pieces of links.

We consider the effects of dimensions to compare the backward-direction link prediction algorithms abbreviated as DDMLP with classic methods such as decision tree and Bayes. The experimental results are shown in Fig. 241. 2.

From the results, we can draw a conclusion that accuracy in DDMLP is higher than the classic methods of both decision tree and Bayes. However it should also be noted that execution time of DDMLP is longer than the other two algorithms.

241.5 Conclusions

In this paper we put forward a link prediction method which not only predicts future possible links but also predicts existing links that might disappear in the future. The experimental results show that it can provide better effects in link prediction of multi-dimension weighted networks. Further work mainly includes optimizing the algorithms and improving their efficiency.

Acknowledgments Supported by the Technology Program of Shandong Province under Grant No. 2012GGB01058; Graduate Education Innovative Projects of Shandong Province under Grant No. SDYY10059.

References

1. Getoor L, Diehl CP (2005) Link mining: a survey. J ACM SIGKDD Explor Newslett 7(2):3–12
2. Lin W, Chao S (2012) Research on link prediction in no-scale networks. Comput Eng 38(3):67–70
3. Allali O, Magnien C, Latapy M (2011) Link prediction in bipartite graphs using internal links and weighted projection. In: IEEE conference on computer communications workshops, pp 936–941

Chapter 242
The Innovation of Information Service in University Library Based on Educational Informationization

Liu Fang

Abstract Information technology has become an important and facilitating role in developing and reforming higher institute during the past 10 years. Higher education informatization has changed the traditional service mode of university library, and it has made information service more flexible and diverse. However, information service is still of low efficiency. Thus, university Library should explore more ways of information service by means of analyzing users, integrating, organizing and making full use of information resources in order to improve the information service of university library and its core competency.

Keywords Education informatization · University library · Information service · Core competency

242.1 Introduction

Higher education informationzation has become an important link in the global education modernization process, and it is an important indicator of measuring a country's level of education and even national competitiveness. Under the impetus of the strategy of rejuvenating the country through science and education, the Chinese government is active in the construction of higher education information technology. In January 13, 2012, the Ministry of Education issued a "Notice of the Ministry of Education to carry out the pilot work on the education informationization (teach skills letter [2012] No. 4)", to start the pilot work and deploy education informationization in nationwide, including 100 pilot undergraduate colleges [1].

L. Fang (✉)
Library of Jianghan University Wuhan Economic Development Zone, Wuhan 430056, China
e-mail: liufang_999@sina.com

As the storage of higher education information resources, university library masters advanced information technology and skills and the ability of information service. It is an inevitable choice to enhance the core competitiveness of the university library in the environment of the educational informationization.

242.2 Educational Information and University Library

242.2.1 The Relationship Between the Education Informationization and the University Library

The own characteristics of university library and the nature of its role determine that it is closely linked with education informationization. The core of education informationization is information technology, which in library has been fully employed. The university library has undergone a revolutionary change in aspects like workflow, service objects, service mode, and social functions. Continuous generation of new information technology, communication and network technology, high-density storage technology, virtual technology, multimedia technology promotes the library to change the traditional service model, and thus to seek information service innovation in depth. That is to say, the emergence and application of information technology has help university library and education informationization develop together and achieve outstanding results.

Information technology connects the university library with education informationization closely. Meanwhile, the support of the distinctive features of professional digital disciplines information repository group assists university library in achieving the effective connection among library resources construction, service innovation and the development of higher education information [2]. Nevertheless, since library information service faces the challenges of network and Information Union, it is necessary for the university library to seek the path of the innovation of the information service for the users' demand [3].

242.2.2 The Significance of Information Services Innovation in Education Informationization

Educational informationization, breaking through the limitation of space and time, provides teachers and students a comprehensive range of information services, a more reasonable distribution of educational resources, and a broadened way to receive information service for their teaching and research. Professional and personalized information service can provide users targeted information services and information support for more extensive and in-depth teaching and research activities.

242.2.3 Six Education Informationization Elements: The Basis and Guarantee of the Actualization of Information Service in University Library

Networks, information resources, the utilization and application of information technology, informationization personnel, informationization industry, informationization policies, regulations and standards are the six elements of the education informationization [4], and also the basis and guarantee of the actualization of the information service in University Library, as shown in Fig. 242.1.

University library must follow the informatization policies, regulations and standards when it offers information technology. It should adapt itself for the promotion and application of information technology, start the digital construction of educational resources using information technology, and make use of it to train a group of specialized talents as an information service reservoir.

242.3 University Library Information Service Innovation Paths

The innovative path of Information service of university library during educational informationization can be summarized as follows: librarians at first carry on the analysis to the user, allocate and integrate the relative educational information resources based on the demand characteristics of educational information of the

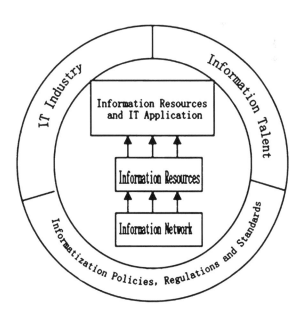

Fig. 242.1 Educational information six elements

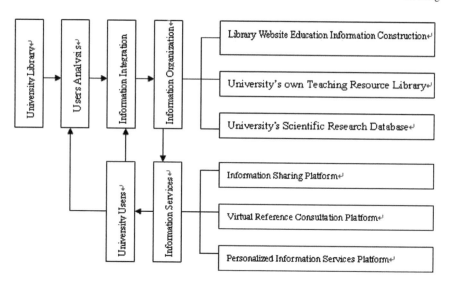

Fig. 242.2 University library information service innovation paths

user. Then, librarians organize information using effective information technology and information means. Lastly, they provide information services to users with information service in an appropriate way (Fig. 242.2).

242.3.1 The Establishment of Users' Information Database

User-oriented information service means that users are regarded as information service innovation co operators and innovation partners. Also, users are encouraged to actively participate in the information service innovation process. It is necessary, therefore, to carry on a preliminary analysis according to users' utilization of education information for different purposes. University Library's users can generally be divided into learning users, application users and research users. Based on the analysis of library user, university library can establish user information resource database, maintain close contact with users according to their specific issues and personalized environment, then establish customer service system in order to provide users with a variety of information service forms such as professional, personalized, diversified, integrated forms.

242.3.2 Information Resources Integration

Integration of information resources is a dynamic process. As time passes by and database is updated, university education resources has made innovation

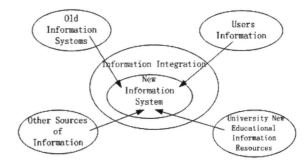

Fig. 242.3 University library knowledge integration modes

continuously with the ongoing teaching activities, Moreover, massive network of educational information resources has emerged. University library must integrate all kinds of educational information resources at any time, discard the useless or outdated information and integrate into the updated information, so that the whole information resources system is clearer, and more complete. When necessary, it can reconstruct the original information system, to form the core of a new information system as well, as shown in Fig. 242.3.

242.3.3 Information Resource Organization

Information resource can be organized favourably by constructing education information resources on library website, building university's own teaching resource library, and constructing university's scientific research database.

242.3.4 Information Services

The level of library's cognition of information needs of readers will directly affect the quality of the construction of information resources, the evidence of service settings, and satisfaction rate of user's demand. As a result, while facing of internal and external diverse user groups and a variety of information needs, the university library should make full use of information technology and information resources to provide a series of personalized information service for teachers and students by means of information sharing platform, virtual reference consultation platform, and personalized information services platform.

242.3.5 Feedback

After finishing such four aspects as the construction of the users database, the integration of the information resources, the organization of information resources and information services, a round of information services reaches an end. University Library shall analyze users' education information access and utilization, users' evaluation to information services and feedback to the librarian in time in order to enrich the education repository, and then begin a new round of user analysis.

242.4 Conclusion

Education informatization is not only the issue on education industry, but has an enormous impact on the development of national education and the enhancement of national quality. The involvement of University Library not only deepens the educational function and service function of libraries, and also makes education resources properly organized and fully employed. It raises the level of information service of university library, enhances the core competency of university library, and is beneficial to the promotion of the development of education.

Acknowledgments This work is partially supported by the National Social Science Fund of "Study on the Core Competency of the Library", China (09BTQ002). The author also gratefully acknowledges the helpful comments and suggestions of the reviewers, which have improved the presentation.

References

1. National long-term Education Reform and Development Plan Working Group Office (2010) National long-term education reform and development plan (2010–2020). China Education Daily, 30 July 2010
2. Chen H (2009) The optimization strategic choice to face the environment of the education informationization for the university library. Acad Libr Info Serv 8(2):1–4
3. Li Y, Sun X (2010) On the practical strategy and mode of library knowledge service. Info Doc Serv 1:74–77
4. Situation and development of China's education information (2013) http://www.it.hc360.com/scyj/zjlt/0108-1.htm. Accessed 18 March 2013

Chapter 243
Speculate the Teaching of Medical Microbiology Network Resource

Wang Hongying, Zhang Tao, Zhang Chuntao, Ma Haimei, Ding Jianbing and Ma Xiumin

Abstract According to the characteristics of medical microbiology, from the inevitability and advantages of network resources, namely, The mission of educates is not only just impart knowledge but more important is teaching students how to use modern measure and tools to acquire knowledge and to guide students to use the obtained knowledge innovation; Modern classroom teaching supplement and perfect sharing of teaching resources, beneficial to the development of the medical students' innovative spirit and quality. Conducive to teacher-student interaction and enhance the emotion between teachers and students. Motivate teachers to promote the improvement of the quality of teaching. We can better understand the medical microbiology knowledge by using network resources.

Keywords Medical microbiology · Network · Speculate introduction

Medical Microbiology is one of the most important subject in basic medicine and study the knowledge of clinical disease etiology, it is also one of the fastest growing disciplines in today's life science field. New knowledge, new theories, new pathogens are emerging and textbook pages are increasing, where as teaching hours are diminishing [1]. Network teaching is a kind of relationship between provider and educator in which use the internet and information technology as a medium and carrier, it has become the most vital mode of out side teaching [2]. To enable students to learn more effectively, review, self-study, as well as to carry out innovative activities. It is necessary to introduce network resources as a brand new teaching methods in medical microbiology.

W. Hongying · Z. Chuntao · M. Haimei · D. Jianbing
Basic Medical College, Xinjiang Medical University, 830011 Urumqi, China

Z. Tao · M. Xiumin (✉)
First Affiliated Hospital, Xinjiang Medical University, 830011 Urumqi, China
e-mail: maxiumin1210@163.com

243.1 Inevitability of Network Resources Teaching in Medical Microbiology

Due to the variety Microbial species are excessive, the individuals are small and knowledge is fragmented and complicated, it is difficult to memory. Now the teacher-centered classroom teaching pattern is used widely, in which teachers speak and students listen. This cause many students are not interested in microbiology study, also affect the enthusiasm of the students' self education innovation ability, in a word this kind of teaching method lack of education advocates the creation ability.

The mission of educates is not only just impart knowledge but more important is teaching students how to use modern measure and tools to acquire knowledge and to guide students to use the obtained knowledge innovation [3]. The powerful function of network technology seep into teaching methods, it also can leads the classroom teaching to the online teaching and can completely change the traditional way of teaching. Teachers are no longer the main part of teaching and should become a guider.

Students are the main part of the learning activities, their participation in the process of activities is the process of learning. The simple transfer of knowledge in classroom teaching converted to a new teaching mode in which teachers guide students how to learn, cultivate their self-learning ability and effectively improve the students' enthusiasm for learning, eventually training their information managing capacity and improve the comprehensive quality.

243.2 The Advantage of Medical Microbiology Network Resources Teaching

243.2.1 Modern Classroom Teaching Supplement and Perfect

Medical microbiology teaching material content is various, it is impossible to complete all the acquired outline teaching within the limited class hours. Classroom teaching as the main and combined network resources teaching after class, provide more flexible learning conditions and more extensibility of rich learning content for students, it is good for students students' self learning active motivation, meet the requirements of the different needs and different levels of students.

243.2.2 Sharing of Teaching Resources

Students can directly visit other domestic and foreign institutions by linking medical microbiology teaching websites, consult with each other and promote learning. Let the institutions to make full use of teaching resources, improve utilization level of teaching resource among colleges and universities rapidly.

243.2.3 Beneficial to the Development of the Medical Students' Innovative Spirit and Quality

Students can understand the latest progress and enrich knowledge of the discipline through the network resource, stimulate their interest in learning; Guide students to identify problems, research issues, self-search problems and summarize the thinking, temper the students' self-learning, analysis, judgment, and reasoning ability, can improve the teaching effect of the microbiology course also helps students to develop problem solving, self-learning and independent innovation ability, it can train information processing capacity and improve the comprehensive quality.

243.2.4 Conducive to Teacher–Student Interaction and Enhance the Emotion Between Teachers and Students

Teaching is a process of communication, positive interaction and common development between teachers and students. The communication and emotion participation between teachers and students in the teaching process is advantageous to the development of student non-intelligence factor, helps students to broaden their horizons, teachers can understand students' learning effect in time.

Students can take advantage of the network online BBS, expand intense discussions with schoolmates and teachers, give full play to students masters of spirit and mobilize students' learning enthusiasm, make teachers turn into a guider from just a knowledge imparter, provide conditions to develop students thinking ability and makes the classroom learning to continue and extend.

In the traditional classroom teaching, teachers exchange emotions through words, expressions, body movements, classroom communication, however, is limited by the teaching content and class hours. The QQ network platform, e-mail create the opportunity for teachers and students emotion cultivation. On QQ platform, in addition to discussion of learning, teachers and students can also exchange their own ideas, employment considerations and ideals, the emotional distance between teachers and students become closer with communication network.

243.2.5 Motivate Teachers to Promote the Improvement of the Quality of Teaching

On the network, such as micro-channel, QQ, MSN, E-mail, students will ask some questions they want to know, which is often related to clinical medicine, preventive medicine, laboratory diagnostic medicine and many other disciplines. Therefore as a professor of medical microbiology courses, in addition to mastering the expertise, should also grasp the relevant professional knowledge, in order to meet the expectations of students and learning needs. With the social progress and the development of education, every teacher should promptly grasp and track the dynamic modern educational thinking and technology, constantly update their own educational philosophy. In order to meet the needs of students, the community, the era, to become qualified teachers, they should posses comprehensive knowledge and overall quality.

243.2.6 The Effects of the Using the Teaching of Medical Microbiology Network Resource

See Table 243.1

243.3 How to Take Advantage of Network Resources

243.3.1 Use of Network Information

A wealth of network information resources, as well as a powerful search function, enables us to collect information through the network. By searching the relevant information, make students acquire the ability of judgment, screening with exercise. Through search engines (Google, Baidu, etc.), Searching for the information

Table 243.1 The result of the questionnaire survey in the using the teaching of medical microbiology network resource(%)

The questionnaire content	good	common	bad
Modern classroom teaching supplement and perfect	75.2	14.2	10.6
Sharing of teaching resources	89.6	10.8	0
Beneficial to the development of the medical students' innovative spirit and quality	67.2	25.3	7.5
Conducive to teacher-student interaction and enhance the emotion between teachers and students	70.4	20.6	9
Motivate teachers to promote the improvement of the quality of teaching	86.2	10.8	3

you need, Such as do not understand the concept, a biochemical reactions, microbial picture, teaching PPT courseware, the new progress of research, the discovery of microbes, microbial story, make it a new classroom resources and the auxiliary means of learning after school.

243.3.2 Use of Excellent Courses Network Resources

The Microbiology is a excellent course in our school. We have established "a microbiology of excellent courses website", in college network, many domestic colleges and universities have Excellent Courses website. Usually include course introduction, meeting times, details, the syllabus, courseware, teaching videos, experimental teaching, electronic lesson plans, self-test exercises and so on. Students can make use of access to relevant content of these sites, also playback PPT pictures after class which teachers teaching in the classroom, related to the teaching content and operation videos, illustrations, image explain, convenient and intuitive.

243.3.3 Use of Domestic and Foreign Related Websites

In addition to the Excellent Courses website, there are many professional and comprehensive websites contains the contents of Microbiology, the professional news, forums, online courses, foreign lectures resource, English microbial readings etc.; the foreign Microbiology network resources are richer, including the websites such as the department of microbiology in the university, the immune association comprehensive website etc. These sites update fast, can provide the latest information, results of the teaching and research of the microbiology. It also has a rich multimedia information and pictures available for download, convenient for the teachers and the students to learn the foreign microorganisms teaching experience.

243.3.4 Use of Network Interaction Platform

Teachers can use the modern method such as QQ, MSN, microblog, micro-letters and E-mail etc. publish their own teaching resources, each student can be arranged learning according to their actual situation, can make students easily do the followings: ① Students will sent the encountered problems in the learning to the teacher and teachers can also give a reply in time; ② They can share their knowledge and experience with netizens and discuss some hot issues, seek help or find what you want from learning materials. ③ They also can write their own learning experience, inspired ideas into the blog and share with friends. Therefore take advantage of the interactive features of the network, and a variety means of communication, can express their views on a particular issue, the exchange of learning, widely absorb the beneficial views, recognize from different perspectives, stimulate students' interest in the learning of medical microbiology; Teachers can also get feedback at any time, reduce teaching blindness, to achieve interaction between teachers and students, truly individualized and teaching and learning, continue to improve teachers' teaching level.

243.3.5 Use of Microbial Forum

The professional medical forum is a very useful tool, according to the different needs can obtain corresponding resources, such as teaching courseware, video, maps and literature resources. It also can be accessed online or download preservation viewing, students can, flexible and convenient to arrange their own learning time, which is the traditional teaching methods can not match.

In short, the use of network resources can improve the students' learning enthusiasm and broaden their horizons, stimulate students' potential innovative thinking, students can study in the practice, seek knowledge in the exploration, change the teachers "chalk and talk", to encourage students to independent learning, to better grasp the knowledge of medical microbiology.

Acknowledgments This work was supported by the fund project: teaching reform project of Xinjiang Medical University (YG2011051,YG2011036, YG2008006); National Basic Medical Experimental Teaching Center Teaching reform project of Xinjiang Medical University (201016,201004).

References

1. Cao, M, Pan W, Qi, Z (2007) Combination of traditional teaching and multimedia technology for medical microbiology. J. Shanxi Med. Univ.(Preclinical Medical Education Edition) 9:712–714
2. Wang W, An Y, Wen M et al (2011) Construction of a new e-learning teaching model of immunology by using network. China Med Equip 8:43–46
3. Yang C, Hou C (2010) Reform on opened surgical nursing experimental teaching based on the "network". Chin Nurs Res 24:2710–2712
4. Huang, X, Mo, B, Li, F et al (2010) The exploration and practice of network course in medical microbiology. J Xinjiang Med Univ 33:91–94
5. Wang, L (2005) Promoting english teaching by the affective education. J Inner Mongolia Agric Univ (Social Science Edition) 7:277–279
6. Zhang, X, She, F (2009) Application of QQ network platform in the teaching of medical microbiology. J Fujian Med Univ (Social Science Edition) 7:277–2

Chapter 244
Clinical Significance of the Detection of Serum Procalcitonin in Patients with Lung Infection After Liver Transplantation

Juan Guo, Wei Cao, Xiao Yang and Hui Xie

Abstract To investigate the clinical diagnostic value of procalcitonin after liver transplantation in patients with bacterial pneumonia. We divided 49 patients who operated liver transplantation into two groups, which were bacterial pneumonia infection group and non-bacterial pneumonia group. Extracted serums to detect procalcitonin and C-reactive protein, the difference of results were compared by ROC curve. PCT detection in patients after liver transplantation who complicated bacterial pneumonia showed a statistically significant difference ($P < 0.05$). CRP detection in patients after liver transplantation who complicated bacterial pneumonia showed no significant difference ($P > 0.05$), compared with patients with non-bacterial pneumonia. With the development of pneumonia, PCT of bacterial pneumonia group increased significantly, sensitivity and specificity difference were statistically significant ($P < 0.05$), compared with CRP. Procalcitonin was more sensitive to detect the development of patients after liver transplantation with bacterial pneumonia, compared with C-reactive protein, and provided better and rapid clinical diagnostic.

Keywords Liver transplantation · Pneumonia · Procalcitonin

J. Guo (✉)
People's Hospital of Zhengzhou, Zhengzhou, Henan 450003, People's Republic of China
e-mail: cynthiagj@163.com

W. Cao · X. Yang · H. Xie
Department of Clinical Laboratory, People's Hospital of Zhengzhou, Attached to Southern Medical University, Zhengzhou, People's Republic of China

244.1 Introduction

In recent years, the lung infection after liver transplantation is still a common complication after liver transplantation and the infection rate in early stage of transplantation centers abroad can reach over 80 % [1], which is a main reason for death in early stage after transplantation of the receptors. Once the infection happens, it is very difficult to control the infection, and multiple infections from bacteria, virus and fungi are likely to happen, causing difficulties in the choice of antibiotics in clinical practice [2–4].

Therefore, the diagnosis of bacterial infection in the early stage, to judge the seriousness of infection and to monitor the clinical treatment results is significant to raise the survival rate of the patients. Through monitoring the Procalcitonin (PCT) density in the serum of bacterial pneumonia patients after liver transplantation, and comparing it to the C-reactive protein (CRP) density, to discuss the clinical diagnosis value and significance of PCT monitoring in liver transplantation complicated with bacterial pneumonia.

244.2 Data and Methods

244.2.1 Clinical Data

Two hundred and sixty seven cases of allograft liver transplantation patients operated in our hospital from 2005 to 2011, including 49 cases of liver transplantation complicated with bacterial pneumonia. Common symptoms of patients with lung infection include fever, coughing, anhelation, chest distress, lung rale, or with low blood oxygen saturation from assisted mechanical ventilator in early stages after liver transplantation. With the development of the disease, all cases are with image diagnosis, that the chest X-ray or chest CT plain scanning all display flake or plaque invasive shadows of different levels, with or without pleural effusion. The pathogen diagnosis standard of bacterial infection of lungs is based on the clinical diagnosis, and in accordance with one of the following conditions: (a) the same pathogen bacterium is separated in selected sputum twice continuously, (b) pathogen bacterium $\geq 10^8$ cfu/ml is separated by pollution prevention sample brush or bronchoalveolar lavage in the bronchoscope or artificial airway, (c) the density of quantitative sputum culture $\geq 10^9$ cfu/ml.

244.2.2 Detection Method

The PCT detection is through electrochemiluminescence assay quantitative detection, using Roch 6000 automatic luminiferous instrument and the original reagents. The results are based on the assumption that from 0.00 to 0.49 ng/ml are negative and >0.50 ng/ml for bacterial infection. The CPR detection is through latex agglomeration tests, applying biochemical analyzer to test quantitatively.

244.2.3 Statistical Analysis

Using SPSS15.0 to analyze statistically, the statistical data form is mean ± variance. The comparison between statistical data groups is through t test of the two dependent samples, U-test for sensitivity and specificity comparison, χ^2test for enumeration data and statistically significant if $P < 0.05$.

244.3 Results

244.3.1 PCT and CRP Detection Results of the Patients Complicated with Pneumonia After Liver Transplantation

The detection difference of PCT of the patients complicated with bacterial pneumonia and non-bacterial pneumonia after liver transplantation is statistically significant ($P < 0.05$). The detection difference of CRP of the patients complicated with bacterial pneumonia is not statistically significant ($P < 0.05$) (Table 244.1).

244.3.2 ROC Curve of the Bacterial Pneumonia After Liver Transplantation Group

In order to judge the prognosis of the patients, receiver operator characteristic curve (ROC) is applied, to get the area under the curve and the 95 % confidence interval (CI). The first hemospasia is bordered with PCT 1 ng/ml, and

Table 244.1 Comparison of PCT and CRP in serum between two groups

Group	PCT(ng/ml) (t = 0)	CRP(mg/L) (t = 0)	PCT(ng/ml) (t = 48 h)	CRP(mg/L) (t = 48 h)
Bacterial pneumonia (n = 18)	1.45 ± 0.42[a]	41.8 ± 26.2[b]	2.80 ± 0.63[ca]	47.8 ± 28.9[bd]
Non-bacterial pneumonia (n = 11)	0.21 ± 0.07	36.2 ± 20.7	0.28 ± 0.09	37.8 ± 19.6

[a] $P < 0.05$
[b] $P > 0.05$ in the comparison of PCT in two groups
[c] $P < 0.05$
[d] $P > 0.05$ in the comparison of CRT in two groups

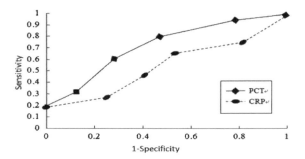

Fig. 244.1 ROC curves of PCT and CRP of bacterial pneumonia patients's first hemospasia after liver transplantation

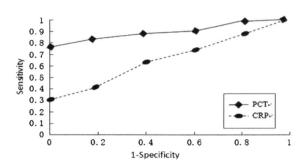

Fig. 244.2 ROC curves of PCT and CRP of bacterial pneumonia patients's second hemospasia after liver transplantation

the judgments of PCT and CRP for the patients are similar, but both with poor sensitivity and specificity. The second hemospasia is bordered with PCT 1.3 ng/ml, and the ROC curve moves upward significantly, compared with CRP, which displays that the detection of prognosis of PCT is superior to CRP (Figs. 244.1 and 244.2).

244.4 Discussion

The purpose of this experiment is to prove that PCT is a symbol in diagnosis of pneumonia and prognosis of the patients after liver transplantation. Compared with CRP, the difference in detection of PCT in patients with bacterial pneumonia and patients with non-bacterial pneumonia is more statistically significant. With the development of the disease, the rise of PCT levels in the bacterial pneumonia group is more significant. Considering that the sensibility and specificity are only 69 and 62 % for CRP in early stage fever of bacterial pneumonia, CRP cannot be an index to distinct bacterial pneumonia and non-bacterial pneumonia.

In comparison, the sensibility and specificity of PCT of the same stage reach 78 and 77 %, which is consistent with the Chinese and international literature. The sensibility of PCT in early stage of fever from bacterial pneumonia patients reaches 78 and 100 % after 48 h. As a result, PCT is superior CRP, in detecting bacterial pneumonia and non-bacterial pneumonia, and PCT can be applied as an index for the diagnosis and monitoring of bacterial pneumonia. The PCT level can evaluate the severity of the infection and inflammation, and to monitor the development, because it is an indication of severity of reaction from the immune system and the continuous existence of systemic inflammatory response.

If the level of PCT rises continuously in bacterial pneumonia, which means the inflammation is in the rising period, or the exacerbation occurs, and it is necessary to access further medical examinations such as pathogenic examination. If it is necessary, the treatment protocols shall be altered. On the other hand, if the level of PCT is lowered, the patient is on recovery and the inflammation and infection are controlled effectively, which is proved by experiments in this paper.

PCT levels can provide evidence for the empirical treatment of infection in early stage, and lower the misuse rate of antibiotic, in order to lower the death rate of the infected patients, thus to raise the survival rate of transplantation receivers. CRP has similar results, but the sensibility and specificity is not as good as the PCT. To conclude, the level of PCT in serum is valuable to the differential diagnosis of pneumonia, and is related to the severity of pneumonia, which can be applied to diagnose the patients of pneumonia after liver transplantation, and to guide clinical doctors in medication. In addition, it can be used as an index in early stage of judge the prognosis of the patients with pneumonia after liver transplantation and the observation of curative effect.

References

1. Schuetz P, Albrich WC, Mueller B (2011) Procalcitonin for diagnosis of infection and guide to antibiotic decisions past present and future. BMC Med 9(1):107
2. Broek MA, Olde Damink SW, Winkens B et al (2010) Procalcitonin as a prognostic marker for infectious complications in liver transplant recipients in an intensive care unit. Liver Transpl 16(3):402–410
3. Wang DM, Zhu B, Ding LC et al (2011) Usefulness of procalcitonin in the diagnosis of pulmonary infection in patients after renal transplantation. Zhonghua Ji Zhen Yi Xue Zazhi 20(5):524–527
4. Suberviola Cañas B, González Castro A, Holanda Peña MS (2009) Usefulness of procalcitonin in the diagnosis of infection in lung transplant patients. Med Intensiva 33(7):358–359

Chapter 245
Exploration of Teaching Strategies in Medical Network Teaching

Bing Li, Jian Tan, Zhi Dong, Chen Xu, Zhaohui Zhong and Xiaoli He

Abstract Medical network teaching, a new teaching mode combining network technology and modern medicine, has speed up the pace of training medical talents and promoted the development of medical education with the development of medical science and technology. This study aimed to explore the network teaching mode in higher medical education, to detect deficiencies in the current network teaching mode and to propose effective teaching strategies suitable for the situation of higher medical teaching network in China, thus further promote the development of the network teaching in higher medical education in china.

Keywords Medical education · Online education · Teaching strategies · Blended learning · Online learning

245.1 Introduction

As a new teaching method, online education has become a teaching mode of various colleges and universities generally adopted and extended gradually. Online education applied in medical education, has become a new form and important means of medical talent training, facilitating the development of medical education. However, as the Medical network teaching in our country has a lot of deficiencies, to explore and structure effective teaching strategies suitable for medical education which emphasis on both teaching and learning, and to improve the quality of online education meeting the requirements of the times, are important task of medical education in the new period [1].

B. Li · J. Tan · Z. Dong (✉) · C. Xu · Z. Zhong · X. He
Dean's office, Chongqing Medical University, No. 1 YiXueYuan Road, YuZhong District, Chongqing 400016, People's Republic of China
e-mail: dclibing@sina.com

245.2 The Characteristics of Medical Network Teaching

Besides the characteristics of autonomy, openness, sharing, interactivity, flexibility in online education, other outstanding features include: ① abundant medical teaching resources [2] the students can learn as much as possible through the multimedia teaching information as text, image, video etc. ② Virtual teaching environment [3] students' learning interest can be aroused by describing some of the boring content vividly and intuitively, allowing them to master the contents of human anatomy and the pathophysiological procedure of disease. Virtual teaching environment can also provide operating skills in physical examination and surgery, and so as to bring along qualified doctors.

245.3 The Form of Medical Network Teaching

Currently, the main forms of network teaching applied to medical education are the following in our country [2]: First, entering the class for medical academic education. Second, assisting experiment and practice teaching to improve the effect of experiment and practice teaching. Third, providing favorable conditions for continuing medical education and skills training. Fourth, building the sharing platform of medical research information through online exchanges. In specific practice, medical teaching mode through network teaching platform could be summarized as [4, 5]: teachers' leading mode, students' autonomous learning mode and problem-based inquiry teaching mode.

245.4 The Problems of Medical Network Teaching in our Country

245.4.1 The Problem of Building Teaching Network Platform

Firstly, it is the network teaching infrastructure issues, such as the very slow speed of network transmission. Secondly, autonomic learning resources are not relatively enough and the medical network courses or courseware development is not enough. Thirdly, it's the teachers' team issue that we need to cultivate some excellent teachers and technical management teams who can understand and adapt to the Internet culture and meet the teaching content, student needs and network technology. Finally, curriculum development is emphasized while ignoring the role of information technology teaching platform and the navigation system is not strong.

245.4.2 The Defects of Teaching Mode

Currently, the prevailing problems in network teaching are the followings: ① the teaching mode is single, ② the simplifying teaching content overemphasizing the present and interpretation is mainly a repeat of the specified teaching material content in the network [4], ③ the network teaching result in a lack of emotional interaction between teachers and students as well as students in the teaching, which is not beneficial to teaching emotional objectives and the cultivation of students' interpersonal skills [6], ④ lack of reasonable learning monitor and evaluation. Students' learning processes and learning effect are short of supervision. Evaluation is generally in the form of examinations or assignments, stressing the evaluation of the students' basic knowledge, and ignoring other capacity evaluation. The evaluation of teachers to students is more, lacking in students' self-evaluation and peer assessment among students.

245.5 Effectively Network Strategy on Medicine

245.5.1 Guiding Ideology and Theory

In new era, the training objective is to develop medicine talents processing comprehensive capacities for independent, critical and innovative thinking. At the same time, the request for medical training is establishing innovate scientifically long-term evaluation systems through building more free and harmonious inclusively environment for teaching and scientific research, which play a leading role in innovation culturing [7].

For guaranteeing and promoting the quality of online education, we come up with "effective teaching" should be our guiding ideology, so as to direct online education to be most widely application in medical education. "Effective teaching" is that the instructors abide by objective rules on teaching activities and achieve more teaching performances though fewer investment in time, material and financial resources, consequently, realize specific teaching goals and finally satisfy the need of social and personal education value [8]. The teaching theory of "dominant-principle", proposed based on behaviorism and constructivism theory, contends that we should incarnate both the didactically leading role from teachers and the cognitively main role from students and combine the merits of these two theories, and thus gradually become the main guiding ideology of online education [9]. The nature of online education which is equal priority on instruction and learning is a dialogue teaching respecting and developing subjectivities of teachers and students. In the process of online teaching, we should arouse the enthusiasm and initiative of teaching and learning and thus construct effective strategy which is equal priority on instruction and learning and ultimately stimulate the innovation and initiative of teachers and students, which is just a reflection of theory of "dominant-principle" and "effective teaching" and the demand for adaptation medical education in new era, simultaneously, the guarantee of promoting the quality of online medicine teaching.

245.5.2 The Strategy of "Effective Teaching" Equal Priority on Instruction and Learning

In conclusion, in the process of online medicine teaching, the strategy of "effective teaching" equal priority on instruction and learning can be summarized that we should take the theory of "dominant-principle and "effective teaching" as our guidance, and then make a reasonable integration of three kinds of teaching modes including teachers dominant mode, students autonomous learning mode and inquire mode based on problems and finally culture medicine talents fitting the need of medical training goal in the new period by means of blended learning making a combination of traditional teaching and online teaching. In this teaching strategy, the pedagogical practices can be performed through serious interactivities including among learners and teachers, learners and learners, learners and learning resources, teachers and teaching resources; interactivities among learners and teachers can be realized through making a combination of asynchronous interaction and synchronous interaction, the teachers leading role must be reflected by students subjectivity, which can be embodied at the same time, via the teachers leading role in the process of teaching [10].

In the study of network teaching at home and abroad, Coomey and Stephenson [11] summarized different learning strategies, they think that the network teaching can be related to four characters: dialogue, involvement, support, control and suggest a paradigm grid for online learning, there are four basic perspectives or approaches : ① learner-managed specified learning activities; ② teacher-controlled, specified learning activities; ③ teacher-controlled, open-ended or strategic learning; ④ learner-managed, open-ended or strategic learning. One can take in regard to network teaching and net online learning. According to the method of the first module: learner-managed specified learning activities, Jönsson [12] developed a web-based distance course in medical physics held for school teachers of the upper secondary level, achieved good results. It is suggested that the basic approach taken can also have applicability to the training of medical and nursing students. It most can manifest the strategy of "effective teaching" equal priority on instruction and learning that we have described. Combining with Jönsson's method and the specific situation of the network teaching of medicine in our country, we put forward the following implementation flow chart for effective strategy (Fig. 245.1).

Although it is not a simple matter to decide what strategy to adopt in planning medical network teaching and how to develop it, the paradigm system described above may make this task easier. The strategy of "effective teaching" equal priority on instruction and learning, has the characteristics of comprehensiveness,

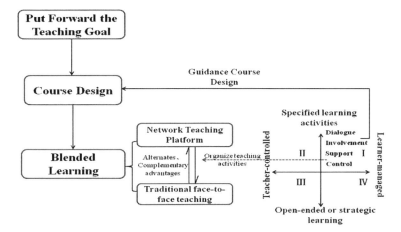

Fig. 245.1 A summary of the "online paradigm grid" for online courses suggested by Coomey and Stephenson [11]. In the first quadrant (*I*), the learning tasks (e.g. case studies) and perhaps also the learning goals are specified but learners have control of how they work towards and achieve the set. *Dialogue*: The teacher sets out the general responsibilities and procedures, but not participation. *Involvement*: Task-focused self-managed groups. The learner is able to relate or adapt tasks to his or her own circumstances and aspirations. *Support*: The tutor provides advice on the nature of the task, learning goals and so forth. *Control*: learner conducts tasks, variety of sources. T*eacher role*: Coach

operability, and flexibility, there should be a lot of ways to make it manifest, and each kind of model the implementation process, conditions are different. In the medical network teaching, how to organize teaching to give full play to the advantages of the strategy and to explore a set of optimization teaching mode which suitable for network teaching of medicine, still need educate workers to in-depth study.

References

1. Zhang L, Liu X (2010) Present situation and reflections on the teaching mode of college network in China. Mod Distance Educ 3:46–49
2. Sheng G, Yang R (2005) Application of network teaching in medical education. China Adult Educ 9:81–82
3. Ouyang Q (2008) Development of medical network-based teaching. China Med Educ Technol 1(22):28–30
4. Peng M, Zhang W, Xie B (2005) Design and realization of multifunctional web instructional platform based on three patterns. China Med Educ Technol 19(4):284–287
5. Zhang Liguo Liu Xiaolin (2012) Meta-analysis of the network teaching pattern research in colleges and both at home and aboard. Online Educ Distance Educ 4:40–46
6. Xu X, Yang X (2008) Present situation of network teaching in colleges and universities and countermeasures. China Adult Educ 7:132–133

7. Tang J, X Hu, Yao Y (2010) Characteristics of the times of medical education in the new century and the main features and trends. Mod Med Health 26(22):3513–3514
8. Jia L (2008) The enlightenment to college english teaching from effective instruction. J Taiyuan Univ 9(4):111–113
9. He K, Li K, Xie Y, Wang B (2000) Theoretical basis of "teacher-led-learner-centered" teaching mode. Audiov Educ Res 2:3–9
10. Li Y, Hu L, Shen Y, Liu G, Chang J (2010) Study on the evaluation system of teaching mode and teaching effect based on network environment. Northwest Med Educ 18(5):876–878
11. Coomey M, Stephenson J (2001) Online learning: it is all about dialogue, involvement, support and control—according to research. In: Stephenson J (ed) Teaching and learning online pedagogies for new technologies. Kogan Page, London, pp 37–52
12. Jönsson BA (2005) A case study of successful e-learning: a web-based distance course in medical physics held for school teachers of the upper secondary level. Med Eng Phys 27(7):571–581

Chapter 246
The Application of Information Technology Means During Clinical Medical Education in China

Ying Xing, Shu-lai Zhu and Chun-di Chang

Abstract In recent years, with the development of multimedia and network technology, the application of information technology means in teaching medical students and their learning is more and more widely used, but how to make the medical education informatzation working more effectively is still worthy to be discussed. In this paper, we discuss the present situation of clinical medical education in our country and the application of the clinical medical education informatization, emphasize on the role of information technology means in clinical teaching, in order to further promote the development of medical education and improve the quality of personnel training.

Keywords Clinical medicine · Informatization · Education · Application

246.1 Introduction

With the development of computer network technology and multimedia technology, the increasingly means of modern education technology provides the convenience for the higher medical colleges and universities to implement the teaching reform. Introduction of modern education technology in medical education can effectively solve the defect of traditional medical teaching means, such as deficiency of interesting and visual, simple of medical teaching methods, it is the implementation of student-centered teaching concept that can strengthen the cultivation of students innovation ability [1]. Today podcast, blogs, social network services, and social media are considered to be the update tool of clinical doctor education and the innovation of knowledge [2]. Therefore, it is of great importance

Y. Xing (✉) · S. Zhu · C. Chang
Department of Neurology, China-Japan Union Hospital of Jilin University, 130033 Changchun, China
e-mail: xingying1970@163.com

to promote the development of medical education and cultivate high quality medical talents by realizing the application of information technology in medical education. In this paper, we summarized the application of the current information technology means in clinical medical education in our country—China.

246.2 The Concept of Higher Medical Education Informatization

Higher medical education informatization is an important part of education informatization. In order to adapt to social requirement during teaching, scientific research, learning, management, logistics service, the institutions of higher learning using computer, multimedia and network communication which based on the modern information technology contribute to realizing the education information of the whole teaching process by building information application environment, integrating education resources, promoting and deepening the reform of the education teaching [3]. As an essential stage of the higher medical education, the core of the informatization of clinical medical education is the clinical application of information technology means and the essence is to enhance the quality of medical education, realize of the informatization of clinical medical knowledge, its final aim is to cultivate higher quality of medical talents.

246.3 The Application of Informatization in Clinical Medical Education

246.3.1 The Application of Education Informatization in the Theory Teaching

The part of the theoretical knowledge in clinical teaching need basic knowledge, such as anatomy, physiology, pathology, and so on. Through information networks, information collecting and organizing the related information can be produced to the multimedia way, combination of audio, video and graphic information transforms the teaching content of the abstract to a more intuitive information, on the premise of highlighting priorities, expounds related content from various angles, this way can interact with students and make them become the leader of the study, which breaks through the traditional model to achieve good teaching effects [4]. At present the ratio of clinical application of multimedia teaching are more than 95 % of the whole teaching [5]. With the help of the education informatization means, teachers have transformed their role from traditional knowledge to learning organizer and coordinator, they pay more attention to cultivate students' ability of self-study and access to information and knowledge. Besides that, teachers can make use of the Internet to virtual targeted design diseases, realistic scenarios, any changes in advance through the animation and demonstrate the whole process of disease development. Its advantage is the flexibility of time and space, it is a good way to follow the teaching train of thought, digest and think of the teaching content, at last to expand students' thinking ability. Combined with theory of actual treatment, plan is designed by students and the prognosis is put forward through the analysis of the illness. This approach greatly improves the students' interests in learning, get a more active advantage for students, and cultivate the ability to autonomous learning, expand their subject knowledge.

246.3.2 The Application of Education Informatization in Difficult Cases

In clinical works, we often face difficult cases. It is often time-consuming and sometimes can't get the right answer if just simply to find books, documents and other materials, small range of experience. But now, we encourage students to professional medical web site such as "clove garden", garden "image", on difficult cases discussion platforms, everyone can submit characteristic of detailed cases, results of relevant inspection, organize case discussions in the relatively wide range of areas through multiple nodes interconnected, learn the experience, opinion from different regions, the personage inside course of study at home and abroad, this can not only solve the problem, constantly improve related knowledge in the process of discussion, but also increase experiences, achieve resource sharing, greatly contribute to the information transfer [6]. In 2012, with this method, we confirmed several difficult cases and published in magazines which indexed by SCI.

246.3.3 The Application of Education Informatization in Clinical Practice

Clinical practice is an important part of clinical medicine education, it is the important period for students to integrate theory with practice, bridge basic medical knowledge and clinical practice and transform the state from students to doctors. The skilled operation skills, medical technology and the formation of the correct clinical thinking is closely related to clinical practice, therefore, clinical practice teaching quality is directly related to the cultivation of medical students quality. Based on a digital teaching auxiliary platform, Nanjing gulou hospital applied information management for clinical practice, greatly improving the students' learning efficiency [7]. However, current medical colleges with this condition is still few.

246.4 Insufficient Practical Application of Education Informatization in Our Country at Present Stage

There is no denying the fact that in recent years, informatization construction in Chinese clinical medical teaching has made a great achievement, there are a growing number of schools, teachers and students getting benefits from the informatization teaching. But due to various aspects reality factors and restriction, medical education in China still exist many problems and gaps compared to the development of higher medical education informatization degree of the western developed countries [8]. For example, at present, the proportion of domestic medical colleges and schools which can provide the complete online course is very low. The students access to knowledge link through several limited opened database in the school library, resource sharing between intercollegiate hasn't completely achieved. At the same time, in the wireless network, infrastructure networking technology, network transmission ability and coverage are still very low. Development imbalances between urban and rural areas, regions, schools still exist. There is a big gap in medical colleges and universities teacher's information technology application level, so the application ability of information technology teaching still needs to be improved, and so on.

246.5 Conclusion

In conclusion, in order to apply informatization technology to the teaching of clinical medical education better, the government needs to perfect network management system construction step by step, and gradually establish information feedback system, introduction of equipment and talents; establish a good network teaching system and network repository; it is necessary to cultivate large number of talents possess both a relatively high level of medical knowledge and better information technology. With the dominant of modern information technology, it is very important for the reform of medical education and the future development of the medical education in China, so as to build up a complete information system with technology diversity, digitization, networked, totalization, establishment of cooperatives and standardization.

References

1. Weidong C, Xuefeng H, Jing W et al (2009) Research on the construction of higher education informatization under the vision of scientific concept of development. Mod Distance Educ 12(6):24–27
2. Santoro E, Caldarola P, Villella A (2011) Using web2.0 technologies and social media for the cardiologist' education and update. G Ital Cardiol (Rome) 12(3):174–181

3. Guo-chao S, Lian-hong L, Shao-wu W et al (2009) Research and practice on clinical practice teaching mode of medical education. China High Med Educ 8:11–12
4. Jing-yang S, Wen L, Yuan-zhen Q (2011) The application of network teaching in higher medical education. China High Med Educ 11:111–113
5. Jun-li Y (2006) Discussion of the application of the network in medical teaching. J Shanxi Med Univ (Preclinical Med Educ Ed) 8(3):283–285
6. Chang-ming Z, Xiao-yan Z, Zhu Z (2006) Status of network teaching in medical education. China High Med Educ 3:43–44
7. Jianxun Z, Qi Z, Lin Z (2012) Present situation and the countermeasures of information technology support teaching in medical colleges. Northwest Med Educ 20(2):368–372
8. Wei-hua Z, Ya-li H, Yan S (2011) Implementation clinical practice based on curriculum and information. Acta Univ Med Nanjing (Soc Sci) 11(3):212–213

Chapter 247
Research Hotspots Analysis of Hypertension Treatment by PubMed

Hou Jinjie, Chen Lianqun and Li Ruiyu

Abstract The papers about hypertension in Pubmed were retrieved, and Medical Subject Headings (MeSH) in retrieved papers were analyzed (word frequency analysis, clustering analysis, co-word network graph), it suggested that the current hypertension treatment research hotspots had focus on angiotensin, vasodilator agent, calcium channel blockers, etc., also the most importance of which was the angiotensin.

Keywords Hypertension · Treatment · Word frequency analysis · Clustering analysis · Co-word network graph · Angiotensin

247.1 Introduction

Hypertension is a major public health problem worldwide, there are approximately 1 billion individuals suffer from high blood pressure worldwide [1], at present the research of hypertension treatment is mainly related to the research of various vasodilator agent, it has a great significance to pathogenesis and treatment of hypertension. We hope that through this research the analysis of the Medical Subject Headings (MeSH) can draw the outline of hypertension treatment research hotspot. Therefore this research retrieved the hypertension papers of PubMed

---

H. Jinjie · C. Lianqun
Xingtai Medical College, No. 618 Gangtiebei Road, Xingtai, Hebei Province, China
e-mail: wein871@sohu.com

L. Ruiyu (✉)
Second Affiliated Hospital of Xingtai Medical College, No. 618 Gangtiebei Road, Xingtai, Hebei Province, China
e-mail: liruiyu651021@163.com

(http://www.ncbi.nlm.nih.gov/pubmed) within recent 5 years, got 79,825 papers, and analyzed MeSH of above papers using Co-word Analysis [2].

247.2 Materials and Methods

First, we retrieved PubMed papers with publication dates between 1 January 2008 and 15 November 2012. Second, search terms was "hypertension" [MeSH Terms] OR "hypertension" [All Fields] OR "high blood pressure" [All Fields]. Third, using Microsoft Excel we recorded All MeSH terms of above papers, and sort and filter the terms, and looked for the high frequency terms (occurrences), and we also counted occurrences of two high frequency terms together in the same paper, setting up the original co-word matrix. Fourth, the statistical analysis: we made MeSH term's clustering analysis using SPSS13.0 statistical software, draw the co-word network graph of the high frequency terms using Cytoscape software [3].

247.3 MeSH Terms Analysis of Papers About Hypertension

247.3.1 MeSH Terms Word Frequency Analysis

We retrieved 79,825 papers, among them we got 68,183 papers with MeSH terms, we extracted MeSH terms and established the MeSH terms database. We got 22 MeSH terms of treatment which occurrences frequency was over 390 (including 390). From Table 247.1, we can infered some ideas: the relevant research of hypertension treatment hotspots mainly concentrated in the angiotensin, vasodilator agent, calcium channel blockers, etc., it also suggests that angiotensin has become hypertension treatment most major research hotspots.

247.3.2 Clustering Analysis of the High Frequency MeSH Terms

This research used hierarchical clustering analysis which is one of the most commonly used Classify analysis to analyze the above 22 MeSH terms, drew a dendrogram, and the results were shown in Fig. 247.1.

From Fig. 247.1, in addition to individual MeSH term as "Amides; Vasodilator Agents; Natriuretic Peptide, Brain; Patient Education as Topic", we could seen the other high frequency MeSH terms could be divided into the following five groups. Group 1 contains MeSH terms (Tetrazoles; Imidazoles; Angiotensin II Type 1

Table 247.1 The top 22 MeSH terms about hypertension treatment

Ranking	MeSH terms	Occurrences frequency (times)
1	Angiotensin-converting enzyme inhibitors	1782
2	Angiotensin II type 1 receptor blockers	1611
3	Angiotensin II	1267
4	Vasodilator agents	1135
5	Calcium channel blockers	1080
6	Tetrazoles	1036
7	Adrenergic beta-antagonists	909
8	Diet	770
9	Diuretics	750
10	Nitric oxide synthase type III	700
11	Sodium chloride, dietary	655
12	Amlodipine	640
13	Antioxidants	636
14	Benzimidazoles	630
15	Natriuretic peptide, brain	563
16	Losartan	520
17	Hydrochlorothiazide	506
18	Imidazoles	496
19	Alcohol drinking	479
20	Patient education as topic	469
21	Amides	428
22	Angiotensin receptor antagonists	390

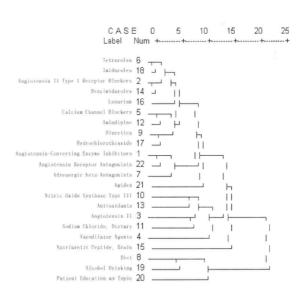

Fig. 247.1 Hierarchical clustering analysis dendrogram of MeSH terms

Receptor Blockers; Benzimidazoles; Losartan; Calcium Channel Blockers; Amlodipine; Diuretics; Hydrochlorothiazide), it suggests that angiotensin receptor blockers (mostly as imidazoles antihypertensive drugs, a representative of the Losartan, Eprosartan, benzimidazole), and calcium channel blockers (amlodipine), diuretic (hydrochlorothiazide) are commonly antihypertensive drugs. Group 2 contains MeSH terms (Angiotensin-Converting Enzyme Inhibitors; Angiotensin Receptor Antagonists; Adrenergic beta-Antagonists), it suggests that angiotensin converting enzyme inhibitors (ACEI), angiotensin receptor antagonist and adrenergic beta receptor antagonists are antihypertensive drugs about Renin-angiotensin System. Group 3 contains MeSH terms (Nitric Oxide Synthase Type III; Antioxidants), it suggests that Nitric oxide synthase [4] and antioxidants (vitamin C, E) [5] are new kind antihypertensive drugs. Group 4 contains MeSH terms (Angiotensin II; Sodium Chloride, Dietary), it suggests that High nacl diet can increase angiotensin [6]. Group 5 contains MeSH terms (Diet; Alcohol Drinking), it suggests that Long-term drinking is bad for hypertension. The above clustering results suggest that several MeSH terms within one group have certain inherent logic connection between eachother; If there are no known correlation between the MeSH terms, it indicates we find a new research hotspot.

247.3.3 Co-word Network Graph of the High Frequency MeSH Pair

By analyzing MeSH terms of the top 12 (word frequency), we got the top 5 MeSH terms pair (A and B, see Table 247.2) and co-word network graph of the MeSH terms pair (see Fig. 247.2). Especially the first MeSH terms pair of Angiotensin II Type 1 Receptor Blockers and Tetrazoles appeared 1,168 times in the same paper, it was far higher than that of the second MeSH terms pair (545 times, Angiotensin-Converting Enzyme Inhibitors and Angiotensin II Type 1 Receptor Blockers).

Table 247.2 The top 5 MeSH terms pair

Ranking	MeSH terms A	MeSH terms B	Co-word occurrences frequency (times)
1	Angiotensin II type 1 receptor blockers	Tetrazoles	1168
2	Angiotensin-converting enzyme inhibitors	Angiotensin II type 1 receptor blockers	545
3	Angiotensin-converting enzyme inhibitors	Calcium channel blockers	349
4	Calcium channel blockers	Amlodipine	276
5	Angiotensin II type 1 receptor blockers	Calcium channel blockers	264

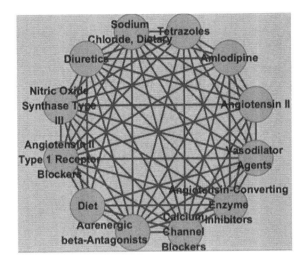

Fig. 247.2 Co-word network graph of the high frequency MeSH terms pair

In Fig. 247.2 the edge represents the concurrence relationship between MeSH terms pair and if the edge between one MeSH term to other MeSH term, it suggests that the one MeSH term is more important, it is in the center of the research hotspots. So we could infer that Angiotensin receptor blockers (Tetrazoles: losartan and Eprosartan as a representative) are the research hotspots now.

247.4 Concluding Remarks

By analyzing MeSH terms (word frequency analysis, clustering analysis, co-word network graph) of PubMed papers about hypertension, we could infer that the current Hypertension treatment research hotspots had focus on angiotensin, vasodilator agent, calcium channel blockers, etc., also the most importance of which was the angiotensin.

References

1. Chobanian AV, Bakris GL, Black HR et al (2003) The seventh report of the joint national committee on prevention, detection, evaluation, and treatment of high blood pressure: the JNC 7 report. JAMA 289(19):2560–2572
2. Viedma-Del-Jesus MI, Perakakis P, Muñoz MÁ et al (2011) Sketching the first 45 years of the journal Psychophysiology (1964–2008): a co-word-based analysis. Psychophysiology 48(8):1029–1036
3. Lopes CT, Franz M, Kazi F et al (2010) Cytoscape web: an interactive web-based network browser. Bioinformatics 26(18):2347–2348

4. Kayhan FE, Koldemir M, Cagatay P et al (2013) Prevalence of endothelial nitric oxide synthase E298D polymorphism in Turkish patients with essential hypertension. Diabetes Metab Syndr 7(1):12–16. doi:10.1016/j.dsx.2013.02.001
5. Vasdev S, Stuckless J, Richardson V (2011) Role of the immune system in hypertension: modulation by dietary antioxidants. Int J Angiol 20(4):189–212
6. Castañeda-Bueno M, Gamba G (2012) Mechanisms of sodium-chloride cotransporter modulation by angiotensin II. Curr Opin Nephrol Hypertens 21(5):516–522

Chapter 248
Research Hotspots Analysis of Hepatitis Receptor by PubMed

Hou Jinjie and Li Ruiyu

Abstract The papers about Hepatitis in Pubmed were retrieved, and Medical Subject Headings (MeSH) in retrieved papers were analyzed (word frequency analysis, clustering analysis, co-word network graph), it suggested that the current Hepatitis receptor research focus had focus on Programmed Cell Death Receptor, Tumor Necrosis Factor Receptor, Interleukin Receptor, also the most important of which was the Programmed Cell Death Receptor, the current hypertension ligand research focus had focus on making Antiviral Agents (Interferon-alpha) by Recombinant Proteins.

Keywords Hepatitis · Receptor · Word frequency analysis · Clustering analysis · Co-word network graph · Programmed cell death receptor

248.1 Introduction

There are about two billion people around the world who have been infected with the hepatitis b virus, including more than 350 million people suffering from chronic infection, 500,000–700,000 people each year die from hepatitis b virus infection. About 130–170 million people have been infected with chronic hepatitis c virus (HCV), an estimated 350,000 people have died of liver disease associated with hepatitis c [1]. At present the fundamental research of Hepatitis is mainly related to the research of receptor and ligand, it has a great significance to pathogenesis and

H. Jinjie
Xingtai Medical College, No. 618 Gangtiebei Road, Xingtai, Hebei, China
e-mail: wein871@sohu.com

L. Ruiyu (✉)
Second Affiliated Hospital of Xingtai Medical College, No. 618 Gangtiebei Road, Xingtai, Hebei, China
e-mail: liruiyu651021@163.com

treatment of Hepatitis. We hope that through this research the analysis of the Medical Subject Headings (MeSH) can draw the outline of Hepatitis receptors research hotspot. Therefore this research retrieved the hepatitis papers of PubMed (http://www.ncbi.nlm.nih.gov/pubmed) within recent 5 years, got 21,786 papers, and analyzed MeSH of above papers using Co-word Analysis [2].

248.2 Materials and Methods

First, we retrieved PubMed papers with publication dates between 27 February 2008 and 27 February 2013. Second, search terms was "Hepatitis"[Mesh] AND ("2008/02/27"[PDat] : "2013/02/27"[PDat]). Third, using Microsoft Excel we recorded All MeSH terms of above papers, and sort and filter the terms, and looked for the high frequency terms (occurrences), and we also counted occurrences of two high frequency terms together in the same paper, setting up the original co-word matrix. Fourth, the statistical analysis: we made MeSH term's clustering analysis using SPSS13.0 statistical software, draw the co-word network graph of the high frequency terms using Cytoscape software [3].

248.3 MeSH Terms Analysis of Papers about Hepatitis

248.3.1 MeSH Terms Word Frequency Analysis

We retrieved 21,786 papers, every paper has MeSH terms, we extracted MeSH terms and established the MeSH terms database. We got 11 MeSH terms of receptor which occurrences frequency was over 23 (including 23), We also got 11 MeSH terms of ligand which occurrences frequency was over 431 (including 431), which self and which derivatives may do ligand, and was a specific chemical or drug name. From Table 248.1, we can infered some ideas: the relevant research of hepatitis receptor hotspots mainly concentrated in the Programmed Cell Death Receptor, Tumor Necrosis Factor Receptor, Interleukin Receptor, etc, it also suggests that Programmed Cell Death Receptor has become hepatitis receptor most major research hotspots.

248.3.2 Clustering Analysis of the High Frequency MeSH Terms

This research used hierarchical clustering analysis which is one of the most commonly used Classify analysis to analyze the above 20 MeSH terms (Receptor

Table 248.1 The top 11 MeSH terms about receptor

Ranking	MeSH terms	Occurrences frequency(times)
1	Programmed cell death 1 receptor	76
2	Receptors, tumor necrosis factor	57
3	Interleukin-2 receptor alpha subunit	49
4	Toll-like receptor 4	46
5	Toll-like receptors	43
6	Receptors, virus	33
7	Receptor, interferon alpha–beta	30
8	Toll-like receptor 2	26
9	Receptors, KIR	25
10	Interleukin-7 receptor alpha subunit	24
11	Receptors, CCR5	23

Table 248.2 The top 11 MeSH terms about ligand

Ranking	MeSH terms	Occurrences frequency(times)
1	Antiviral agents	5,579
2	Interferon-alpha	2,729
3	Ribavirin	2,322
4	Recombinant proteins	2,267
5	Polyethylene glycols	2,022
6	Alanine transaminase	1,040
7	Interferons	620
8	Immunosuppressive agents	589
9	Organophosphonates	514
10	Adenine	511
11	Interleukins	431

related MeSH terms top 10 and ligand related MeSH terms top 10), Table 248.2 drew a dendrogram, and the results were shown in Fig. 248.1.

From the Fig. 248.1, in addition to individual MeSH term as "Receptors, KIR; Receptors, Virus; Polyethylene Glycols; Ribavirin", we could seen the other high frequency MeSH terms could be divided into the following five groups. Group 1 contains MeSH terms (Organophosphonates; Adenine; Alanine Transaminase), it suggests that Organophosphonates and Adenine are relate to reducing Alanine Transaminase [4]. Group 2 contains MeSH terms (Receptors, Tumor Necrosis Factor; Immunosuppressive Agents), it suggests that Tumor Necrosis Factor α antagonist is new Immunosuppressive Agents [5]. Group 3 contains MeSH terms (Recombinant Proteins; Interferon-alpha; Antiviral Agents), it suggests that Interferon-alpha and Antiviral Agents are usually made by use of recombinant protein technolog. Group 4 contains MeSH terms (Receptor, Interferon alpha–beta; Interferons), it suggests that Interferon Receptor can specifical combined with interferon. Group 5 contains MeSH terms (Toll-Like Receptor 4; Toll-Like Receptor 2; Toll-Like Receptors), it suggests that they all are same Kind of

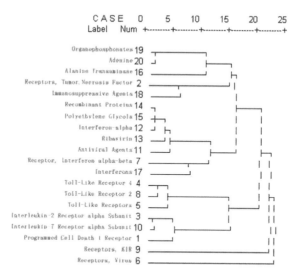

Fig. 248.1 Hierarchical clustering analysis dendrogram of MeSH terms

receptors. Group 6 contains MeSH terms (Interleukin-2 Receptor alpha Subunit; Interleukin-7 Receptor alpha Subunit; Programmed Cell Death 1 Receptor), it suggests that Interleukins factors are key regulators of cell apoptosis [6]. The above clustering results suggest that several MeSH terms within one group have certain inherent logic connection between eachother; If there are no known correlation between the MeSH terms, it indicates we find a new research hotspot.

248.3.3 Co-word Network Graph of the High Frequency MeSH Pair

By analyzing receptor MeSH terms of the top 10 (word frequency) and ligand MeSH terms of the top 10 (word frequency), which totalled 20, we got the top five MeSH terms pair (A and B, see Table 248.3) and co-word network graph of the

Table 248.3 The top five MeSH terms pair

Ranking	MeSH terms A	MeSH terms B	Co-word occurrences frequency (times)
1	Antiviral agents	Interferon-alpha	2,403
2	Antiviral agents	Ribavirin	2,154
3	Interferon-alpha	Recombinant proteins	2,133
4	Antiviral agents	Recombinant proteins	2,005
5	Interferon-alpha	Polyethylene glycols	1,969

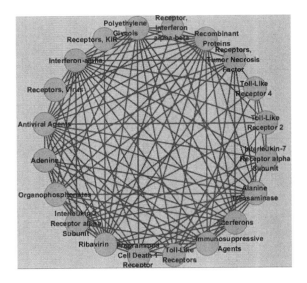

Fig. 248.2 Co-word network graph of the high frequency MeSH terms pair

MeSH terms pair (see Fig. 248.2). Especially the first MeSH terms pair of Antiviral Agents and Interferon-alpha appeared 2,403 times in the same paper, it was far higher than that of the second MeSH terms pair (2,154 times, Antiviral Agents and Ribavirin).

In Fig. 248.2 the edge represents the concurrence relationship between MeSH terms pair and if the edge between one MeSH term to other MeSH term, it suggests that the one MeSH term is more important, it is in the center of the research hotspots. So we could infer that making Antiviral Agents (Interferon-alpha) by Recombinant Proteins is the hypertension ligand research hotspots now.

248.4 Concluding Remarks

By analyzing MeSH terms (word frequency analysis, clustering analysis, co-word network graph) of PubMed papers about hepatitis, we could infer that the current Hepatitis receptor research focus had focus on Programmed Cell Death Receptor, Tumor Necrosis Factor Receptor, Interleukin Receptor, also the most important of which was the Programmed Cell Death Receptor, the current hypertension ligand research focus had focus on making Antiviral Agents (Interferon-alpha) by Recombinant Proteins.

References

1. Marcellin P (2009) Hepatitis B and hepatitis C in 2009. Liver Int 29:1–8
2. Viedma-Del-Jesus MI, Perakakis P, Muñoz MÁ et al (2011) Sketching the first 45 years of the journal Psychophysiology (1964–2008): a co-word-based analysis. Psychophysiology 48(8):1029–1036
3. Lopes CT, Franz M, Kazi F et al (2010) Cytoscape web: an interactive web-based network browser. Bioinformatics 26(18):2347–2348
4. Tang Z, Liu P, Ma C et al (2011) Molecular beacon based bioassay for highly sensitive and selective detection of nicotinamide adenine dinucleotide and the activity of alanine aminotransferase. Anal Chem 83(7):2505–2510. doi:10.1021/ac102742k
5. Mahlmann A, Pfluecke C, Ouda A et al (2012) Combined immunosuppressive therapy including a TNF-alpha blocker induces remission in a difficult to treat patient with Takayasu arteriitis and coronary involvement. Vasa 41(6):451–457. doi:10.1024/0301-1526/a000236
6. Yin Y, Liu W, Ji G et al (2013) The essential role of p38 MAPK in mediating the interplay of oxLDL and IL-10 in regulating endothelial cell apoptosis. Eur J Cell Biol pii: S0171-9335(13)00019-8. doi: 10.1016/j.ejcb.2013.01.001 (Epub ahead of print)

Chapter 249
The Application of Information Technology in Modern Sports Teaching

Xiao Hong Li and Tuan Ting Zhang

Abstract The development of education depends on the support of science and technology. The development of information technology brought a profound change to education thought patterns and methods. With the development of information technology, multimedia technology provides a new means of teaching in physical education teaching for the school, which not only deepen the students' understanding of techniques, but also have obvious promoting effect on students' sports skills, thinking ability and learning interest. So under the environment of the increasing popularity of the information technology, school sports teaching should continuously strengthen the application of information technology, improve the level of informationization, which can promote the further development of college PE teaching management.

Keywords Information technology · Sports teaching · Intuitive feelings · Interest · Application

Informationization is an important trend for the world's economic and social development. Since the 1990s, with the rising popularity of multimedia technology and Internet, information technology is changing the human society production mode, working way, life and learning style. The application ability of information acquisition, analysis and processing will serve as one of the most basic quality symbols of modern people. In the field of education teaching, changing with the development of information technology, teachers and the students' thinking [2], behavior mode (including education teaching mode, learning mode) and so on are deep affected, at the same time, information technology also affects the reform of

---

X. H. Li (✉) · T. T. Zhang
Department of Physical Education, Xi'an University of Architecture and Technology,
Xi'an 710055, China
e-mail: lxh112130@163.com

T. T. Zhang
e-mail: hxztt718@126.com

school physical education teaching. Now the application of modern information technology in sports teaching in colleges and universities, has become a hot spot of school physical education teaching reform. Physical education is not an exception, through the multimedia images, animation, video, voice, etc., intuitive display, which not only deepen the students understanding of techniques, but also can learn more basic knowledge in the limited time, which has played a good role in improving students' sports skills, developing thinking ability and inspire their learning interest and arousing the learning enthusiasm. Therefore, reasonable use of information technology in sports teaching can make the students keep the nervous system excitability in different stimulus, and grasp sports skills, improve the quality of teaching, broaden students' vision, and promote students' development of personality in a relaxed and lively atmosphere.

249.1 Reflect the Teaching Content Intuitively

Traditional sports teaching means teachers' demonstration, students' imitation, which make the sports teaching dull, and the use of information technology will bring a brand-new teaching environment to physical education teaching. In sports teaching software transformation of the teaching scene, superposition of sound effect, the processing of animation effect, which will immediately make the students energetic and active in high spirits, arouse the students' strong desire of seeking knowledge. Such as in indoor class we can let the students enjoy some wonderful sports games or courseware through two-way control system of the information electronic teaching, make silent teaching materials audio and visual, static and dynamic, take students into a pleasant atmosphere; in practice part, such as learning basketball technology [1], we can organize students to watch the VCD album "Flying Jordan" in indoor gym class, in which Jordan' unusual bounce, quick cuts, long time action in the air, pretty dunk and rapid aerial intercepting, make students dizzying and cheerful. By appreciating that they know Jordan's successful experience, they will understand that if you want to accomplish something in some field you have to pay hard, this has inspired students to love basketball and take interest in sports. Bright images, vivid picture and wonderful sound in multimedia can effectively arouse students' visual senses, arouse the students' learning enthusiasm, and make students get the pleasure of body and mind, experience the fun of sports, enjoy the lofty "sports spirit", easy to stimulate students' interest, to guide students to take part in sports activities actively. Using information technology to assist teaching in the process of sports teaching [6], in essence, is a kind of novelty stimulus to students, aiming at inducing students to explore the reflection of extraneous stimulus, in other words, to use novel teaching methods to stimulate students' learning interest.

249.2 Help to Regulate Technical Action

Clear action image is the important foundation of forming ability, which comes from the teacher's explanation, demonstration. Some techniques in sports teaching process are difficult to use words to describe clearly, especially some the instantaneous technology is more, detail explanation is difficult, demonstration effect is unsatisfactory. If Information technology assisted teaching is used in teaching, with the aid of teaching courseware the whole technical movement, including complete action and decomposition action pre-recorded by teachers will be shown beside the corresponding action in text interpretation on screen. According to teaching needs teachers can choose repeat play and repeated interpretation. In this way, students can form clear and complete technical movements in the brain. They will be more active to practice and grasp the behavioral essentials faster.

For example, in the teaching of the goat straddle vault, the teacher's demonstration is only a complete and consecutive technique action [6], which can not stay in the air to let the students see the action in the air. For beginners, such a demonstration in the brain can only be broken fuzzy impression, which is bad for their learning. And the use of multimedia courseware can satisfy what the students need. They can establish clearer action images. Practice shows that using this technology can fully improve the learning efficiency. Therefore, the use of information technology in teaching can stimulate learners' multiple senses to make their brain in a positive working state. With the modern audiovisual media network teachers can introduce the advanced technology of outstanding athletes in the world to the students to help students establish a correct, complete technical action concept and a good grasp of technical movements.

249.3 Help Highlight the Emphasis and Difficulty of Technical Movements

The use of information technology can effectively make up for the inadequacy of traditional teaching, which can turn abstract into concrete, mobilize students' visual intuitive features and create good atmosphere for breaking through the difficulties. For example: when teaching " diving forward roll", it is hard for most of the students to understand and grasp the feeling of "jump", and teachers cannot do decomposition of movement in the teaching demonstration, and the use of multimedia courseware makes it simpler [2]. The cartoon of "Diving forward roll" based on Flash animation, divide actions into leaping, hand hold down, and turn and squat stand four coherent actions, and add the failure actions and special music into every step of the animation, students can judge what action is correct or not just by listening. So, when teaching the students are asked to watch the animation, and the contrast actions of success and failure are demonstrated step by step. Students are asked to carry on the comparison, analysis, action concept is formed in the brain. Then they will have a desire to have a try in practice. In practice, the teachers just give a little explanation or demonstration, which can have an obvious effect compared with the traditional teaching. These technical movements are small, the strength needed is also small, exquisite skills are demanded, so teachers have certain difficulties in interpretation model. Because teacher's demonstration is fleeting, which is difficult for students to observe carefully, and the multimedia courseware in the modern education technology can use a space design such as 2 d and 3 d, turning texts to images and dynamic to static, fast to slow, and demonstrate every subtle change of the technology, show the key points, analyze the difficulties, coupled with the affectionate explanation of teacher, students can understand tacitly, which can play a positive role in the students quick learning technology.

249.4 Help to Correct Mistakes in Time

In order to reduce and avoid the errors produced by students in the practice, it is better to point out the causes and mistakes which easily are made when the teacher demonstrate a right action, with modern information technology, correct action as well as the wrong action can be shown in courseware, let students think by watching them, in this way they can avoid many common wrong actions. When having Wushu theory class [5], for example, the teacher show the action pictures which can be hard to show in demonstration action, at the same time, make how the students practice Wushu into a video by the movements from different angles, with functions of a pause, replay, slow play, let the student watch action process and key technology clearly, adopt heuristic teaching, discussing while playing, make the students fully understand their mistakes and insufficiency, which can enhances their learning efficiency.

249.5 Help Teachers Change the Teaching Concept

The outstanding characteristics of the information age are openness and beyond the time and space. The use of modern information technology is a new challenge for all regions, schools, and everybody, PE teachers only by studying hard and constantly enriching himself can stand in the forefront of the times, meet the challenge of the new era, become a vital force to achieve the leap development of modern education [4]. The key to the cultivation of the students' sports interest is physical education teachers. The change of teachers' education conception not only is the symbol of times development but also plays a vital role in the development of education. By correct, reasonable and efficient utilization of information resources, teachers can cultivate students' ability to acquire and update knowledge, such as school sports scheduling and preparation is a big workload for physical education teachers, the use of computers can greatly reduce the work burden of PE teachers. We can use ACCESS database create a school sports teaching system, which includes the educational research group management, teacher preparation system, the students physical training, physical education grades management, sports team management, sports equipment management, this can greatly relieves the workload of PE teachers.

In short, through classroom practice, the application of multimedia technology in the sports teaching achieve the effect which conventional teaching methods cannot do However, multimedia is not a substitute for the teacher's explanation, demonstration, presentation and discussion. Teachers still play a leading role in the teaching process. Different teaching media has its own characteristics, the teaching effect can be optimized with the reasonable use. Therefore, that information technology is applied in sports teaching is well worth trying, exploring and promoting.

References

1. Bing C, Jie L (2002) The role of physical education in quality education. Social science of Henan, China
2. Tao J (2010) How to use modern education technology innovation education. China's adult education, China
3. Hui L (2010) The information age the ordinary university sports teaching research. Education and professional, China
4. Hu zhen S (2010) Reasonable use modern education technology, improve the efficiency of classroom teaching. Education and exploration, China
5. Du yan X (2001) Network era and sports. Physical education and science, China
6. Chun fang Z (2004) Informationization and development of physical education. J Wuhan Inst Phys Educ 38(6):54–56

Chapter 250
How to Use Multimedia Technology for Improvement of the Teaching Effect of Medical Immunology

Ding Jianbing, Wang Song, Zhou Xiao Tao, Fulati Rexiti, Dilinar Bolati, Wei Xiaoli and Xu Qian

Abstract Medical immunology is a basic course, difficult to understand but fast speed of knowledge updating. Multimedia computer assisted instruction, can make the teaching content imaginary, rich, stimulate students interest in learning. Combined with our teaching practice, this paper explores how to improve the teaching effect of medical immunology by making full and reasonable use of multimedia and network technology.

Keywords Medical immunology · Multimedia technology · Teaching effect

The rapid development and wide application of computer multimedia and network technology, teaching methods and means even schools have undergone a fundamental change in the structure. Whether computer multimedia and network technology can be used in the field of education and teaching is a measure of the education to be a basis for the future. This will have a profound impact on the education and the teaching process. Medical Immunology is the study of the organizational structure of the immune system, the physiological function and pathological role, immunology theory and methods of application, such as science, is a basic course in medical colleges. Its rich content, involving a wide range of disciplines developed rapidly, fast updating of knowledge, and the contents of the abstract, boring and difficult to understand. To vividly introduce essence of content

---

This work was supported by Grant of Xinjiang Medical University (YG2013001, YG2013017) and by Grant from Xinjiang key laboratory in China (201301 and XYDXK50780328).

D. Jianbing (✉) · W. Song · Z. X. Tao · F. Rexiti ·
D. Bolati · W. Xiaoli · X. Qian
Department of Medical Immunology, Xinjiang Medical University, Urumqi, China
e-mail: djbing002@sina.com

to the students in the limited class and to raise the level of curriculum teaching and learning, we try to use multimedia computer aided instruction from 1999, has achieved rapid development in the years, has been formed with discipline characteristics of multimedia application system.

250.1 The Guiding Ideology of Multimedia Applications

To provide students with a more direct, efficient, highly informative learning environment, in multimedia application system, we use computer and network as media, through the interaction with students, to achieve the purpose of teaching. "Interactivity, instantaneity, vivid, pertinence and flexibility" are its most prominent feature. During the teaching time, teachers lead and students orient. Teaching environment does not adhere to the traditional classroom, the classroom, through the network and multimedia technology platform, teachers can provide students with a real-time interactive curriculum to meet the individual needs and characteristics, and is conducive to the students' self-learning and review.

250.2 Collection and Compilation of Teaching Materials

Enriching multimedia teaching materials is an important link to better play the advantages of multimedia computer-aided teaching and to improve teaching quality and efficiency. Teachers downloaded teaching-related material from the Internet at home and abroad related website, to remain part of colorful pictures and sketches in the purchased foreign language original materials and Chinese textbooks via scanning in computer to make the gallery. With the use of digital cameras, digital cameras we record operation and its results on the usual experimental research, teaching, or with video capture system we kept teaching video for editing after conversion, made of rich digital image data. Meanwhile attention to the collection of relevant immunological history of the development and some of the important characters and story pictures, sound, animation, video, and so on. These data application courseware can highlight teaching points, breaking the difficulty of teaching, so that visualize the abstract concept. We have completed the construction of our hospital Youth Foundation Medical Microbiology and Medical Immunology multimedia teaching material library, waiting for acceptance.

250.3 Making Electronic Lesson Plans and Multimedia Courseware

250.3.1 Electronic Lesson Plans

Since 2000, teachers have started production of electronic lesson plans, and continue to improve with the update of the teaching material. In the production process of the electronic lesson plans, it emphasizes closely linked to the syllabus, makes the focal points stand out, clarifies the difficulty and reflects teaching ideas. Over years of accumulation, every teacher gradually formed a set of different students, electronic lesson plans have their own style, and be correct in constant use, enrich, and laid a foundation for the improvement of the standard teaching.

250.3.2 Multimedia Courseware

When teaching assignments were arranged, courseware produced separately by the teachers according to textbooks, teaching profession, teaching mode (theoretical lectures, workshops, experiments, problem-centered self-teaching). The different modes of different design ideas, and then integrate the courseware through collective classes, lectures observation and evaluation, personal communication to revise and improve the form of courseware. During courseware making process, we adhere to the following principles.

250.3.2.1 Scientific and Correct

Scientific errors can not be involved in the courseware content, according to the students' understanding of the law, make full use of the advantages of multimedia, and effectively improve the performance of the learning activities; In addition, make full use of the modern theory of classroom teaching, optimizing the organization of classroom teaching and implemented in accordance with the rules of teaching.

250.3.2.2 Simple and Intuitive

The design of multimedia courseware should pay attention to this principle. Take the basic concept, important principle, the basic methods and ideas to solve practical problems in the most concise way to teach their students. Avoid a pile of simple text, the courseware made of textbooks projection. For this, teachers should conscientiously study materials, and study professional knowledge and modern teaching theory, rational use of the multimedia space–time expressive abstract knowledge simplistic, concrete, make the students understand and remember. For example, when you explain the immune response, as it involves the monocyte-macrophage cells, dendritic cells, T cells and B cells and other cells and cell surface molecules interaction, the process can not be observed. In the past students only imagine from the teachers' explanation of the introduction, and often feel difficult to understand and remember. Now the use of animation to reflect the interaction of cells and cell surface molecules, its vivid visually demonstrate to students, and finally use the simple flow chart of the entire response process to be summed up, to extract the main points of knowledge, accelerate students understand speed, to deepen the level of understanding, the students learn to understand, remember, and to achieve a multiplier effect.

250.3.2.3 Beautiful and Rich

Prevent only the courseware as "electronic projection", we can take advantage of Excel, Photoshop, Flash and other software tools, timely and appropriate to insert charts, 3D modeling, video and sound playback to make teaching content multi-faceted, vivid, overcome previous teaching description and abstract understanding, to improve the students' interest in learning and learning efficiency. For example, a short animation display of famous scientist in the history of immunology typical contribution and add a classic experiment that students can not operate, with the form of video to the courseware to give students pleasant learning environment, multi-sensory comprehensive stimulus, that are conducive to the holding of the students' attention.

250.4 Correctly Grasp the Link of Teaching

With the continuous improvement of teaching conditions, the theoretical and experimental teaching of our college has been used in all the multimedia computer assisted instruction. Multimedia is modern teaching tool significantly improving the effectiveness of teaching in the teaching, but with the increased use of multimedia its ills gradually revealed. Therefore, in teaching should pay attention to the following points.

250.4.1 The Dominant Status of Teachers Can't be Ignored During Teaching Process

Teachers not only act as narrators, but should be by design and flexible operation of the teaching process, strengthen the interaction with students, and to keep abreast of teaching effectiveness and students' learning situation to get the best of multimedia teaching. At the same time, from the relations between people and multimedia, teaching content and multimedia, to explore basic teaching of the law and the requirements of multimedia in teaching the operation, to make multimedia take targeted effects via a role in teacher mastery.

250.4.2 Multimedia is not a Substitute for the Experimental Teaching

In experimental teaching, multimedia can demonstrate some operations of the experiment that are dangerous, difficult to observe and no conditions for doing, a multiplier effect as the finishing point. But the problem can be resolved by experiment, teachers never use multimedia simulation for students to understand, so that students learn to understand, remember, to achieve a multiplier effect. Students through experimental observation, study to gain knowledge, to faithfully reproduce the process of change, a strong persuasive means of teaching, but also the important aspects of students' ability to observe and develop.

250.4.3 Implementation of Multimedia Teaching Can't be Flashy

Multimedia teaching makes some of the teaching difficulties that have long plagued teachers solved. But sometimes improper use of sound, video, animation will become the source of the interference of teaching, and dispersed the students' attention. Therefore, the use of multimedia teaching must not be flashy, grandstanding, should be used with purpose and plan.

250.4.4 Multimedia Teaching Can't be Completely Replaced to Make the Teaching of Writing on the Blackboard

Multimedia technology has a vivid picture of the frequent changes of the pleasant sound, powerful role at the same time. Lots of information and long screen may enable students to psychological pressure and visual fatigue. At this time, if teachers can briefly outline some of the reasoning process and summarize the contents using the writing on the blackboard, not only to better reflect the teaching process, and can also interact with students, regulating students' emotions, relieve stress, get better teaching effect.

250.5 Guide the Students to Learn to Use the Network

While teaching in the classroom, we opened up a teaching garden of medical microbiology and immunology campus network, including the introduction of basic immunology course syllabus, courseware, exercises, etc., so that students can have a general curriculum understanding, and targeted previewing and reviewing. While taking advantage of the interests of the students on the network, and collected a lot of recent literature related to classroom content and website resources, introduced to the students, to narrow the distance of the classroom teaching and academic frontiers, greatly stimulate students' interest in learning.

In the past two years, the five-year undergraduate students design experimental teaching, we ask students to collect relevant information online, topic selection, experimental design, turned over to the experimental application by e-mail, implementation adjusting modified by the teachers. Students' multimedia tools for self-learning and cooperation on the network in a timely manner, doubts answering, become popular among students.

In the all, making full use of modern educational technology, updating teaching methods, enriching the teaching content are the inevitable requirements of the reform and development of higher education. How to actively promote the new teaching mode of medical immunology, make teaching forms various, stimulate students' interest in learning, improve the overall quality of students and the actual ability to work, every teacher is concerned it as a challenge and promotion. That needs teachers to explore from all aspects, seek experience, and continuously improve, to make it constantly improve and update in running, play a long-lasting role.

References

1. Yuan S, Zhang L (2010) Optimization of classroom teaching assistant is one of the modern educational technologies. Chin Mod Educ Equip 92(4):44–45
2. Li W, Du W (2007) Experiment teaching with modern educational technology. Sci Technol Consult Herald 4:205–206

Chapter 251
Application of Mind Map in Teaching and Learning of Medical Immunology

Song Wang, Jianbing Ding, Qi Xu, Xiaoli Wei, Qi Xu and Bolati Dilinar

Abstract As a new teaching and learning method, Mind map has the advantages that it enhance the visibility and logic correlation among knowledge points. Mind map gives a good solution to the problems existing in medical immunology learning, it also helps student's divergent thinking and their innovation ability.

Keywords Mind map · Medical immunology

Medical immunology in recent decades has been a frontier subjects crossing with molecular biology, biochemistry, pathology and genetics. It is developing a backbone course for the undergraduates major in medicine. Immunological theory is growing rapidly, its increasingly important position in public health poses a new challenge to Immunology teaching.

Most students think Immunology is difficult to learn for its abstract theory and the obscure concept, even many senior teachers agree with them. Modern medical education requires new education pattern through visual, vivid and interactive teaching to transfer initiative and enthusiasm which the student studies. As a consequence, mind map has been introduced to learn immunology.

Mind map is an organizational thinking tool which was put forward by an Englishman called Tony Buzan in the 1970s [1]. He believes that the traditional linear notes which may cover up me keywords is difficult to memorize and is a waste of time. Also, it cannot stimulate the brain effectively. He tries to open a graphics-oriented approach to the human brain's potential and his idea leads to the coming of mind map. Mind map is able to stimulate the cerebral cortex skills such as languages, images, numbers, logic, rhythm, colors and spatial awareness, and so on. Mind map can be applied to all aspects of life, improving learning and clear thinking so that people's performance can be greatly improved.

S. Wang · J. Ding (✉) · Q. Xu · X. Wei · Q. Xu · B. Dilinar
Department of Medical Immunology, Xinjiang Medical University, Urumqi, China
e-mail: djbing002@sina.com

There are two obvious advantages of mind map, it enhances the visibility and logic correlation among knowledge points. And both of them are exactly why students feel that medical immunology is difficult to learn—the subject is not visible and has wider internal correlation although it was develop from a medical morphological subjects, microbiology. Immunology does not emphasize the morphological features of immune organs and cells but their physiological and pathological functions, though these organs and cells can be seen under microscope or by our eyes. For example, we cannot distinguish T cells from lymphocytes only through a morphological detection, we must use some specific antibodies such as anti-CD3, -CD4 or -CD8 to detect them, and what are CD3, CD4 and CD8? they are special trans-membrane proteins on T cell surface, and they cannot be observed. That is difficult to be understood by students when teachers introduce the chapter of T cells. Students have to transfer their "imagination" in order to remember these molecules which they never see in daily life. At this time, if teachers give a map, T cell is the only keyword in it, and other important topics including the development of T cell in thymus, CD molecules about T cell-mediated response, T cell subsets and their functions around the keyword, teacher use the sub-maps or movies to indicate intuitively these CD molecules expression and their structure on T cells, we are certain it can help students to decrease their learning difficulty.

Some students reflect that it's so difficult to remember large amount of knowledge points and feel not fully understood when they finish the immunology learning. We think they neglect the internal relationships of these points. Immunology learning is based on the mechanism of an immune response. When an antigen exists, tens of immune molecules and cells become involved in the innate or adaptive response to the antigen. That is very complex process, there are extensive interactions among lymphocytes and other effect cells in vivo. However, in class, the cells is isolated by chapters, teachers have to introduce different cells according to the teaching contents. As a result, the teaching in previous sections have to mention some knowledge of later sections. For example, "antigen" must be introduced in the first lecture according to the schedule, in fact, some points such as antigen's classification, clinical significance of antigens are ahead for learning at this moments. It's belong to the innate difficulty of immunology, and immunology teaching is impossible to take account of all contents. Just like the story of "An Elephant and Blind Men", students play the blind men, they are instilled with the knowledge chapter by chapter, and do not know the complete picture of an immune response. The segmentary learning brings incomplete, even wrong cognition sometimes. All people have known T cells mediate cellular response, B cell mediates humoral respone when they are High school students. But that is not true, both of responses need the interactions between T cells and B cells, modern immunology think respneses have complex correlation and cannot be described so partially. The mind map is good at showing the relationship of knowledge, it trains the logical and divergent thinking ability of students.

We did an experiment with some students, asked them for drawing different mind-maps after each chapter's learning, defining the conceptions only with some words or one sentence, using some icons and arrows to indicate the relationships among different knowledge points, then let them improve the maps continuously and intergrate them as a complete map at the end of session. These students said immunology were so interesting and they felt the learning-road opened up suddenly. Compared to other students who taught with traditional teaching method, their average scores of the subject was six points higher than other students, especially for some comprehensive questions which related to different knowledge points, they got 26 % higher accuracy than others. This test proved that teaching with a mind map is indeed a good way and suited to immunology learning.

With the rapid development of network and information technology, the computer has almost been deeply applied to every field, including the education. There are lots of software to draw a mind map, such as mindmanager, imindmap, xmind, freemind, etc. They help us to sort our thought more conveniently and efficiently. Mind map is no longer composed of just text information that it was several decades ago, it still contains voice, movies, pictures and hyperlinks to internet or other maps, it is complex and beautiful, of course, make a mind map is not easy. In fact, it spends a lot of time and energy and need cooperation. During making a mind map, students communicate with teachers, it help teachers to keep abreast of student's study situation. Sometimes student finds new problems which enlighten his teachers and classmates. This is an example, a student asked me a question when he made a mind map about mast cell, "Why anaphylactic shock is not induced by immunoglobulin G but by immunoglobulin E?" He found in textbook that there are two receptors on mast cell which bind IgE and IgG separately. IgE can mediate shock, why IgG cannot. His question is real quality, now he is a PhD candidate, and his project is the relationship between anaphylactic shock and immunoglobulins.

In conclusion, mind map is able to let us know the logic correlation among knowledge point more intuitively, it can help teachers get the thread of textbook, enhance students motivation for learning, help students get the main points and improve their efficiency. Mindmap also make students think in a way of problem-based learning, and its advantage in training up divergent thinking could also develop student's innovation ability [2].

As we enter the 21st century, people's living standards are being improved in general. However, at the same time, people are facing the rapid growth in human diseases and the development of modern medicine is facing many new problems and challenges, too. One important way to solve the problem is to train more high quality medical professionals. Having many advantages, mind map must be widely applied in immunology teaching and learning, and in other medical courses as an important complement of the traditional education mode.

Acknowledgments This work was supported by Grant of Xinjiang Medical University (YG2013017, YG2013001) and by Grant from national key laboratory in China (201011 and XYDXK50780328).

References

1. Wikipedia Mindmap, http://en.wikipedia.org/wiki/Mind_map, Cited 20 March 2013
2. Li L, Hu X (2011) On applying mind mapping toreduce cognitive load in college english classes. J Anhui Sci Technol Univ 24:83–87

Chapter 252
Electron Microscopy Technology and It's Application in the Morphology

Caili Sun, Xiaohong Li, Zhou Li and Tuanting Zhang

Abstract *Objective* To observe the influence of different load on the rat gastrocnemius muscle spindle of shape and structure. *Methods* Adopt swimming training model. Medium load group swim 60 min each day. Over load group, loaded with the weight of 5 %, swim 60 min each day, 6 days a week. Adopt muscle spindle of Faworky's display and electron microscopy techniques; observe changes of different load training on the rat gastrocnemius muscle spindle shape and structure. Results show that gastrocnemius muscle spindle form is smaller, while muscle spindle structure is normal. In medium load group muscle spindle structure is integrate, spindle extrinsic is aligned, muscle spindle in neural myelin structure are clear and complete, nuclear bag fiber, nuclear chain fiber diameter than the control group significantly increases. In over load group spindle body increased obviously, inside and outside is separated by capsule seriously. Muscle fibrils quantity is less, sac cells are swollen, axis clearance increased obviously, spindle in neural axis lining and myelin has separated. These preliminary findings indicate medium load movement could significantly improve muscle spindle shape and structure, while over load sports training could lead to pathological changes of muscle spindle structure.

C. Sun (✉) · X. Li · Z. Li · T. Zhang
Department of Physical Education, Xi'an University of Architecture and Technology, Xi'an 710055, China
e-mail: hxztt718@126.com

X. Li
e-mail: lxh112130@163.com

T. Zhang
e-mail: hxztt718@126.com

Z. Li
Talent Fund of Xi'an University of Architecture and Technology, RC1017,
Fund of Shaanxi Provincial Sports Bureau, Xi'an T11088, China

Keywords Load · rat · Gastrocnemius · Muscle spindle · Electron microscopy techniques

252.1 Introduction

The muscle spindle is the special sensory devices within the skeletal muscle, skeletal muscle and muscle spindle on (shuttle muscle) have the same origin and the same blood supply, their relationships are parallel in structure, in function the muscle spindle is the receptors, while skeletal muscle is the effector, both belong to different portions of the reflex arc. By gravity traction, muscle spindle impulse constantly into central nervous system, creating and maintaining muscle tension, and involve in the coordination of voluntary movement. The impact of exercise on muscle spindle morphology has an important value to improve the work efficiency of muscle and athletic performance. In this term, the study of the muscle spindle mainly focus on the distribution of the muscle spindle in muscle and muscular atrophy of muscle spindle morphology, the study of exercise on muscle spindle morphology spindle. Institutions has not been reported. So, this model of different load swimming training is established to study the impact of exercise on muscle spindle structure to reveal the effect of exercise on muscle.

252.2 Materials and Methods

Healthy male SD rats were 30 (Xi'an Fourth Military Medical University Animal Management Centre), 2 months of age, body weight 180 ± 20 g, rats were randomly divided into control group, moderate load group and heavy load group. All animals were reared in accordance with the national standard rodent standards, free food, activities. Adaptability of animal feeding 1 week after training, during which a large load group daily 15 min adaptation training, the control group without any training.

Moderate load group daily swam 60 min, trained 6 days weekly, and trained a total of 8 weeks. Heavy load group, weighted 5 % of the weight, swam 60 min a day, 6 days a week, 1 day, and trained a total of 8 weeks [1, 2].

Draw materials in 24 h after the last training session, the control group and trained group is drawn on the same day. All of rats were injected Intraperitoneal of sodium pentobarbital (50 mg/kg body weight) anesthesia, stripped rats' muscle, quickly took the gastrocnemius into the fixative to make the slice of electron microscopy and light microscopy.

252.3 Results

The control group can be seen in microscope, the gastrocnemius muscle spindle and the muscle fibers parallel arrangement, small form. Electron microscope, visible capsule surrounding the muscle spindle by spindle, nuclear bag fibers, nuclear chain fibers, intrafusal nerve, blood vessels and other structures, normal muscle spindle structure (Fig. 252.1).

Moderate load group, light microscopy showed that the muscle spindle structure is complete, the extrafusal neat, close, brown, muscle spindle capsule a slight expansion, but the difference was not significant. Intrafusal muscle is clearly visible, no increase in the number of intrafusal intrafusal nerve was spiral wrapped around the intrafusal muscle, nervous clear and neat. Electron microscope, the muscle spindle structural integrity of the axis week gap widened, but the nuclear bag fibers and nuclear chain fiber diameter was significantly increased compared with the control group, significant differences ($P < 0.05$), myelin structure within the muscle spindle is clear and complete (Fig. 252.2).

Large group of load under the light microscope, significantly increased the shuttle body, inside and outside the tunicate serious separation, the intrafusal nerve derangement. Load of the group electron microscopy equatorial diameter increased significantly, compared with middle-load group significant difference ($P < 0.05$); the intrafusal diameter increased significantly ($P < 0.05$, $P < 0.01$), intrafusal backpack discontinuous, a fracture. The perinuclear rich mitochondria, some swelling of mitochondria, the small number of myofibrils, the follicle cells swelling the axis week gap increases significantly increased the intrafusal nerve cross-sectional, and the control group, medium-compound group, the difference is very significant ($P < 0.01$), but the intrafusal axonal intima and myelin serious separation (Fig. 252.3).

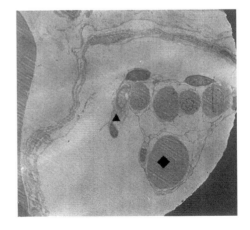

Fig. 252.1 The control group gastrocnemius muscle spindle crosscut (ultrastructure 15 × 100 times). *Note* ▲ intrafusal nerves, ◆ intrafusal muscle, ★ spindle capsule cell

Fig. 252.2 Medium load group gastrocnemius muscle spindle crosscut (ultrastructure 15 × 100 times). *Note* ▲ intrafusal nerves, ◆ intrafusal muscle, ★ spindle capsule cell

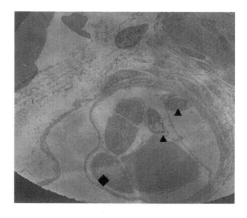

Fig. 252.3 Over-load group gastrocnemius muscle spindle crosscut (ultrastructure 15 × 100 times). *Note* ▲ intrafusal nerves, ◆ intrafusal muscle, ★ spindle capsule cell

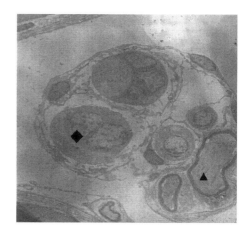

252.4 Discussion and Conclusion

Muscle spindle attached to the skeletal muscle on the long axis and parallel to the skeletal muscle, in the middle named slightly enlarged spindle-shaped. Feelings of skeletal muscle length, tension, movement direction, speed, and speed the rate of change of the stretch reflex receptors [3], mainly by intrafusal nerve shuttle capsule and the composition of tiny blood vessels. Intrafusal nerve with the spindle capsule, and other factors to determine the functional status of the muscle spindle [4].

252.4.1 The Change on Rats' Gastrocnemius Intrafusal Muscle

Muscle fibers (skeletal) muscle spindle the outer surface of the coating by the connective tissue capsule, known as the spindle capsule, so that separate the muscle spindle and the surrounding muscle fibers in the muscle fibers of the spindle capsule known as intrafusal muscle located in the spindle capsule called extrafusal muscle. Usually intrafusal muscle fibers are divided into two categories [5]: the nuclear bag fibers and nuclear chain fibers. Nuclear chain fibers were stripes like, with the contractile function of the nuclear bag fibers in the middle of multi-core ministry, but not systolic function, but this is part of the distribution of sensory nerve endings, to feel the stimulation of muscle spindle inside and outside the tension and stress, muscle spindle stretch reflex receptors. This study found that the medium-load group intrafusal muscle arranged in neat rows and the structural integrity of the nuclear bag fibers and nuclear chain fiber diameter was significantly increased compared with the control group. From the central point of view, stretch the muscles can change the excitability of the corresponding central block and through the negative role of the stretch reflex spasm caused by excessive muscle spindle excitement, and to improve local tissue ischemia caused by spasm, thus improving muscle blood flow, to promote the rehabilitation of the damaged tissue and further damage received. Muscle spindle changes due to disease, can lead to muscle changes [2]. Yuan Zenong found an increase in patients with idiopathic scoliosis convex side of the paravertebral muscle contraction increase, acting to increase, and thus the convex side of the paraspinal muscle spindle stimulation felt their structure and function of the corresponding changes in the performance of intrafusal muscle fiber number and cross sectional area increase. The impulse of the muscle spindle afferents central reflex caused by the increase in muscle tension, muscle metabolic activity increased, the performance of muscle fiber hyperplasia or hypertrophy. These results suggest that the medium-load can cause the enhancement of muscle activity and increase in force a few. Although the decrease in myofibril number of heavy load group cross-section was significantly increased, suggesting that the large load exercise stimulus may make the extrafusal the acting to increase and contraction of the enhanced muscle activity increesed intrafusal muscle cross-sectional area increases, but the number of myofibrils decreased significantly, this may be the intrafusal a compensatory response, which may affect the regulation of voluntary movement of body muscle spindle.

252.4.2 The Change on the Nerves in Rat Gastrocnemius Intrafusal

Each intrafusal fibers are subject to both motor and sensory nerve fibers control [6]. Muscle spindle afferent generally constitute I and II class of nerve fibers. I a class of fiber as the primary sensory nerve endings, thicker, faster conduction velocity of their peripheral spiral around the central nuclear region in the nuclear chain fibers and nuclear bag fibers; II fibers secondary sensory nerve endings, small diameter, slower conduction velocity was squid-like distribution in the nuclear chain fibers. This study found that moderate load group, the structural integrity of the muscle spindle intrafusal nerve clear neat spiral around intrafusal myelin structure is clear and complete. Serious lesions of neural structures within the spindle of the heavy load group, nerves obscure, the intima of intrafusal axon and myelin sheath separation, prompted the exercise load increases muscle spindle suitable stimulate disappear, forced to stimulate the increase, resulting in muscle spindle afferent impulses to reduce the intrafusal the structure and innervation changes, structural changes in muscle spindle muscle spindle afferent input to further reduce, thereby enabling the ability to reduce or change spinal anterior horn motor neuron activity, which decline caused by the muscles ability to work.

252.4.3 The Change on the Gastrocnemius Muscle Spindle Capsule

Muscle spindle outer surface of the coated capsule of connective tissue called the shuttle capsule spindle capsule at the equator of enlargement, the muscle spindle to spindle-shaped. Shuttle capsule is divided into outer and inner layers, the inner layer by a thin layer of flat cells, showed a small tube surrounding the muscle fibers within each shuttle, the outer layer of the myelin sheath of nerve fibers enter the muscle spindle is continuous from a few layer flat into fiber cells constitute the outer layer of swelling in the muscle spindle equator within about 2 mm, so that the inner and outer layers have a larger gap, this gap is called the axis week gap, the gap containing nerve fibers. This study found that moderate load group muscle spindle structural integrity of the axis week gap widened significantly, nuclear bag fibers and nuclear chain fiber diameter was significantly increased compared with the control group, the myelin structure within the muscle spindle is clear and complete. Therefore, by the large load after exercise the muscle spindle capsule cell swelling axis week gap significantly increases the intima of intrafusal axonal and myelin separation, the movement of large loads can lead to muscle spindle structure and function change, which affects muscle improvement of force and muscle to do work. Infer the movement of large loads can result in muscle spindle morphology of pathological changes, changes in the structure of muscle spindle muscle spindle afferent impulses to reduce changes, and then induced central parts, the latter caused by complex neurohumoral regulation mechanisms intrafusal change in the structure, metabolism and function of muscle, causing muscle tension, reduce, and eventually lead to muscle atrophy [7], which is not conducive to the improvement of skeletal muscle function. Muscle spindle activity in skeletal muscle output, abnormal muscle spindle discharge, abnormal skeletal muscle output, this output exception can be offset by the high-frequency vibration muscle, while the high-frequency vibration can be excited muscle spindle [8]. To sum up the middle load to improve the structure of the rat gastrocnemius muscle spindle intrafusal nerve clearer arranged in order, myofibril diameter increases, indicating that the appropriate exercise has become a positive stimulus on the muscle spindle, the muscle spindle structure and function changed. Due to gravity traction, muscle spindle continue to payment of the impulse to the incoming center, to produce and maintain muscle tension, and to participate in fine-tuning of voluntary movement. According to the movement of large loads intrafusal muscle morphological and functional changes in correlation analysis, we believe that changes in muscle spindle overload movement caused by changes in muscle structure and function of great significance, is likely to be the initial muscle lesions one of the reasons. In the movement under the conditions of heavy load, due to the excessive increase of the force of muscle long-term overload and forced to shrink, the suitability of the muscle spindle stimulation disappeared, resulting in the change of the metabolism, structure and function of muscle spindle, so that the hub of muscle spindle afferents reduce the impulse to induce the central parts of the change, the latter through the complex neural, humoral regulation mechanisms cause intrafusal muscle structure, metabolism and functional changes caused by reduced muscle tension, excitability, resulting in (or increase) of extrafusal muscle metabolism, structural and functional changes, eventually leading to (or increase) muscle lesions and loss of function.

Moderate exercise can significantly improve muscle spindle morphology to improve the muscle to do work, to improve muscle strength; the heavy load exercise training can lead to structural lesions occurred in the muscle spindle, normal muscle function play.

References

1. Ning-chuan L, Qi-guan J, Xin-rong S (2000) The effect of exhaustive swimming training on the establishment of a model for overtraining in rats. Sports Sci 21(1):53–55
2. Wang W (1997) The research progress of muscle spindle morphology. Chin J Clin Anat 15(1):71–73
3. Yang-rong S, Feng G (2003) Structure and function of muscle spindle. J Yanan Univ (Medical Sciences) 1(2):148–151
4. Ro JY, Capra NF (2001) Modulation of jaw muscle spindle afferent activity following intramuscular injections with hypertonic saline. Pain 92:117–127

5. Birznieks L, Burton AR, Macesield VG et al (2008) The effects of experimental muscle and skin pain on the static stretch sensitivity of human muscle spindles in relaxed leg muscles. J Physiol 586(10):2713–2723
6. McCall GE, Grindeland RE, Roy RR et al (2000) Muscle afferent activity modulates bioassayable growth hormone in human plasma. J Appl Physiol 59(12):2137–1141
7. Bin T, Xiaoli F, Sudi W et al (2003) Influence of stimulated weightlessness on the morphology of nerve endings of muscle spindle in rat soleus muscle. Space Med Medical Eng 16(3):162–164
8. Hagbarth KE, Macefield VG (1995) The fusimotor system its role in fatigue. Adv Exp Med Biol 384:259–270

Chapter 253
Empirical Study on the Relationship Between Financial Structure and Economic Growth: An Example of Zhejiang Province

Songyan Zhang

Abstract This paper uses the time-series data from 1978 to 2009 of Zhejiang province to make an empirical analysis on the relationship between financial structure and economic growth. The results show that: There is long-term stable equilibrium relationship between financial structure and economic growth in Zhejiang Province; Rapid economic growth is one of the reasons for the rapid development of the financial industry, while the rise of the financial sector in turns promotes economic growth in Zhejiang Province. At last, the author gives some suggestions based on the above analysis.

Keywords Financial structure · Economic growth · Cointegration tests · Granger causality tests

253.1 Introduction

Financial development theory is based on the theory of economic growth. The relationship between financial development and economic growth has been the research field of economists. As early as 1911, the Austrian economist Joseph Schumpeter expounded a well-functioning financial system can promote long-term economic growth. In 1969, Goldsmith supported this assertion through empirical research, he thought that there was a rough parallel relationship between the economic and financial development. In 1973, McKinnon and Shaw put forward the theory of "financial repression" and "financial deepening". Kapoor et al. developed static analysis of McKinnon and Shaw, they further clarified the important role of financial deepening that plays on economic development of

---

S. Zhang (✉)
School of Economics and Management, Zhejiang University of Science and Technology, Hangzhou 310023, People's Republic of China
e-mail: syzh201@163.com

developing countries by the method of dynamic analysis. Endogenous financial theory that has been developed since 1990s emphasizes the improvement of capital efficiency is benefited from the key role that financial intermediaries and financial markets distribute capital to the best possible uses. After that, Diamond, Levine, Beck and many famous scholars had carried out a variety of theoretical and empirical researches on the relationship between financial development and economic growth.

In addition, the domestic and foreign scholars mainly focus on the national level when they study the relationship between financial development and economic growth, while the district level is relatively rare, and it is especially uncommon on the study of Zhejiang Province. Since the reform and opening policy has been carried out, Zhejiang Province is one of provinces to realize rapid economic growth in eastern area of China. Therefore, the study of relationship between financial development and economic growth in Zhejiang Province makes great theoretical and practical significance.

253.2 Variables Selected

Finance-related rate (FIR) is the ratio of a country's total value of financial assets and the country's economic total activity at a specific date. Finance-related rate (FIR) formula is expressed as M2/GDP, which holds the economic meaning and function that you can use it to illustrate the degree of monetization of the economy. In this paper, we use the amount of the proportion of total financial assets in Zhejiang Province to measure Zhejiang Finance-related rate (FIR). Kuznets considers that a country's economic growth can be defined as the long-term rising ability to provide economic products for the residents. Most scholars take the indicator of GDP growth when they study economic growth. As the finance-related rate (FIR) is the total indicator, we take the total indicator of economic growth in the traditional sense.

The basic data are derived from the "Zhejiang Provincial Statistical Yearbook 2010", we use the GDP of Zhejiang Province in 1978–2009 (GDP1978 = 100); FIR is equal to the sum, which is the sum of balance of RMB deposits and outstanding loans of all financial institutions, divided by the GDP of the province (no price adjustment).

253.3 Empirical Analysis

Using the sample data from 1978 to 2009 of Zhejiang Province, we consider the relationship between financial structure and economic growth by unit root test, cointegration test and Granger causality test. All empirical analysis figures and forms are analyzed by Eviews software.

253.3.1 Unit Root Test

At first, we use Expansion Dickey-Fuller (ADF) test to measure the stationarity of time series before we take the cointegration test on the time series of GDP and FIR.

The test results show that the sequences of GDP and FIR can not reject the null hypothesis, which means unit root exists; we use ADF test to first-order differential of these two sequences, they also reject the null hypothesis, so there is a unit root; then, we use ADF test to second-order differential of these two sequences, the test results indicate that GDP second-order differential sequence accept the null hypothesis at the 5 % significant level, which means there is no unit root, and GDP and FIR second-order differential sequences are steady.

253.3.2 Cointegration Test

In this paper, we do unit root test on the residuals of the regression equation by using the two-step method of Engle-Granger. In order to weaken the heteroscedasticity problem, we analyze logarithmic time series. Through logarithmic, the first-order differential of the two time series is stationary.

The first step is to establish the following regression equation:

$$LNGDP = a + b\ LNFIR + u \qquad (253.1)$$

The results are as follows through OLS estimation:

$$LNGDP = 5.657571 + 2.280434\ LNFIR + u \qquad (253.2)$$

$$t = 127.2485 \quad 41.96829 \quad R = 0.9645 \quad F = 815.2623$$

Overall explanatory power of the equation is relatively strong, each coefficient is also significantly. Coefficient 2.280434 in the equation denotes elastic, which shows that when financial related rate increases 1 %, the actual GDP increases 2.28 %.

The second step, we do the residual of the regression results for the unit root test, the results (see Table 253.1) show that ADF equals −3.069101, the critical value at 1, 5, 10 % are −3.670170, −2.963972, −2.621007 respectively, the residual of the equation is stable at 5 % level. By comparing these critical value, it indicates that there exists cointegration relationship between lnGDP and lnFIR.

Table 253.1 Residuals unit root (ADF) test results

Series	(C T k)	ADF values	1 %	5 %	10 %	Conclusion
Residuals	(C 0 1)	−3.069	−3.670	−2.963	−2.621	Steady

Table 253.2 Granger causality test results

Null hypothesis	The number of samples	Lag	F statistic	Significance level	Conclusion
LNGDP does not granger cause LNFIR	30	2	8.8652	0.00123	Refuse
LNFIR does not granger cause LNGDP	30	2	4.2102	0.02655	Refuse

253.3.3 Granger Causality Test

Through empirical methods, we need to verify whether FIR causes change in GDP, or GDP causes FIR changes, or they are both changed by other common reasons. The regression analysis can neither test the existence nor the direction of causal relationship. Granger causality test is a commonly used method for solving such problems. According to the AIC criterion, we determine the number of lags of each variable is 2, the results of Granger causality test for each variable are as shown in Table 253.2.

Strickly speaking, as the null hypothesis is there exists no causal relationship, we may call this test Granger noncausality test. From Table 253.4, we can conclude that GDP and FIR have a causal relationship to each other. This result indicates that the economic growth of Zhejiang Province plays a significant role in promoting the development of financial markets, strong economic growth is an important condition for the development of financial markets. Conversely, the latter can also promote the former. But the effect of former is notable than the latter.

253.4 Conclusions and Recommendations

253.4.1 Strengthening the Financial System

As finance plays an important role in the development of national economy, Zhejiang should vigorously strengthen the financial system, and promote the development of the insurance industry, the securities industry and other financial industries. There are a large number of small and medium enterprises in Zhejiang Province, we should encourage SMEs to expand business scale and provide more jobs for the province.

253.4.2 Strengthening the Financial Risk Prevention and Regulatory System

Financial development can play a positive role in promoting economic growth, but excessive expansion of the financial industry will cause economic recession.

The risk of the financial industry can easily spread to the real economy. Therefore, the prevention of financial risks is the most important task of the financial regulatory agencies. Local financial regulators should strengthen the monitoring and analysis in the financial operation.

253.4.3 Promote Positive Interaction of Financial Development and Economic Growth

Zhejiang local financial institutions should focus on supporting the most vigorous parts of economic growth in the region actively. Moreover, strengthening the SMEs credit and consumer credit in order to expand demand and promote economic growth are also necessary. At the same time, we should exert the promoting role of economic growth that plays on financial development, and guide these two to make a positive interaction so as to promote sustainable economic growth.

Acknowledgments This research was financially supported by the National Natural Science Foundation of China (Grant No. 11171306) and the Natural Science Foundation of Zhejiang Province (Grant No. LY12A01024).

References

1. Brown B, Aaron M (2001) The politics of nature. In: Smith J (ed) The rise of modern genomics, 3rd edn. Wiley, New York
2. Goyal SK (1977) An integrated inventory model for a single supplier-single customer problem. Int J Prod Res 15:107–111
3. Banerjee A (1986) A joint economic-lot-size model for purchaser and vendor. Decis Sci 17:292–311
4. Goyal SK (1988) A joint economic-lot-size model for purchaser and vendor: a comment. Decis Sci 19:236–241
5. Hill RM (1997) The single-vendor single-buyer integrated production–inventory model with a generalized policy. Eur J Oper Res 97:493–499
6. Kim SL, Ha D (2003) A JIT lot-splitting model for supply chain management: enhancing buyer–supplier linkage. Int J Prod Econ 86:1–10

Chapter 254
The Teaching Design of Digital Signal Processing Based on MATLAB and FPGA

Xiaoyan Tian, Lei Chen and Jiao Pang

Abstract Due to the wide-ranging contents, abstract concepts and complicated designs involved in Digital Signal Processing (DSP), this paper proposed a technology scheme that incorporated MATLAB and FPGA into the theoretical and practical teaching. The scheme developed a multimedia teaching system based on VC++ and MATLAB which gives full play to the advantages of visual graphics, consequently achieved the purpose of stimulating interests of learning, reducing the difficulty of understanding and improving the quality of teaching. In order to improve the ability of engineering application, also designed a comprehensive experiment based on the combination of MATLAB DSP Builder and FPGA instead of the previous experiment methods using the MATLAB tools for the single simulation. The results show that this scheme achieved anticipated goals.

Keywords Digital signal processing · MATLAB · VC++ · Field programmable gate array

254.1 Introduction

In the past half-century, with the development of computer and microelectronics technology, the strong theoretical and engineering discipline DSP has been a leap in the development. Its status and influence are becoming more and more important, turning into the theoretical and technical basis of communications, radar, sonar, electro-acoustic, TV, monitoring and control, biomedical engineering and many other subjects. However, on account of the DSP features of involving many contents, abstract concepts and complicated designs, there is a phenomenon that many students are afraid to learn and feel weariness for this course, even they

X. Tian (✉) · L. Chen · J. Pang
College of Electronic and Information Engineering, Hebei University, Baoding 071002, China
e-mail: tianxiaoyan_1999@163.com

cannot understand it. At the same time, DSP algorithm implementation is based on numerical calculation of the computer, manual calculation is much more complicated, even impossible to achieve. As a result, assignments are generally not easy for teachers which leads to certain restrictions for students' after-school practice and affects the teaching effect at a large extent.

In the current domain of domestic and international signal processing and system design, MATLAB is one of the most popular engineering simulation software. MATLAB teaching demonstration covers all the DSP teaching contents, such as signal and system Fourier analysis, convolution calculation, filter design, signal filter etc. Using the MATLAB graphical visualization advantages and graphics to explain the theory, we turn the abstract theory into the close combination of theory and application, which can greatly improve the teaching effect.

In the meantime, as a result of its reconfigurability and parallel computing, programmable logic device FPGA/CPLD is widely adopted, and it is an important branch in the field of electronic design.

254.2 Multimedia Teaching System Based of MATLAB

In order to make full use of the advantages of MATLAB visualization, and to meet the need of multimedia teaching, the task group has developed a multimedia teaching system based on MATLAB to arouse interest in learning, improve understanding and strengthen the capability of the combination of theory and practice. Because this course involves too much content, it cannot be described in detail. The teaching process basically takes the "analog signal digital transmission" as the main line, "discrete Fourier transform and digital filter design" as two cores to unfold, focusing on the basic concepts, basic theory and basic methods of DSP, weakening complex operation and formula derivation, emphasizing the physical meaning and engineering concepts behind the formula. The teaching system is accomplished according to the design of this concept which consists of two parts—lectures and demonstrations.

The teaching system architecture is shown in Fig. 254.1.

The system develops the main operating window based on Basic Class Library MFC provided by Microsoft VC++. Using ActiveX controls and COM interfaces to achieve entrying and displaying content of the course of PPT, alleviating the tedious process of the contents entrying, making modification more convenient. With MATLAB GUI, by changing the different design parameters, we can obtain different calculation results to carry out comparative analysis and understanding.

Deploy Tools use MFC compiler to generate the corresponding C language files and data files according to the M file, and then call C/C++ compiler to compile. MATLAB project is compiled into an executable file, so that the system can be operated out of the MATLAB environment, which mean it is not necessary to install MATLAB on the machine.

Some demonstration pictures are shown in Fig. 254.2.

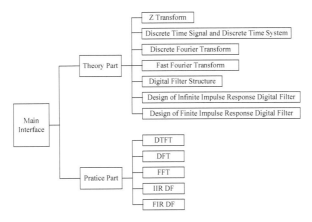

Fig. 254.1 Structure of multimedia teaching system

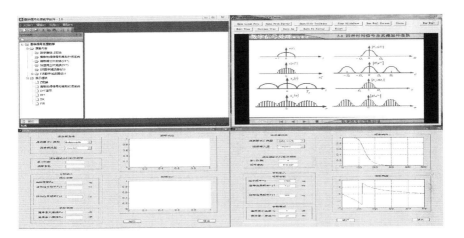

Fig. 254.2 Multimedia teaching system

254.3 Development of Comprehensive Experiment Based on MATLAB and FPGA

Currently, there are two ways for the experiment on the course of DSP in our colleges: One is MATLAB simulation. With its built-in functions, powerful plotting and GUI to make the problems quite simple and clear. Although it can make for a better understanding of the theoretical knowledge, that no hardwire implementation details are involved is a severe weakness. Another is use DSP experiment box to conduct the test. This method is characterized by application

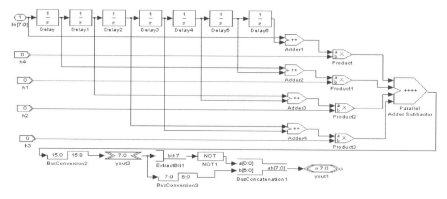

Fig. 254.3 Design of 7-order linear phase FIR DF in DSP Builder

and complicated, unreadable program for a certain DSP chip. It hardly has anything to do with the context of DSP though the results are obvious.

Programmable FPGA/CPLD is widely used with its capability of reconfigurability and parallel computation so that it is an important branch of electronic design field. Increasingly, FPGA becomes a substitute of ASIC and DSP chips for the development of DSP system. Hence we integrate the experimental teaching system of single MATLAB simulation into coordination between MATLAB and FPGA so that much more all-around design experiments can be performed. With the platform students can finish the design and simulation using MATLAB and implement on FPGA.

Take the "FIR filter design based on MATLAB and FPGA" as a example. With the help of FDATool in MATLAB, we can easily design our filters, quantify and normalize the coefficients. After that a model can be devised in DSP Builder graphical interface using the quantitative and normalized coefficients with two available simplified implementation structures-Direct and Linear phase. In our experiment, a filter employed in coherent demodulation is considered. We will obtain it and validate the correctness by simulation in MATLAB with automatic generation of corresponding VHDL files and Quartus III project files using SignalCompiler to be followed. After that a waveform file will be created for simulation and we will go on to implement the design in FPGA if the result is right. The main process is shown in Figs. 254.3, 254.4, and 254.5.

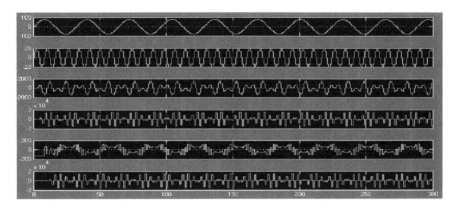

Fig. 254.4 Simulation result in MATLAB

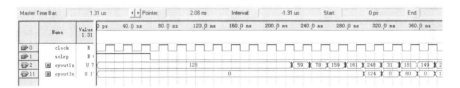

Fig. 254.5 Simulation result in Quartus II

254.4 Conclusions

MATLAB is a numerical and visible calculation language which has remarkable features of powerful, efficient, high interactivity. It provided with a big advantage in digital signal processing. The combination of VC++ and MATLAB improves the teaching effect. Comprehensive experiments based on MATLAB and FPGA fuses advanced software simulation with hardware implementation, which is consistent with engineering practices and can boost students' engineering application abilities.

Acknowledgments This project supported by Science and Technology Research Project of College and University in Hebei Province(Z2012126, Z2011252); educational reform project JX07-Y-36 of Hebei University; educational reform project JX2010006 of Industrial and Commercial College, Hebei University.

References

1. Cheng P (2007) Digital signal processing. Tsinghua University Press, Beijing
2. Lou S, Yao R, Shen J (2006) MATLAB7.X programming language. Xidian University Press, Xi'an

3. Wang Y, Zhang X (2012) Application of the Matlab practice in the teaching reform of digital signal processing course. Exp Sci Technol 10(5):108–110
4. Shen Y (2009) The comprehensive experiment design of digital signal processing based of Matlab. Res Explor Lab 28(8):60–61,73

Chapter 255
The Design of an Management Software for High Value Medical Consumables

Zhou Longfu, Hu Yonghe, Fan Quanshui, Zhao Ming, Zhang Chaoqun and Li Zheng

Abstract In this paper, an software, which is written in C# program language based on ORACLE and .NET Frame Work, for high value medical consumables management is introduced. Using client–server model as system structural, data structure and the data flow are defined according to hospital information systems (HIS) database. In the software, indexed by patient ID number, the patient information and the high value medical consumable they used in the treatment process is made up as a whole in the process of the warehousing operation. Then, a two-dimension code including information of patient and material is built, which can be added in medical record automatic. In the end, by using the software, management consciousness and working efficiency is raised.

Keywords High value consumable · Hospital management · Hospital information system · Traceable · Identification system

Since 1990s of the last century, accompanied with widely clinical application, the management of high value medical consumables has became one of hot topic in the hospital manage. Xu et al. [1] uses bar code to integrate high value consumables physical distribution, financial information and clinical information into an information chain for convenient analysis and management. ERP management software is used in [2] to manage medical consumable material in the hospital. By ERP, standard technological process for medical consumable material management is established. Based on the analysis of the current management state of hospital high value consumables, a comprehensive trace management system of high value medical consumables by bar code is developed and designed in [3].

Z. Longfu · H. Yonghe (✉) · Z. Ming · Z. Chaoqun · L. Zheng
The Department of Medical Engineer, The General Hospital of Chengdu, No.270, Rongdu Road, Chengdu 610083 Sichuan, People's Republic China
e-mail: huyonghe@vip.126.com

Z. Longfu · H. Yonghe · F. Quanshui
Center for Disease Control and Prevention of Chengdu Command, No.118,Daguan Road, Kunming 650032, China

Bar code recognition technology was introduced into the management of high-value medical consumables in [4]. Dynamic management of high value medical consumables resulted in higher efficiency and quality than static one.

255.1 HIS and High Value Medical Consumables

Hospital information systems (HIS) [5] is massive, integrated systems that support the comprehensive information requirements of hospitals, including patient, clinical, ancillary and financial management. The aim of an HIS is to achieve the best possible support of patient care and outcome and administration by presenting data where needed and acquiring data when generated with networked electronic data processing. Hospitals are becoming more reliant on the ability of HIS to assist in the diagnosis, management and education for better and improved services and practices.

High value medical consumables generally refer to those productions which are very important to sufferers, must be strictly controlled, limited to some special use and the price is relatively higher. It mainly belongs to a medical specialist treatment material, such as cardiac intervention, peripheral vascular intervention, artificial joint, other organ involvement of alternative and other medical materials. Economic benefit and social effect can be more exerted through the usage of management techniques of high value medical consumable materials, and more full scale service can be provided.

Nowadays, HIS becomes the foundation of hospital and high value medical consumable has become a most important part in clinical works too. Although many methods had been introduced in the management of high value medical consumables in hospital, the question on how to improve the management efficiency and ensure the safety is still open. In this paper, an management software is designed and introduced which binds the information of high value medical consumables with the identity of patient.

255.2 System Architecture

255.2.1 Structural Design

The client-server model [6, 7] (C/S) is an approach to computer network programming developed during the 1970s. It is now prevalent in computer networks. The model assigns one of two roles to the computers in a network: client or server. A server is a computer system that selectively shares its resources; a client is a computer or computer program that initiates contact with a server in order to make use of a resource. Clients and servers exchange messages in a request-response messaging pattern. The server is a centralized system. The more simultaneous clients a server has, the more resources it needs.

In the design, the system architecture with five layers is adopted shown in Fig. 255.1. The database of HIS is used as data source of the designed software, which achieve the query, update, delete and persistent preservation operation of underlying data. Then, the execution results are returned to the layer of "Data Persistence". In this layer, all function are finished by Oracle general database operation class "OleDbHelper.cs". The SQL statement sent by domain is executed and the results are returned afterwards. Next, those packaged business operation in the layer of domain is assembled accordance with the actual business processes and data are sent to layer "Presentation" from layer "Controller/Mediator". Through data, format and data type conversion, the processed data is shown in the user interface finally.

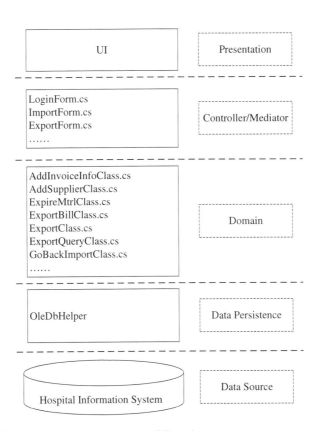

Fig. 255.1 The system architecture based on C/S mode

255.2.2 The Relationship with HIS

Nowadays, HIS has become the foundation of digital operation in hospital. Therefore, good compatibility with HIS is the basic demand in any software aimed to use in hospital. In the software, all data structure and the data flow are according to the definition of HIS database.

Through maintenance the comparison table between "material price" and "HIS price list", the valuation relationship of the high value consumables and patient relationship between departments and patient are built in the designed software. At same time, only those authorized users in HIS can achieve the distribution of the corresponding authority. In the end, details of high value consumables supplied to patient will be shown in electronic medical records in the form of a two-dimensional code.

255.3 Main Functions

In the software, around the management of high value consumable, four major function modules including inventory, dictionary maintenance, query statistics and data modification are designed. In the module of inventory management, warehousing, bookkeeping and return of high value consumable are deal. Name, inventory and price of high value consumable are defined in the module of dictionary maintenance management. Dynamic multiple conditions query is supported and query results can be output into Excel. In the module of data modification, the time of warehousing and the information of invoice can be revised.

255.3.1 Main Interface

After verification by HIS database, authorized user is permit to open the management software. The main interface is shown as in Fig. 255.2. The software is inserted four toolbar buttons in the drop-down menu. Users can choose the drop-down menu of options to do some relevant manipulation.

255.3.2 The Module of Inventory Management

In the module, the operations including storage, warehousing, bookkeeping and return of high value consumable are deal.

During the warehousing operation, as shown in Fig. 255.3, patient information is combined with those high value medical consumable though patient ID number,

255 Management Software for High Value Medical Consumables 2119

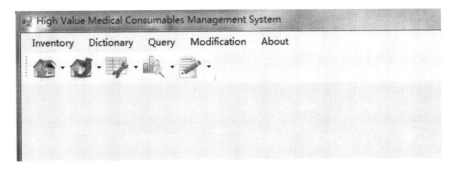

Fig. 255.2 Main interface

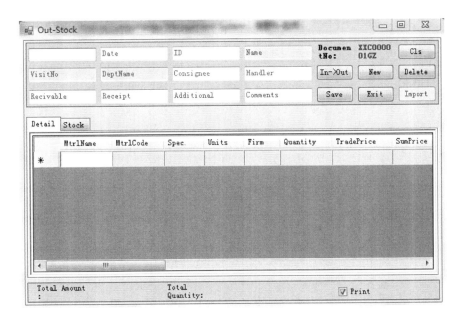

Fig. 255.3 Warehousing interface

which is the only characteristic of a patient in HIS database. Then, the material is rationed out directly to the end user rather than clinical department in hospital.

In the tradition working mode, warehousing staff keep account according the application of clinical department in hospital. The user and usage model of the high value medical consumable depend on the statistics of clinical department, which cause inconsistent information. Through this new working mode, the relationship between material and user get clear. Data in the software becomes the only information source.

255.3.3 The Module of Dictionary Maintenance

A high value medical consumable's property includes name, inventory level and price, which need manual definition in the module. Then, material code and input code are automatically generated.

In order to enhance the working efficiency, to each class of material, a two-dimension code in Fig. 255.4 is built in the definition process. During the process of entering-warehouse, through scanning the two-dimension code, the information of material can be input into the system. By this way, error rate in entry is reduced and working efficiency can be obviously raised.

255.3.4 The Module of Query Statistics

Five sub-modules are designed here. They are recently stock inquiry, entering-warehouse inquiry, out-of-warehouse inquiry, expired material inquiry and using record inquiry. The details about all high value consumables can be inquiry and counted.

255.3.5 The Module of Data Modification

Sometimes, invoice cannot be provided with consumable at same time. In such condition, staff unable to feed the whole information into system. The function of modification offers the possible to perfect data.

Fig. 255.4 Two-dimension code of material

255.4 Conclusion

The management of high value consumable is one of hot topic in hospital, which related medical safety and the doctor-patient relations. As the cornerstone of modern medical work, the function of HIS also needs continuous improvement. To meet the requirement of hospital management team, so as to realize the comprehensive trace and control for purchase, supply, use as well as management of high value medical consumables, management software for high value medical consumable is designed and introduced in the paper, which can enhance management consciousness, raise working efficiency, avoid flaw and waste and gain good economic and social benefits.

Because patient information is combined with those high value medical consumable though patient ID number, by using the software, a two-dimension code, not only including the information of material but containing the primary identity information of user, can be built. Written the two-dimension code in medical record, the mistake made by band-kept can be efficiently avoided.

References

1. Xu Z-R, Wang Z-Z, Li T-J, et al. (2012) Analysis of difficulty in management of high value consumables based on bar code technology. China Med Equip, 9(6):25–27.
2. Li X, Zhao Y-H, Wang S, Li W, Han S-Q (2010) Medical consumable material management with ERP. Chin Med Equip J 31(2):85–87
3. Fei X-L, Jin P (2010) Construction and practice of management information system for medical high value consumable. China Med Equip 25(7):11–13
4. Lv M, Hao Y-W, Gao Y (2012) Applied research of bar code technology in high-value medical consumables management. Chin Med Equip J 33(8):119–121
5. 2011 International conference on social science and humanity [C]
6. Randolph N, Gardner D (2008) Professional visual studio [M]. WROX PR/PEER Information INC
7. Pedersen JH (2010) Beginning microsoft visual C#[M]. 2010, WROX PR/PEER Information INC

Chapter 256
Libraries Follow-Up Services in the Era of Fragmentation Reading

Lu Yanxiang

Abstract The advance of technology changes the way people read. Mobile Internet develops quickly. Digital publication grows swiftly. Reading terminal changes everyday. Readers get used to reading digitally through reading in a new environment. Things people read have become more and more fragmented. In order to adapt the change, libraries start to contribute more digital resources, to increase notification service, to use social media to promote, interact and share, to buildup mobile library, and to provide ubiquitous service on the basis of traditional service. The resource and the service of a library should be updated frequently to fit the way in which readers get information.

Keywords Fragmentation reading · Library · Digital resources · Media sharing · Mobile library

256.1 Introduction

The Development of Information Technology Brings Fragmentation Reading. As the latest report from China Internet Network Information Center says, the number of Internet users in China has reached 538 million, and the internet penetration is 39.9 %. Moreover, the number of internet users via mobile phone to access the internet has reached 388 million in the first half year of 2012.

According to a report released by the Ninth National Reading Survey, the online rate of adult internet users was with more than 50 % for the first time in the national region of China in 2011, and the online rate is 54.9 % for the users aged from 18 to 70 years old. Generally speaking, the online rate is more than 50 %

L. Yanxiang (✉)
The Library of Jianghan University, Wuhan 430056, China
e-mail: 327579500@qq.com

(specifically 50.6 %) for computer users, and 25.4 % for mobile users. Compared the increase rate of 16.6 % in 2010, the mobile online rate won a significant increase, that is, it has an increase of 53 % [1].

Diversified terminals promote composite publishing. Along with the big sales growth in the three largest mobile digital reading terminals, that is, e-reader, tablet computer and smart mobile phone, it as well created nice hardware foundation and reading conditions for digital publication.

According to the result released by the Ninth National Reading Survey, the contact rate of 2011 national digital reading methods (online reading, mobile reading, e-reader reading, CD reading, PDA/MP4/MP5 reading etc.) is 38.6 %. The daily mobile reading time is 13.53 min, while the daily e-reader reading time is 3.11 min for each person.

The publishing of electronic publications is 11,154 in total, and the total profit is 13 billion RMB, which won an increase of 28 % compared to 2010. In 2011, the digital publishing achieved 137.78 billion RMB in operation revenue, and 10.67 billion RMB in total profit, which won an increase of 19.1 % compared to 2010. The readers' digital reading habits have been cultivated gradually [2].

256.2 Readers' Fragmentation Reading

Alwin·Toffler, the famous futurologist in the U. S., noted in his book of The Third Wave "This is a fragment era, information fragmentation, audience fragmentation, media fragmentation."

Reading content is fragmented. After the birth of e-reading, operators decidedly adopted focus strategy in the face of hundreds of millions reading contents, which therefore made the reading contents get into pieces. The fragmented reading content made readers get access to fragmented knowledge [3].

We have discussed that the content spread by communicators is fragmented in the era of e-reading. Conversely, being the recipient, they received the fragmented knowledge as well. Under the internet environment, we often got lost in fragmented digital reading due to poor understanding on the digital world, which brought incoherent thinking and reflection from reading, thus caused the fragmented crisis in knowledge and ideas.

Reading carrier is fragmented. The popularization of various mobile terminals has also accelerated the development of fragmentation reading. Different types of e-book reader, MP4, mobile phone, computer and other carriers co-exist with traditional books, newspapers, and magazines. BLOG, MICRO-BLOG, Video and Spaces are all characterized by fragmentation.

Reading time is fragmented. As life rhythm speeds up, time is fragmented, accompanied by fragmentation reading. For this, people have to enter the era of fragmentation reading [4]. They can get access to a great quantity of information from mobile phone, internet or other electronic terminal receivers every day. Reading is so easy, it seems all the information and knowledge can get without the least difficulty [5]. Diversified channels for information transmission make the traditional way of reading being not the only way for people to acquire knowledge and information any more.

256.3 Characteristics of Fragmentation Reading

The characteristics of digital publishing, that is, high popularization, low cost, mobility, interaction and sound with pictures set up a brand-new era of digital reading. This new digital reading refreshed the reader's reading experience, and meantime met their multiple reading desires to the maximum extent.

The biggest characteristic of digital reading is skip reading, micro reading, light reading, and extensive reading. The fragmented language, platter-type content, led people to "know more" instead of "know-how". Simple straightforward and fast reading guides people to do fast reading [6]. To some extent, this way of reading will lead more skip reading and less deep reading.

The information is lack of stability, reliability and system. Just as Baudrillard said, "Information dispels significance and society as an illegible status, which would not bring excessive innovation, while the contrary disorder's full increase." Under the unstable internet space time, people can not read in a smooth and natural way while read in the features of disorders and fragmentation.

256.4 Library Follow-Up Service and Innovation

256.4.1 Integration of Fragmentation Reading

Massive information easily leads to read blindly, distract people's attention to the normal information. Disordered information may add difficulty to understand specific things. Then it will require professional operator to both integrate information and offer services with specific target audience and unique pattern of product's processing services so as to meet different demands for focus services.

One is to organize, classify, index, reveal and map the information resources. Massive information may easily lead to reading blindly. If capacitated content can be carefully selected, it will mean opportunities. The other is to offer abundant, complete and comprehensive resources to enrich the database structure platform. Digital reading platform has abandoned the traditional methods which listed as date resource type to directly integrate the specific content into the platform so that users may link to related resources in one key and smoothly read all resources straightly. Such a way of reading can also support the access to PC, iPad, IPod touch, mobile phone, handheld reader, and other terminal access equipment. To set up the principle as reader-centered, to sort and classify mass information, to fully develop the functions of hyperlink and search will allow readers to enjoy the process of reading. They may read the key information without losing any interest; meantime, it will bring readers convenience of acquiring comprehensive knowledge by using different terminals during fragmented time.

256.4.2 Use Media to Extend, Interact and Share

The method has been changed from passively waiting for readers into positively giving publicity to readers, such as introducing the information resources and services of library to readers, communicating with readers by MSN, QQ, and etc., or offering virtual consulting services to pass information or eliminate confusion for readers [7]. More than the above, we try to expand the channels of information interaction with readers through BLOG and WIKI.

Second is social media. Nowadays, with the further integration of traditional Internet and mobile Internet, social media has been developed rapidly, which is as well widely used in library. According to the survey of Metropolitan Library Committee, three fourths of libraries is in the use of social media, 89 % of them are using FACEBOOK, 80 % are using Twitter, 76 % develop BLOG information services. Network video conference is also popular in the world of library. According to the statistics from China Internet Network Information Center, there are a total of 250 million MICRO-BLOG users in China by the end of 2011, which made China as the biggest MICRO-BLOG user in the world. The application of MICRO-BLOG has been quite popular in library, which is not only conductive to the promotion of library, but also an effective way of communicating with readers.

256.4.3 Mobile Phone Library-Services at Anywhere and Anytime

According to the result from the Ninth National Reading Survey newly released by China Research Institute of the News Publishing, we have 27.6 % users who aged from 18 to 70 years old in China used mobile phone reading in 2011. They spent about 40 min on mobile reading every day, and their annual cost on it is about 20 RMB. And you may see the detailed information as the following chart 2.

National Library of China, Shanghai Library, Shenzhen Library and some public libraries and university all have established mobile library. Via short message platform, web message platform, mobile reading platform to offer services like book search, book renewal and book reservation, return alert, reader's card management, reference consulting, lecture reservation, new books' notice, reader's recommendation, news' release, personalized customization, mobile reading to users. Therefore, users may timely share resources and services from library by mobile phone movement (Fig. 256.1, Table 256.1).

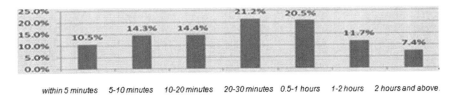

Fig. 256.1 Reading time length of daily mobile reading

Table 256.1 Form of digital publications in 2011 Unit: 100 million RMB

Category	Operation revenue	Increase value	Output	Total profit
Mobile publication	367.34	103.81	367.34	28.44
Mobile music	282.00	79.69	282.00	21.83
Mobile reading	45.74	12.93	45.74	3.54
Mobile game	39.60	11.19	39.60	3.07
Internet game	428.50	121.09	428.50	33.17
Digital periodical	9.34	2.64	9.34	0.72
E-book	16.50	4.66	16.50	1.28
Digital journal (Online edition)	12.00	3.39	12.00	0.93
Internet advertising	512.9	144.95	512.9	39.71
Internet comic and animation	3.50	0.99	3.50	0.27
Online music	3.80	1.07	3.80	0.29
BLOG	24.00	6.78	24.00	1.86
Total	1377.88	389.38	1377.88	106.68

256.5 Conclusion

The third generation wave is the "Mobile Internet", which has brought great changes to people's reading and even way of life, way of thinking. People can obtain resources at any time, any place, to make use of odd moment to have fragmentation reading [8]. The new mass media information and fragmentation reading becomes more popular, which as well poses a severe challenge to the traditional library. Mobile phone screen can be books. Library keeps pace with the times, which brings quality library information resources and services access to Apple, Samsung, and other terminal products. Obviously, it plays the role of library to help readers form reading habits and cultivate the reading market.

Acknowledgments This work is partially supported by the National Social Science Fund of "Study on the Core Competency of the Library", China (09BTQ002). The author also gratefully acknowledges the helpful comments and suggestions of the reviewers, which have improved the presentation.

References

1. Ninth national reading survey preliminary results released, [EB/OL]. http://www.chuban.cc/ztjj/yddc/mtjj/201204/t20120420_105469.html.[2012-04-20]
2. 2011 Press and publication industry analysis report (Summary), [EB/OL]. http://data.chinaxwcb.com/zgcb/bktg/201207/24333.html.[2012-07-30]
3. Xiaoyuan Li (2011) On the fragmented reading under internet environment. Info Documentation Serv 6:84–87
4. Haiyan Hu, Ruiqing Jian (2011) New reading trends challenge reading guidance of the library. New Century Libr 5:14–17
5. Peters Tom (2009) The future of reading. Libr J 123(18):18–22
6. Enis M (2012) Pew: younger Americans reading more. Libr J 137(19):12
7. Haslam-Odoardi Rebecca (2010) Gifted readers and libraries: a natural fit. Teach Librarian 37(3):32–36
8. Weinberger David (2008) Everything is miscellaneous: the power of the new digital disorder. Henry Holt and Company Inc, New York

Chapter 257
Research on Construction of Green Agriculture Products Supply Chain Based on the Model Differentiation

Bo Zhao

Abstract According to the basic ideas of green agriculture products supply chain, focusing on the comparative analysis of the general structure, the advantages and disadvantages of the traditional supply chain and modern closed supply chain of green agriculture products, on the basis of the traditional supply chain optimization, we construct the closed supply chain system based on the modern logistics center, thus to ensure the quality of green agriculture products, and to realize the sustainable development of agriculture and rural.

Keywords Differentiation · Supply chain · Green agriculture products · Logistics center

257.1 Basic Ideas of Green Agriculture Products Supply Chain

Green Agriculture Products Supply Chain (GAPSC) makes the concept of "green, health and environmental protection" throughout the agriculture products supply chain, in the product life cycle process from agriculture products design, production, packaging, warehousing, transportation, consumption and waste recycling processing, through green design, green material, green production, green manufacturing, green logistics, green marketing and green recycling and other technical means, produce high yield, high quality, efficient green agriculture products, and advocate green consumption, to ensure quality and safety of agriculture products.

B. Zhao (✉)
Research Center of Rural Economy and Management, College of Economics and Management, Southwest University, 400715 Chongqing, China
e-mail: zhbo323@swu.edu.cn

257.2 Disadvantages about China's Traditional Agriculture Products Supply Chain

Agriculture products supply chain in developed countries is the earliest supply chain model in the logistics industry, but in our country is still at the primary stage of construction. China's traditional agriculture products supply chain structure is shown in Fig. 257.1.

For the green agriculture products, at present, China's regional and national green agriculture products logistics system has not yet been formed, green agriculture products circulation is still too dependent on traditional marketing channels. As with common produce, a large number of green agriculture products sold through the farmers market and multi-level wholesale market, not only the logistics efficiency is low, product loss is big, but there is no guarantee that the circulation of agriculture products in the process of "green" features, which cannot satisfy the demand of green agriculture products logistics.

The disadvantages of China's traditional agriculture products supply chain are shown in Table 257.1.

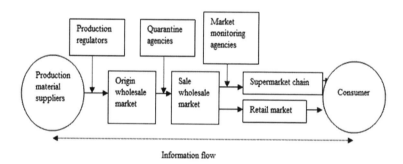

Fig. 257.1 Traditional agriculture products supply chain structure

Table 257.1 The disadvantages of traditional agriculture products supply chain

The disadvantages of traditional agriculture products supply chain
1 The traditional farmer-based agricultural production method is difficult to achieve green production requirements
2 The traditional supply chain technology is backward, which is difficult to guarantee product safety and quality in the logistics process
3 The multi-link and open structure of traditional supply chain is not conducive to reduce the cost
4 The traditional supply chain is lack of supervision system, and has not formed the perfect agriculture products safety information monitoring system
5 Traditional agriculture products market is not conducive to the establishment of green agriculture products brand

From the above we can see, the traditional agriculture products supply chain is associated with lower levels of economic development, it is difficult to adapt to the requirements of green produce industrialization development. In order to promote green agriculture products industry health development, we must establish a unique green agriculture products proprietary supply chain to ensure the quality and safety, and to reduce the logistics cost.

257.3 Construction of Modern Green Agriculture Products Supply Chain System

Considering the traditional agriculture products supply chain has many drawbacks, we constructed a modern closed supply chain of green agriculture products, which form a set of management main body, information chain, the core enterprise and tracing system—Green agriculture products closed supply chain based on the logistics center (as shown in Fig. 257.2).

This closed supply chain is composed of the following parts: agriculture products logistics center, is mainly composed of agricultural products processing enterprises, warehousing distribution and marketing enterprises; the production base, is mainly composed of modular standardized planting base, new agricultural cooperation organization, rural area economic cooperatives, farmer brokers and the farmer; the production material suppliers; the retailers, is mainly composed of

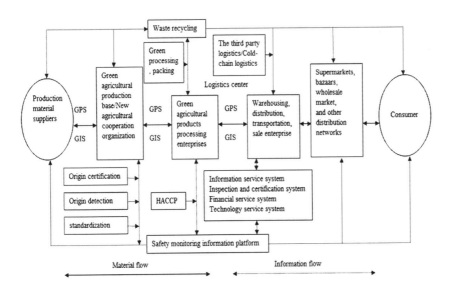

Fig. 257.2 Closed supply chain of green agriculture products general structure

the fresh supermarkets, wholesale mall and other distribution network; the consumers.

The model has realized the optimization of green agriculture products closed supply chain based on the traditional supply chain model, specifically in the following 4 aspects.

Firstly, expression of green agriculture products definition and basic requirements.Agriculture products include green pollution-free agriculture products, green food and organic food, according to international and national laws and standards, the operation must strictly implement the management system, certification system, detection system and production system.

Secondly, expression of the basic characteristics and basic requirements of agriculture products supply chain. The model has realized the integrity of the supply chain process including production management, warehousing, distribution and consumption of green agriculture products, containing the logistics, business flow, information flow and cash flow.

Thirdly, expression of the common characteristics of logistics system and supply chain and its particularity—green and closed. It is mainly manifested as "green logistics", "the circular logistics", strict access management system, a unified operational norms and technical standards, the real-time monitoring and dynamic tracking and traceability.

Finally, expression of the exclusive strategic cooperative partnership between the supply chain subjects. Comparing with the traditional open supply chain, the controllability, coordination and the ability to resist risk of closed supply chain is stronger. Closed supply chain concept embodies the whole process control about production, exchange, distribution and consumption, to ensure the quality and safety of agriculture products; By using the closed marketing channels, integrating the advanced information technology and modern logistics technology, relying on e-commerce platform operation efficiency advantage, closed supply chain has realized the real-time tracing, effective control and management of the entire process, and led the development of agriculture industrialization.

In general, comparing with the traditional agriculture products supply chain, green agriculture products closed supply chain has the following features (as shown in Table 257.2):

Table 257.2 The features of green agriculture products closed supply chain

The features of green agriculture products closed supply chain
1 The closed, few links and unique business model
2 The tracing system realizes the comprehensive monitoring of green agriculture products quality
3 The cold-chain logistics system effectively ensures the product quality, safety and reduces the logistics cost
4 The standardized operation of closed supply chain system

257.4 Conclusion

At present, with the development of economic globalization, the traditional tariff and non-tariff barriers have been gradually weakened, green barriers is gradually on the rise. Especially in recent years, the cases about China's agriculture products encountered green barrier in the international market have occurred from time to time. Closed supply chain of green agriculture products with advanced technology and management mode, strict monitoring system and strict testing standards, can maximize the green agriculture products quality. Therefore, the development of closed supply chain of green agriculture products is to improve China's agriculture products competitiveness in the international market, break the foreign agriculture products export green barriers, and participate competition in international market. At the same time, because the closed supply chain of green agriculture products operation reduces the decay in the process of agriculture products logistics, reduce logistics costs, therefore, will become the strategic choice of our country agriculture synergism, promoting agricultural and rural sustainable development.

Acknowledgments The paper was supported by 2011 Chongqing Social Science Foundation Youth Project(NO:2011QNGL66), 2010 Chongqing Arts Key Research Base Project(Research on Citizenization Behavior of Migrant Workers,NO:1010006) and the Fundamental Research Funds for the Central Universities(NO:SWU1309003; NO:SWU1309383).

References

1. Lorice S, Allan G, Allan S (2005) The UK food supply chain-an ethical perspective. Food Res Int 37:23–40
2. Gnaeshna R, Terry PH (2006) An introduction to supply chain management in third part logistics providers. Eur Journey Oper Res 5:332–356
3. Terry M, Gilian B (2000) Food supply chain approaches: exploring their role in rural development. European Soc Rural Sociol 10:424–439
4. Lambert DM, Cooper MC (2000) Issues in supply chain management. Ind Mark Manage 29:65–83
5. Samir KS(2007) Green supply-chain management: a state-of-the-art literature review. Int Journey Manage rev 9:53–80
6. Gunnar S (2005) Business-to-business data sharing a source for integration of supply chains. Int J Prod Econ 7:165–180
7. Fearne A, Hughes D (2000) Success factors in the fresh produce supply chain. Br Food J 102:760–772

Chapter 258
Visualization Analysis and Research of Scientific Papers and Thesis in University

Jiangning Xie, Xueqing Li, Lei Wang and Ye Tao

Abstract The study about visualization of paper has been developed abroad in the recent few years. To analysis the thesis status and track research hotspots in universities, we propose an effective visualization method based on some techniques and utilities. A combined method of the data integration, data mining and visualization analysis is applied to analyze thesis keywords and citation. We use model-driven approach to design and build the scientific data integration and data mining platform. And a visible data analysis method is outlined to reveal research hotspot and conceptual graph.

Keywords Information visualization · Model-driven · Thesis hotspots

258.1 Introduction

With the year-to-year growth in domestic graduate students, the quality of postgraduate training is becoming a key issue for colleges and universities to enhance their teaching and research level. How to train the high-level personnel of the academic with the strong research ability and the good academic literacy has

---

J. Xie (✉) · X. Li
The Department of Computer Science and Technology, Shandong University,
Jinan 250101, Shandong, China
e-mail: xjn@sdu.edu.cn

X. Li
e-mail: xqli@sdu.edu.cn

L. Wang
Weifang University, Weifang, Shandong, China

Y. Tao
Qingdao University of Science and Technology, Qingdao, Shandong, China

became the most important aim for the graduate education in various countries. Postgraduate training includes the processes of the admissions, teaching, research, thesis writing and defence, and how through assessment analysis of the formation of the related link analysis and support of decision-making culture training model innovation key issues [1]. In particular, the key evaluate data is the Graduate Thesis Topic and writing. We can quickly access the valuable information and data through the systematic research and analysis for the graduate research projects status, and improve the academic quality of graduate education.

Extraction and analysis of key data, we can more accurately grasp the development of cutting-edge issues of domestic and international technology and current research focus. And the decision management department is able to obtain accurate data to support the understanding the current execution policies meet the needs of the development and timely adjust for individual colleges and domain-specific.

258.2 Related Work

With the continuous development of the education level of information technology, the system provides quantitative data sources for the analysis of the quality of graduate education. So the quantitative analysis combined with the actual data for the training quality has become the core of graduate education quality research methods. Data analysis and data visualization analysis method provides the intuitive and effective visual effects for papers [2]. The purpose of the visualization analysis is the analysis and interpretation of the results with our ability to obtain the model and structure in visual situation [3]. The approach combining data mining and visualization techniques effectively solve the problem that we can't quickly and efficiently analyze the information because the huge amount postgraduate training data. The visual mining analysis provides a communication interface between the users and the computers [4]. The interface helps the users to discover the method, theory and technology from unknown, potential and valuable information.

Therefore, for the assessment of quality of graduate education described herein, we propose a visual analysis method based on the graduate thesis. And for visual analysis research of graduate thesis data, we propose a combination of methods based on data integration, data mining and visualization analysis. First, for university research data analysis, we use the model-driven approach to design and build the scientific data integration and data mining analysis platform. Then, for the thesis topic and research hot spot problem related to training quality analysis, we propose the analysis method of data showing based on the research focus and concept maps in the overall data analysis platform.

Analysis of university research means the system analyzes and displays the information including graduate thesis information, academic information, the research directions and hotspots in colleges. Currently, the universities have been established various information management systems including research institutions management, faculty information management, scientific research information management, academic information management, business information management system and etc. The problem is that the decentralized business management systems can't provide the valid data and can't effectively put information into knowledge. So In order to solve the above-mentioned problems, we design and implement the research and scientific data analysis platform which unifies the data integration, data analysis and presentation. And the design idea is based on model-driven development.

The data platform consists of four functional modules including multidimensional data modeling module, data integration module, data analysis module and visual display modules. Before data analysis and visualization display, we need build a visual modeling of business data and establish a multi-dimensional data model. Then using the established multidimensional data model to extract, clean and transform the data and obtain the analysis and display of the data set. Finally, the interactive display tools analyze and display data.

The platform can help customers quickly building a complete multi-dimensional data analysis system. It will not only be able to connect business systems in real-time data, but also connect to the warehouse data for decisions. The users can query the information based on the real-time business data and analyze deeply based on the historical data. The overall design of the structure diagram is shown in Fig. 258.1.

258.2.1 Date Layer

In the data analysis platform, the first part is the integration platform of the entire data. Design and implementation process combine with a description of the data based on the metadata model, described methods, data extraction and conversion. This layer gets the data from different business database analysis and show data. ETL process is the key process establishing the data warehouse, in ETL [4], data in various business databases are integrated into the data warehouse. Metadata storage supplies the standard and the basis for conversion mapping and integrated load data. Metadata description and ETL data processing form the data warehouse of overall research and data analysis. And the data warehouse supplies the all data for the data analysis layer.

258.2.2 Data Analysis Layer

Data analysis layer is mainly composed by two components for data modeling and query analysis. The data modeling component complete the multi-dimensional data description modeling including the various topics cube and dimension

Fig. 258.1 The structure diagram of data analysis platform

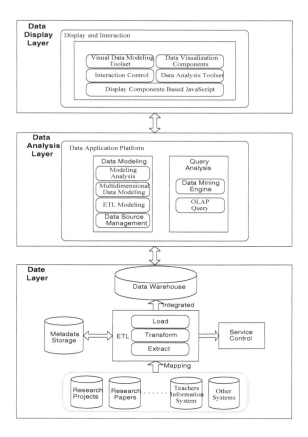

modeling. The components mainly create the metadata modeling for data extraction and display. Query analysis components include the interface of data mining algorithms and the query parser based on OLAP, the components mainly perform data mining algorithms, parse and execute OLAP query language.

258.2.3 Data Display Layer

The data display layer supplies the operating interface and display interface for users. The users can easily complete the visual analysis of data modeling and data display. This layer is mainly composed by the visual data modeling tools, interactive control components, and the display component library based on the JavaScript. In this paper, the display component library uses the multidimensional data demonstrate component platform based D3 [5]. By D3, we get the parallel to the axis, scatter plots, concept map and other multidimensional data display components.

258.3 Multidimensional Data Analysis and Display

By applying the above-mentioned data integration process, we get the corresponding data warehouse which could be used for university scientific data analysis [6]. It is necessary to clarify the target of the data analysis based on the requirements of the postgraduate training and discipline construction in colleges and universities. Therefore, the overall data analysis processes include requirement analysis, feature extraction from multi-dimensional indicators from and the corresponding data processing. The detailed flowchart of multidimensional data analysis is shown in Fig. 258.2. Firstly, we analyze the requirement and establish the corresponding indicators for multi dimensional data. Secondly, the data collection for the overall analysis is determined by the indicators obtained in the previous step. Thirdly, data collection is processed by applying various analyzing processes, e.g. data clustering, classification and regression operations. Finally, common multidimensional data manipulation processes (e.g. up-drills, down-drills, slice and etc.) and visualization techniques are together applied to the data collection, to get a visual representation of the final data collection.

According to the problem of data visual analysis of university's scientific research, this paper adopts the visual analysis of data research based on the above data analysis platform and multidimensional data analysis platform. Combined with the practical teaching and cultivating situation of Shandong University at present, the rest of this paper mainly obtains the research hot spots of institutes and the relationship between college scientific research personnel and research hot spots through the analysis of graduates' papers.

1. We have finished fetching every college graduate thesis project and its related information through the data integration platform, thus established the overall research papers analysis data warehouse.

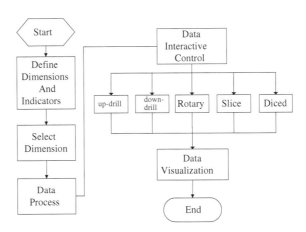

Fig. 258.2 Flow chart of multi-dimensional data analysis

2. We analyzed business for graduate thesis established the overall analysis of the dimension information, mainly including the keywords of graduate thesis dimension, the student dimension and the college dimension.
3. By establishing corresponding graduate thesis analysis dimensions, main dimensions for keywords of the corresponding data analysis and processing. In the corresponding research focus in the extraction process, this paper adopted symbiosis based and similarity calculation method for data clustering and dimension of operation, finally obtain the corresponding college research hot spot and correlation analysis.
4. After obtaining the relevant information of research focus, it gets a subset of the whole data through the corresponding interaction control research including the choice of college and hot spot specified degree of other related information
5. In the process of data show, this article realizes the final data show based on the D3 multidimensional data presentation layers.

As shown in Fig. 258.3, on the basis these multidimensional data to show the process analysis, obtained the keywords of graduate thesis dimension tables through the data integration and the data analysis, then, through the co-occurrence matrix analysis to get the corresponding medical research focus in the current study including prognosis, diagnosis, treatment and other related information.

After acquiring the research focus of each college, management department can analysis the work of several aspects, including staff arrangement, according to the research focus and its relevant researchers involved. Therefore, in order to take advantage of research focus and some other information efficiently, this article combined with conception figures implements the relationship between relevant tutor's research direction and research focus. And in the meanwhile, it can analyze the core tutors staffs that have the same research direction by relevant relation. As is shown in Fig. 258.4, it presents the core researchers mentioned above who are related to the key research focus.

Fig. 258. 3 Research focus tag cloud

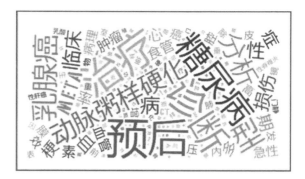

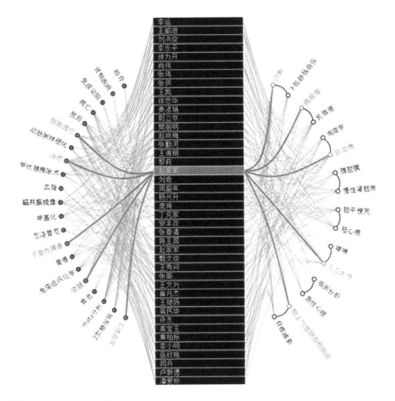

Fig. 258.4 The associated hotspot analysis

258.4 Conclusion

This paper proposed a data based visible analysis method to analyze the master degree student research status in university, through analyzing the issues about master degree student cultivation, hotspot of research aspects and etcetera. In particular, based on analyzing the data used in thesis of master students, this paper established an analysis method which combined data integration, data mining and visualization analysis method. Firstly, the paper created a data analysis platform on data integration and data mining, through analyzing college research data and the model driven method. Afterwards, based on this platform, the authors propose a visible data analysis method to reveal research hotspot and conceptual graph.

References

1. Chen X, Dong Z (2009) Analysis of the constituent elements of the post-graduate training mode. Acad Degrees Graduate Educ 11:4–7
2. Robertson GG, Mackinlay JD, Card SK (1997) Cone trees: animated 3D visualizations of hierarchical information.Conf Human Factors Comput Syst 189–194
3. Mizoguchi F (2000) Anomaly detection using visualization and machine learning. In: Proceedings of IEEE 9th international workshops on 14–16 June 2000, pp 165–170
4. Zhang N, Jia Z, Shi Z (2002) ETL in database system. Comput Eng Appl 38(24):213–216
5. Bostock M, Ogievetsky V, Heer J (2011) D3: data-driven documents. IEEE Trans Vis Comp Graph (Proc Info Vis)
6. Chen C (2005) Measuring the movement of a research paradigm. Vislization and data analysis (VDA 2005), San Jose, (5669), pp 63–76
7. Iyengar S (2001) XML METADATA interchange(OMG XMI) distributed metadata interchange for the WEB generation. Meta Data Conf 5(4):19–22

Chapter 259
Multimedia Assisted Case-Based Teaching Application in Intercultural Communication

Huang Fang and Zhao Chen

Abstract Human-computer interaction of multimedia technology provides an innovative platform for foreign language education. Assisted by multimedia technology, case-based teaching is widely applied to teaching intercultural communication, a new area in English curriculum system. This pedagogy increasingly arouses great concern for its effectiveness of theory input and students' criticality development. According to a survey result of 100 sophomores from intercultural communication class in Qingdao Agricultural University, 95 % of them positively approve it helpful and effective in theory explanation; 90 % of them believe it can better stimulate students' learning motivation. Some teaching practices are also suggested in the paper.

Keywords Multimedia · Case-based teaching · Intercultural communication

259.1 Multimedia Assisted Case-Based Teaching

Multimedia teaching is popularized along with the computer development in hardware and software and is accelerated with promotion of the Constructivism theory [1]. Multimedia technology plays the best role in creating an authentic learning context. Case-based teaching is a popular pedagogy in areas of law and economy education, which was firstly advocated in Harvard University. It embodies a task-based principle, a widely advocated in language learning practice [2, 3]. Learners' learning motivations and interests are caused and sustained by

H. Fang · Z. Chen (✉)
Qingdao Agricultural University, Qingdao 266109, China
e-mail: zhao918chen@163.com

H. Fang
e-mail: huang311fang@163.com

task explorations in authentic learning environment, which is also in line with constructivism theory. For achieving a given communicative purpose, six elements, goals, input, activities, teachers' roles, learners' roles and settings can be displayed in task-based learning combining cases [4]. Case-based teaching activities typically call for collaboration and communicative interaction based on a designed task.

Multimedia assisted case-based teaching is widely used in teaching intercultural communication. Different from traditional exemplification, it values the specially designed task involvement and teacher-student interaction based on the learning targets. Besides, it strengthens students' analyzing abilities, their introspection and critical thoughts that are important evaluating criteria for students in Intercultural Communication. Therefore, this pedagogy is widely accepted as the most effective, attractive and desired teaching method in intercultural communication [5].

259.2 Intercultural Communication Study in China

Intercultural communication is a new area of research in the communication discipline [6], and it was offered as a course in American universities in 1970s. Since then, intercultural communication has been arousing great concerns worldwide, setting the stage for academic exploration of not only culture and communication, but pedagogical research. Comparatively, the history of intercultural communication teaching and study in China is much shorter. With China's reform and opening up initiatives and the entry into WTO, foreign language teachers gradually took interest in it. The globalization of economy and culture and people's frequent interaction put intercultural communication education in an urgent place. Chinese scholars began to engage in intercultural communication study, especially after *The China Association for Intercultural Communication* had been founded in 1995.

Compared with the theoretical appeal, education practice in intercultural communication is not optimistic in China. Lin [7] investigated that only five universities in China opened intercultural communication course, and the course is especially for English majors, indicating it only benefits a minority of college students. However, study in relationships between language and culture has been putting increasing emphases. China's *Medium and long-term development plan for educational reform (2010–2020)* explicitly puts forward the strategies of international talents cultivation. It defines talents are supposed to have international views, understand international rules, participate in international businesses and competitions. This plan calls for a new challenge in English education, and particularly puts intercultural communication to an unprecedentedly important position. Nowadays, more and more universities in China opened intercultural communication as a course for students of different majors. Even so, intercultural communication study has not been a mainstream of academic research in China, teaching pedagogy is still at an exploring stage.

259.3 Multimedia Assisted Case-Based Teaching Suggestions in Intercultural Communication

The effectiveness of multimedia assisted case-based teaching has been proved by an interview survey of 100 sophomores who study intercultural communication in Qingdao Agricultural University. According to the survey result, 95 % of them positively approve it helpful and effective in demonstration and explanation of the IC theory and knowledge. Eighty six percentages of them believe this teaching method is better helpful for understanding than traditional teachers' verbal description. In addition, 90 % of them believe it better stimulate students' learning motivation, trigger their curiosities. Therefore, the teaching effectiveness can be guaranteed. Here are some teaching suggestions.

259.3.1 Preparing Case-Based Multimedia Courseware

Teachers are highly motivated, but admittedly, lack of overseas self-experience for most teachers is the biggest difficulties at that time. Confronting the status quo, teachers who are interested in intercultural communication and who have overseas experiences organize an academic group, and discuss intercultural theories and facts in scenarios twice a week. Before the scenario, a case-based task is determined. Teachers preparation include: proper understands of the theory; how to teach and explain it in a limited time; how to test students' learning outcome. Based on the task, teachers are required to collect and explore materials by making use of internet. They usually download authentic videos and pictures, and make the movie clips if necessary to manifest the given theory. In the discussion, teachers are required to effectively explain intercultural theories using multimedia. Other teachers may claim their advices or suggestions, even criticisms to improve multimedia courseware. After revision, they share multimedia courseware with other teachers.

259.3.2 Case Analysis in Multimedia Courseware

Traditional case-based teaching is usually confined to linguistic description, which is not vivid and attractive. Learning outcome is highly influenced by students' linguistic abilities. Multimedia course integrating human–computer interaction, digitization and instantaneity helps to surpass linguistic limitation.

In the teaching process of intercultural communication, teachers are supposed to apply case analysis to multimedia-aided instruction to improve theory input. Take teaching social practice theory for example, teachers are supposed to produce multimedia courseware. The teaching objective including definition input and how the unawareness of social practice leads to serious communication failure. Teachers are required to produce courseware according to the objective. Practically, the difficult part is the abstract theory understanding. Therefore, teachers are suggested to resort to Internet materials. Here is a real case showed in a video clip: the American young man was invited to be a guest in an India family. He was very welcomed and warmly treated. Later, the India parents asked him "married? Have children?" his facial expression turns to be embarrassed. When the pizza was ready, the young man takes the pizza with his left hand and bite. His behavior instantly irritated the India family, but they do not say directly until the American young man kept eating with his left hand. Later he felt the strange atmosphere around them and asked "what happened? Did I do something wrong?" The India grandpa couldn't restrain his angry and stood up, and use his left hand to touch his own ass from top to bottom repeatedly. Watching this, the American young man was suddenly enlightened. India parents said, "we do not eat with left hand, we regard left hand be unclean...." In this teaching process, the authentic case is demonstrated by a video clip, students are totally attracted by the plot and the learning objective is easily approached. As for evaluation of the learning outcome, teachers can also design a task that calls for the integration of case and multimedia technology. Students' critical thoughts are important in evaluation.

259.4 Conclusion

English learning and education in China has been characterized by emphasis on rote memory and passive acceptance. Intercultural Communication, a new English course, has to adopt a new pedagogy, for students' critical reflection on values, beliefs, and behaviors through a comparative study Byram 2009. In teaching practice, multimedia assisted case-based teaching best inspires students' learning enthusiasm compared with traditional teaching method. It is of great reference for intercultural communication teaching and study.

References

1. Chen X (2004) Problems and countermeasures for multimedia-assisted college English reformation. J Beijing Univ Technol (Social Science Edition)
2. Ellis R (2005) Instructed second language acquisition: a literature review. Ministry of Education, Wellington
3. Nunan D (1989) Designing tasks for the communicative classroom. Cambridge University Press, Cambridge
4. Shouguo Y (2002) Task based language teaching: summary, motivation and application. Foreign Lang Teach Res 5:36–364
5. Fang H (2012) Case-based teaching application in teaching intercultural communication. Master

6. Gudykunst WB (2007) Cross-cultural and intercultural communication. Shanghai Foreign Language Education Press, Shanghai
7. Lin D (1999) Intercultural communication study. Fujian People's Publishing House, Fujian
8. Byram M (1997) Teaching and assessing intercultural communicative competence. Multilingual Matters, Clevedon

Chapter 260
The Informatization Reform and Practice of the Humanities Courses in Nursing Profession

Ying Wang

Abstract According to the changes in the Medical (Nursing) pattern and the needs in social development, we analyze the status quo of humanities courses in the nursing colleges of domestic and explore the ways and basic ideas to reform the humanities courses in nursing colleges, to cultivate applied nursing talents with human spirit and innovation capacity, capable of nursing, education, health care and rehabilitation at the same time.

Keywords Nursing education, Humanities courses, Information technology

260.1 Introduction

Nursing is a human health-centered care, with objects including patients and healthy person and service areas including hospitals, families as well as communities [1]. Therefore, higher requirements are put forward to the courses offered and objectives of the nursing colleges. Excellent nursing talents not only need to have a higher level of expertise, but also need to have good professional ethics and psychological qualities, otherwise it is difficult to adapt to the needs of rapid social development. The purpose to give nursing majors Humanities and Social Science Education is to improve students' thinking ability, psychological and social adaptability, to enable students to better understand the psychological and social factors in health and disease, to master some sociology and psychology theory contacted with professional nursing, and to study the humanities and social factors in health and disease. The amount of obtained knowledge has a close relationship with the application of information technology.

Y. Wang (✉)
College of Nursing, Henan University, Kaifeng, China
e-mail: hdywy@henu.edu.cn

260.2 Overview on the Humanities Courses of Nursing Profession

Currently, humanities courses in domestic nursing colleges generally include compulsory and elective courses such as political and ideological class, ethics, culture and arts, education and psychological, and so on. Judging from the total credits of the nursing profession, the curriculum is unreasonable. There is a big difference between professional courses and humanities courses in the degree of attention and too little practical operation lesson, moreover, the electives are not standardized. From nursing education law, the appropriate proportion of humanities and social sciences courses is 20 % [2]. The United States and Germany has the highest proportion reached 20–25 %, and 15 % in the United Kingdom and Japan, but in our medical colleges, humanities and social sciences courses account for only about 8–10 % of the total period [3]. The ratio of limited period and credits affect the learning outcomes, so it is difficult to achieve the requirements of training objectives.

260.3 Teaching Information Reform of Humanities Courses in Nursing Profession

"Nursing development plan in China (2011–2015)" point out that the education of nursing students should adapt to the development needs of modern medicine and internationalization, carry out all-around quality education [4]. In the survey of courses setting for nursing colleges in Henan province, we found that, generally, the mode of professional knowledge preference and humanities education at naught has not fundamentally changed [5]. What's worse, affected by the market economy and the existing health management system, the pragmatism trend of undergraduate nursing students is more serious, they take nursing humanities courses as soft courses and pay little attention, which directly affect the effectiveness and quality of nursing education. So, we must strengthen the teaching methods reform of nursing humanities and social sciences.

260.3.1 Teaching Methods Reform

260.3.1.1 Actively Introduce Problem Based Learning

The PBL shift the center from imparting knowledge to cultivating capacity [6], from discipline-based professional courses to a quality-purposed comprehensive curriculum, from teacher-centered to student-centered, from class teaching system to steering group discussions system. Its teaching process as follows: put forward the problem-establish assumptions-collect information-demonstrate assumptions-summarize the discussions. In this way, students seek answers to the problems with access to information, encouraging students to change from "learned" to "capable of learning", from study for the exam to for solving the problem, and thus helping students develop good study habits.

260.3.1.2 Application of Case-Based Teaching

Teachers offer teaching-related cases, and students use the Internet to look up information according to the case and teaching requirements, then the teacher organizes students to discuss and makes assessment and assumption, at last students carry out the final drill. Sometimes, students enumerate widely disseminated health care cases on the Network, expressing their views in class in a warm atmosphere. Case-based teaching not only allows students to acquire knowledge, but also enables students to understand the industry rules, capable of the ability to apply knowledge and create knowledge.

260.3.1.3 The Use of Information Technology Teaching Means

In the teaching process, teachers make full use of modern information technology to conduct network teaching and multimedia teaching. Teachers take advantage of Network teaching platform to give students personalized guidance, and use multimedia technology to make multiple senses stimulated multimedia courseware containing graphic audio and video, graphically teaching professional knowledge. For example, network multimedia courseware like "Western Religious Culture" and "Medical Ethics", with application of video, audio, images, animation, text, and other means, making abstract contents to be specific and dynamic.

260.3.2 The Combination of Theory and Practice

Humanistic knowledge and theory come from continuous learning, but the shape of the human spirit and the improvement of the overall quality depend on a positive life experience and behavior to develop. Therefore, nursing humanities courses can't only focus on classroom teaching, but practice should be more stressed. We make full use of opportunities arranged by school teaching plan like the military training, social surveys and professional internship, and we design necessary professional activities at the same time. For example, using online media to expand the influence of the annual 5.12 Nurses Day commemoration, carrying out health counseling activities through an online survey, following teachers to do free clinic and sympathy performance in orphanages and nursing homes, sublimating students' outlook on life and values in practice.

260.3.3 To Create and Take Advantage of Favourable Environment

We should pay attention to the effects of the environment while emphasizing on curriculum system and teaching methods. Enhance spiritual civilization construction, the construction of campus culture as the center, and students' daily behavior norms and major events as the carriers, put the humanities and social sciences into the campus cultural environment, make full use of the campus network, database, and a range of network resources, so that students can have comprehensive and coordinated developments of their abilities in good campus cultural environment.

260.4 Effect Evaluations

Evaluation methods include: classroom observation, questionnaires, short-term teaching effect (feedback from students' assignments and discussions). We conduct a survey mainly for 2010–2012 students in Nursing College of Henan University: the results aimed at course settings, teaching means and the reform effect of humanities courses see in Table. 260.1, Table. 260.2 and Table. 260.3 respectively.

The information-oriented reforms of the humanities and social science courses can teach students new ways of thinking and help broaden their horizons, let them understand more health care-related social knowledge, which laid a foundation for the establishment of the new concept of health and the large concept of medical. Humanities and social sciences courses inspire students' interest to learn health

Table. 260.1 Preliminary evaluation from students on nursing humanities courses settings

Courses setting	Frequency/N	Effective percentage/%	Cumulative percentage/%
Reasonable	102	82.3	82.3
Relatively reasonable	20	16.1	98.4
Not so reasonable	2	1.6	100.0
Total	124	100.0	

Table. 260.2 Evaluation from students on the degree of informatization of teaching means

Informatization	Frequency/N	Effective percentage/%	Cumulative percentage/%
Higher	80	64.5	64.5
High	34	27.4	91.9
General	10	8.1	100
Total	124	100	

Table. 260.3 Evaluation on the teaching effects of humanities courses (%, N = 124)

Investigation content	Completely sure (%)	Basically sure (%)	Not quite sure (%)	Not sure (%)
Increase knowledge and broaden horizons	36.1	47.9	14.4	1.6
Improve professional pride	58.1	37.3	3.6	0.8
Improve learning interest in professional courses	34.0	51.0	13.2	0.8
Cultivate ability to analyze problems comprehensively	30.2	60.8	8.0	0.8
Improve the level of artistic accomplishment	38.8	42.6	17.0	1.6
Improve interpersonal communication skills	30.4	53.6	15.2	0.8
Promote solidarity and collaboration between students	46.4	50.4	3.2	0
Cultivate the ability to use modern information technology	46.2	47.8	5.2	0.8
Improve the ability to solve practical problems	22.0	61.2	15.2	1.6

care-related and non-nursing expertise and social and cultural knowledge, thus changing its original knowledge structure and professional attitude, enhancing the humanistic quality.

Changes in teaching methods, make full use of the resources associated with the courses, expand students' horizons, stimulate students' interest in learning, change the traditional teaching model fundamentally that students receive knowledge passively, improve the learning efficiency, train students' self-learning ability and problem-analyzing and problem-solving skills. Meanwhile, in the course of the discussion, through students' open mind like questioning, summarizing and analyzing, developing their organizational skills and language expressing skills.

References

1. Jiang A, Shi Q (2003) New fundamentals of nursing. Higher Education Press, Beijing
2. Liang L, Yu D (2005) Thinking about the present condition of medical humanity education in ordinary medical college. Med Philos 17:1–6
3. Zou Z (2010) Analysis of causes and countermeasures for lagging quality education of medical students. Chin Med Mod Distance Educ China 8:15–17
4. Ministry of Public Health (2011) Nursing development plan in China (2011–2015). Ministry of Public Health, Beijing
5. Zhang G, Chen J, Chen Y et al (2012) Reflection of China's higher nursing education mode. Edu Forum Mag 33:26–29
6. Luan P (2011) Interpretation of PBL medical teaching mode. S Med Edu 2:50–53

Chapter 261
A Modified Minimum Risk Bayes and It's Application in Spam Filtering

Zhenfang Zhu, Peipei Wang, Zhiping Jia, Hairong Xiao, Guangyuan Zhang and Hao Liang

Abstract To settle the problem of the flood spam, a spam filtering algorithm based on AdaBoost algorithm and minimum Risk Bayes algorithm is created by the combination of the latter two after in-depth analysis and research of them. Experiments have been run to apply it to spam filtering, the result of which shows that this algorithm can better the performance of spam filtering system by improving the accuracy of mail filtering.

Keywords: Mail filtering · Minimum risk bayes · AdaBoost

261.1 Introduction

Minimum Risk Bayes algorithm [1] could calculate posterior probability explicitly, in most cases, it has the equal performance with other algorithms, and even better in some situations, so it is used as the measure of optimal decision. However, in practical application, the prior probabilities of categories are unknown, and the calculating cost of Minimum Risk Bayes to determine the optimal decision is large [2, 3].

AdaBoost algorithm [4, 5] is put forward by Freund and Schapire in 1995, which based on online distribution algorithm. Weak classifier could be promoted

Z. Zhu (✉) · Z. Jia
School of Computer Science and Technology, Shandong University, Jinan 250100, China
e-mail: zhuzhfyt@163.com

Z. Zhu · H. Xiao · G. Zhang · H. Liang
School of Information Science and Electric Engineering, Shandong Jiaotong University, Jinan 250357, China

P. Wang
School of Accountancy Shandong management University, Jinan 250100, China

to a strong classifier by AdaBoost algorithm, and won't have a overfitting problem. But there are also some defects [6], that is, it has a over dependent on data and weak learners, is sensitive to noisy data, and it couldn't reach high accuracy of any if weak learner is too weak. So the search of weak learner is the point, the algorithm couldn't perform well if there is not a good weak learner. To originally solve the problem, this article chooses a quite strong learner—minimum Risk Bayes.

261.2 Minimum Risk Bayes Algorithm

Minimum Risk Bayes algorithm [7] is proposed by Maron, the main thought is, regard article as an independent words collection, according to training set, obtain the probabilities of every word in different categories by bayes theory, and then construct the model of Bayes. Minimum Risk Bayes Algorithm is based on Bayes algorithm and Naïve Bayes algorithm to solve the problem of false discretion, besides, it would bring users huge loss if a normal mail is identified as spam. Minimum Risk Bayes Algorithm is a rule, which takes all classification errors into account and minimizes the risk and loss of false discretion in the greatest degree.

261.3 Adaboost Algorithm

Adaptive Boosting (AdaBoost) is a kind of classic integrated learning algorithm [8–11], its main thought is, for one training set, train different classifiers and then assemble the classifiers to build a final stronger classifier. Suppose that, given training sample set $S = \{(x1, y1), (x2, y2)), \ldots, (xl, yl)\}$, where X and Y correspond to positive sample and negative sample, T is the maximum iteration number of training; The sample weight of initial is 1/n, that is the initial probability distribution of training sample.

261.4 Minimum Risk Bayes Based on Adaboost

Based on the two algorithms presented above, we apply AdaBoost algorithm as the framework of classifier training and replace weak classifier with minimum Risk Bayes algorithm as the base classifier of AdaBoost thus realize combination of the two algorithms. The specific algorithm is:

(1) Input data in the form of matrix: $S = \{(x1, y1), (x2, y2)), \ldots, (xi, yi), \quad xi \in X, \quad yi \in \{-1, +1\}\}$;
(2) Initialize weight: $\omega_i = 1/n$, $i = 1, 2, \ldots, n$

(3) Execution cycle: $m = 1, 2, ..., M$
Substitute ω_i into AdaBoost and train minimum Risk Bayes classifier, then we get the hypothesis of learning machine $P : X \in yi$;
(4) Apply classifier P to the whole data set, mark correct and incorrect samples classified by P separately and judge the number of incorrect samples according to quantity of population samples, caculate the classification error rate α_m of P.
(5) Update the weights of all training samples's by α_m,

$$D_{m+1}(i) = \frac{D_m(i) \exp(-\alpha_m y_i p_m(x_i))}{Z_m} \quad (261.1)$$

(6) Do the next iteration, until the end of M iterations. Through iterations, the minimum Risk Bayes algorithm based on AdaBoost boils down to M classifiers P_m,

$$P(x) = sign\left(\sum_{m=1}^{M} \alpha_m P_m(x)\right) \quad (261.2)$$

$P(x)$ is the final classifier obtained by the combined algorithm through m learnings.

261.5 Experimental Results and Analysis

According to Symantec's observation [12], at present, three spam mail types: (1) network related type (shopping online, computer related products, making money online), which occupies 27 %; (2) product related type (daily essentials, services), which occupies 20 %; (3) health related type (health related products, health care), finance related type, which occupy 17 % [6, 13]. On the basis of spam mail types above, this paper contrasts the two algorithms. But due to restrictions of time and manpower, we just collect 300 mails of various types, there are 50 spam mails on shopping online, 30 on electronics promotion, 40 on daily essentials, 50 on health care, 50 on politically sensitive information, 30 on educational training and 50 normal mails, which are mainly used to test the spam filter capacity of minimum Risk Bayes classifier based on AdaBoost.

Minimum Risk Bayes algorithm has better performance on closed test, but its accuracy and recall rate would reduce sharply on open test. Because spam filtering should be applied to Internet in real time, experiments in this paper are all coducted in open environment. From the experiment result we also found that modified algorithm has higher accuracy rate than the rest two algorithms on shopping online and health care. Although it is inferior to rest two algorithms on politically sensitive information, it has better integral stability. The integral stability of the rest two algorithms are worse.

261.6 Flow-Distribution and Filtering Thought

Plenty of experimental results show that the filter capacity and effect of different algorithms in different domains are distinctive. So according to mails' content, we separate mails into different types then divide them into module which is expert in filtering this type, in this way, we could utilize different algorithm to filter accordingly [14–17]. The shunt filter's brief flow chart is shown as follow (Fig. 261.1).

A few questions should be noticed:

(1) After segmentation and feature selection, text categorization needs to be conducted again in the back, so text classifier should be simple when the first text categorization is in progress, so that filtration rate could accelerate.
(2) Estimate text types after categorization then divide them into different category modules according to text content.
(3) The classifier used by second spam filtering is trained in advance.

Flow-distribution and filtering idea is realized as above. Each algorithm has different content filtering effect, flow-distribution and filtering would make each algorithm give full play to respective advantages thus filter could be conducted effectively. Moreover, flow-distribution and filtering is also a parallel filtering method, when data are mass, it could show better capacity than common classifiers.

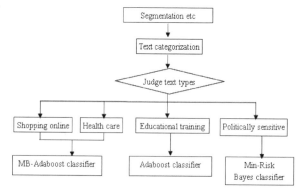

Fig. 261.1 The flow chart of shunt filter

261.7 Conclusion

To settle the problem that spam filtering effect of single traditional algotithm is unsatisfactory, a spam filtering algorithm combine AdaBoost Algorithm with minimum Risk Bayes algorithm is proposed after in-depth analysis of the two algorithms. The result of experiments shows that this algorithm could better the performance of spam filter. The next step we would effectively combine spam's flow-distribution and filtering with feedback mechanism and reflect mail filtering situation through feedback mechanism, thereby achieve better filtering effect.

References

1. Wang L, Lin Y-P, Peng Y et al (2004) An algorithm of filtering junk mails based on cognition-learning and minimum risk naive bayes. Acta Simulata Systematica Sinica 32:69–85
2. Bedi P, Vashisth P (2011) Interest based recommendations with argumentation. J Artif Intell 4:119–142
3. Muda Z, Yassin W, Sulaiman MN, Udzir NI (2011) A K-Means and naive Bayes learning approach for better intrusion detection. Inf Technol J 10:648–655
4. Yoav F, Schapire RE (1999) A short introduction to boosting. J Japanese Soc Artif Intell 5:771–778
5. Chang HL, Yue TW (2011) Entropy-directed AdaBoost algorithm with NBBP features for face detection. Inf Technol J, 10:1518–1526
6. Lee LH, Wan CH, Yong TF, Kok HM (2010) A review of nearest neighbor-support vector machines hybrid classification models. J Appl Sci 10:1841–1858
7. Li XY, Ye F (2006) Method of spam filtering based on multi-bayes algorithms. Comput Eng Appl 9:114–116
8. Zhen L, Liang T, Ming-Tian Z (2008) Research on spam classifier based on features of spammer's behaviours. Inf Technol J 7:165–169
9. Jing-ping J, Fei-zhou Z, Yan-mei C (2009) Adaboost object tracking algorithm. Pattern Recogn Artif Intell 3:477–478
10. Jiang Y, Ding XQ (2008) AdaBoost algorithm using multi-step correction. J Tsinghua Univ Sci Technol 10:1610–1611
11. Hammoud D, Maamri R, Sahnoun Z (2011) Machine learning in an agent: a generic model and an intelligent agent based on inductive decision learning. J Artif Intell 4:29–44
12. Stambouli TB, Keche M, Ouamri A (2010) Iterative feature selection for classification. J Appl Sci 10:1015–1018
13. Wang T, Qiu GY, He JH, (2008) New bayes e-mail filtering model based on risk minimization. Appl Res Comput 4:1147–1149
14. Su S, Hongfei L, Ye Z (2009) Character-based language modeling approach for spam filtering. J Chin Inf Process 2:41–47
15. Sebastini F (2002) Machine learning in automated text categorization. JACM 1:1–47
16. Li L (2006) Data complexity in machine learning and novel classification algorithms. Ph.D. Thesis, California Institute of Technology, California
17. Wang B, Pan WF (2005) A survey of content-based anti-spam email filtering. J Chin Inf Process 5:1–6

Chapter 262
Research of CRYPTO1 Algorithm Based on FPGA

Zhang Haifeng, Yang Zhu and Zhang Pei

Abstract The Mifare Classic card is the most widely used contactless smart card in the world. The internal encryption algorithm and security attract more and more people's attention recently. This paper studies three-pass authentication and gives the design procedure of CRYPTO1 algorithm. The design uses FSM method based on FPGA to implement this algorithm. Test results show that the system of encryption and authentication runs fast and correctly. The research builds the foundation to research and estimate the security of the smart card.

Keywords Mifare classic · CRYPTO1 encryption algorithm · LFSR · FPGA

262.1 Introduction

Contactless smart card is based on RFID (radio frequency identification) technology. The card consists of a small piece of memory that can be accessed wirelessly. The most widely used card is NXP Mifare smart card. There are four different types: Standard, Ultralight, DES-Fire and SmartMX. They are mainly used in payment field, transport system and access control. Mifare Classic [1] is compliant with the protocol of ISO14443. The part 4 of ISO14443 defines the high-level protocol. Mifare Classic uses a proprietary and undisclosed protocol [2], it differs from the ISO standard, and this is the key point. Mifare Classic uses the CRYPTO1 encryption algorithm in three-pass authentication protocol. Nohl and

---

Z. Haifeng (✉)
Study on RFID and embedded system Xiasha Higher Education Zone,
Hangzhou 310018 Zhejiang, China
e-mail: hfzhang0811@hdu.edu.cn

Y. Zhu · Z. Pei
College of Electronics Information, Hangzhou Dianzi University, Hangzhou, China

Plötz [3] declare that they have revealed CRYPTO1 encryption algorithm. Since then, people pay more attention to the security of Mifare Classic. This Paper analyzes the three-pass authentication process and designs the system based on FPGA to run CRYPTO1 algorithm.

262.2 Authentication Protocol

Once the tag enters the RF field of the card reader, it uses inductive coupling to get energy from the reader antenna, then the tag starts the anti-collision protocol by sending its UID (unique identifier). The reader selects this tag according to the commands specified in ISO14443-A [4].

According to the card documentation, the following step is three-pass authentication. The reader sends an authentication request for a specific block. The tag sends a challenge nonce n_T to the reader. Then the reader sends its own challenge nonce n_R together with the answer a_R to the tag. The tag finishes authentication by replying a_T to the challenge of the reader. Starting with n_R, all procedures of communication have been encrypted. This means that n_R, a_R and a_T are XOR-ed with the key stream ks1, ks2, ks3 [5].

The pseudo-random generator in the tag used to generate n_T is a 16-bit LFSR (linear feedback shift register). The generator polynomial [5] is as below.

$$f(x) = x^{16} + x^{14} + x^{13} + x^{11} + 1 \tag{262.1}$$

In brief, three-pass authentication flow can be described as follows: the tag sends 32-bit plain text pseudo-random nonce n_T to the reader. Both the tag and reader initialize the cipher generator with the shared key K, uid and the nonce n_T. The reader sends cipher text n_R and updates LFSR state to generate cipher a_R to the tag. The tag updates LFSR state in the same way, sends cipher a_T to verify the authenticity of the reader.

262.3 Algorithm Flow

The core of CRYPTO1 algorithm used in three-pass authentication is a 48-bit LFSR with this generating polynomial [6].

$$g(x) = x^{48} + x^{43} + x^{39} + x^{38} + x^{36} + x^{34} + x^{33} + x^{31} + x^{29} + x^{24} + x^{23} + x^{21} + x^{19}$$
$$+ x^{13} + x^9 + x^7 + x^6 + x^5 + 1. \tag{262.2}$$

On every clock edge, the register shifts one bit from right to the left. The leftmost bit has been discarded and the input bit of LFSR is also XOR-ed with the feedback bit. There are two levels filter function in the cipher generator. The

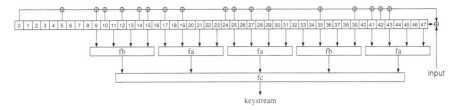

Fig. 262.1 The structure of CRYPTO1 cipher generator

system puts the odd bits of LFSR in at the first level, and then five outputs in at the second level. The key stream is generated at the second level (Fig. 262.1).

It is appropriate to let this algorithm running in FPGA while FPGA has a large number of register resources. The system uses verilog HDL to realize this algorithm. The core is a FSM (finite state machine). Figure 262.2 is the state transition diagram. The word in bracket means the cipher text in the context. FSM is a design common method of FPGA. The system divides three stages to implement FSM: update current state of state machine, judge the following state, produce the output of state machine according to current state. At first, the system defines the state value and coding scheme (such as Gray, One-Hot), using One-Hot coding scheme.

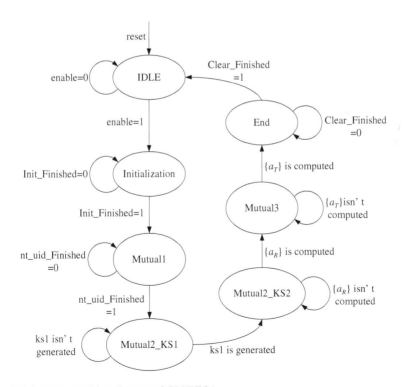

Fig. 262.2 State transition diagram of CRYPTO1

The synthesizer can easily find the state machine while the code style is standard. Pay attention to consider each state seriously and the perspective of code readability.

There are seven states. State machine is idle while the system reset. Once enable signal is valid, the state machine goes into initialization state. In the state mutual1, n_T and uid are fed into LFSR. Mutual2_ks1 state generates key stream ks1 and mutual2_ks2 generates cipher text $\{a_R\}$. When cipher text $\{a_T\}$ generates, state machine goes into END state and clears some registers, then returns to IDLE sate.

262.3.1 Initialization

In this period, the input data enters into corresponding registers. The data includes shared key K, uid, n_T and $\{n_R\}$. The system defines 48-bit LFSR and 32-bit PRNG register. 48-bit LFSR is the core register, it generates key streams. 32-bit PRNG register generates the pseudo-random a_R and a_T.

262.3.2 First Mutual Process

This step finishes the initialization of CRYPTO1 cipher generator. Firstly, $n_T \oplus$ uid gets into LFSR. Figure 262.3 depicts this process. 48-bit LFSR produces key stream following two level filter functions. First level has five registers and second level has one register. The outputs of second level register depend on first level registers. The system uses sequential logic to implement algorithm, the valid outputs of key stream will delay two clock periods because of two level filter functions.

The result of nT $\oplus$ uid is 32-bit. The LSB of each byte enters into LFSR firstly. CRYPTO1 generates 32-bit key stream after 32 clock periods. The non-blocking assignment is used to update the rightmost bit of LFSR.

Fig. 262.3 Initialization of CRYPTO1

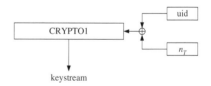

Fig. 262.4 Diagram of ks1 generation

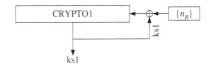

262.3.3 Second Mutual Process

The tag verifies cipher text $\{a_R\}$ according to cipher text $\{n_R\}$ the reader sends to the tag. This step emulates computation process in the tag. There are two states in this step: Mutual2_ks1 and Mutual2_ks2. Cipher texts $\{n_R\}$ are XOR-ed with ks1 to compute plain text n_R. Figure 262.4 shows this process. 32-bit pseudo-random nonce a_R and a_T also generates during this state. The nonce n_T in register PRNG shifts 64 times and 96 times. The feedback bit is also wire type. The system uses non-blocking assignment to finish this operation.

The second state generates key stream ks2. 48-bit LFSR shifts 32 times to generate ks2 without loading external inputs at this time. This is different from mutual2_ks1 state. The cipher text $\{a_R\}$ is the result of a_R XOR-ed with ks2.

262.3.4 Third Mutual Process

This state generates key stream ks3. When the tag verifies the validity of cipher nonce $\{a_R\}$, it sends $\{a_T\}$ to the reader. LFSR doesn't load external inputs. The system shifts 32 times to generate ks3. Then it computes cipher text $\{a_T\}$. Once $\{a_T\}$ generates, state machine goes into the END state. The system resets registers and goes into the next idle state. At this moment, the system finishes the process of CRYPTO1 encryption algorithm.

262.4 Algorithm Verification and Result Analysis

The system uses the software ModelSim to emulator MIFARE Classic 1 K authentication data which is snooped by Proxmark3 RFID instrument. The snooped data shows in Table 262.1.

The time between messages shows in etu (elementary time unit). Known key is 0XFFFFFFFFFFFF. In the Table 262.1, tag challenge nonce n_T = 0X254391b1, reader challenge nonce $\{n_R\}$ = 0X48686182. Figure 262.5 shows the emulation result. The emulation shows that $\{a_R\}$ = 0X523e7a1b, $\{a_T\}$ = 0X78280638. This result is the same as Table 262.1. Additionally, we can see the 48-bit LFSR data state at each clock. Key stream ks1 = 0X1d292810, ks2 = 0X394e85a2, ks3 = 0X082daf14. Plain text n_R = 0X55414992, a_R = 0X6b70ffb9, a_T = 0X7005a92c.

Table 262.1 Authentication data

etu	Seq	Sender	Bytes
+0:	01:	Reader:	52
+236:	02:	Tag:	04 00
+0:	03:	Reader:	93 20
+452:	04:	Tag:	6c 32 95 18 d3
+0:	05:	Reader:	93 70 6c 32 95 18 d3 18 75
+308:	06:	Tag:	08 b6 dd
+0:	07:	Reader:	60 05 58 2c
+428:	08:	Tag:	25 43 91 b1
+0:	09:	Reader:	48 68 61 82 52 3e 7a 1b
+380:	10:	Tag:	78 28! 06 38!

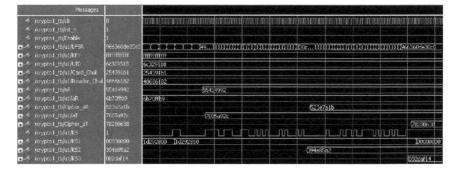

Fig. 262.5 Emulation result

The input clock is 50 MHz. Time is less than 5 microsecond before $\{a_T\}$ generates.

At last, we test the CRYPTO1 algorithm with the FPGA EP2C5T144C8. The system sends the result to the Mega32 MCU over serial transmitter at 9,600 kbps speed. Encrypted results display on 84*48 dot matrix LCD. Synthesized results show that the whole design occupies 524 logic cells and accounts, ten percent of system logic cells. The top design schematic shows as Fig. 262.6. U1 and U2 module make up the serial transmitter. U3 is the CRYPTO1 algorithm module.

After many groups of data tests, the simulation data encryption result is the same as the actual result. Experimental results show that the design of the realization of the CRYPTO1 encryption algorithm can meet the expected requirement. The time of the system per data CRYPTO1 encryption is about 270 us.

Compared with other methods, such as CRYPTO1 encryption based on the DSP, or only on MCU platform. Design based on FPGA and MCU has obvious advantages, like fast running speed and short encryption time, high performance-cost ratio, flexibility, and human-computer interaction. The system in this paper is faster than other methods at least 20 %.

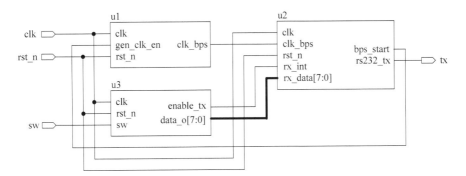

Fig. 262.6 Top design schematic

We test lots of data from different MIFARE classic card. The results show that this algorithm can meet the timing requirements, the design can make good use of the resource of FPGA and implement CRYPTO1 encryption algorithm correctly in three-pass authentication.

262.5 Summary

MIFARE Classic card is one of the most widely used cards in the world. This paper introduces three-pass authentication as well as the CRYPTO1 algorithm encryption implementation procedure. And design the system based on FPGA. Experimental test shows that the encryption result is completely correct.

The encryption process of MIFARE Classic card is clear and known, the decryption is very easy. The cipher key has been broken out. MIFARE Classic has serious security and vulnerability problems. This research builds the foundation for future researchers to study and estimate the security of MIFARE Classic card. People can do further research on the basis of this paper, aiming at improving the system security of the MIFARE Classic card. Reduce the risk of using MIFARE Classic card. Prevent the card from being copied, tampered or cracked. Improve the CRYPTO1 algorithm or put forward more advanced encryption algorithm.

Acknowledgments This work has been supported by the Zhejiang Open Foundation of the Most Important Subjects under grant GK110204003-10.

References

1. NXP semiconductors Mifare standard 4 K byte card IC functional specification. http://www.nxp.com/documents
2. de Koning Gans G (2008) Analysis of the Mifare Classic used in the ovchipkaart project. Radboud University Nijmegen, Netherlands

3. Nohl K, Plötz H (2007) Mifare little security, Despite obscurity. In: Presentation on the 24th congress of the Chaos Computer Club, Berlin
4. ISO/IEC 14443. Identification cards—Contactless integrated circuit card—Proximity cards
5. Garcia FD, de Koning Gans G, Ruben M, van Rossum P, Roel V, Wichers Schreur R, Jacobs B (2008) Lecture notes in computer science, vol 5283. Springer, Berlin, pp 97–114
6. Nohl K, Evans D, Starbug S, Plötz H (2008) Reverse-engineering a crypto-graphic RFID tag. USENIX Security
7. Finkenzeller K (2006) RFID-Handbuch. Publishing House of Electronics Industry, Beijing

Chapter 263
Change of Plasma Adrenomedullin and Expression of Adrenomedullin and its Receptor in Villus of Normal Early Pregnancy

Lihong Ruan, Zhenghui Fang, Jingxia Tian, Yan Dou, Wenyu Zhong, Xiue Song, Wei Shi, Aiying Lu, Lizhi Sun, Guihua Jia, Haifeng Yu, Shuyi Han and Hongqiao Wu

Abstract *Objective* To study the role of adrenomedullin (ADM) in normal early pregnancy. *Method* Plasma concentrations of ADM were measured in 30 normal early pregnancy and 30 non-pregnant women (control group) by radioimmunoassay. The expression of ADM, ADM mRNA and ADMR mRNA in villi of normal early pregnancy were determined by immunohistochemistry and in situ hybridization respectively. *Results* The Plasma concentration of ADM in normal early pregnancy was significantly higher than that of control group (22.735 + 2.382 ng/l vs. 15.800 + 3.142 ng/l, $P < 0.05$). The expressions of ADM, ADM mRNA and ADMR mRNA in villi of normal early pregnancy were found in the cytoplasm and cell membrane of the syncytiotrophoblast and cytotrophoblast. *Conclusion* During human normal early pregnancy, plasma ADM was involved in the regulation of maternal homeostasis, and villus ADM might contribute to trophoblasts invasion and vasculogenesis.

Keywords Early pregnancy · Adrenomedullin · RNA · Messenger

263.1 Introduction

Adrenomedullin was first isolated from pheochromocytoma tissue as a novel vasodilative peptide in 1993 [1]. There were many reports that adrenomedullin level changed in cancer [2], sepsis [3], mutiply pregnancy [4] and other conditions. Adrenomedullin and its receptor in normal early pregnancy were not revealed

---

L. Ruan · Z. Fang · J. Tian · Y. Dou · W. Zhong · X. Song · W. Shi · A. Lu · L. Sun · G. Jia · H. Yu · S. Han · H. Wu (✉)
Jinan Central Hospital, Shandong University, Jinan, Shandong, China
e-mail: alice6620@163.com

when the villi vascular system had not been established. The expression of ADM and its receptor were detected in the early pregnancy by radioimmunoassay, immunohistochemistry and in situ hybridization to investigate them possible roles in normal early pregnancy.

263.2 Materials and Methods

263.2.1 Subject

We collected samples of maternal plasma and villus from 30 singleton pregnancies with live fetuses at 45–50 days of gestation. These pregnant women requested suction termination of pregnancy for psychosocial indications. Thirty cases of normal non-pregnant women in the proliferative phase were recruited as controls. All participants were examined at the Department of Obstetrics and Gynecology, Jinan Central Hospital affiliated to Shandong University, China. The study was approved by the local Research Ethics Committee, and written consent was obtained from all participants.

The 4 ml maternal blood was obtained in all cases before the induction of anesthesia and the control group. The samples were placed in tubes with 10 % EDTA.Na2 40 μl and 500 IU aprotinin, put at 4 °C for 10 min, and centrifugated with $3000 r \cdot min^{-1}$ for 10 min. The plasma was separated and stored at −70 °C until assayed. The parts of the villi in early pregnancy were taken after suction termination of pregnancy, which were divided into two parts respectively. One parts were fixed with 10 % buffered formaldehyde solution for 24 h, embedded with paraffin, selected 4 μm consecutively and prepared for immunohistochemistry. The other parts were fixed with 4 % formaldehyde/0.1 MPBS (pH 7.0–7.4), containing 1/1000 DEPC for 2 h. Then embedded, the 8 μm consecutive slices were taken for in situ hybridization.

263.2.2 Detection Methods

263.2.2.1 Radioimmunoassay Determination of Plasma ADM

Every plasma sample was thawed at room temperature, mixed 500 μL 1 % trifluoroacetic acid (TFA), centrifugated with $3500 r \cdot min^{-1}$ for 20 min in 4 °C, and the supernatant was taken into Sep-PakC-18 column (Waters, Inc., Massachusetts, USA).

Every Sep-PakC-18 column was eluted with 5 ml 1 % TFA at a flow rate of 1 ml/2 min, then eluted with 60 % methyl cyanides 2 ml +1 % TFA 3 ml at a flow rate of 1 ml/3 min. The above eluent was collected into 10 ml vial, frozen and dried at −42 °C, then dissolved into 250 μl 0.05 mol/L (pH 7.4) PBS, and oscillated in the oscillator for 3 min. 100 μl solution were taken to determined ADM concentration by using radioimmunoassay technique. Radioimmunoassay kit was purchased from the Beijing Huaying Biotechnology Institute. The detection equipment for the productions was GC-911 fully automated radioimmunoassay gamma counter from industrial company affiliated to University of Science and Technology, China. All procedures were performed according to the manufacturer's instructions. All samples were determined with the same batch of reagents in the same experiment.

263.2.2.2 Immunohistochemistry Assay (Streptavidin Biotin Complex, SABC) for Detecting ADM Expression in Villi

Rabbit anti-human polyclonal antibody of ADM and SABC kit were purchased from Wuhan Boster Biological Engineering Company. Primary antibody dilution of 1:200 was used. Normal rabbit serum instead of primary antibody was used in negative control. Nucleus was stained with hematoxylin. The ADM positive results showed brown particles in the cytoplasm and cell membrane.

263.2.2.3 In Situ Hybridization Assay for Detecting ADM mRNA and ADMR mRNA in Villi

Digoxigenin labeled oligonucleotide probes matching to target genes (ADM mRNA and ADMR mRNA) were used with in situ hybridization. The probes and in situ hybridization detection kit were purchased from Wuhan Boster Biological Engineering Company. No probe was used in negative control. Nuclei were stained with hematoxylin. Positive results of ADM mRNA and ADMR mRNA showed brownish-yellow coloring in the cytoplasm and cell membrane.

263.2.3 Statistics

The data were expressed as average ± standard deviation (x ± s). Significant statistical significance was assessed by Mann–Whitney U-test and P values less than 0.05 were considered significant.

263.3 Results

1. The maternal age was 26.6 + 3.2 years. The age of control group was 26.1 + 3.7 years. There was no significance between ages of two groups. The concentration of ADM in maternal plasma was significantly higher than that of control group (22.735 ± 2.382 ng/l vs. 15.800 ± 3.142 ng/l, $P < 0.05$) (Table 263.1).
2. ADM proteins in the villi located in the cytoplasm and cell membrane of the syncytiotrophoblast and cytotrophoblast (see Fig. 263.1).
3. ADM mRNA and ADMR mRNA of normal early pregnancy located in the cytoplasm and cell membrane of the syncytiotrophoblast and cytotrophoblast. ADM mRNA stained more significantly than the ADMR mRNA in normal early pregnancy (see Fig. 263.2).

263.4 Discussion

263.4.1 Function of the Plasma ADM During Early Pregnancy

The results of this study showed that plasma ADM was significantly increased in normal early pregnancy. Pregnancy was a normal physiological process, and the maternal hemodynamics changed significantly in this process. In early pregnancy, maternal blood volume increased, but blood pressure was not significantly higher.

Table 263.1 Comparison of ADM of non-pregnant women and normal early pregnancy (X ± s)

Group	N	ADM (ng/l)
Normal early pregnancy	30	22.735 ± 2.382*
Control group	30	15.800 ± 3.142

*$P < 0.05$ compared with control group

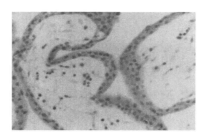

Fig. 263.1 Immunohistochemistry of ADM protein in villus (×400)

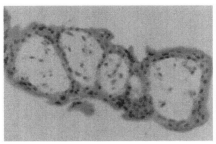 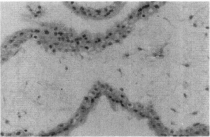

Fig. 263.2 In situ hybridization. *Left* ADM mRNA in villus (×400). *Right* ADMRmRNA in villus (×400)

The maternal organs of many systems changed adaptively, especially the blood vascular. Under the intricate regulation, a variety of vasoactive factors such as endothelin (ET), Thromboxane (TXA2), angiotensin (Ang II) nitric oxide (NO), prostacyclin (PGI2), atrial natriuretic peptide (ANP) were synthesized and released appropriately, which interacted to maintain maternal homeostasis during early pregnancy. Adrenomedullin is a new polypeptide discovered by Kitamura (1993, Japan) [1] in human chromaffin cell tumor. Human ADM gene was located on chromosome 11 [5], which coded and produced the ADM protein containing 52 amino acid residues. 16th and 21st cysteine of ADM protein formed a disulfide bond to become a ring structure [1]. Because of mild homology with the calcitonin gene-related peptide (CGRP), it belonged to the calcitonin gene-related peptide (CGRP) family. Studies had shown that ADM was widely distributed in the body, which concentrations were higher in the adrenal medulla, pituitary, stomach, brain, lung, heart, kidney than others. Plasma ADM comes primarily from vascular endothelial cells and vascular smooth muscle cell.

The studies on vasodilatory mechanism of ADM had been partly shown. The majority of scholars believed that it acted on the receptors of vascular smooth muscle, activated adenylate cyclase, increased cAMP levels, and resulted in vascular smooth muscle relaxation [6]. Secondly it stimulated NO synthesis and activated K^+ channels [7]. NO was a necessary factor to maintain adequate uteroplacental blood flow, which was also an important material to maintain maternal vascular tone. In addition, it was reported that ADM inhibited the releasing of ET-1 [8] and Ang II [9], and antagonized their roles. The latter two were the more strong vasoconstrictor, which played an important role on the stability of blood pressure and cardiovascular system.

The reason that plasma ADM significantly increased in early pregnancy might related to increasing synthesis and releasing of ADM in human organs, including the lung, heart, kidney, and uterine. As a circulating hormone the plasma ADM regulated maternal homeostasis and involved in maintaining normal early pregnancy.

263.4.2 Roles of ADM and its Receptor in Villi of Early Pregnancy

This study had shown that the syncytiotrophoblast and cytotrophoblast in the villi of normal early pregnancy had ADM protein, ADM mRNA and ADMR mRNA. In addition to the vasodilator, ADM had the role on regulation of cell growth. It had been reported that ADM could stimulate DNA synthesis and cell proliferation of Swiss3T3 fibroblast, and induct the cell from G0 phase into the G1 phase [10]. It expressed in human tumor cell lines from multiple sources, including lung, colon, prostate, ovarian and skin, which could promote tumor cell growth [11]. Hypoxia induced ADM expression [12]. Hypoxia response element [13] were found in the ADM gene promoter region. ADM not only promoted cell growth as the regulator of cell growth, but also was angiogenic factor [14].

This study showed that localization of ADM and its receptor were same. ADM mRNA and ADM protein had high levels in trophoblast cells of early pregnancy. It suggested that ADM regulated trophoblast cells in the physiological state by self-secretion and (or) paracrine. Prior to the establishment of blood vessels into villi of early pregnancy, trophoblastic invasion into the endometrium was not deep enough, so the villi revealed ischemia and hypoxia state, which might cause a large number of ADM gene expression and corresponding expression of its receptor gene. On the one hand ADM directly combined with the receptor on the trophoblast cells to promote trophoblastic cell growth and further invasion in order to guarantee the supply of nutrients and oxygen to embryo before the effective maternal–fetal circulation was established. On the other hand ADM might promote the establishment of the vascular system in the villi as the angiogenic factor. In addition, ADM highly expression in the villi might be one of the causes of increasing maternal plasma ADM.

References

1. Kitamura K, Kangawa K, Kawamoto M et al (1993) Adrenomedullin: a novel hypotensive peptide isolated from human pheochromocytoma. Biochem Biophys Res Commun 192:553–560
2. Evans JJ, Chitcholtan K, Dann JM et al (2012) Adrenomedullin interacts with VEGF in endometrial cancer and has varied modulation in tumours of different grades. Gynecol Oncol 125:214–219
3. Kotsovolis G, Kallaras K (2010) The role of endothelium and endogenous vasoactive substances in sepsis.Hippokratia 14:88–93
4. Shinozaki H, Aoki H, Kasahara Y et al (2010) Plasma adrenomedullin levels during multiple pregnancy.Gynecol Obstet Invest 69:169–173
5. Ishimitsu T, Kojima M, Kangawa K et al (1994) Genomic structure of human adrenomedullin gene. Biochem Biophys Res Commun 203:631–639
6. Ishiyama Y, Kitamura K, Ichiki Y et al (1993) Hemodynamic effects of a novel hypotensive peptide, human adrenomedullin, in rats. Eur J Pharmacol 241:271–273

7. Terata K, Miura H, Liu Y et al (2000) Human coronary arteriolar dilation to adrenomedullin: role of nitric oxide and K(+) channels. Am J Physiol Heart Circ Physiol 279:2620–2626
8. Hillier C, Petrie MC, Love MP et al (2001) Effect of adrenomedullin on the production of endothelin-1 and on its vasoconstrictor action in resistance arteries: evidence for a receptor-specific functional interaction in patients with heart failure. Clin Sci 101:45–51
9. Troughton RW, Frampton CM, Lewis LK et al (2001) Differing thresholds for modulatory effects of Adrenomedullin infusion on haemodynamic and hormone responses to angiotension Iigand adrenocorticotrophic hormone in healthy volunteers. Clin Sci (Lond) 101:103–109
10. Isumi Y, Minamino N, Katafuchi T et al (1998) Adrenomedullin production in fibroblasts: its possible function as a growth regulator of Swiss 3T3 cells. Endocrinology 139:2552–2563
11. Miller MJ, Martínez A, Unsworth EJ et al (1996) Adrenomedullin expression in human tumor cell lines. Its potential role as an autocrine growth factor. J Biol Chem 271:23345–23351
12. Marinoni E, Pacioni K, Sambuchini A et al (2011) Regulation by hypoxia of adrenomedullin output and expression in human trophoblast cells. Eur J Obstet Gynecol Reprod Biol 154:146–150
13. Garayoa M, Martínez A, Lee S et al (2000) Hypoxia-inducible factor-1 (HIF-1) up-regulates adrenomedullin expression in human tumor cell lines during oxygen deprivation: a possible promotion mechanism of carcinogenesis. Mol Endocrinol 14:848–862
14. Hague S, Zhang L, Oehler MK et al (2000) Expression of the hypoxically regulated angiogenic factor adrenomedullin correlates with uterine leiomyoma vascular density. Clin Cancer Res 6:2808–2814

Chapter 264
A Summary of Role of Alveolar Epithelial Type II Cells in Respiratory Diseases

Xueliang Li, Yiqin Wang and Zhaoxia Xu

Abstract This paper summarized the structure and functions of alveolar epithelial type II cells (AEC II) as well as its role in some kinds of lung diseases. AEC II is one of the important structures in lung and plays an important role in many kinds of lung diseases. There are more studies on the relationship between AEC II and acute lung injury (ALI), pulmonary edema or pulmonary fibrosis than studies on relationship between AEC II and asthma. And the study on the role of AEC II in the treatment of asthma with Chinese medicine is even fewer. Strengthening the study on its role in the treatment of disease with Chinese medicine, may provide new ideas for explaining the pathogenesis of asthma.

Keywords Alveolar epithelial cells type II · Lung injury · Pulmonary fibrosis · Pulmonary edema · Asthma

Alveolar epithelial type II cell (AEC II) is one of the important structures in lung and plays an important role in many kinds of lung diseases. The further study of AEC II will help to explain the pathogenesis of many lung diseases. In this paper, we reviewed the studies on AEC II in recent years.

264.1 Structure and Function of Alveolar Epithelial Type II Cells

AEC II are small, cubical cells. Radiation autoradiography and immunohistochemistry show that their protein precursors are synthesized by AEC II

X. Li · Y. Wang (✉) · Z. Xu
Basic Medical College of Shanghai University of Traditional Chinese Medicine,
Shanghai 201203, China
e-mail: wangyiqin2380@vip.sina.com

endoplasmic reticulum, transformed into glycoprotein by the glycosylation of Golgi complex, and then combined with phospholipid in the lamellar body. The mature AEC II contains lamellar bodies whose limiting membrane is fused with membrane. Secreting contents by exocytosis, the lamellar bodies are places where the pulmonary surfactants (PS), which can reduce the alveolar surface tension and maintain gas–liquid equilibrium, are synthesized, stored and secreted. The function of the AEC II depends on the structure integrity of AEC II [1–4].

The important functions of AEC II cells include: (1) to synthesize, store, and secrete surfactant, thus reducing surface tension and preventing collapse of the alveolus; (2) to transport ions from the alveolar fluid into the interstitium, thereby minimizing alveolar fluid and maximizing gas exchange; (3) to serve as progenitor cells for AEC II cells, which is particularly important during reepithelialization of the alveolus after lung injury; and (4) to provide pulmonary host defense by synthesizing and secreting several complement proteins including C3 and C5 (1–3) as well as numerous cytokines and interleukins that modulate functions of lymphocyte, macrophage, and neutrophil [5].

264.2 Alveolar Epithelial Type II Cells and Acute Lung Injury

A study suggested that apoptosis is a way for AEC II to maintain normal physiological function and dynamic equilibrium and that all the three pathological phase (exudative phase, proliferation phase and fibrosis phase) of acute lung injury and acute respiratory distress syndrome (ALI/ARDS) are accompanied with apoptosis of AEC II [6]. AEC II apoptosis is one of the major causes of the widening gap between the alveolar epithelial cells and the loss of their barrier function, which may lead to acute lung injury (ALI) [7]. In addition, Zhang et al. found that during ALI the amount of osmiophilic lamellar bodies in the cytoplasm of apoptotic AEC II decreased, the mitochondria swelled, pseudoinclusion body formed, and cell membrane microvilli decreased or disappeared. The integrity of the respiratory membrane was damaged, resulting in dysfunction. At the same time, the inflammation caused by removing the damaged AEC II aggravated the existing impairment in lung tissue [8]. In a study of endotoxin-induced lung injury, Giraud et al. found that AEC II cells can be activated by LPS to release a large amount of inflammatory mediators, whose role in the occurrence and development of ALI cannot be ignored either [9]. AEC II cells are the main stem cells of lung and their proliferation and transdifferentiation to AEC I is the only way to repair the lung injury, so that the alveolar wall can be re-epithelized to restore barrier, especially in the lung repair process of ALI and chronic obstructive pulmonary disease (COPD) [10–12]. The apoptosis of alveolar epithelial cells play an important role in ALI/ARDS and the inflammation can promote the development of this process. AEC II is the major target organ, while AEC II can aggravate lung injury by its secretion of inflammatory cytokines and chemokines [13, 14]. Another study showed that AEC II is a key factor in the development of fetal lung as well as in the process of acute or chronic lung injury and its reparations [15]. Moreover, studies have found that the significance of the proliferation and differentiation of AEC II cells is to maintain the integrity of the alveolar cells and the barrier function of alveolar epithelium, which plays a key role in the occurrence and development of ALI and restoring the normal structure and function of lungs [16, 17].

264.3 Alveolar Epithelial Type II Cells and Pulmonary Edema

The studies on AEC II have changed the conventional understanding about the mechanism of pulmonary edema. The change of pressure difference across pulmonary alveoli was thought to be the direct cause of pulmonary edema previously. The studies in recent years, both domestic and abroad, however, showed that AEC II has a strong capacity in liquid transport and it plays an important role in the generation and removal of alveolar fluid in alveoli during pulmonary edema. Saldias et al. found that the active transport of water and sodium by AEC II is the main mechanism of removing lung water and AEC II is the main target cell [18]. Furthermore, some researchers believe that besides secreting endogenous PS, AEC II is also the main location of Na^+-K^+-ATPase which has a very important role in AEC II repair, sodium and water transport, and maintaining the dryness of normal alveolar space [19, 20]. Johnson et al. found that the reabsorption of water by AEC II is a key step in the repair of lung injury in early stage of pulmonary edema [21]. Another study found that AEC II not only secretes the surfactant and transforms it into AT I in lung injury but also transports liquid [22].

264.4 Alveolar Epithelial Type II Cells and Pulmonary Fibrosis

The apoptosis of AEC II is closely associated with pulmonary fibrosis. Some studies have found that overapoptosis of AEC II in pathological condition may be the key factor of fibroblast activation by promoting the onset and development of pulmonary fibrosis [23, 24]. Another study found that the impairment of AEC II and proliferation of fibroblast are the key factors of pulmonary fibrosis and that the impairment of epithelial cell is the initial step of pulmonary fibrosis [25]. Overapoptosis of AEC II can eliminate the inhibitory effect on fibroblast cells and activate the fibrosis process [26], while the transforming growth factor $\beta1$ can induce the transformation from AEC II to mesenchymal cell and fibroblast by up-regulating phosphodiesterase 4, thus promoting the process of pulmonary fibrosis

[27]. Another study showed that alveolar epithelial injury is an important feature of hyperoxia-induced lung injury and its repair mainly depend on proliferation and differentiation of its stem cell, AEC II. AEC II function damage and loss of its repair capacity is an important mechanism of the development of pulmonary fibrosis [28, 29].

264.5 Alveolar Epithelial Type II Cells and Asthma

With the development of modern immunology and molecular biology, it is believed that AEC II is not only the affected cell, but also one of the cells that participate in the process of asthma. Its involvement in the occurrence of chronic inflammation and increased reactivity of airway through PS indicates a close relationship with asthma, which has attracted wide attention since the 1990s [30]. As the target cells of acute inflammatory injury in airway, the acute attack of asthma hypoxia may induce the energy metabolism dysfunction of AEC II, resulting in the change of morphology and structure; meanwhile, besides aggravating the AEC II injury, a series of cytokines and inflammatory mediators can also promote the apoptosis of AEC II, eventually leading to decreased production and activity of PS, which may affect the defense function of lung and intensify the development of airway inflammation and airway obstruction [31–35].

264.6 Discussion

AEC II apoptosis is one of the important causes of the widening gap between the alveolar epithelial cells and the loss of their barrier function, thus may lead to ALI; AEC II has a strong capacity in liquid transport, which plays an important role in the generation and removal of liquid in alveoli during pulmonary edema; overapoptosis of AEC II may be one of the key factors for fibroblast activation which may initiate and promote the development of pulmonary fibrosis; AEC II involves in the chronic inflammatory process and airway hyperreactivity in asthma through PS.

At present, there are more studies on the relationship between AEC II and ALI, pulmonary edema or pulmonary fibrosis than studies on relationship between AEC II and asthma. And the study on the role of AEC II in the treatment of asthma with Chinese medicine is even fewer. Asthma is a common disease in clinic and its pathogenesis is still unknown very clearly. Strengthening the study on the relationship between the AEC II and asthma, especially its role in the treatment of disease with Chinese medicine, may provide new ideas for explaining the pathogenesis of asthma.

Acknowledgements This study is supported by the National Natural Science Foundation of China (No.81072787), the National Natural Science Foundation of Shanghai (No.10ZR1429900).

References

1. Li H, Liu Y, Hao H et al (2012) Relationship of epidermal growth factor receptor in lung development. Hereditas 34(1):27–32
2. Li R, Wang J, Ju X et al (2007) Effect of long-term smoking on the histomorphology in rat lung tissues. Acta Academiae Medicinae Weifang 29(2):97–100
3. Mao B, Qian G, Chen Z (2002) Acute respiratory distress syndrome. People's Medical Publishing House, Beijing, p 58
4. Shu L-H, Wei K-L, Shang Y-X et al (2008) Relationship between alveolar epithelial type II cells and pulmonary surfactant protein A levels in young rats with acute lung injury. Chin J Contemp Pediatr 10(4):504–508
5. Wang D, Haviland DL, Burns AR et al (2007) A pure population of lung alveolar epithelial type II cells derived from human embryonic stem cells. Proc Natl Acad Sci USA 104(11):4449–4454
6. Li T, Yin M, Feng L, et al (2002) The research status of the apoptosis mechanism of the alveolar type II cells in the acute lung injury. Chin Crit Care Med 3(14):185–187
7. Mason RJ (2006) Biology of alveolar type II cells. Respirology 11(Suppl):S12–S15
8. Zhang S, Chen RK, Lin M et al (2004) Dynamic change of apoptosis of alveolar cells in ischemia-reperfusion induced pulmonary injury: an experimental study with rats. Zhonghua Yi Xue Za Zhi 84(19):1597–1600
9. Giraud O, Molliex S, Rolland C et al (2003) Halogenated anesthetics reduce interleukin-1 beta-induced cytokine secretion by rat alveolar type II cells in primary culture. Anesthesiology 98(1):74–81
10. Yu W, Fang X, Ewald A et al (2007) Formation of cysts by alveolar type II cells in three-dimensional culture reveals a novel mechanism for epithelial morphogenesis. Mol Biol Cell 18(5):1693–1700
11. Wang H, Chang L, Li W et al (2006) Temporal expression of notch receptor in lungs injury of preterm rat exposed to hyperoxia. J Appl Clin Pediatr 21(6):328–330
12. Shi X, Zhang H, Xiong S et al (2008) Primary culture of alveolar epithelial type II cell and its bionomics study. Chin J Pathophysiol 24(11):2282–2284, 2288
13. Perl M, Lomas-Neira J, Chung CS et al (2008) Epithelial cell apoptosis and neutrophil recruitment in acute lung injury-a unifying hypothesis? What we have learned from small interfering RNAs. Mol Med 14(7–8):465–475
14. Hengarther MO (2000) The biochemistry of apoptosis. Nature 407(6805):770–776
15. Wang H, Chang L, Lu H et al (2008) Effect of gamma-secretase inhibitor on notch signaling pathway in alveolar epithelial type II cells of preterm rat. J Appl Clin Pediatr 23(6):457–459
16. Ma H, Ye Y, Huang Y et al (2007) Hepatocyte growth factor in endotoxin-induced injury of alveolar epithelial type II cells. Guangdong Med J 28(10):1601–1603
17. Guan X, Wang D (2012) Progress of research on apoptosis of type II alveolar epithelial cell in acute lung injury. J Clin Pulm Med 17(6):1101–1103
18. Saldias FJ, Lecuona E, Comellas AP et al (2000) Beta-adrenergic stimulation restores rat lung ability to clear edema in ventilator-associated lung injury. Am J Respir Crit Care Med 162(1): 282–287
19. Ware LB, Matthay MA (2000) The acute respiratory distress syndrome. N Engl J Med 342(18):1334–1349
20. Matthay MA, Folkesson HG, Clerici C (2002) Lung epithelial Fluid transport and the resolution of pulmonary edema. Physiol Rev 82(3):569–600

21. Johnson MD, Bao HF, Chen XJ et al (2006) Functional ion channels in pulmonary alveolar type I cells support a role for type I cells in lung ion transport. Proc Natl Sci USA 103(13):4964–4969
22. Zhou W, He L, Li T et al (2009) Epithelial sodium channel subunit mRNA expression in acutely isolated rat alveolar type II cells. J Southern Med Univ 29(1):54–56
23. Uhal BD, Joshi I, Hughes WF et al (1998) Alveolar epithelial cell death adjacent to underlying myofibroblasts in advanced fibrotic human lung. Am J Physiol 275(6 Pt 1):L1192–L1199
24. Kuwano K, Kunitake R, Kawasaki M et al (1996) P21Waf1/Cip1/Sdi1 and p53 expression in association with DNA strand breaks in idiopathic pulmonary fibrosis. Am J Respir Crit Care Med 154(2 Pt 1):477–483
25. Huang Y, Ye Y, Shi J et al (2008) Effects of pulmonary fibroblasts on type II alveolar epithelial cells in the rat model of pulmonary fibrosis induced by pingyangmycin. Med J Wuhan Univ 29(4):467–471
26. Bardales RH, Xie SS, Schaefer RF et al (1996) Apoptosis is a major pathway responsible for the resolution of type II pneumocytes in acute lung injury. Am J Pathol 149(3):845–852
27. Kolosionek E (2009) Expression and activity of phosphodiesterase isoforms during epithelial mesenchymal transition: the role of phosphodiesterase 4. Mol Biol Cell 20(22):4751–4765
28. Uhal BD (2002) Apoptosis in lung fibrosis and repair. Chest 122(6 Suppl):293S–298S
29. Selman M, Pardo A (2002) Idiopathic pulmonary fibrosis: an epithelial/fibroblastic cross-talk disorder. Respir Res 3:3
30. Li H, Ye R, Shangguan W et al (2010) Effects of herbal application on lamella body and pulmonary surfactant secretion in lung tissues of asthma guinea pig. Acta Universitatis Traditionis Medicalis Sinensis Pharmacologiaeque Shanghai 24(6):67–69
31. Turhal NS, Erdal S, Karacav S (2000) Efficacy of treatment to relieve mucositis-induced discomfort. Supp Care Cancer 8(1):55–58
32. Babu KS, Woodcock DA, Smith SE et al (2003) Inhaled synthetic surfactant abolishes the early allergen-induced response in asthma. Eur Respir J 21(6):1046–1049
33. Malmstrum K, Pelkonen AS, Malmberg LP et al (2011) Lung function, airway remodeling and inflammation in symptomatic infants: outcome at 3 years. Thorax 66(2):157–162
34. Liu C (2009) Infant lung function testing and its application in wheezing diseases. Chin Pediatr Emerg Med 16(2):101–103
35. Borrego LM, Stocks J, Leiria-Pinto P et al (2009) Lung function and clinical risk factors for asthma in infants and young children with recurrent wheeze. Thorax 64(3):203–209

Chapter 265
Application of Inquiry Teaching in Econometrics Course

Songyan Zhang

Abstract In this paper, from the econometric development and teaching situation, we describe the need for the introduction of inquiry teaching mode, point out the basic conditions for the implementation of the inquiry teaching mode and some problems that should be paid attention to in specific organizational implementation process.

Keywords Inquiry teaching · Econometrics course · Innovation and practice

265.1 Introduction

Inquiry Teaching is also known as discovery method or research method, it refers that teachers just give students some examples and problems when students learn the concepts and principles, and let students inquiry independently and discovery the corresponding principles and conclusions by reading, observating, experimenting, thinking, discussing, listening and other ways. Its guiding principle is that under the guidance of teachers, let students be the subjects, and let them explore consciously, actively and master and understand problem-solving methods and steps to study the properties of objective things, find the cause of the development of things and relations of the internal of things. As a result, they can find out the law and form their own concept.

S. Zhang (✉)
School of Economics and Management, Zhejiang University of Science and Technology, Hangzhou 310023, People's Republic of China
e-mail: syzh201@163.com

265.2 The Necessity for Inquiry Teaching Methods in the Teaching of Econometrics

Econometrics is an economic discipline combined by economics, statistics and mathematics. Economics provide the theoretical framework of quantitative analysis. Statistics provide economic statistics information. Mathematics provide means of model solution. In the process of traditional teaching, we always too much emphasize on theory, so it is not easy to let the students receive econometrics. By way of inquiry teaching, we can eliminate the gap between theory and practice, and then will enable students to receive this course.

265.2.1 Inquiry Teaching Methods Can Improve the Students' Initiative and Participation of the Teaching

Currently, new methods of econometrics are emerging, course content system is increasingly rich. However, due to the limit of lessons, teachers mainly teach model estimation methods and test methods, and take the traditional chalk and talk in teaching. While taking research teaching methods, teaching content will be extending to the outside of classroom. Teachers design problems or propose a topic for students to collect relevant informations, understand the Econometrics methods and application status so as to improve students' learning initiative and participatory teaching.

265.2.2 Implementation of Inquiry-Based Teaching is Help in Training Students the Ability to Collect and Process Information

Writting application cases and course papers are important means for the implementation of inquiry-based pedagogy. On one hand, it requires students to learn to collect relevant informations, master and make use of certain information-search methods to search relevant bibliographies and databases in order to know about the development of the discipline and learn the application of econometric methods, or make use of the method of scientific investigation to conduct actual surveys to obtain relevant informations and data; On the other hand, we must learn to process information, especially considering the requirements based on the purpose of establishing the econometric models and estimation methods, we should select appropriate processing methods and software for statistical data processing.

Therefore, the inquiry teaching method can train students the ability to collect and process information.

265.2.3 Implementation of Inquiry-Based Teaching Methods Can Help Students to Improve the Ability of Analyzing and Solving Practical Problems

Currently, teachers pay more attention to theoretical lectures but less on practical application in the teaching of econometrics. Teachers focus on teaching a variety of model estimation and testing methods in class, and students mainly familiar with and master the econometric analysis software when they have computer courses. When inquiry-based teaching methods are adopted, teachers supervise the students to combine with professional features and real economic hot issues to write cases and papers, and act these as important aspect of assessment. This will not only help students understand and master the model estimates and inspection methods, but also train students using professional knowledge and econometric analysis to solve real-world economic problems.

265.2.4 Implementation of Inquiry-Based Teaching Methods Will Help to Develop Students' Innovation and Ability

Cultivating students' innovation and ability is one of the important goals of higher education talents training in new era. Higher education should focus on training top creative talents, and actively create a favorable environment of encouraging students to think independently, explore freely and create boldly. When inquiry-based teaching methods are adopted, by allowing students to write related research and applied overview, teachers may encourage students to understand the developments of subject and train students' ability of discovering and analyzing problems.

265.3 The Basic Conditions for the Implementation of Inquiry Teaching Mode

Inquiry Teaching Method is a more advanced teaching method, it requires more for teachers and students, in order to better achieve the goal of teaching, we should pay attention to the following aspects in the application of this method.

265.3.1 Teachers Should Have a Strong Research Capability

Using Inquiry Teaching Method in "Econometrics" teaching, teachers should not only familiar with the course content system, grasp the focus and difficulty of the course content correctly, express the basic principles and knowledge of econometric methods accurately, but also have a certain ability to research, such as: having a strong literature search and data collection capabilities with a solid economic theory; grasping the real economy hot issues of the relevant field expertise and academic developments; familiaring with the meaning of statistical indicators on economic and data processing methods; being able to write teaching cases; having a rich experience in the subject developed. The research capacity of teachers is a prerequisite for the implementation of inquiry teaching methods.

265.3.2 Rational Assignment of Teaching Hours

The inquiry teaching should be used as part of the entire econometrics teaching methodology, it can not completely replace the doctrines taught and hands-on experiments. Because the total teaching time is limited, we want a reasonable division of the proportion of the three kinds of teaching time among the doctrines taught, experiments on the computer and inquiry teaching. Inquiry teaching plan should not be more than 20 % of the total number of teaching plan hours. In fact, the inquiry teaching time can be extended to extra-curricular, teachers should led students to use their spare time for inquiry learning. In the classroom, teachers do the case discuss and papers analysis.

265.3.3 Improve the Assess Way of Courses Grading

There must be a course grade assessment method matches for the implementation of inquiry teaching. At present, students are assessed econometric basic principles and the assessment form of the method is relatively simple. This will be the hinder for students' ability to express. Writing course papers should be acted as an important part in students' curriculum assessment. Teachers should assess the final grade comprehensively combined with the classroom tests, hands-on and essay writing.

265.4 Organization and Implementation of Inquiry Teaching

265.4.1 Write a Literature Review

The literature review is an integral part of scientific research, it is the basis of scientific research and innovation. A literature review can reflect on a topic and its research process, analysis methods, main ideas and research trends and shortcomings, so it can discover new perspectives of these thematic studies and determine the new starting point. Teachers should teach the general method, the basic format and problems of needing attention for writing economics literature review. The literature review can be used as an important part of the course work. After teaching about the inspection and application method, teachers should let students to collect sample data and write course papers based on the literature review.

265.4.2 The Combination of Cases Teaching and Experimental Teaching

Case teaching and experiment teaching are two components complemented in economics courses. In the teaching schedule, we should co-ordinate the planning. We can complete a paper theory teaching in 2 weeks, so it is more appropriate to arrange 2 h for experimental teaching every 2 weeks. In addition, based on the actual situation, teachers can also led students to find and identify problems from socio-economic phenomenon, read books and collect relevant data, and according to the knowledge econometric models, to analysis and research by using software. Through this part of practice, all aspects of students' ability can be improved.

265.4.3 Writing Course Papers

Writing course papers is an effective way to develop students' research skills and the spirit of innovation. More than half of the courses are taught in econometrics. Teachers should ask students to prepare for course paper writing and introduce the writing methods. Trough writing course papers, students can train general ability such as self-study, literature review, analysis application of theoretical, model construction and software using.

265.5 Conclusion

Implementation of the inquiry teaching in econometrics course should be paid more attention to teaching methods. Teachers should accumulate teaching cases material, handle the knowledge relationship among mathematics, statistics and economics. At the same time, we should improve the assessment system. We will assess student achievement combining with the theory teaching, course work and experiments teaching. Through teaching practice, we believe that it is feasible to carry out inquiry teaching in econometrics course.

References

1. Zhang S-Y (2010) Mathematical method applied in the logistics management. In: The 2010 international conference on management science and information engineering, 2010, 12
2. Xie Z-Z (2004) Econometrics 2nd edn. Higher Education Press, Beijing
3. Shan Y-B (2004) Teaching Case selection and design. Stat Educ 2000(4)
4. Li Z-N, Pai W-Q (2005) Econometrics. Higher Education Press, Beijing

Chapter 266
Extract Examining Data Using Medical Field Association Knowledge Base

Li Wang, Yuanpeng Zhang, Danmin Qian, Min Yao, Jiancheng Dong and Dengfu Yao

Abstract The electronical medical record incorporate a significant amount of information, which is useful for medical study. The examining data is the results of patients' inspection. In order to extract examining data from huge amount electronic medical record. A new method is utilized in our research. The start point of the research is the whole process that human recognize the examining data in the text. The presented method takes use of medical field association knowledge. In the experiment, the value of recall and precision is 81 and 83 % respectively. The satisfied experiment values prove that the presented new method can avoid weak point exiting in the traditional methods, at the same time, can extract the examing data efficiently.

Keywords Examining data · Field association · Knowledge base

266.1 Introduction

The contents in the electronical medical record (EMR) include disease history, symptoms, and examining data, etc. In Chinese EMR text, sentences are represented as strings of Chinese characters (hanzi), plus some English characters, words, numbers, and symbols are often included, without natural delimiters between them. Fig 266.1 presents an example text in the EMR system used in our research.

L. Wang (✉) · Y. Zhang · D. Qian · M. Yao · J. Dong · D. Yao
Department of Medical Informatics, Nantong University, Qixiu Road #19, Nantong 226001, China
e-mail: wangli@ntu.edu.cn

患者两年前出现发作性胸痛，诊断为"冠心病"，后于15月前行CABG手术。既往有高血压病史，最高血压190/130mmHg，平时口服"缬沙坦"控制血压。15月前有CABG手术史，术中有输血。T36.4℃，P58次/分，R18次/分，Bp140/80mmHg。心脏相对浊音界不大，Hr：58次/分。

Fig. 266.1 An example medical text in the EMR system

Table 266.1 lists the seven most common kinds of examining data expression.

Nowadays, the prevalent methods in medical text information extraction are all based on the natural language processing, including two important aspects: based on rules and machine learning.

The main idea in rule based on method is that the limited rules can support unlimited phenomenon. Therefore, in the ideal cases, if the perfect and limited language rule system is established, all the unlimited phenomenon can be solved. However, in the real situation, the examining data is expressed in the varied styles, as shown in Table 266.1. Collecting all the rules is almost impossible. In addition, due to the inputter's habits differences and mistake, some spaces and symbols are mixed among the data. All the mentioned language phenomenon bring troubleness to the rule based method obviously.

Another empirical method is based on statistical machine learning. The main idea in this method is "the more is the truth". That is to say, if the amount of corpus is sufficient and the structure is reasonable enough, all the language phenomenon can be understood through statistical method. To this method, enough corpus is the key point. However, in the real EMR text, the examining data is normally recorded within one or two sentences, even scattered in the disordered sentences. All these cause a series of problems, for example, the training data is too sparse, then, the feature is not so obvious.

One another important problem exiting in the two mentioned traditional methods is that the transplant is not so well. The constructed rules and training data model can not give good performance when facing totally new medical texts.

Table 266.1 Common examining data expression and examples

	Examining data expression	Examples
(1)	Number and Chinese	心率78次
(2)	English and number	*Bp* 145/90 mmHg
(3)	English and symbol	*NS* (−)
(4)	English, number and Chinese	*P*78次/分 , *R*18次/分
(5)	Number and symbol	腹部移动性浊音 (−)
(6)	English, Chinese and symbol	*Murphy's*征 (+)
(7)	English, number and symbol	*AST* 179 u/L

266.2 Research Method

In our research, we take use of medical field association knowledge, which can solve the exited problems in the traditional methods.

266.2.1 Medical Field Association Knowledge

The field association knowledge research is based on the fact that, we human can usually recognize the fields like "sports" or "economy" by finding some specific words without reading the whole document [1]. Field association terms are single or compound words appearing in related field documents that enable the fields of document identification [2, 3]. For example, when field association terms "NBA" and "Yao Ming" appear in a document, humans can understand the document that is talking about field <basketball>.

Field association knowledge is constituted by field association terms, which can record, perform, communicate and store the knowledge of phenomenon in the specific field.

The medical field association knowledge research is established on the general field association knowledge research foundation [4], the study of the idea is the same based on people's cognitive processes. When we human recognize the examining data in the medical text, we focus on the number, letter, and symbols, plus some words around the target examining data [5]. All the number, letter, symbols, and words are medical examining field association terms.

In the hospital, patients have the same examining items even in the different departments, such as body temperature, heart rate, breathing rate, and blood pressure (T:36.9 °C, P:64 次/分, R16次/分, BP:142/98 mmHg), at the same time, department of infectious diseases usually checks liver function (ALT 782U/L, AST 452U/L, TBi 11 umol/L), department of endocrinology cares the blood glucose (16.1 mmol/L).

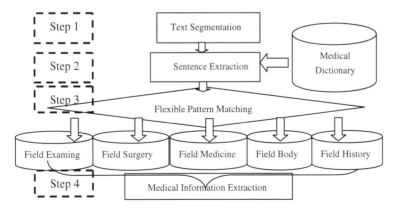

Fig. 266.2 Main steps in examining data extraction

266.2.2 Experimental Method

Four main steps are used to extract examining data from medical text as shown in Fig. 266.2.

- Step 1 The text is segmented according to the punctuation in the sentences. In the test, method I takes use of comma, method II takes use of full stop.
- Step 2 Extract sentences that contain number, symbol and English character. In this step, all the extracted sentences can be classified into three type.

  Type 1: The sentence contains the examining data.
  Type 2: The sentence contains English characters, however, English characters are not the examining item. For example, "CABG" is a surgery name.
  Type 3: The sentence contains number, however, the number is not examining result. For example, "75 mg qd" is used to indicate dosage.

- Step 3 Extract terms in the sentences using flexible pattern matching. A huge medical dictionary, covering 200,000 terms, is used to select the terms. All the extracted terms are classified into five fields, including examining, surgery, medicine, body and history fields. Since medical term has different scope to associate with a field, assigning proper weight is necessary. If the term only appears in one field, that is to say, this term has a strong distinction ability, weight eight is assigned. If the number of the fields that the word appearing in is increasing, the corresponding distinction ability becomes weak. Weight 6, 4, 2 and 0 is assigned to the term, if it is related to 2, 3, 4 and 5 fields respectively.
- Step 4 Using medical field association terms to judge the related field of the sentence belonging to. Calculate the value of the weight of all the terms extracted from the sentence. If the maximum value belongs to field examining, the examining data is extracted.

266.3 Results and Evaluation

The medical texts in 10 departments (200 pieces in each department) are collected, including, infectious, endocrine, and neurology, etc. 100 pieces are utilized to collect medical field association knowledge, the left 100 pieces are utilized to make test.

Two values, precision and recall, are used to evaluate the experimental results.

Table 266.2 Experimental results using two methods

	Method I (%)	Method II (%)
Recall	79	81
Precision	80	83

Precision = (the number of correct answers)/(the number of tested examining data)

Recall = (the number of correct answers)/(the number of all examining data)

Experiments are carried using two segmentation methods in step 1. Table 266.2 presents the experimental results. The value precision and recall is 79 and 80 % respectively using method I. Both two values increase slightly 2 and 3 % respectively using method II. The main reason is, the field weight can be calculated more precisely when using the all terms appearing in the whole sentence. Overall, the satisfied experiment results can show the efficiency by using the new method.

In the future, the most important work is that more field association terms will be added into the field association knowledge base.

Acknowledgments This work is supported by Nantong social undertakings technology innovation and demonstration program (No. HS2012045) and China Postdoctoral Science Foundation (No. 2012M521108).

References

1. Fuketa M, Lee S, Tsuji T et al (2000) A document classification method by using field association words. Int J Inf Sci 126(2):57–70
2. Lee SS, Shishibori M, Sumitomo T et al (2002) Extraction of field-coherent passages. Int J Inf Process Manag 38(2):173–207
3. Atlam E-S, Fuketa M, Morita K et al (2003) Document similarity measurement using field association term. Int J Inf Process Manag 39(6):809–824
4. Wang L, Yata S, Atlam E-S et al (2009) A Method of building Chinese field association knowledge from wikipedia. In: Proceeding of the 5th international conference on natural language processing and knowledge engineering (IEEE NLP-KE'2009), Dalian
5. Wang L, Fuketa M, Morita K et al (2011) Context constraint disambiguation of word semantics by field association schemes. Int J Inf Process Manag 47(5):560–574

Chapter 267
The Analysis and Research on Digital Campus Construct Model

Liu Xiaoming and Jiang Changyun

Abstract The digital campus construct is the foundation and core of education informatization. This paper introduces the idea of the digital campus, analyzes the existing problems of the construct, discusses the digital campus construct based on the business model and service-oriented model, then analyzes the influence of the different models to the digital campus construct.

Keywords Digital campus · Informatization · Business mode · Service mode

267.1 Introduction

Education informatization is the trend of current education development. The standard of the college digital campus construct embodies the application of education informationization. Education informationization provides requirements and supports for studying and teaching. The digital campus continuously moves forward, and raises education informatization levels. The digital campus is a digital space which is formed by all kinds of digital resources on the traditional campus, using advanced information techniques.s. It is based on the college network infrastructures, including the environment (such as equipment and classrooms), resources (e.g., books, notes, images and courseware), and instructional activity (including teaching, learning, management, service and office). College network and application system structure, being the nervous system of the campus, fulfills the information transfer and other information services. The digital campus means, with the support of information technology, achieving "network omnipresent, data omniscient", application universality, business universality, and

L. Xiaoming (✉) · J. Changyun
Huaihai Institute of Technolgoy, Lianyungang 222005 Jiangsu,
People's Republic of China
e-mail: liuxm029@gmail.com

finally realizing the "wisdom school" in the digital environment. This ideal environment would be based on cable for the integration of wireless networks; a variety of access methods for terminal with wireless intelligent security and protection, digital broadcast for the integration of a green, low-carbon and intelligent digital network environment; digital management systems shared data center and unified identity authentication and authorization; uniform information portal platforms and various application information platforms; building work flows and collaborative management information systems; On the basis of digital teaching and research, and centralized educational administration, it constructs resource platforms for teaching and learning in cloud computing centers. It provides convenient conditions for teaching and learning, with a variety of scientific research resources and management, digital resources, and experiment platforms. The digital campus provides a convenient and efficient digital environment and e-commerce service platform, using the IC card system, and monitoring school resource utilization, payments, identity authentication, access control, etc. The digital campus integrates all sorts of data and application system functions into one-stop services, data mining and decision support.

267.2 The Problems of the Ideal Digital Campus

Investment and development in information systems has brought about the network office system, network teaching, and some network services, but there are still some outstanding problems:

1. Leadership understanding and appreciation of information technology.

Leadership in the age of Internet is different from the industrialized era. Perceptions on investment in informatization seriously affect progress in the construct of the digital campus. In the information environment, information technology provides a powerful information acquisition ability that changes the leader's knowledge structure, and changes the nature of the leadership in the process of informatization Construct.

2. The management system and operational mechanism

Development of information systems and development of management systems is an organic whole. Typically, after development the informatization tasks of each business unit are fragmented, the teaching information and engineering data on operation and maintenance are not unified, and a lagging informatization management mechanism leaves the decision makers unable to get valid data.

3. The lack of integration system

Due to the rapid development of information technology and the limitation of resources, the college currently has a variety of operating systems and system architectures. The low efficiency of information sharing and non-uniform data standards creates a serious problem of "information islands" which must be addressed with the advancement of education informationization process. There is a need to integrate all kinds of education information resources, databases and application systems. A "large system" uniform platform will be the next step of education informatization development

4. Poor business flexibility and extensibility

Various business systems belong to different departments and data cannot be shared amongst them. Some application systems are inflexible, of limited application outside individual departments, and require expensive, ongoing maintenance

5. Data security mechanism

Because the systems are independent and deployed in scattered locations, unified control and maintenance is difficult to realize. Security solutions are unable to ensure that individual application systems are adequately served with virus protection, network security, or data security.

267.3 The Needed Perspective

Informatization process will encounter more complex problems, but must remain global, system-wide and long term in perspective in planning and execution. Here we introduce two models for the development of the digital campus: the business model and the service model.

267.3.1 Business Model

As shown in Fig. 267.1, the key points in the reality map for a virtual campus are composed of learning, content, resource support, management schemes, and people. In the digital campus design, by adopting the method of the Business Process Management System (BPM) and workflow technologies, we build for students and teachers, scientific research, financial, assets, and resources management—a core business of the digital campus URP system.

College service activities are driven by people. It is important to record the changing activities of the "people" and to support the people. The teaching and scientific research of colleges and universities are built around people's learning behavior; teaching, scientific research and social service are the three major functions. Structured resources, life cycle management evaluation standards and various elements are the import determinants of the business mode. According to the different application environments, service goals and service needs, the digital campus application and information system, from the bottom to the top, must consist of a high-speed, stable physically secure network, various management

Fig. 267.1 Business model for function levels

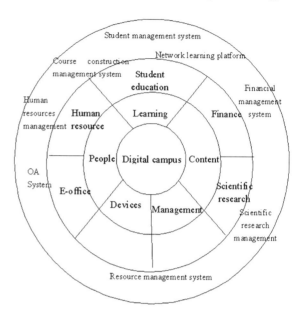

information systems based on business and functional integration, e-commerce, planning and decision-making services, and other personalized services, all on the basis of data fusion.

267.3.2 Service Mode

The purpose of digital campus construct is to provide services for students and teacher staff, for study, for research, and for life. The schematic diagram of Fig. 267.2 is based on the service system pattern. Information technology services are seen as an indispensable part of the process of teaching, learning and management. Figure 267.2 shows a focus on academic affairs, human resource management, college students' services, major logistics, security information, and the financial system in the service mode. In the development of colleges and universities, the service oriented model focuses on the cultivation of talents. Teacher development is the foundation, and efficient management is the guarantee. Under this service system, anyone who has simple access can be connected to the campus digital service system, to retrieve content to satisfy his or her needs. The system of service functions needs to be enriched constantly according to the requirements of users; that is to say, the small business system development, and the overall system must be highly integrated and unified to provide users with a public platform and convenient access. It must provide a comprehensive information system with public data sharing and data integration as part of a unified public data platform. The new systems should be on a platform which reduces data conflicts and incompatibilities.

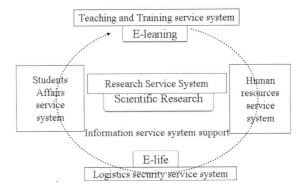

Fig. 267.2 Service-oriented structure mode

Table 267.1 Construct mode comparisons

Mode type	Object	Architecture	Access point	Data	Expandability
Business mode	Application	Function	Multi-application	Independent unshared	Weaken
Service mode	Personnel	Service	Single-platform	Integrated shared	Strong

267.3.3 Mode Comparison

In the service model, data, resources, and information systems are all based on the network infrastructure, but the business-oriented functions are relatively independent. It primarily meets the needs of teaching, learning, research, management, and establishes different management information systems for people, study, equipment, and content. As Table 267.1 show, the business model does not consider the system in terms of data integration, sharing, exchange, and system integration. The framework of the service-oriented model for the primary business and micro businesses can satisfy the digital campus construct along with advancing college development, advancing technology, and enriching business needs.

It also solves the problems of heterogeneous data, and with sharing and exchanging information. It provides users with a unified integration interface, reduces the difficulty of user access, and reduces the impact of new online business systems on all users.

267.4 Conclusion

Digital campus Construct is a complicated system engineering task. The design, data requirements, and technology all have high requirements. The emergence of new technologies such as cloud computing and the Internet of things (IoT) brings new technology tools. IoT provides data mining and knowledge discovery. Cloud storage meets the needs for processing, and securely storing, huge amounts of data. These new technologies provide new opportunities to unify and integrate education resources and develop a new kind of digital campus.

References

1. Zhou J (2011) The research on the higher education informatization and the digitalization campus construct. Manufact Autom 3:218–210
2. Zongshan W Fei L (2011) Exploration and practice on construct of digitalization campus. Lab Res Explor 10(5):162–164
3. Peng L (2012) Public service platform design based on the pattern of "cloud + agent" in digital campus. E-education Res 10:64–68
4. Mingguang Z (2011) The strategy and practice to promote Ningbo campus digitalization construct of education informatization. Chin Educ Technol (4):39–42
5. Zhonglin L (2012) The problems and countermeasures based on university digital campus construct. Vocat Techn Educ Forum 26:49–50

Chapter 268
Emotional Deficiency in Web-Based Learning Environment and Suggested Solutions

Cai Li-hua

Abstract Emotion is one of the key elements influencing language learning, but the phenomenon of emotional deficiency has arisen with the widespread application of web-based autonomous learning platforms. This paper, based on the author's own teaching experiences and some other studies, discusses the importance of emotional factors to language learning, explores the main causes of emotional deficiency in autonomous learning in web-based environment and offers some suggested solutions as to how to ensure students' subjective status in autonomous learning and how to improve their performance.

Keywords Emotional deficiency · Web-based learning environment · Solution

268.1 Introduction

As is defined in Wikipedia, "emotion is the generic term for subjective, conscious experience that is characterized primarily by psychophysiological expressions, biological reactions, and mental states."

With the widespread application of web-based learning platforms in colleges and universities, autonomous learning online becomes more and more popular, which has brought students problems as well as benefits, especially the problem of emotional deficiency. Emotion is of great significance to language learning, and it can improve learning effect. It is hard for students with negative feelings, such as uneasiness, frustration, self-doubt and tension, to learn a language well. Therefore, some measures must be taken to deal with students' emotional deficiency in autonomous learning online.

C. Li-hua (✉)
University of Science and Technology, Anshan 114051 Liaoning, China
e-mail: clh9972@163.com

268.2 The Importance of Emotional Factors to Language Learning

The function of emotion in language learning used to be neglected, while cognition has been laid more emphasis on for long. However, according to Arnold [1, p. 1], "the affective side of learning is not in opposition to the cognitive side. When both are used together, the learning process can be constructed on a firmer foundation."

Emotion is considered the driving force behind motivation, either positive or negative. Positive emotion may enhance learning effect, while negative emotions such as anxiety, fear, stress, anger or depression may obstruct the learning process. Foreign language learners are liable to be affected by these emotional factors.

"Studies show the negative correlation of anxiety with grades in language courses, proficiency test performance, performance in speaking and writing tasks, self-confidence in language learning, and self-esteem, i.e. the judgment of one's own worth" [1, p. 61]. From some studies,

J. Arnold and H. D. Brown have found that second language learning process is the process in which cognition and emotion interact with each other.

Neural scientist LeDoux [5] sees emotion and cognition as partners in the mind. He notes how, after years of behaviourist dominance, cognitive science once again made it respectable to study mental states; and he insists that it is time 'to reunite cognition and emotion in the mind'. LeDoux even goes so far as to say that 'minds without emotions are not really minds at all'.

Studies on emotion are of great importance to language learning, which may improve language learning effect. Learners with positive feelings usually devote to their learning enthusiastically, while negative feelings such as uneasiness, tension, fear, anxiety or disgust may prevent learners from learning efficiently.

268.3 Emotional Deficiency in Web-Based Environment and Causes

Platforms equipped with computers and network with multilevel linguistic data in various forms provide a learning environment totally different from that of the traditional classrooms. On the platform, language learners can talk to the computer with the help of some software, or communicate with teachers or other students online. Owing to these advantages of network platforms, English autonomous learning on network has gradually become a new trend in more and more Chinese universities.

However, with the widespread use of web-based learning platforms, problems have arisen, among which are unbalanced development of cognition and emotion, lack of autonomous learning awareness, much anxiety and lack of affective interaction between students and teachers.

268.3.1 Unbalanced Development of Cognition and Emotion

Studies in social psychology and psycholinguistics show that emotion and cognition, which are inseparably connected, are important factors influencing knowledge acquisition. Nevertheless, more importance has long been attached to cognition than emotion, which is a common phenomenon in China as well as abroad.

According to American linguist Krashen [4], language input is not the only thing to decide whether language learning is successful or not. What differentiates one learner from another can be attributed to either their amount of comprehensible language input or their different emotional factors like motivation, self-confidence and anxiety, the so-called affective filter. Students who are emotionally disturbed may suffer from high affective filters so that they will acquire very little of a second language, while those who are relaxed, comfortable and at ease will experience low affective filters and thus acquire the most of the language.

However, most students do not have the integrative orientation, "a desire to learn the language in order to relate to and even become part of the target language culture" [1], and so they may lose their interest and motivation after the "honeymoon" period, in which their curiosity about the new language learning mode has been satisfied.

268.3.2 Lack of Autonomous Learning Awareness

When having autonomous learning online, students are not restricted by time and place, and so they can arrange their own studies at a proper level and pace, which is very good for learners' self-study.

However, students in China, from pupils to adult students, have been used to the practice of passing on knowledge from teachers to students since ancient times. Almost no courses have ever been delivered on how students learn knowledge and skills by themselves, i.e. they don't know how to 'fish' on their own. With foreign language learning network platforms equipped in more and more colleges and universities, autonomous learning on network has been popular. Students have to make their own learning plan and arrange their own schedule, which they haven't done in their previous learning experience. For those who come from rural or remote areas, it is even harder to adapt to the new learning mode since computers are almost not available in their home and schools. Quite a few students, especially those in ordinary universities, do not have enough self-monitoring abilities and they want to relax themselves after having experienced the strain of the college entrance examination. In addition, there are too many interesting things online, and students are likely to be distracted from what they are supposed to learn.

Based on a survey done by Liu [6] among some freshmen and sophomores in a key university, a conclusion can be drawn that "under the internet circumstances, students' self-monitoring level is low on the whole." The situation is even worse in ordinary universities according to the author and some other teachers.

Therefore, it can be concluded that quite a number of college students are lacking in autonomous learning awareness, to be specific, they are poor at plan-making, self-evaluation, initiative and learning strategy application, etc.

268.3.3 Much Anxiety

Anxiety is one of the emotions influencing language learning. Language anxiety ranks high among factors influencing language learning, regardless of whether the setting is informal (learning language 'on the streets') or formal (in the language classroom) [1].

Researchers such as Zhang and Guo [12], Zeng and Liu [11] and Sui [9], etc. have found in their studies that the Internet-based learning environment helps to reduce students' anxiety to some extent. However, Zeng and Liu [11] has also found that freshmen learning in the web-based environment suffer from more anxiety than their counterparts learning in the traditional classrooms.

Different environments and teaching and learning styles in university itself may take most freshmen quite a while to get accustomed, not to mention the completely new Internet-based learning environment. Being unable to operate computers and use some programs skillfully makes students rather frustrated. Unfamiliarity with teachers, students and network multi-media technology makes students less confident and more anxious unavoidably. Besides, the large quantity of learning materials available online makes students confused about what they should choose to learn.

Another fact should never be neglected that in almost every university quite a few students come from rural or remote areas, and they have never got access to computers and Internet. So they must have difficulty in computer operation, which may cause a great anxiety about the totally new learning mode. Many a student is introverted and shy, due to which they might not ask for help from teachers or other students when they have questions. They may be afraid of being laughed at by others because of their accent or incorrect pronunciation.

Some students feel at a loss in a virtual classroom, but teachers are usually unable to find out the students' problems in time and help them out, which may cause a greater degree of anxiety. Sometimes long waiting owing to network fault or low speed of computers may cause students' boredom and loss of interest in the learning mode and even the course.

268.3.4 Lack of Affective Interaction

Herczeg [3] once compared web-based education to "knowledge assembly line", which emphasizes knowledge transmission more than its special product—learners' affection. With the unification of web-based education in teaching methods, learning process, multimedia authoring tool, learning environment, evaluation strategy, etc., learners, especially younger ones or extroverts are likely to lose their interest in such structured and unified learning mode.

In the Internet-based environment there exist different phenomena, among which two are representative—"sheep herding style", in which students get too little control and are free to do whatever they like online, watching movies, playing games, chatting in their mother tongue other than studying foreign language, and "captive style", in which students are given too little freedom and they have to study under strict control of teachers via internet technology. Students have to learn the required materials within certain time, thus may lose their initiative and creativity, for they have little time to get access to the large quantity of learning materials online. Although students can communicate with teachers via MSN, QQ or BBS, they are probably not online at the same time. If teachers do not answer some student's questions in time, the student's enthusiasm may increasingly decline after anxious and impatient waiting.

According to Luo et al. [7] and others, learners seldom ask for help from teachers or classmates via E-mail or BBS when they come across problems in learning online. The reasons why many people choose to be content with superficial understanding are that they are too shy or just reluctant to ask for help from others especially those they are unfamiliar with.

It is hard for students to resonate with their teachers due to separation of time and space. Unable to see teachers' smiling faces or encouraging nodding, some students are not used to talking to the cold computer screen. Visual, physical and mental fatigue, caused by too much exposure to computer screen, may bring about students' resistance to screen, loss of initiative, even suspicion or hatred for English autonomous online learning [2].

According to some researchers, learners' emotions directly affect their learning process and results. Positive feelings improve cognition, memory and creative thinking, while negative feelings may inhibit learners' potentials and creativity.

268.4 Suggested Solutions to Emotional Deficiency

In view of the harmful impact of emotional deficiency in web-based autonomous learning environment on language learners, some suggested solutions are offered here and it is hoped that they might be of some help to improvement of autonomous language learning practice.

268.4.1 To Improve Students' Cognitive Ability Through Emotional Help

American futurist John Naisbitt once expressed his original idea "High Tech/High Touch" in *Megatrends 2000: Ten new directions for the 1990s* to show that the development of technology should be combined with humanity. By the vivid expression "High Touch", he emphasizes the importance of emotion, i.e. people should communicate with one another more.

Students' autonomous learning online should not be totally independent; they need teachers' help and support as their 'scaffold'. When having autonomous learning online, students need to have teachers' attention and guidance, because "stimulating the different positive emotional factors, such as esteem, empathy or motivation, can greatly facilitate the language learning process"[1]. Teachers should be available whenever they are needed, for their presence is the emotional support of students and the guarantee of students' effective learning. Only when students have a sense of safety, great motivation and initiative, can they exert their cognitive ability to the greatest extent.

268.4.2 To Promote Interaction and Reduce Anxiety

In Internet-based autonomous learning environment, anxiety can't be avoided owing to different levels of students' computer operating skills, lack of autonomous learning strategy, inadequate instructional monitoring of teachers and less communicative interaction, which has a great impact on students' learning effect.

According to Krashen's [4] affective filter hypothesis, those who are emotionally disturbed or distracted will employ high affective filters and will acquire very little of the language, while those who are relaxed, comfortable and at ease will present with very low affective filters and thus will acquire the most of a second language.

Teachers should try to make up for the emotional deficiency of students in online learning. At the initial phase, students should receive systematic training about how the web-based learning platform works. Teachers should be at hand whenever students come across any problems. Teachers have to be observant of those students, who are more anxious and need detailed instruction, and give them timely help to reduce their anxiety.

By promoting the interaction between teachers and students, a harmonious learning atmosphere will be created and if teachers try every means to lower affective filters and turn debilitating anxiety into facilitating anxiety which will improve concentration and creative thinking, students will acquire more knowledge and skills.

268.4.3 To Strengthen Monitoring

To guarantee the learning effect and cultivate students' autonomous learning ability and creativity, teachers should have appropriate monitoring means, neither leaving students alone nor controlling them too strictly. Learners should not be

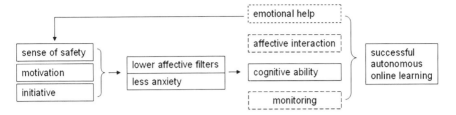

Fig. 268 1 Ways to improve autonomous online learning

imposed too much pressure or expectation; instead, they should be left enough free time to learn what they like after finishing the required tasks so that they will have a sense of achievement. Teachers need to offer them advice on how to choose appropriate materials in the sea of resources in order to improve their learning efficiency.

Various measures should be taken to ensure the successful operation of autonomous learning. Whenever there are students learning on the platform, there should be a teacher available to help students who have problems or confusion either about computer operation or the learning subject. Teachers should be around to make sure that students are learning the language instead of chatting, and that every student finishes the required tasks by themselves rather than by someone else. Only by strengthening monitoring, can autonomous learning serve its real purpose.

As is shown in Fig. 268.1, teachers' emotional help, monitoring and interaction (shown in boxes with dotted line frames) are essential to improving learners' performance (shown in boxes with real line frames) in autonomous learning in a web-based environment.

268.5 Conclusion

It is said that it is emotion rather than intelligence that determines students' future and destiny. Sun [10] believes that advanced technology is not the whole picture of teaching, but a beneficial supplement of classroom instruction. Web-based learning platform should not become the means for electronic cramming, which may cause emotional fatigue among students.

It's not easy to get rid of the strong influence of traditional education mode within a short time. Enough time should be allowed so that students will be accustomed to the new way of learning in web-based environment. Effective measures should be taken so that teachers and students can take advantage of web-based learning platforms and students' subjective status is ensured.

The problem of emotional deficiency can be solved or alleviated by improving students' cognitive ability through teachers' emotional help, promoting interaction between teachers and students and strengthening monitoring of students' autonomous learning. Thus students will have better performance in self-discipline, goal-setting, plan-making, and more importantly, creative thinking. Still, more studies need to be conducted to achieve successful autonomous online learning.

References

1. Arnold J (2000) Affect in language learning. Foreign language teaching and research press, Beijing
2. Chen D-Y (2009) Emotional concerns and training in college English network self-study. J AnHui Sci Technol Univ 23(5):46–50
3. Herczeg M (2004) Experience design for computer-based learning system: learning with engagement and emotions. http://www.eduweb.com/likelearn html
4. Krashen S (1982) Principles and practice in second language acquisition. Pergamon press, Oxford
5. LeDoux J (1996) The emotional brain. Simon and Schuster, New York
6. Liu Z (2010) Influence of learners' emotional factors on self-monitoring learning behavior under the Internet circumstances. J High Educ Sci Technol 29(4):134–138
7. Luo H-W, Wang Y-M, Zhu Z-T (2008) Research on emotional deficiency in the multimedia learning system of open English. Open Educ Res 14(3):74–78
8. Naisbitt J (1990) Megatrends 2000: ten new directions for the 1990s. William Morrow & Co, New York, pp 156–157
9. Sui X (2012) The study on anxiety problems with English learners under the Internet-based environment. Comput-Assist Foreign Lang Educ 143:78–80
10. Sun Y-D (2007) A study on the web-based English teaching model. J KaiFeng Univ 21(2):41–42
11. Zeng X-S, Liu Q-Y (2012) A study of English learning anxiety of science and engineering college students under multimedia environment. Comput Assist Foreign Lang Educ 147:50–55
12. Zhang H-X, Guo H (2012) A study on foreign language learning anxiety in computer and network environment and relevant countermeasures. J HeBei Univ Sci Technol (Soc Sci) 12(1):107–111

Chapter 269
Mapping Knowledge Domain Analysis of Medical Informatics Education

Danmin Qian, Yuanpeng Zhang, Jiancheng Dong and Li Wang

Abstract This research analyzes the mapping knowledge domain of the medical informatics education through the program CiteSpaceII. The data sample is downloaded from the SCI-E. The research takes the words that related to the field of the medical informatics education as the search terms, articles are searched from the Web of Science search engine. Through the visualization of the downloaded articles using CiteSpaceII, the research frontiers, countries (regions) in the area medical informatics research and education are found. At last, in order to improve the development of the medical informatics education, several suggestions are given.

Keywords Medical informatics education · CiteSpaceII · Mapping knowledge domain

269.1 Introduction

Medical Informatics is a new subject which across several disciplines including medicine, information and management science, etc. [1]. Nowadays, though bibliometrics and survey are popular in research field, the two methods can not give good performance of visualization. This research takes use of the CiteSpaceII, which is a Java program for co-citation analysis, especially for visualizing co-citation networks, to analysis the education of medical informatics ("EMI" in short).

D. Qian · Y. Zhang · J. Dong · L. Wang (✉)
Department of Medical Informatics, Nantong University, Qixiu Road #19, Nantong, 226001China
e-mail: wangli@ntu.edu.cn

269.2 Research Methods

269.2.1 Data Source

This research takes the SCI-EXPANDED as the data source. The number of 544 records are retrieved through the search strategy as follows:

- Topic = ("Medical Informat *") AND Topic = (educat * OR teach *).
- Time Span = 2003-01-01–2012-12-31.

269.2.2 Research Methods

In this research, the program CiteSpaceII is utilized to visualize the data in the articles. According to the different perspective, the Node Type is set as Keyword, Institution and Country. Other relevant parameters are set as following:

- Time Slicing = 2003–2012.
- # Years PerSlice = 1 year.
- Term Source = Title, Abstract, Author Keyword (DE), Keyword Plus (ID).
- Term Type = Noun Phrases.
- Mode of threshold setting = Threshold Interpolation (c, cc, ccv), and the threshold values are set or adjusted in the whole process of the visualization map generation.

269.3 Mapping Knowledge Domain Analysis

269.3.1 From the View of the Keywords Co-occurrence

Figure 269.1 is the visualization of the mapping knowledge from the view of the keywords co-occurrence, which is shown in the value of the centrality. Table 269.1 shows the statistical information from the view of the keywords co-occurrence. In this table, the frequency of these keywords is not less than 40 or the value of the burst is relatively large.

In addition to "medical informatics", "medical information" and "education", there are some other keywords are also attractive. For example, "internet", "information" and "communication", etc. These keywords indicate that EMI also involves in the following fields: Internet, information, communications and so on. The keywords "care", "patient education" and "health information", etc. show that EMI is not only for the professional students, but also for the students in other majors including medical care and public health. The keywords "attitudes" and "quality" have a higher burst value or frequency. This phenomenon indicate that

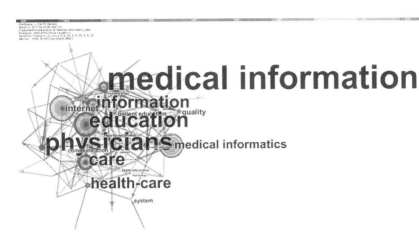

Fig. 269.1 Mapping knowledge domain of keywords co-occurrence in EMI

Table 269.1 Keywords with frequency >= 40 or larger burst value

Freq	Burst	Centrality	Keyword
120		0.15	Medical informatics
117		0.11	Internet
104		0.25	Education
63		0.21	Care
59		0.20	Information
53		0.39	Medical information
50		0.09	Quality
47		0.07	Patient education
46		0.03	Health information
37	2.54	0.07	Communication
24	3.14	0.04	Knowledge
14	2.93	0.00	Attitudes
13	2.76	0.00	Randomized controlled-trial

the doctors are improving their own medical information literacy gradually in the recent years, and they have begun to focus on the study of EMI quality, at the same time, they also propose their opinions in the field of the EMI development.

269.3.2 From the View of the Institution Cooperation and Country (Region) Distribution

The visualization of institution cooperation and country (region) distribution are shown in Figs. 269.2 and 269.3, the statistical information is shown in Table 269.2.

Fig. 269.2 Mapping knowledge domain of national (regional) distribuition in EMI

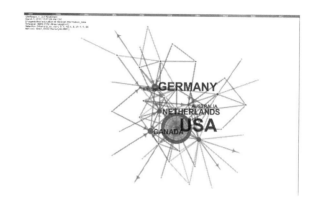

Fig. 269.3 Mapping knowledge domain of institutional cooperation in EMI

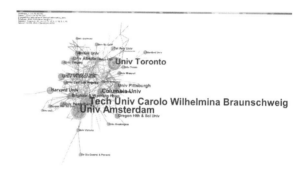

Table 269.2 Institutions with frequency in the top 7

Institution	Freq	Centrality	Sigma	Years
University of Amsterdam	15	0.08	1.00	2004
Technical University Carolo-Wilhelmina at Brunswick	15	0.00	1.00	2006
University of Toronto	13	0.01	1.00	2004
Columbia University	9	0.02	1.00	2003
University of Wisconsin Madison	7	0.00	1.00	2007
University of Pittsburgh	7	0.01	1.00	2004
Harvard University	7	0.04	1.00	2006

Following the information in Fig. 269.2, we find the leader of EMI is United States, German, Canada and other western developed countries, this maybe related to their research earlier in this field and their stronger information technologies.

Following the information in Fig. 269.3 and Table 269.2, we check the structure of the departments in these famous universities, and we find all of them have set up Medical Science Schools or Life Sciences Schools. The cooperation among famous university is close [2, 3], for example, Technical University Carolo-Wilhelmina at Brunswick cooperates with Stanford University, University of Toronto, and Zhejiang University, etc.

269.4 Summary

The presented research focuses on the visualization of the EMI Mapping knowledge domain analysis. Our work starts from two aspects, including the keywords co-occurrence, institutional cooperation and country (region) distribution. From the view of the keywords co-occurrence, we find the EMI research is active in the recent years, and the EMI research will pay more attention to the study of medical information risk and security technology. From the view of the institution cooperation and country (region) distribution, the most EMI research reports and paper published from famous universities and the affiliated hospitals, the attendance of the medical research centers and the health executive departments can supply more medical information, therefore, can promote the development of the EMI research.

Acknowledgments This work is supported by Jiangsu Province modern technology education project (No. 2013-R-24890), Nantong social undertakings technology innovation and demonstration program (No. HS2012045), Nantong University high education project(No. 03060224).

References

1. Xu YX, Ying J, Dong JC (2006) The development of medical informatics. Chinese Hosp Manage 26(3):30–32
2. Mantas J, Ammenwerth E, Demiris G et al (2010) Recommendations of the International Medical Informatics Association (IMIA) on education in biomedical and health informatics first revision. Methods Inf Med 49(2):105–120
3. Hasman A, Bergemann D, McCray A T et al (2006) Triangulation applied to Jan H. van bemmel Methods Inf Med 45(6):656–667

Chapter 270
Negation Detection in Chinese Electronic Medical Record Based on Rules and Word Co-occurrence

Yuanpeng Zhang, Kui Jiang, Jiancheng Dong, Danmin Qian, Huiqun Wu, Xinyun Geng and Li Wang

Abstract In order to extract negative terminologies in Chinese Electronic Record. Many methods have been developed. One popular and simple method is based on rules. However, the negative predictive value drops significant if the sentence contains several kinds of punctuation. In our research, a new method is used to solve the problem. The new method combines rules with word co-occurrence. In the experiments, 200 medical texts including 150,865 Chinese characters are used to test the new method. The negative predictive value is 99.85 %, which is 7.85 % higher than the rule-based method. That is to say, this method can tolerate various kinds of punctuations existing in the sentences. Therefore, the value of false-positive probability drops obviously.

Keywords Word co-occurrence · Mutual information · Negation detection

270.1 Introduction

Negation is common in Chinese Electronic Medical Record (EMR). The negation in Chinese is an important source of poor precision in automated indexing system.

International studies in this domain have developed for several years. But the study based on Chinese EMR is almost blank. Only one research paper is reported by Li Haomin et al. They design a negation detection algorithm based on the simplified syntax pattern matching in clinical documents. The positive predictive

---

Y. Zhang · K. Jiang · J. Dong · D. Qian · H. Wu · X. Geng · L. Wang (✉)
Department of medical informatics, Nantong University,
Qixiu Road #19, Nantong 226001, China
e-mail: wangli@ntu.edu.cn

value is 100 % and the negative predictive value is 98.99 % [1]. Although this algorithm can give good experimental results, but the false-positive problems caused by punctuation can not be solved. In our research, this difficult is overcome by using a new algorithm which combines rules with words co-occurrence.

270.2 Pretreatment

270.2.1 Negative Words in Chinese EMR

We collect 40 EMRs randomly from different departments in the hospital used as statistical samples. The number of negative words is 1312. The most 6 used words are as followings, "无", "未", "不", "否认", "阴性", and "排除".

270.2.2 Terminology Extraction

Classical Forward Maximum Matching (FMM) method can detect terminologies with high sensitivity [2]. However, there are too many overlapping ambiguities existing in EMRs. In order to overcome the ambiguous results caused by overlapping ambiguities, mutual information is introduced to modify the terminology extraction results. The mutual information of two random variables is a quantity that measures the mutual dependence of the two random variables in probability theory and information theory.

Definition 1
Formally, the mutual information of two discrete random variables X and Y can be defined as:

$$I(X,Y) = \log_2 \frac{P(X,Y)}{P(X)P(Y)} \tag{270.1}$$

$$\begin{cases} P(X,Y) = \dfrac{f(X,Y)}{N} \\ P(X) = \dfrac{f(X)}{N} \\ P(Y) = \dfrac{f(Y)}{N} \end{cases} \tag{270.2}$$

where P(X, Y) is the joint probability distribution function of X and Y, and P(X) and P(Y) are the marginal probability distribution functions of X and Y respectively.

Steps of extract terminology are explicitly described as follows.

Step 1: Split the EMRs into clauses using recursive algorithm. This procedure should follow two principles.
1. Clauses contain negative word.
2. Split the EMRs only using the punctuations including ".", ";" and "Enter".

Step 2: Extract terminologies by the FMM and mutual information algorithm using a dictionary that combines UMLS with ICD-10 (Chinese version).

Step 3: Tag the speech of terminologies using ICTCLAS [1].

270.3 The Rule-Based Negation Detection Algorithm

After the pretreatment in Sect. 270.2, terminologies have been extracted and tagged speech. Now, all the terminologies are to be detected negative or not by the rule-based method.

According to the 6 negative words in Sect. 270.2.1, 9 rules are established as shown in Table 270.1. All the rules must obey the following conditions:

1. Clause must contain negative words and terminologies.
2. The coverage area of the negative words can not exceed the clause.

The extracted examples using rule-based method are shown in Table 270.1. We can find most of the negative terminologies can be detected. However, the terminologies are missing when several kinds of punctuations existing in the clause.

Table 270.1 Rules and examples

Negative words	Rules	Examples	Detection
无	<[1]无+<术语>>	无乏力、纳差、尿黄等症状	yes
		无乏力,纳, 差尿黄等症状	no
	主语+无+<术语>	唇无紫绀, 牙龈无渗血	yes
	无 + *[2]+动词+<术语>	无明显诱因出现咳嗽、咳血	no
未	未+动词+<术语>	未闻及干、湿啰音	yes
	未+动词+*+动词+<术语>	2d后体温仍未下降并开始咳嗽	no
否认	否认+<术语>	否认高血压、冠心病、糖尿病等	yes
不	不伴+<术语>	不伴关节疼痛	yes
排除	排除+<术语>	排除SARS后以"老年性痴呆"住院	yes
阴性	<术语>+阴性	腹部移动性浊音阴性	yes

1 The contents in the "<>" are paratactic elements connected by conjunctive words or "、"
2 "*" represents any word but is not null

270.4 The Negation Detective Algorithm Based on Rules and Co-occurrence

It is normal that some certain clauses are used to describe the diagnosis and symptom of the same disease. We calculate the word co-occurrence times in the 40 EMRs used in the Sect. 270.2.

270.4.1 Co-occurrence

Definition 2

Word co-occurrence refers to two words appearing in the same context which ignore the position and the order of each other. Suppose T_i and T_j are two terms, $P(T_i, T_j)$ is the co-occurrence rate of T_i and T_j. The value of $P(T_i, T_j)$ is calculated through formula (270.3):

$$P(T_i, T_j) = \frac{||Segment(T_i, T_j)||}{l} \qquad (270.3)$$

where $||Segment(T_i, T_j)||$ refers to the number of clauses containing T_i and T_j. l refers to the total number of clauses [3].

270.4.2 Present New Algorithm

The new method takes use of word co-occurrence, the details of the algorithm are given as follows:

Suppose "$W_{negative}$ T_1 T_2 ... T_k ... T_n" is a serial of words in one clause.

"$W_{negative}$" refers to the negative word in the clause.

"$T_{1 \text{ to } n}$" refers to the terminologies in the clause and T_1 is the closest terminology to the negative word.

"n" refers to number of the total terminologies.

```
New Algorithm :
for(int j=2; j< =n; j++)
{
  if( P(T₁, Tⱼ)> threshold)
    Tⱼ is a negative terminology;
  else
  {
    Tⱼ is not a negative terminology;
    Tⱼ₊₁ ₜₒ ₙ is also not negative terminology;
    break;
  }
}
```

270.5 Experimental Results and Evaluation

Two hundred EMRs including 150,865 Chinese characters belonging to 4 departments (Infectious Disease, Endocrinology, Neurology and Cardiovascular) are used as the test samples.

The negative predictive value is used to evaluate the final experimental results, which is defined as following,

$$\text{Negative predictive value} = \frac{\text{the number of the detected negative terminologies}}{\text{the total number of negative terminologies}} \quad (270.4)$$

Table 270.2 gives the finial experiment results. The negative predictive value is 99.85 % by using the new algorithm, which is 7.85 % higher than the rule-based algorithm.

By using the word co-occurrence rate, the area of the negative word can cover the whole clause. Therefore, the new method can tolerate various kinds of punctuations existing in the sentence.

Table 270.2 Experimental results

Detect algorithm	Negative predictive value
Rule-based algorithm	92.00 %
The New algorithm	99.85 %

270.6 Conclusions

This research proposes a new algorithm combining rules with word co-occurrence. This new method takes use of the phenomenon that terminologies describing the same disease co-occur in the same clause with high probability, the area of the negative word can cover the whole clause. Therefore, all the terminologies can be detected.

Acknowledgments This work is supported by Nantong social undertakings technology innovation and demonstration program (No. HS2012045) and Natural Science Foundation of Nantong University (No. 11Z010) and Jiangsu Province modern technology education project (No. 2013-R-24890).

References

1. Haomin Li, Ying Li, Huilon Duan et al (2008) Term extraction and negation detection method in chinese clinical document. Chin J Biomed Eng 27:716–734
2. Yinghong Liang, Wenjing Zhang, Youcheng Zhang (2010) Term recognition based on integration of c-value and mutual information. Comput Appl Soft 27:108–110
3. Bullinaria JA, Levy JP (2012) Extracting semantic representations from word co-occurrence statistics: stop-lists, stemming, and SVD. Behav Res Methods 44:890–907

Chapter 271
Design and Implementation of Information Management System for Multimedia Classroom Based on B/S Structure

Xian Zhu, Yansong Ling and Yongle Yang

Abstract Informationalized management of multimedia classroom occupies extremely significant position in university teaching management. In this paper, we propose a system model aiming to implement concentrated classification management and decentralized processing of a vast number of data of multimedia classroom. The technical support solutions and requirements from two aspects (functional and non-functional) are discussed. In addition, a comprehensive system design structure is given. By adapting this system, working efficiency can be stimulated. Based on B/S structure, this system is oriented to different levels of users of each department in university which enables the teachers, students and educational administrators to obtain the data no matter when and where in diverse roles. The system dramatically enhances the capacity of information sharing and simplifies the work process of classroom searching and reservation in writing and being busy running about the Dean's Office, which has tremendous practical meaning.

Keywords B/S structure · Multimedia classroom · Information management · Classroom reservation

---

X. Zhu (✉)
School of Economics Trade and Management, Nanjing University of Nanjing University of Traditional Chinese Medicine, No.138, Xianlin Avenue, Nanjing 210023, China
e-mail: shellezhu@hotmail.com

Y. Ling
Centre of Educational Technology, Nanjing University, No. 22, Hankou Road, Nanjing 210093, China

Y. Yang
School of Computer Science, Nanjing University, No. 22, Hankou Road, Nanjing 210093, China

271.1 Introduction

As the significant role of computer network being realized by most education institutions, the application of network permeates into nearly every nook and corner inside or outside the campus in order to support innovation of higher education [1]. Nowadays, digitalization of teaching resources, informatization of teaching management and networking of teaching process have obtained major breakthrough.

Since multimedia classroom is applied in most universities which directly affects the healthy process of teaching and management, the importance of Information management of it cannot be ignored. At present, in most universities, if teachers intend to make classroom reservation or carry out teaching activities, they have to go to the Dean's Office to apply and wait for the notification after the office staffs' searching the classroom arrangement records in writing [2]. This pattern not only wastes time, but also has long-term problem of data decentralization, processing delay and high error rate etc.

This system intends to integrate the various data information of multimedia classroom, executes centralized management and maintenance which is in order to solve the long-stand problem of decentralized data, non-timely data processing, high error rate in classroom management process. This system is based on B/S (Brower/Server) three layer distributed application mode which benefits the application logic implementation, maintenance and update. In addition, with the capability of high speed information sharing and the convenience it brings from network, the system breaks up the limitation of former classroom management system [3].

In the following sections, we will discuss the whole system developing procedure, including requirement analysis, system structure design, database design and system implementation in practical work.

271.2 Requirement Analysis

271.2.1 Functional Requirement Analysis

The users of multimedia classroom information management system include students, teachers, educational administration and system maintenance personnel. According to the diversity of users on using this system in different purposes, the system should assign different permissions for users. Administrative privileges of the system are divided into four levels:

- Student level. Query multimedia classroom information, view the announcement and multimedia presentations.

- Teacher level. Register and login to manage personal information, query multimedia classroom information, view the announcement and multimedia presentations, and make appointment of classrooms.
- Educational administrator level. Publish announcement and multimedia specification, manage information of teacher users, deal with the appointment of the classrooms, and own ability to add, modify and delete multimedia classroom information.
- System administrator level. Maintain and update multimedia classroom information management system and guarantee the security of the system, as well as the security of the database. Have the authorization to enter any sub-module of the system, assign the permissions of administrators, teachers and students, and process information (e.g. query, modify, delete). Conduct code maintenance and data maintenance, provide the functions of code data query, enter, modify, delete etc. of administrator-level and public-level's information. Establish effective disaster avoidance plans and disaster recovery plans including data redundancy and remote storage.

271.2.2 Non-Functional Requirement Analysis

- Operating environment. Since student and teacher users are dispersed with non-uniform platforms, the system requires distributed application based on B/S model. The client only needs a Windows XP/2000/NT environment through a browser (e.g. Firefox, Chrome, IE) to complete all application requirements. It is conducive to implementation of application logic of the system as well as system maintenance and upgrade. In order to facilitate the educational administrator and system maintenance personnel to get adapt to this system, we use the Windows XP platform as Server, and Access 2007 as database.
- User interface. User interface should be friendly and precise, so that the structure and usage of the system are clear at a glance to users. Furthermore, the misuse of user should be prompted. Meanwhile, the interface of the system should be artistic, and the tone of each page should be uniform without gaudy. As the users uses this system as teaching assistance, the interface should be simple and generous, but without losing the aesthetics.
- System security. For Internet application, security is critical. In generally, in order to ensure the security of the users and data of this system, we should meet the following aspects [4]:
  - Network security. In all security issues, the network is most likely to lead to security problems. As network provides internal to external physical channel, technology experts or hackers can easily break through the network security settings, and trespass the system. Based on the general rule of thumb, in the following areas we consider to strengthen network security: Firstly, physical isolation. For example, use a gatekeeper. Secondly, multi-firewall. Implement different security policy to each firewall. Thirdly, rigorous network security

management institution can avoid the occurrence of conventional security issues.
- System security. It includes the operating system, web software, database software and other system-level software's security. In normal circumstances, the system security is influenced by two aspects: system management (e.g. default security configuration of Windows system, user account management strategies). Loopholes of the system itself. To establish appropriate security policies (including account strategy) and update system patches to fix the loopholes timely can avoid such security problems.
- User security. On the network, the user security mainly refers to the counterfeiting of the user's identity. This system uses the account password to ensure the security of users. The administrator can view the users' information to verify their identities are legal or not. It prevents unauthorized users from accessing the system and meanwhile, assigns user roles (e.g. the general user does not have system administrator's permission to publish bulletins).

271.3 System Structure Design

271.3.1 B/S Structure

When we develop a software system based on network, system computing model being applied should be considered first. Network computing model (also be called network model) refers to the method of processing computer information on networks [5]. Different network models with personal diversity offer different services which users should select the appropriate one based on the application they implement.

From mid-1990s, with the extensive application and popularization of Internet, people have obtained more convenient, fast and diverse information from the Internet without understanding the network internal implementation details [6]. B/S structure is generated in this context. In B/S structure, all applications of the system are integrated to the server, eliminating the development of individual client program. All applications on the server can be executed on the client through a Web browser.

In B/S structure, we only need to install a browser (e.g. Internet Explorer, Chrome), and a small support library (e.g. Java or VB dynamic link library). The middle layer on the client uses Web server to accept the client's request and convert it to SQL statement, then passes it to the database server via ODBC or other means. At last, the results returned from database server are transmitted to client in HTML file format. Therefore, the client is actually an interpreter to convert standard language into the interface. The application is installed on the Web server, and its operation is also carried out there.

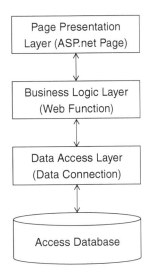

Fig. 271.1 System architecture

According to the needs of the actual multimedia classroom information management and design philosophy, the system uses a three-tier structure (Fig. 271.1). As shown in Fig. 271.1, the architecture includes page presentation layer, business logic layer and data access layer. The page presentation layer is on the client which is equivalent to the user interface (e.g. IE browser). This layer shows users a friendly, efficient data manipulation interface. Through the layer, the user can call a business method provided by the business logic layer to conduct operations such as classroom information query, classroom appointment, etc. The business logic layer as the core part of this system is mainly responsible for the business logic processing tasks [7], which plays the role of the bond. When the use layer requests the operation, the page presentation completes the operation of data through the corresponding method of business logic layer. As to data access layer, it is the initiator of the action which directly communicate with data access layer, finally show, submit, return the database' data to the page presentation layer. The data access layer is located in the lowest level, which is mainly used to interact with the database, complete the actions of query, insert, modify and delete of database' data. We can use a server to implement all the functions, or can divide the functions into the Web server and database server so that we can reduce the burden on the server and improve the efficiency of the implementation.

Multimedia classroom information management system mainly consists of foreground general module and background management module. Foreground user module includes three sub-modules: user management, classroom reservation and information browsing. Background management module includes five sub-modules: teacher information management, classroom information management, reservation information management, announcement information management and multimedia information management (Fig. 271.2).

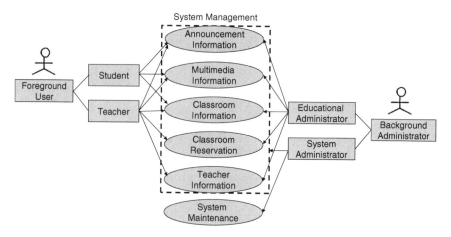

Fig. 271.2 System function structure (use case)

271.3.2 Foreground General Module

The main users of foreground general module are teachers and students. This module takes full account of flexibility and convenience of human–computer interaction and is able to meet the needs of different users. Meanwhile, teacher login function is designed to make their authority higher than the students (e.g. can make classroom reservation, manage personal details).

- User management module
  Functions: teacher users can register, login, manage personal information (after login), including personal information change (department, name, email address etc.), password change, etc.
- Classroom reservation module
  Function: teacher users can select, search the information of multimedia classroom, submit classrooms reservation application. When searching the classroom, two options are given as 'choose by the classroom' and 'choose by the multimedia'. According to the location of classroom teachers need, the multimedia equipments or the capacity of classroom they require, they select the ideal one and make an appointment. If no proper classroom is in their choice, prompt will be shown.
- Information browsing module
  Functions: all users can browse the timetable, announcement, multimedia information to check the timetable arrangement of this semester, read news, introduction and specification of multimedia.

271.3.3 Background Management Module

In order to provide convenience to educational administrators (even the staff without computer experience), the user interface of background management module needs to be clear and simple. The operation process of different data should be convenient, unified and similar. Initial system creates a default system administrator who is named 'admin'. It is added to the database manually by the system designers. After the educational administrator login the background management system, they can manage teacher users information, classroom information, reservation information, announcement information, multimedia information etc.

- Teacher management module
  Functions: educational administrator can do query, modify, and delete operations of registered teacher information, and is able to add new teacher users.
- Classroom management module
  Functions: educational administrator can do query, modify, and delete operations of classroom information (e.g. room number, location, capacity, multimedia equipment), and is able to add new classrooms.
- Reservation management module
  Functions: educational administrator can view all classroom reservation application information and approve the application or not.
- Announcement management module
  Functions: educational administrator can publish new bulletin, search, modify and delete the published announcement.
- Multimedia management module
  Functions: similar to announcement management module, educational administrator can add new multimedia introduction and search, modify and delete the outdated ones.

271.4 Database Design

Database is the core and basis of an information system. It organizes the large amount of data in the information system by a certain model, and provides the features of retrieve, storage and maintenance of data, making the system easily, accurately, timely obtain the required information. A good designed database will greatly reduce the redundant data and improve the effective utilization of the data [8]. Therefore, the database design is a crucial part of development and construction of this multimedia classroom information management system.

The basic principles of database design are under the guidance of the overall scheme of the system. Each library should serve for the management it supports [9]. When considering the design of this system, we follow the following principles:

- Naming convention. All the database name, table name, domain name follow a uniform naming rules. And necessary instructions are added to facilitate design, maintenance and query. In addition, taking into full consideration of the need of transplantation, with good scalability and scalability, the system application is adapt to different databases.
- Control field. When designing, we select the appropriate database design and management tools to facilitate the design and management. We adopt a unified naming convention. If design field already exists, it can be directly invoked; otherwise, it should be redesigned.
- We use integrated approach to organize data, to ensure the highest possible access efficiency. In design process, the use of the index can improve query speed.
- Concurrency control. We consider concurrency control to make data process effectively and timely. For instance, for a same database table, only one person at the same time has the authority to modify data while other people can query.
- We consider the consistency and integrity of the data, using constraints (Check) and rules (Rule) to enhance the association between the tables and reduce data redundancy.
- In order to prevent legitimate or unlawful users adding non-semantic data to the database, the database audit and restraint mechanisms are used to ensure data integrity, security, and reliability.

E-R (Entity-Relationship) model is a problem-oriented conceptual model. According to the function modules above, various entities are designed to meet the needs of users. The information entities in this system are administrator, teacher user, classroom, announcement, multimedia information entity. The E-R diagram which describes the main entity information is shown (Fig. 271.3):

271.5 System Development and Implementation

The system uses Dreamweaver 8.0 and Visual Studio 2008 as its development platform. Through the combination of Dreamweaver and Visual Studio, we can greatly improve working efficiency in the development, release of database and web, the integration of application server. Dreamweaver includes feature-rich ASP.NET integrated development environment which includes the complete coding, debugging, testing, and publishing capabilities. On the other hand, Visual Studio solves the difficulty in Dreamweaver that it is hard to precisely reach exactly the same visual effect on the browser display to make the system interface more precise and meticulous. Combined with Ajax, XML and other technologies, this system supports comprehensively for the progress of gain, storage, transmission and disposition etc. of multimedia classroom's information. Meanwhile, this system makes the information management of multimedia classroom standard and scientific, the information transmission fast and accurate.

271 Design and Implementation of Information Management System

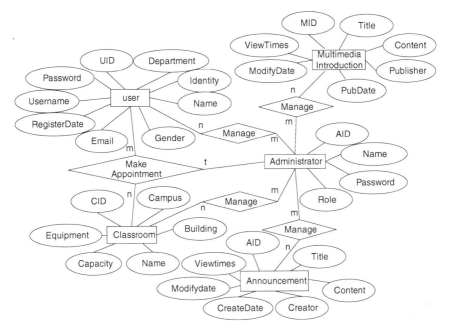

Fig. 271.3 Database E-R diagram

Web server uses IIS 6. IIS, one of the most popular web servers now, is the web server product of Microsoft which allows information distribution on the public intranet or Internet. IIS provides support for dynamic Web pages and Web applications, and provides a graphical interface management tool called the Internet Services Manager to monitor and control the configuration Internet service [10]. In addition, it also provides an Internet Database Connector to achieve query and update functions of the database.

The database server uses the Access 2007. The advantage of Access is that it can use the datasheet and custom forms to collect information. A datasheet is similar to an Excel spreadsheet to make the database clear. In addition, Access allows administrators to create custom report forms for print or export of database information. Moreover, Access provides a data repository. It means you can use the desktop database file to arrange database files on a network file server and share database with other network users. Access owns powerful capacity of desktop database and relational database in a packet, which is very convenient to implement in small size data exchange.

271.6 Conclusion

Currently, there are two methods of educational management system which are implemented in different universities. One is standalone version, which was developed in the 1980s and early 1990s. During this period, the computer hardware's price kept declining which provided a basic condition for its widely application all around the world. Meanwhile, universities purchased a vast number of computers to apply in educational management. However, information management of multimedia classroom have not obtain proper attention and the function of it is simple. Computers are only used to store and record data instead of paper documents record. This method owns a lot of drawbacks, such as poor ability of information exchanging and sharing, prone data losing and system crashes etc. Therefore, this method has left behind the trend and should finally be replaced.

The other method started from the mid-1990s, which is called network version. It takes full advantage of network to construct campus office system. This educational management system appears basically LAN-based. Supported by network technology, modern educational technology and information technology, the developing purpose is to structure a secure, reliable, speedy, open, interactive and sharing educational management environment. At present, as teaching assistance, multimedia is widely applied in a lot of educational institutions. Universities are facing a new situation when various electronic equipments are used in multimedia classroom (e.g. desktops, projectors, speakers). Multimedia classroom information management system is an important part of the educational management system in university. It complements with other systems (e.g. faculty management system, student information management system, archives management system, teaching management system, general logistics management system) to provide service for the university's informationalized management. However, at present, the development of classroom reservations system based on B/S structure is not perfect. In most universities, the teachers who need to apply classrooms have to run back and forth to the Dean's Office, which undoubtedly brings a wide range inconvenience and trouble in information management process.

From the above analysis, we fully understand the necessary to design and develop a multimedia classroom information management system. This design and development of multimedia classroom information management system have achieved the rules and demand of classroom information management of the universities. Meanwhile, it has achieved the operation requirement of convenience, utility, security and aesthetics when we generally consider constructing a software system.

The system uses modular programming method, which benefits both the combination and modification of the system functionality, and brings convenience to complement of the technical maintenance personnel who is not participate in the system development process. Multimedia classroom information management system integrates the information of the entire university's multimedia classrooms, provides comprehensive classroom information to educational management departments. With this system, teachers can apply classroom online efficiently and conveniently. Meanwhile, the information of multimedia classrooms is shared with teachers and students, so that they can browse the information to arrange their schedule. Lastly, as all the universities have similar multimedia classrooms, it also has tremendous promotion value and development potential.

Acknowledgments This project is partial supported by the plan of information educational management innovation of Nanjing University. And many thanks to the Centre of Educational Technology, Nanjing University to provide testing and piloting platform.

References

1. Visscher AJ (1996) Information technology in educational management as an emerging discipline. Int J Educ Res 25(4):291–296
2. Walker A, Townsend T (2010) In: International encyclopedia of education. Peterson P, Baker E, McGaw B (eds) 3rd edn, pp 681–687. Commonwealth Council on Educational Administration and Management, Hong Kong
3. Rytivaara A (2012) Collaborative classroom management in a co-taught primary school classroom. Int J Educ Res 53:182–191
4. Callahan DW, Pedigo RM (2003) Development of an information engineering and management program. IEEE Trans Educ 46(1):111–114
5. Cimino JJ, Socratous SA, Clayton PD (1995) Internet as clinical information system: application development using the world wide web. J Am Med Inform Assoc 2(5):273–284
6. Silver MS (2006) Browser-based application: popular but Flawed. Inf Syst e-Bus Manage 4(4):361–393
7. Stuart LH, Ulrich R, Mills AM (2011) Breaking the ice: organizational culture and the implementation of a student management system. J Cases Inf Technol 13(1):1–14
8. Dominguez C, Jaime A (2010) Database design learning: a project-based approach organized through a course management system. Comput Educ 55(3):1312–1320
9. Mullins CS (2010) Avoiding database design traps to ensure usability. Database Trends Appl 26(4), 37
10. Guo D, Xuan H, Fu X (2010) modern teaching support platform design. Tsinghua Sci Technol 15(3):352–356

Chapter 272
The Application of E-Learning in English Teaching of Non-English Major Postgraduate Education

Qu Daqing

Abstract Application of E-learning in English teaching of non-English major postgraduate education has been a commonly debated issue in English teaching field of higher education. As an advanced and comprehensive learning method, E-learning has demonstrated a great potential in promoting the overall English teaching level in various postgraduate programs, as well as enhancing students' capacity of academic reading, writing and translating. This paper cites the definition of E-learning, then illustrates characteristics of both E-learning and English teaching in higher education, finally point out steps of application of E-learning in Non-English major postgraduate programs.

Keywords E-learning · Non-english major postgraduate education · Bridging function between cultures · Innovativeness

272.1 Introduction

According to English-teaching Outline of Non-English Major Postgraduates promulgated in November 1992, English teachers are required to focus on students' ability of skillful reading, competence of writing and translating and basic listening and speaking skills so that they are capable of utilizing English as a tool for their future professional learning and research. Since introduced, the outline has greatly enhanced the development and standardization of Non-English major postgraduate English teaching steadily. But for recent years, especially with the rapid progress of social education, a national craze of English learning and an improved high school and undergraduate English teaching, the scholars nationwide

---

Q. Daqing (✉)
University of Science and Technology Liaoning, Liaoning, China
e-mail: markqu1969@163.com

realize that general goal of Non-English major postgraduate English education should be revised accordingly so that it can leapfrog from previous framework of teaching objectives to higher levels. But how? The author thinks E-learning, as an advanced method and platform of foreign language learning, can shoulder task in this IT era. Thus, an effective re-evaluation of relationship between the essential characteristics of Non-English major postgraduate education and E-learning will surely propel optimization of course syllabus and teaching reforms.

272.2 The Definition of E-Learning and Its Characteristics

E-Learning refers to learning and teaching activities through the Internet. In recent years, from theoretical to practical context, many scholars have conducted relevant research and analysis on problem of E-learning resources utilization which has been defined as crucial question. Studies on fields as resource pool and its management system, resources transmission technology in the network environment, and E-Learning strategies have turned out to be fruitful and established a solid understanding of its following different characteristics.

1. Multimedia revealed by integration of media modes
2. Digitalization;
3. Non-linearity and inter-activeness
4. Virtuality
5. Sharing, and fertile.

Compared with other network resources, E-Learning Learning resources have revealed its irreplaceable advantages, such as, strict national technical specifications in construction of learning resources; specified teaching objective, contents, learning activities and research tasks; manufactured by co-works of professional teachers and IT staff through teaching design and medium production and integration; relatively stable structure pattern of learning resources and contents (Fig. 272.1).

272.3 Characteristics of English Teaching in Non-English Major Postgraduate Programs

272.3.1 Bridging Function Between Cultures

As the carrier of cultures, the English course taught in Non-English major postgraduates programs should not only be a single portfolio made up of phonetics, grammar and vocabulary, but also a kind of materialized culture phenomenon with its own structure and self-contained specialness, which possesses a strong vitality

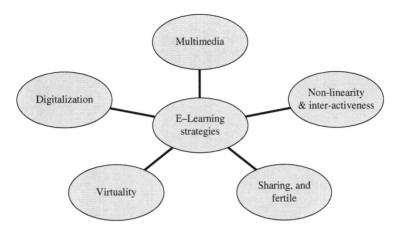

Fig. 272.1 Breakdown of E-learning's characteristics

and social function. The western cultural knowledge reflected by English should be divided into four categories:

1. Material culture, namely materialized knowledge forces consisting of various cultural objectifications;
2. Systematical culture, summation of established human social norms and practices;
3. Behavior culture, behavioral modes authorized through the long-term social practices and complicated inner-communications among people, in some cases, with a national and regional distinction.
4. Spiritual culture is summation of sublimed values in the field of ideology, namely the knowledge systems, aesthetic tastes and ways of logical thinking and so on. In a word, the basic spirit of western cultures is indispensable important content in postgraduate.

272.3.2 Innovativeness

Innovative spirit in English teaching of postgraduates programs should be embodied in the desire of seeking new knowledge and the re-evaluative attitude to the known contents. We should realize that continuous attempts of questioning can serve as motivation and sources of innovation. Innovation ability of postgraduate students in twenty-first century should encompass ability of creative and diverse thinking, agile judgment, and critical learning, as well as the practical ability to solve the problem, to communicate and cooperate with people, to organize affairs and to make decisions. Their innovative personality can be revealed by the psychological and ideological qualities necessary to achieve innovation, it includes self-confidence, optimism, carefulness, dedication,sense of responsibility and perseverance, etc. Non-English major postgraduate English education should not follow the traditional teaching routine of simple repetition, but maximize exertion of students' innovative abilities which are on the basis of comprehensive language activities as listening, speaking, reading, writing and translating, and assisted by their knowledge precipitation.

272.4 The Steps and Illustration of Application of E-Learning in Non-English Major Postgraduate Programs

As graduate students have mastered rich experience of autonomic learning of English, the traditional teaching mode is not conducive to create a good English learning atmosphere and improve the English application ability. E-learning strategy can provide a self-directed study mode which is helpful for their adaptation to the different types of learning materials and construction of the interaction between students' learning efforts and the guidance of teachers. To achieve this goal, following works are needed to be implemented in the process of English education management and monitoring.

272.4.1 Establishment of Supervision Mechanism Under the Network Environment

The time allocation of post-graduate students' English learning should be balanced well, online or in classroom. That is to say, students should spend not less than 16 h online study to digest comprehensive practices in classroom, and at the same time, broaden their mind by surfing other related links in E-learning system. It also can provides teachers with each student's school online records, as well as the records of the teachers' online tutoring. And rules can also be carried out to reward five bonus points any student who successfully complete the online "read and write" and "listen and speak" tasks till the end of academic semester. The two-way supervision mechanism ensures that students can utilize their learning time effectively by obtaining the teacher's feedback and guidance in time. The supervision mechanism is revolutionary when compared with traditional mode, it marked a new stage of the popularization education development, namely, an online popularized education of science and technology with a great respect to individual's personality.

272.4.2 The Information Extension Under the Network Environment

Computer and network set up a platform of fully extended information for English education of postgraduates. In the course of teaching, students should be encouraged to design a learning framework of background information, discussion topics, related knowledge in advance. During the classroom time, students are not only motivated to get access to a combination of large amounts of text, sound, audiovisual material, but also to fully participate in the activities of each topic. Such activities can not only greatly broaden the students' horizon and train of thought, also lower degree of understanding difficulty of written content. Take a difficult piece of passage for example, if students are only supposed to comprehend it literally, a long time is needed. But with a PPT teaching file attached to pictures and video, an open field unfolds before students at once. Teachers should also require students to participate in collecting and organizing information by making it compulsory assignment for every student of an average production of 10 PPTs within each school term. Such activities can not only improve students' English practical ability and enrich their knowledge of English language, and also enhance their language sense and self-confidence.

272.4.3 Illustration of Test Result (Year 2011–2012) of Non-English Major Students in Postgraduate School of USTL

After one-year's implementation of E-learning strategies in Postgraduate School of USTL (University of Science and Technology Liaoning), a striking result of scores leapfrog is viewed at a comparison of experimental classes authorized to a full access to efficient on campus. E-learning system and regular classes which were maintained to a unchanged teaching plan and after-class activities. Clearly, we can draw upon the fact like this: at the end of 1st semester of academic year 2011–2012, the average score of English test for Experimental classes is 11.8 higher than those from regular classes while the gap is widened to 18.2 at the end of 2nd semester. The reason can be attributed to a bettered learning environment, improved efficiency and a highly inspired enthusiasm in English learning (Fig. 272.2).

272.5 Summary

Researches show that the active method of E-learning of postgraduate English education is crucial in improving students' interest and ability of English language

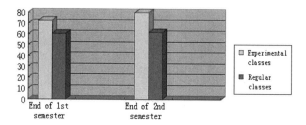

Fig. 272.2 Comparison of average English final test result of experimental classes and regular classes

application. Massive teaching information in network, great convenience of information transmission, efficient inter-activeness, those are all beneficial to develop collaborative teaching, thus train the students to put forth questions and solve them through online learning. At the same time, the network of E-learning platform is the most effective information retrieval tool, so teachers can cultivate students' remarkable ability of information acquisition, analysis, processing by carrying out the network teaching. Proper use of network and multimedia teaching materials actually increase the amount of information, also reduces the difficulty of understanding, so it is generally welcomed by the students and teachers nationwide. But in real practice, it can also be found that some problematic issues concerning E-learning need further exploration.

References

1. Field RF (2008) Identity community and power in bilingual education. In: Hornberger NH (ed) Encyclopedia of Language and education, 2nd edn. Shanghai, China
2. Kaplan RB, Balduf R (2008) An ecology perspective on language planning. In: Hornberger NH (ed) Encyclopedia of Language and education, 2nd edn. Shanghai, China
3. McDonough K, Trofimovich P (2011) Using priming methods in second language research. Beijing, China
4. Ricento T (2008) Researching historical perspectives on language, education and ideology. In: Hornberger NH (ed) Encyclopedia of Language and education, 2nd edn. Shanghai, China
5. Williams G (2008) Language Socialization: a systemic functional perspective. Hornberger, In

Chapter 273
The Construction of Semantic Network for Traditional Acupuncture Knowledge

Ling Zhu, Feng Yang, Shuo Yang, Jinghua Li, Lirong Jia, Tong Yu, Bo Gao and Yan Dong

Abstract Objective: Because traditional concepts of TCM have multiple meanings resulting in the ambiguity of understanding, which restricting the construction and expression of acupuncture knowledge systems. To facilitate the exchange of ancient and modern knowledge, we designed to build a semantic network of traditional acupuncture knowledge. Methods: We use the seven-step method to build traditional acupuncture ontology which could be represented in the form of semantic network. Conclusions: The knowledge system of traditional acupuncture could be re-organization and interpreted by semantic network built on the basis of conceptual terms. Acupuncture ontology is divided into eight categories, acupuncture and moxibustion, Body Constituents and Orifices of Sense Organ, treatment, diseases, meridians, blood and body fluids, acupoints, acupuncture appliances, included 939 terms and 16 semantic relations.

Keywords Traditional acupuncture knowledge · Semantic network

273.1 Introduction

Acupuncture is important part of traditional Chinese medicine, with relative independence, in the earliest extant Chinese classics "Neijing" already [1] basically completed the system of acupuncture theory. Knowledge systems of traditional acupuncture refer to ancient acupuncture books and other medical books (including the unearthed documents) involved in the aspects of acupuncture and moxibustion, which could be manifested by acupuncture terms. The traditional terms have semantic complexity, ambiguity, which restricted the construction and

L. Zhu · F. Yang (✉) · S. Yang · J. Li · L. Jia · T. Yu · B. Gao · Y. Dong
No.16 Dongzhimen Nei Nanxiaojie, Dongcheng, Beijing, China
e-mail: yangfengzhuling@163.com

expression of knowledge systems. Semantic loss is common in semantic networks in the past, resulting in error distortion in semantics network.

Semantic networks [2] is an information organization system, which is an important bridge between user information needs and information resources manifested knowledge. Formally, a semantic network is a directed graph with marks, which used to represent the concept. Arc with identification between nodes with mark used to represent the semantic relations.

The research object is traditional acupuncture knowledge system. Semantic networks f traditional acupuncture should be built by ontology, manifested by JUNG algorithm package, with textual research of the key terms of acupuncture and moxibustion, referred by Chinese medicine language system TCMLS, which could revealed hidden relation between the terms of acupuncture and improve search of the literature of acupuncture and TCMLS.

273.2 Methods

Seven-step method [3] is used to build an ontology of traditional acupuncture, show its semantic network, to lay the foundation for creating the ontology of the related fields.

273.2.1 Acquired Important Knowledge in the Field of Traditional Acupuncture

First of all, a list of all terms and explanations of terms could be filtered from the Medical Subject Headings, Acupuncture materials, dictionaries, standard literature. At this stage, a set of terms should be prepared, which is described by natural language.

273.2.2 To Determine Their Relationships Stages

The previous step has generated a lot of terms, but lack of organization according to certain rules, which requires groups to form a different class in the same class concept, its relevance should be relatively strong.

In addition, the importance of each term should be evaluated in order to pick out the key terms which can express knowledge in the field accurately and streamlined as possible and form a knowledge framework.

273.2.3 Formal Coding

We adopted open source software Protégé4.1 use the formal method to encode these terms in order to let the machine-understandable.

273.3 Results

273.3.1 Filter Out the Key Terms of Knowledge of Traditional Acupuncture

Nine hundred and thirty one terms have been filtered from dictionary and other acupuncture tools. Specific meridians and acupoints should be listed, which have a concise explanation which is not covered in the list of key terms, but considering the relative comprehensiveness of building a semantic network.

273.3.2 Relations between Classes

We created relations between classes referring TCMLS in order to express the relation between specific terms (Table 273.1).

273.3.3 Construction of the Ontology of Traditional Acupuncture Knowledge Systems

The key terms should be filtered out to construct a ontology of knowledge systems of traditional acupuncture with protégé4.1.

Table 273.1 Semantic relationship with "acupoints"

Terms	Semantic relationship	Related terms
Acupoints	Channel tropism	Channels
	Pass through	Channels
	Treatment	Diseases
	Treatment	Syndrome
	The effect of	Function
	Be included	Specific acupoint
	Locate	Physical orifices
	Adjacent to…	Certain acupoints or landmarks
	Prohibit the use of	Therapy

273.3.4 Graphical Display of the Knowledge System

Figure 273.1 is a tree structure display of meridian class. In order to comply with the traditional acupuncture knowledge which is originated from Neijing, Shoutaiyin zhizheng is used as normal term, meridian divergences of lung meridian as a synonym. Xiahexue such as Zusanli Shangjuxu Yanglingquan Weiyang Weizhong Zusanli, were under the specific points, which manifested the acupoints 'therapeutic effect' on corresponding organs. For example, Zusanli tropism Stomach Channel of Foot-Yangming channel, which could treat stomach diseases. This attribute links the expression of knowledge.

Figure 273.2 clearly show the web relationships between terms, which is manifested by JUNG algorithm package For example the original hole contains Taiyuan, Taiyuan normalized by lung meridian, lung meridian corresponding to large intestine meridian, lung meridian connected with the large intestine. Shangjuxu normalized by stomach meridian treat colorectal diseases, which is xiahexue of large intestine. Graphics show the association between the acupoints and meridians achieving a modern expression of the traditional knowledge network.

273.3.5 Comparative Study of Chinese Medicine Language System on Semantic Relations

Semantic network is an important part of Traditional Chinese Medicine language system (TCMLS), which have 126 [4] semantic types and 58 kinds of semantic relations. Semantic types of high-level divided into entities (entity) and events (event) "two categories" [5], and thus expands to form layers of the tree structure. Semantic relationships in addition to the "is a" relationship, others are non-hierarchical relationship, such as physically related, space related, time related functionally related, conceptually related. Expression of the relationship is relatively rich and detailed, but not precise enough in the class description. For example, the name of the source and naming time are two attributes, which did not reflect all properties of class. The concept of graphical only display N terms associated, but the relationship between the unfolded failed to show on the graphics clearly.

Protégé4.1 is mature software of ontology editing [6], more focused on the definition of the class attribute. Attributes of class could be definite freely, while the relations are applied mechanically from united medical language system, which is not applicable to TCM.

There are 16 relations in semantic network of traditional acupuncture knowledge, such as, Connected with, exterior and interior with, Use, have meaning of, Contain, Belong to, Meridian, Treatment, Phenomenon manifestation, prohibit, the use of, Through, Cause, start, ends.

Eleven relationship are common in two systems, such as connected with, exterior and interior with, located, contains, neridian, prohibit the use of,

273 The Construction of Semantic Network

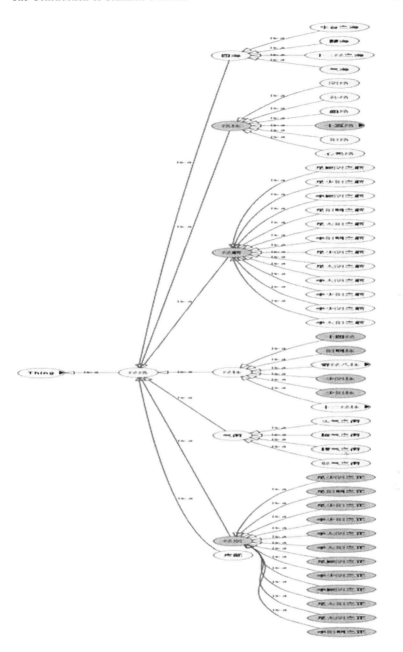

Fig. 273.1 Tree exhibited under the category of "meridians"

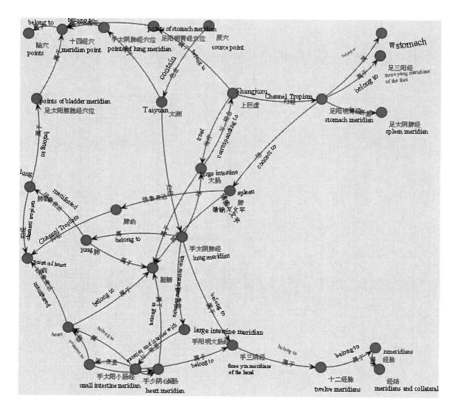

Fig. 273.2 Figure of semantic network

phenomenon manifestation, through, cause, use, treatment. Consistency with, start, ends, belong to, have meaning of, existed only in semantic network of traditional acupuncture knowledge.

The scope of semantic network of traditional acupuncture knowledge is limited, which can not cover all the semantic relations of the ancient language system. But also has its own characteristics. New semantic associations are built in the description of meridian circulation. "Consistency with" should be used to manifest the consistency between Organs and acupoints, such as the large intestine and Shangjuxu consistency, as well as pericardium meridian divergences consistency with such as triple energizer meridian divergences.

"Start" is used to describe the meridians circulation. "Belong" is primarily used to represent the relationship between meridians and organs, such as the lung meridian belong to lung.

"Have meaning of" primarily used to represent polysemy in order to avoid repeated emergence. Quepen belong to blood and body fluids, giant bone defects of Adam's apple, which is belong to the stomach meridian acupoints.

The relationship between the highest frequency is included (337), represented upper and lower relation which cannot be exhibited in left tree structure, such as the ban needle hole contains Shentin and Naohu. Second is meridian, start in, and ends, the first one manifested the attribution between the acupoints and meridians, the latter two manifested the attribution of space and position.

They can be conversed mutually and built on each other [7]. The language system could be the basis of ontology processing; meanwhile reverse conversion is also possible. Ontology can be transformed to the form which thesauri can be utilized.

273.4 Conclusion

The knowledge system of traditional acupuncture could be re-organization and interpreted by semantic network built on the basis of conceptual terms. Acupuncture ontology is divided into eight categories, acupuncture and moxibustion, Body Constituents and Orifices of Sense Organ, treatment, diseases, meridians, blood and body fluids, acupoints, acupuncture appliances, included 939 terms and 16 semantic relations.

In this study, we achieved re-organization and representation of knowledge of traditional acupuncture with the method of combining literature research and semantic network research, which making for managing and utilizing the knowledge and contributing to the acupuncture comprehensive search of the literature, database construction and optimizing Traditional Chinese Medicine language system. To a certain extent, ontology language could be expanded.

Acknowledgments This work is supported by "National Natural Science Fund of China (NO. 81202758)" and the Fundamental Research Funds for the Central public welfare research institutes (ZZ22070328).

References

1. Zhang S (2009) Study on acupuncture theories and concepts in Neijing. Nanjing University of Traditional Chinese Medicine
2. Lijie D (2007) Semantic web, semantic grid and semantic network. Comput Modernization 7:38–41
3. Lijing (2005) The ontology theory in the document retrieval system. Beijing Library Press, Beijing, p 111
4. Jia L, Zhu L, Dong Y et al (2012) Study and establishment of appraisal system for traditional Chinese medical language system. China Dig Med 7:13–16
5. Yin A, Zhang R (2003) Study of methodology about built traditional Chinese medicine language system. Chin J Info Tradit Chin Med 10(9):90–92
6. Ontology development for unified traditional Chinese medical language system. J Artif Intell Med 32(9):15–27
7. Jia J, Wei R (2009) Analysis on the methods of converting thesauri into ontology. Info Sci 27(9):1363–1365

Chapter 274
The New Training System for Laboratory Physician

Rong Wang, Xue Li, Yunde Liu, Yan Wu, Xin Qi, Weizhen Gao and Lihong Yang

Abstract Laboratory medicine is the bridge connecting laboratory and the clinic. Currently, laboratory technicians are expected to provide not only data to the physicians, but also diagnostic information based on the results. Hence, laboratory technicians have to change their role to laboratory physicians. In 2003, the Laboratory Physician Association was established by the Chinese Medical Doctor Association. With this background, the new curriculum system has been established in our university. The aim of the new training system is to educate students with an integration of clinical and laboratory knowledge, and to improve their ability and quality together. This system includes reorganizing course groups, increasing multimedia- and web-based courses, utilizing open book examinations and strengthening clinically practical skills. As a result, students are inspired with learning interests, and trained with the integration of quality and creativity. Professional skills of teachers are correspondingly improved. Therefore, we developed a high-integrated, innovative and rational educational system for laboratory medicine students. While, further exploration in several aspects are demanded to continuously improve our higher education system.

Keywords Laboratory medicine · Laboratory physician · Training system

---

R. Wang · X. Li · Y. Liu (✉) · X. Qi · W. Gao · L. Yang
School of Laboratory Science, Tianjin Medical University, Tianjin 300203, People's Republic of China
e-mail: yundeliu@126.com

Y. Wu
Department of Clinical Laboratory, Tianjin TEDA Hospital, Tianjin 300457, People's Republic of China

274.1 Introduction

Currently, laboratory technicians are expected to provide not only data to the physicians, but also diagnostic information based on the test results. Therefore, laboratory technicians have to change their role to laboratory physicians. Hence how to train highly educated laboratory physicians, who adapt to the latest discipline development, is a hot topic in laboratory medicine [1]. In 1998, Chinese Higher Educational Department of the Ministry of Education stated that the educational goals for a bachelor's degree in laboratory medicine should include the knowledge of basic, clinical and laboratory medicine. In 2003, the Laboratory Physician Association was established by the Chinese Medical Doctor Association. Since then the new curriculum system has been established in our department. The aim of the new training system is to educate students with an integration of clinical and laboratory knowledge, and to improve their ability and quality.

274.2 Materials and Methods

1 Personnel requirement of laboratory medicine covers a wide range of skills, The complicated divisions of the curricular systems should be carefully modified to avoid content repetition among different courses. Therefore, we implemented a novel theoretical teaching model which reorganized all the courses into four main groups. This four-group system reasonably and scientifically combined courses, thus reduced content repeating and improved internal connectivity among different courses. The four groups are:
(a) Medical humanities and basic knowledge group. Humanism is essential to medical students, so we enlarged and extended both social and basic science courses, such as history of laboratory medicine and weekly sciences.
(b) Professional basic course group. Rudimentary knowledge was constructed to broaden background knowledge and to improve self-learning ability in students. We are one of the first groups which established courses of molecular diagnosis and radioactive immunology in China, and compiled the corresponding text books, such as Radioimmunology and labelled technology. "Molecular diagnosis" is a bilingual course (in Chinese and English), consisting of modern conception and the latest progress in this field. The establishment of such courses have positive influence on decision making to build more innovative courses.
(c) Clinical medicine group. The key points of these courses are to increase the connectivity between physician and laboratory. We expanded the content of internal medicine, and added clinical transfusion and infection and antibiotics therapy.
(d) Technical skill and practical training group. One or two optional courses, for instance, Cell culture and Quality control system of Laboratory medicine were

established each year from the start of course reformation, such as laboratory management, medical instruments repair and maintenance, etc.

2. Traditional teaching methods purely depending on texts, classes and teachers should be altered. Our latest educational model focused on novel methods in the education. The new model included two main respects:

(a) Updating curriculum content. In order to encourage students to build up their own optimal approach in learning, curriculum contents were rebuilt and optimized in a more scientific and standard way. A course structure aiming at "Relax" education was constructed. The content of course was extended with the further conception, inter-discipline information and complex knowledge. In all, the content was innovated with breadth and depth. On the other hand, elementary medical knowledge was systematically divided, compressed and integrated. The entire content was divided into blocks and established groups of interrelated courses.

(b) Reform the traditional teaching methods. In order to extent the information content, a number of innovative teaching methods were applied. Multimedia technology and internet-based resources were helpful in contemporary education. We carefully and rationally selected material resources, in order to make complicated conception becoming concrete, vivid and intuitionistic. Additionally, implementation of open book exams resulted in more creative thinking and problem solving skills of the students. All above were favourable to construct an educational environment for quality education and innovation training, thus improved students' adaptability and creativity.

3. Strengthen clinical skills

Experiments were the foundation and soul of laboratory medicine. However, as the rapid advance of modern technology and science, the traditional experiments are not suitable for modern laboratory medicine education. "A laboratory physician" should give an authoritative interpretation of the results. Yet the prerequisite is that the laboratory physician has to know well the principles, procedures and influencing factors in all medical tests, because the laboratory results are influenced by physiology, pathology and clinical treatments, etc. [2]. The diverse training programs, plans and curriculums should consist of the development of medicine. Also the training should base on personal characteristics. The content reformation included: (1) Placing more emphasis on comprehensive experiments and design experiments, and decreasing demonstration experiments and verification experiments; (2) Implementing open experimental teaching, in which students could choose, design and complete the experiments themselves. (3) Encouraging students to participate in teachers' research programs.

4. Paying attention to clinical practice. The internship period is the first fundamental connecting step not only between elementary theory and clinical practice, but also between laboratory and clinical medicine [3]. Internship is the key stage for students to learn professional knowledge, skills and the ability to solve practice problems. Furthermore, it is important to bring up qualified talents of laboratory medicine. The students in school are just like semi-finished products

because they only know the theory. They have to go to clinical practice to become the ultimate masterpiece. According to the details about clinical practices, we take these measures. (1) Add an internship period in medical practice. (2) Choose an comprehensive academic hospital with high quality teachers for this practice. (3) Encourage the students to enter clinical practice as early as possible.

274.3 Results and Discussions

1. Achievements of the new training system.Through curricular reorganization, the curricular system became uniform, systematic and reasonable. The curricular system focused on clinical practice training. Meanwhile, the new system motivated students, thus students had the ability of creative thinking to run through the entire 5 years training.
2. Strengthening of quality education in laboratory students.That is to say: (1) Learning interest of students was inspired. The intellectual passion of students was motivated under the change from dependent-learning to self-study. (2) The new mode benefits student on integrated quality, creative ability and personality development. (3) The new mode was beneficial to teacher as well. The teachers could know the students' condition immediately by interaction between teaching and learning.
3. Clinical practice skills were intensified.(1) Under the innovative interactive educational environment, students became more active. They changed their mind from "have to learn" to "want to learn". (2) The new training system focused more on clinic, which guided the student to think more about patients and diseases instead of traditional book-based thinking mode. (3) Experiments were established in a cycler style. By this approach, students had more chances to practice their technical skills. Moreover, their practice skills were improved step by step. (4) During the training, we integrated theory into practice, which made students closer to the actual clinical job immediately after their graduation.
4. The contents of specialized text books were modified to fit our educational aims. This reformation made the content of course more systematic, rational, scientific and integrated. Subsequently, the reformation made the course not only suitable for class-study but also helpful for self-study. As to selecting text books, we firstly conformed to the guidance of the Ministry of Health. Secondly, we combined with self-compiled teaching materials and references. So, the teachers were encouraged to take part in compiling the relative text-books, from 2003 till now, our teachers have edited or participated in compiling 21 books on professional courses (led by Ministry of Health or Ministry of Education), including "clinical microbiology & examination", "introduction of

laboratory medicine experiments in clinical pathogens", "clinical biochemistry & examination", "medical immunology" and "introduction of laboratory tests in clinical hematology", etc. And Internet courses were setting up as well. Network courses of "clinical microbiology & Examination" were launched.

5. Active teaching and learning. The quality of our students largely improved. And we achieved the organization award and the highest award of single Science and Technology Competition. Meanwhile, we hosted the National Science and Technology Summer camp activities in 2007. Students took part in teacher's research program in their spare time. For example, our laboratory medicine students studied *Helminth* infection in Tianjin college students in 2006, and explored the infection of *Clonorchis sinensis* in the fresh water fish in eight main rivers in Tianjin. Each student finished a research report after investigation. Their articles on infection of *helminth and clonorchis sinensis* were published in Chinese Journal of Health Laboratory Technology and Chinese Journal of Epidemiology, respectively.

274.4 Conclusions

By these new measures, students were inspired with great learning interests, and trained with integrated quality and creative ability. Meanwhile, the professional skills of teachers were correspondingly improved. In practice, laboratory physicians not only provides test results to the clinicians, but also offers consultation, thus actively participates in the clinical procedures, including diagnosis, monitoring and observing prognosis of a disease. Therefore, laboratory physician training is the crucial task for laboratory medical education.

Acknowledgements This program is supported by projects of Ministry of Education of the People's Republic of China ([2005] 21), Tianjin Municipal Education Commission (B02-1002 K) and Tianjin Education Sciences Twelfth Five-Year Plan (HEYP6007).

References

1. Fan Y (2005) To cultivate laboratory physicians who can fit the development of laboratory medicine agent task of Clinical Laboratory physician education. J Diagn Concept Prac 4 (6):35–436
2. Tian Y, Liu C, Zhang X et al (2008) Some relevant issues concerning cultivation of boratory physician in professional course teaching China High Med Educ 2:76–77
3. Yaolei (2006) From laboratory physicians's localization to discuss the clinical practice teaching of undergraduate student. Res Med Educ 5(5):429–430
4. Liu L (2009) Study on the training system of laboratory physician. Guide of China Med 7(13):154–155

Chapter 275
The Investigation on Effect of Tele-Care Combined Dietary Reminds in Overweight Cases

Y.-P. Chen, C.-K. Liu, C.-H. Chen, T.-F. Huang, S.-T. Tu and M. -C. Hsieh

Abstract We evaluated the effect of tele-care combined with dietary education on overweight and obese subjects. Cases with body mass index (BMI) greater than 24 kg/m^2 were enrolled in our 8-week tele-care program, which consisted of clinic visits with physician and dietician upon enrollment and at the end of the study, and dietary education delivered via video conferencing. Real-time interaction between subjects and care providers was made possible through tele-communication and transmission of measurement data. Statistical analysis was performed using one-way variation test. After 8 weeks of participation in the tele-care program, the subjects achieved significant reductions in body weight, waist circumference, and BMI of 6.45 kg, 4.21 cm, and 2.35 kg/m^2 ($p < 0.05$), respectively. Serum cholesterol, triglyceride, systolic blood pressure, and diastolic blood pressure also significantly decreased by 22 mg/dl, 33 mg/dl, 8.52 mmHg, and 13.25 mmHg, respectively ($p < 0.05$). At the end of the study, all subjects became more knowledgeable on the proper selection of food with low fat, adequate fiber and low sugar content. Therefore, by promoting healthy behavior and increasing health knowledge, tele-health management is effective for weight reduction as well as control of blood pressure and lipids in overweight and obese subjects.

Keywords Tele-care · Overweight

Y.-P. Chen (✉) · C.-K. Liu · C.-H. Chen · T.-F. Huang
Long-Distance Health Management Center, Changhua Christian Hospital, Changhua, Taiwan R.O.C
e-mail: 155035@cch.org.tw

S.-T. Tu · M.-C. Hsieh
Division of Endocrinology and Metabolism Department of Internal Medicine, Changhua Christian Hospital, Changhua, Taiwan R.O.C

275.1 Introduction

In recent years, innovations in telecommunication have increased the convenience of healthcare delivery through tele-health services. Transmission of physiologic data and delivery of health education can all be accomplished using electronic medical monitoring equipment and telecommunication devices. Some studies have also indicated the effectiveness of community health service stations which employ video conferencing and Internet technology, combined with multi-disciplinary healthcare teams, in the prevention and treatment of chronic conditions such as diabetes and hypertension [1, 2].

Obesity is another important health problem with increasing prevalence around the world. According to Taiwan's "2005–2008 National Nutrition and Health Survey" [3], 44.1 % of Taiwanese adults were overweight or obese. In particular, the percentage had increased from 33.4 to 50.8 % in men and from 31.7 to 36 % in women since 1993–1996. Moreover, one out of every four children was overweight or obese. Obesity is directly associated with mortality and many chronic diseases, such as heart disease, diabetes, hypertension, stroke, gallbladder disease, sleep apnea, cancer, and arthritis. Since 1997, the World Health Organization has classified obesity as chronic disease [4–7].

In this study, we investigated the effectiveness of a tele-care weight reduction program that combined clinic visits with dietary education through video conferencing and communication of health advices through electronic messaging and telephone calls.

275.2 Method

275.2.1 Subject

This study was conducted in Changhua Christian Hospital Diabetes Health e Institute, Taiwan in collaboration with General Mills Co., Ltd., Taiwan. Subjects were volunteers aged 20–65 years with body mass index (BMI) greater than or equal to 24 kg/m^2. Female subjects must be non-pregnant and non-lactating. Informed consent was obtained from each participant.

Anthropometric measurements and blood biochemistry were obtained from each subject at the beginning and at the end of the study. Subjects must be able to comply with tele-care service requirements such as [1] physiologic measurement data transmission, [2] video conferencing, and [3] on-line dietary education. Measurement data transmitted by the subjects were received by the case managers in the hospital, who may then give immediate response or advice back to the subjects.

275.2.2 Intervention

Every participated were checked the pre-and-post intervention measurements: Height, weight, blood pressure, body fat, blood glucose, lipids, uric acid, and finished questionnaire including quality of life, eating out choose of investigation, mood questionnaire.

Measurements taken from each participant pre- and post-intervention included: height, weight, blood pressure, body fat, blood glucose, blood lipids, and uric acid. Questionnaire survey regarding quality of life, dietary habit, and mood was conducted on each participant. Subjects participated in three 30-minutes video conferences, which provided dietary and exercise instructions, during the 2nd, 4th and 6th week of the program, respectively. Dietary instructions included: (1) eat balanced diet of 1,200–1,300 kcal/day, (2) take two exchange portions of carbohydrate, one portion of protein, and one portion of fruit for breakfast, (3) take two exchange portions of protein, one portion of carbohydrate, and three portions of vegetables for dinner, and (4) drink at least 2,000 ml of water daily. At our health management website, an account was provided for each participant, who may log into record their daily food consumption and weekly body weight and blood pressure measurements.

275.2.3 Statistical Analysis

SPSS.12 program pair-T test was used to detect the differences in biochemical data before and after intervention. Statistical significance was defined as p value of <0.05.

275.3 Result

A total of 12 subjects were enrolled in the program. At the end of the study, all subjects achieved significant reduction in body weight. Mean decrease in weight was 6.45 kg ($p < 0.05$), with total reduction of 77.4 kg among all 12 subjects. On the average, serum total cholesterol level decreased by 22 mg/dl ($p < 0.05$), serum triglyceride decreased by 33 mg/dl ($p < 0.05$), systolic blood pressure decreased by 8.52 mmHg ($p < 0.05$), and diastolic blood pressure decreased by 13.25 mmHg ($p < 0.05$). Waist circumference decreased by 4.21 cm ($p < 0.05$) and BMI decreased by 2.35 kg/m^2 ($p < 0.05$) (Table 275.1). Subjects reported improved quality of life and physical fitness while changes in caloric intake had no negative effect on emotion and mood (data not shown). Proper eating behavior increased from 20 to 91 %, with subjects choosing diet well-balanced for the six food groups that met the daily recommended amount of vegetables and fruits.

Healthy food choices when eating out increased from 22 to 91 %, with reduced consumption of fried food, processed food, and sugar-containing beverages (data not shown).

275.4 Discussion

In this study, we provided dietary education and intervention through our tele-care program at Changhua Christian Hospital Diabetes Health e Institute, which included assessment by physicians, online dietary education by dieticians, and follow up by case managers. After this 8-week program, the 12 cases lost a total of 77.4 kg and their total cholesterol level decreased by 10.4 %, triglyceride by 23.7 %, systolic blood pressure by 6.77 %, and diastolic pressure by 14.79 %. Their waist circumference and BMI likewise decreased significantly.

Diet has been a long-standing issue in the treatment of obesity. There have been various diet recommendation, such as the low-carbohydrate diet (Atkins diet) [8], high-fiber, low fat diet (Ornish diet) [8], low glycemic index diet [9], and high-fiber, high calcium diet (Mediterranean diet) [10]. Nonetheless, to achieve weight loss, caloric intake must be negatively balanced against caloric consumption. In this study, we suggested a caloric intake of 1,200–1,300 kcal/day for each subject. We also recommended physical activity of at least 150 min/week in order to prevent loss of muscle mass and to increase basal metabolic rate.

There have been many studies on tele-care based weight reduction programs. Sherwood et al. have shown that participants lose significantly more weight if they received more intensive follow up through more frequent telephone calls within 6 months [11]. Luley et al. divided 70 obese type 2 diabetic patients into two groups: one group had supervision on caloric intake through tele-care and the other group received usual care. They found the intervention group had significantly greater reduction in body weight (by 11.8 kg) and hemoglobin A1C (by 1.6 %) [12].

A study on obese Asian population has shown that weight reduction of 5–10 % was associated with a decrease in mortality of 20 %. If BMI exceeds 25 kg/m^2, the relative risk of death increases by 9 % [13]. In our study, overall weight reduction was 7.6 % and BMI decreased by 2.35 kg/m2. An Oxford University study found that a reduction of systolic blood pressure by 2 mmHg was associated with a decrease in heart disease mortality by 7 % and a decrease in stroke mortality by 10 %. In our study, the systolic blood pressure was reduced by 8.25 mmHg. We therefore expect our program to effectively reduce mortality and cardiovascular disease risk in addition to achieving weight reduction.

One of the limitations of this study was its short duration of only 2 months. Some studies have shown that 6 months is required to achieve the most significant reduction in body weight. However, weight was regained in up to 80 % after 1 year [14, 15]. Another limitation was the small sample size of only 12 subjects. If this care model is established, we hope to expand our program to include

Table 275.1 Results after 8 weeks of tele-healthcare service

	Initial 0 week	End 8 week	△8–0 week	P value
Body weight (kg)	85	78.5	-77.4	<0.05
Waist (cm)	94.6	90.4	-4.21	<0.05
Cholesterol (mg/dl)	209	187	-22	<0.05
TG (mg/dl)	137	104	-33	<0.05
Systolic pressure (mmHg)	125.83	117.58	-8.52	<0.05
Diastolic pressure (mmHg)	89.58	76.33	-13.25	<0.05
BMI (kg/m2)	31.87	29.52	-2.35	<0.05

subjects from work places or schools. Finally, our participants may be more motivated than individuals who lack encouragement and competition from peers.

In conclusion, we demonstrated that tele-care program incorporating dietary reminders is effective for reduction of body weight, cholesterol and triglyceride levels, blood pressure, and waist circumference. In addition, it increases health knowledge and may effectively reduce risk of cardiovascular diseases.

References

1. Davis RM et al (2010) Telehealth improves diabetes self-management in an underserved community: diabetes telecare. Diabetes Care 33(8):1712–1717
2. Verberk WJ, Kessels AG, Thien T (2011) Telecare is a valuable tool for hypertension management, a systematic review and meta-analysis. Blood Press Monit 16(3):149–155
3. Chuang SY, Lee SC, Hsieh YT, Pan WH (2011) Trends in hyperuricema and gout prevalence: nutrition and health survey in Taiwan from 1993–1996 to 2005–2008. Asia Pac J Clin Nutr 20(2):301–308
4. Chang CP, Lee TT, Mills ME (2013) Abdominal obesity and chronic stress interact to predict blunted cardiovascular reactivity.Ann Epidemiol 31(1):29–35
5. Maskarinec G, Grandinetti A, Matsuura G et al (2009) Diabetes prevalence and body mass index differ by ethnicity: the multiethnic cohort. Ethn Dis 19(1):49–55
6. Okosun IS, Liao Y, Rotimi CN et al (2000) Abdominal adiposity and clustering of multiple metabolic syndrome in White, Black and Hispanic americans. 10(5):263–70
7. Prevalence of metabolic syndrome among adults 20 years of age and over, by sex, age, race and ethnicity, and body mass index: United States, 2003–2006. Natl Health Stat Report. 2009 May 5(13):1–7
8. Dansinger ML, Gleason JA, Griffith JL, Selker HP, Schaefer EJ (2005) Comparison of the Atkins, Ornish, Weight Watchers, and Zone diets for weight loss and heart disease risk reduction: a randomized trial. JAMA 293(1):43–53
9. Spieth LE, Harnish JD, Lenders CM (2000) A low glycemic index diet in the treatment of pediatric obesity. Arch Pediatr Adolesc Med 154:947–951
10. Pérez-Guisado J et al (2008) Spanish Ketogenic Mediterranean diet: a healthy cardiovascular diet for weight loss. Nutr J 7:30
11. Sherwood NE et al (2010) The drop it at last study: six-month results of a phone-based weight loss trial. Am J Health 24(6):378–83. doi: 10.4278/ajhp.080826-QUAN-161

12. Luley C, Blaik A, Reschke K et al (2011) Weight loss in obese patients with type 2 diabetes: effects of telemonitoring plus a diet combination-the active body control (ABC)Program. Diab Res Clin Pract 91(3):286–92
13. Pronk NP, Crain AL, Vanwormer JJ et al (2011) Are Asians at greater mortality risks for being overweight than Caucasians? Redefining obesity for Asians. Int J Telemed Appl 2011:909248. doi: 10.1155/2011/909248. Epub 15 Jun 2011
14. Stunkard AJ, McLaren-Hume M (1959) The results of treatment for obesity. Arch Int Med 103:79–85
15. Kassirer J, Angell M (1998) Losing weight—an ill-fated new year's resolution. N Engl J Med 338:52–54

Chapter 276
A Training System for Operating Medical Equipment

Ren Kanehira, Hirohisa Narita, Kazinori Kawaguchi, Hideo Hori and Hideo Fujimoto

Abstract There are continuously increased new possibilities for the application of computer-added learning-education systems as the result of highly developed information communication technology (ICT). In this study, a computer-added training system was proposed for the education of clinical engineers. As the first step, problems in operating medical equipment are made clear, and research subjects are focused accordingly with their solutions clarified.

Keywords Information communication technology · Support for education · Skill science · Computer training system · Medical equipment

276.1 Introduction

There have been recently increased demands towards the use of more and more medical machines in hospitals, needing clinical engineers (CE) as specialists, covering a wide range of works including operation, management, maintenance and repairing. However, it is very difficult to train students to become a CE mastering so many techniques within limited period of time. As the results, the CEs quite often feel the lack of knowledge and skill when working in a hospital. As a solution, it is largely expected to use the ICT in a computer-added education system for clinical engineers.

On the other hand, it has been attracting much attention to use computer technology in e-learning system. Similarly, it has been considered to support the clinical medicine with high technologies in the information and engineering fields,

R. Kanehira (✉) · H. Narita · K. Kawaguchi · H. Hori · H. Fujimoto
FUJITA Health University, 1-98 Dengakugakubo,
Kutsukake-cho, Toyoake 470-1192, Japan
e-mail: kanehira@fujita-hu.ac.jp

though, there is still not any total education system in clinical medicine using operating information as well as the visual one.

In this study, aiming the goal of a computer-added training system which is with low cost, simulated experiences, and good repeatability, we proposed a training system for clinical engineer using the up-to-now technologies in our sequential researches on computer-added skill-training system. The study was done for the undergraduate medical education in university, in order to construct a computer-added training system for the education of clinical engineers.

276.2 Education and Training for Clinical Engineers

276.2.1 Clinical Engineer

With the introduction of clinical engineering as a new field of science and technology, medical technologies have got dramatic progress. Technologies of the clinical engineering have been widely applied to wherever concerning the human life and health. In Japan, the qualification of Clinical Engineer was nationally institutionalized in 1988.

The "Clinical Engineer" is such a person who works in operating and maintenance medical machines and systems for the life of patient under guidance of doctor. He is a technician mastering and applying knowledge in electronics and mechanics, and an engineer for the improvement of clinical engineering science and technology.

There is a closer relationship in the modern society between medical and engineering, as the result of increased demands for high-tech medical machines being more and more applied in therapy. At the same time, any mistake or misuse

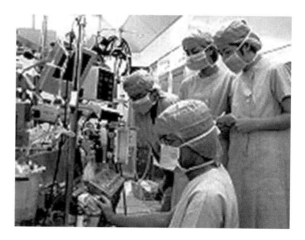

Fig. 276.1 Operation of CE on medical systems

of such medical machines would be closely related to the human life. The responsibility of the clinical engineer is ever higher, and his job contents change with the times. Figure 276.1 shows an example of clinical engineers at work.

276.2.2 Problems from Investigation

There arise several problems in the state-of-the-art of clinical engineering education. For example, CE is shallow history compared with co-medical of Radiological technologist, Medical laboratory technician. Institutions capable of educating CE includes 1 year graduate course to 4 year University, resulting in large variability in their techniques. It is of course equally important to be further trained in hospital after graduation.

It is necessary to master at the same time knowledge from medical and engineering. It is always a pressure to have to fulfill large sum of knowledge and techniques and to pass the national qualification test before graduation within a short period of time. Therefore, it becomes much more important to build up a computer-added training system for CE to match the increased need, and the importance is increasing with time.

However, it is very difficult to train students to become a CE mastering so many techniques within limited period of time. As the results, the CEs quite often feel the lack of knowledge and skill when working in a hospital.

We did a questionnaire last year on the 4th grade students in our university by a question "did you forget the operation sequence of heart–lung machines after you have become the 4th grade student (before hospital practice). Surprisingly, all 31 students regardless of gender answered with "yes, I forgot"! The reasons may be multiple, but "no chance to touch and operate the system" becomes the dominant (Fig. 276.2).

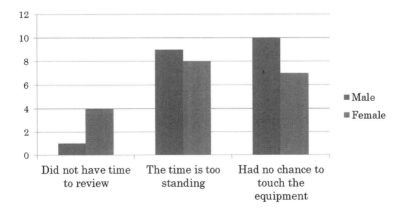

Fig. 276.2 Questionnaire result (1)

We take such problem as the research subject for the development of multi-media text, towards a computer-added CE training system focusing on the skill-up practice using computer simulation.

276.3 Subjects and Proposal in Education System

276.3.1 Focusing the Skill-Up Training in Education

Another questionnaire was pout upon the 4th grade students by a question "do you want to use a computer simulation system capable of simulated experience in preparation and review of your text. The answers divided into different training items are shown in Fig. 276.3, in which 90 % of students answered "yes".

Textbooks cannot answer all questions from students because of the complexity and variety in different operations, different systems and even different hospitals. Recently due to some medical accidents reported, safety education has been taken into considerable account in CE education. In this study for first of all, accidents from system troubles or operation mistakes most popularly related to CEs are confirmed, with related education and training methods provides (Table 276.1).

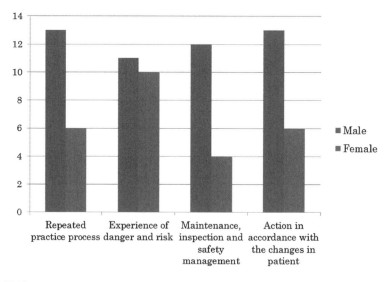

Fig. 276.3 Questionnaire result (2)

Table 276.1 Hope of experience in the computer simulation

Contents	Male	Female
Operation sequence and repeated practice	13	6
Danger or risk experience	11	10
Maintenance, inspection and safety management	12	4
Remedy in response to changes from patient	13	6

276.3.2 Integrated Education with Visual and Operative Operations

CEs are mainly appointed works of managing and operating medical systems, which requiring techniques from repeated practices. Furthermore, such techniques can be mastered not only from textbooks, but by operation exercises using multifunctional system with convenient database and e-learning capabilities.

The computer-added training system proposed in this study applies repeatable exercises and real-time true-or-false judgments characteristic of a computer-added system. The training was carried out using knowledge from textbooks and experience from simulated operations, towards a useful education for skilled CEs.

It is important to provide correct operation for true-or-false judgment for the students. First of all, operations from very skilled CEs are measured, recorded and quantified as standards. The construction of the system is shown in Fig. 276.4.

276.3.3 Problems to be Solved

In learning operation of medical machines, it is considered difficult to master skills from textbook and some operations within a short period of time because the medical machines differ from each other in makers and production time. To solve this problem, comments from experienced CEs are taken into consideration to

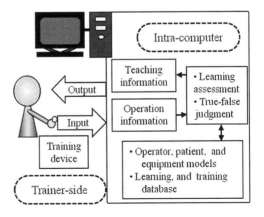

Fig. 276.4 The construction of the system

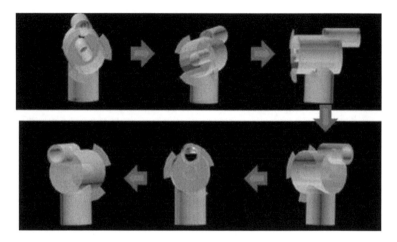

Fig. 276.5 Understanding of installation by rotating the 3D model

make the complex operations into a database which can be indexed and linked to the network.

3D model of the medical machine was constructed in the system, which presents easy-for-understanding information on the structure, position and installation sequence of the machine. Furthermore, software was developed for a real-time presentation of and operation on the inner parts, which is usually invisible and unoperational for a real machine, using such technologies such as computer graphic (CG), see-through modeling, and animating. As an example, a 3D model of parts of the Mechanical ventilator was constructed for its individual parts for training installation and understanding the operation mechanism of the machine. Figure 276.5 demonstrates the representation of inner parts of the machine from universal directions by rotating the 3D model.

276.4 Summary

This study presents as the first step problems in the training of medical machine operation for CEs, with focused research subject and detailed proposal for solution.

References

1. Watanabe K, Kashihara A (2010) A view of learning support research issues based on ICT genealogy. Jan J Educ Technol 34(3):143–152
2. Education IT solutions EXPO. E-learning Japan (2013). http://www.edix-expo.jp/el/
3. Sueda T (2010) Development of a training simulator for extracorporeal circulation with a heart-lung machine. Hiroshima University. http://hutdb.hiroshima-u.ac.jp/seeds/view/3/en

4. Kanehira R et al (2008) Development of an acupuncture training system using virtual reality technology. In: Proceedings of 5th FSKD, IEEE press, pp 665–668
5. Chen LY et al (2007) Basic experiment for analysis of acupuncture technique. In: Proceedings of 6th EUROSIM, pp 1–6
6. Kanehira R et al (2010) Insertion force of acupuncture for a computer training system. Lect Note Comput Sci (LNCS) 6320:64–70
7. Kanehira R, Yang WP, Narita H, Fujimoto H (2011) Acupuncture education system with technique-oriented training. In: Proceedings of FSKD'11, IEEE, pp 2524–2528
8. Kanehira R et al (2012) Education and training environments for skill mastery. In: Multimedia and signal processing. Springer, pp 451–458

Chapter 277
The Essential of Hierarchy of E-Continuing Medical Education in China

Tienan Feng, Xiwen Sun, Hengjing Wu and Chenghua Jiang

Abstract The level gap among different hospitals which exists in China is leading to a situation that doctors in different level hospital share uneven continuing medical education (CME) environment cause the diagnosis divide of doctors. The number of patients seen and guidance from experts had a strong correlation with improvement of the doctors' clinical ability. The implementation of CME needs to consider the two factors. After a primary survey, this study made a systematic and detailed analysis about the current CME situation in different level hospitals. Hospitals are classified into 3 levels. CME patterns via information technique corresponding to different levels were proposed. With this hierarchy continuing medical education, it's hoped that the diagnosis level of doctors in different level hospital should be similar so that each individual can acquire high quality medical service.

Keywords Hierarchy e-continuing medical education · Case quantity of personal experience · Guidance from expert nearby · High quality medical service · Information technique

277.1 Introduction

Though great advance in economics has been made, the inequality of Chinese public medical service is still a national issue. In current, eastern and some central developed regions occupy more resource than other regions, such as fund, experts [1]. Eighty three percentage of 3A hospitals which are the proxies of the top medical level in China are located in key city spread over eastern coastal and some central regions [2]. From the enthusiasm and momentum for a healthy living, most

---

T. Feng · X. Sun · H. Wu · C. Jiang (✉)
Collage of Medicine, Tongji University, Shanghai 200092, China

of patients prefer to see a doctor in 3A hospitals, even though they don't suffer from serious illness. They think that doctors of 3A hospital are more skillful and can make an accuracy diagnosis. In face of the excessive patients, hospital managers and also directors of all medical departments are always trying their best to offer high quality medical service to patients. But the final effort is still far from patients' requirements. It's not practical to require 3A hospital to treat all patients. Hospitals of other level should take their responsibility, attracting patients they can treat. It can be foreseen that the gap among hospitals will be the difference among staff in hospital. Two factors are crucial in the improvement of one doctor, case quantity of personal experience and guidance from expert nearby. Staff in 3A hospital has natural advantages. They can experience high quantity of cases, some of which are very complicated. With the help from some expert nearby, new staff can treat complicated cases. Staff in 2 level hospitals still has opportunity to experience a number of case, but less complicated and less experts who are brought in by manager. Staff in 1 level hospital has shortage both in these two factors. It's very hard to improve them unless they can share some extra resource.

277.2 Self-Improvement Problems of Different Level Hospitals

3A hospital is the symbol of high quality medical service. They are not only serve local residents but also the people over the nation. Most of them also are affiliated to university. Therefore, besides the regular diagnosis and treatment, they also take charge of scientific research and medical education. Abundant and complicated medical records, first-class expert, the latest scientific achievements and the advanced software platform are positive factors to develop doctors' and intern's knowledge and skill. The general way in 3A hospital to help self-improvement of doctors is to let them read all kinds of patient records and ask them write clinical reports. After the reports are finished, key staff should check reports and tell them where the error is and what is needed to be improved and remind them what have been missing. Hence, high quality medical service can always be offered to patients. But in the other side, it requires excess workload to keep in the forefront of science, especially for the key staff of the department. Therefore, little time can be distributed to teach. Teaching is also a burden work, for the reports from fresh doctors are in a mess. There is not standardized template in fresh doctors' mind; and reports written by fresh ones are hard to read. This is a habit-related problem. Habit-corrected is a slow and laborious procedure. Tools of auto habit-corrected are very expected to enhance the work of check reports. High efficiency data-manage tools are also needed to assist scientific research, enhancing the efficiency of researching work to share achievements.

Two level hospitals also have many cases. After the introduction of the experts, fundamental elements of doctor Self-improvement become adequate. Shortages of

2 level hospitals includes: (1) the educational of fresh doctors is less than 3-level. Teaching work requires more effort; (2) the software platform is not less advanced, tutors have to spend more time to prepare teaching documents for the daily teaching as the important work content of doctor self-development; (3) the case recording coverage of disease classification is less than 3A hospitals. Without the addition of new case recordings the doctor self-development is very hard, even if the new educational materials are bought instead. Because real case always different to the same disease in the textbook. The problem based learning (PBL) has more advantages [3–5], but it is hard to be carried out. Despite having the expert and abundant case, some more tools and more widen disease coverage are required to build the time-saving doctor self-development platform.

The doctors' self-development of 1 level hospitals or rural doctor meets the very serious source shortage nearly in all aspect such that self-development nearly cannot be done in local. Though much effort has done by local government, the problem is far from resolved. Considering the duty of 1 level hospital or rural doctor, one of the main training aims is to cultivate doctors' sensitive to the signal of major diseases, especially in early time. If major disease was diagnosed at early time, patient suffered less, so do time and the cost. Because the average educational level of rural doctor is low, the explanation of theory is nearly useless. Practical skills are more expected. To let them have practical skills, we think one of efficient ways is to read the real symptom from real case, write report under the guidance of standard template and receive the review from experts without interruption. Some tests have been done in our institution. When trainees arrived, the score of their test were low. Through the training of read case for some time, the score increased. Trainees became familiar to the special symptom of disease. But their ability retrogressed after they returned to the local hospital. 3 points have been concluded for this situation: (1) rural doctor's low educational level can't make them mapping special symptoms into their deep memory in a short time; (2) they cannot experience the similar case frequently in local hospital; (3) almost no expert can tell them the change of disease. Thus, self-development of doctor in bottom level hospital should add the 3 factors: (1) the training place had better be located in hospital or nearby; (2) uninterrupted self-development should be absolutely necessary; (3) the assistance of expert should be offered in a regular interval of time.

277.3 Hierarchy Continuing Medical Education

The key to improve public medical service is mainly on narrow the gap among doctors' skill on the premise that doctors in 3A hospital keep improvement. Therefore, the solution to this problem is to design different CME strategies matching requirements of each level. Based on the analysis of Sect. 277.3, the information technique is used to enhance the efficiency of self-development

The advantages of 3A hospitals are case-abundant and experts-abundant. How-to manage cases in hospitals is a very critical problem. The realistic situation is disappointed. Little work has done to utilize the abundant case to build a self-development system, let alone how to use real case to design scenario, in which intern, fresh doctors even other doctors can improve themselves without medical risk. Once these conditions are met, CME in 3 level hospitals will be promising. To achieve it, work must be done in 2 parts below:

1. The design of the case database

   In current, the structure of database is designed to serve the daily work in hospital. Though a great number of cases are store in the server, it is not an easy work to use it for CME. Therefore, new data structure should be design to simplify the output of anonymous data, contain the essential information. Each kind of data in one case is with label which reflects data's feature. For instance, the data contain symptom information is labeled with Symp. Through the label, the feature of data is recognized by computer. When case is transformed to terminal computer, the data of each kind are displayed under the order of the trainee or tutor.

2. The design of scenario

   It is a very positive factor to let trainees think. We design a training flow to stimulate the mind of trainee to improve personal diagnosis (Fig. 277.1). At the first step, symptom of the case selected by tutor is displayed to trainee. According to the symptom, trainees diagnose the preliminary disease or list the apparatus to make a further check to support diagnosis. Then his/her performance is assessed. The result is sent to personal learning portfolios. Secondly, based on the check results by apparatus, trainees make the diagnosis results. The performance is also assessed and sent to personal learning portfolios in database. Given the personal characteristic is different tools in server are required to analyze them; and select the proper case to enhance the improvement. All reports written by trainees must follow the standard template. With this platform, many works are done by computer. The training process is similar the true situation. The burden of experts will be weakened. In idea situation, discussions for problem in self-development are held on regular intervals to answer questions. The platform ensures the CME in 3 level hospitals sustainable.

Besides self-improvement, 3A hospitals undertake the obligations to help other doctors' self-development. After modified, this CME platform is appropriate for other level hospital. For level 2 hospitals, a data-transferred interface is designed following the proposed protocol, so that data in level 3 is compatible to level 2 and improves the coverage of disease kinds in local database in level 2 hospitals. Because there are still a number of experts in level 2, it is available that CME in level 2 hospital runs in the similar flow in level 3. With the abundant cases, experts in level 2 also improve themselves. For level 1 hospital or nearby rural doctors, another functional module is added in, letting the performance of doctors in level 1 assessed by experts in high level hospitals.

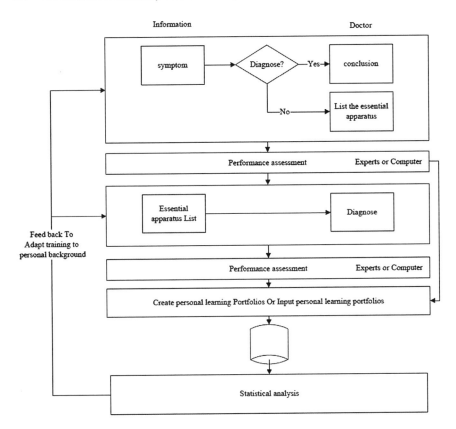

Fig. 277.1 The training flow

277.4 Conclusion

This study proposed the hierarchy of continuing medical education to help doctors in different level hospital self-development. All level of continuing medical education strategies seize two key factors case quantity of personal experience and guidance from expert nearby. The hierarchy comes from the different resource condition of hospitals. CME patterns of respective level hospital aim to give doctors the access to these two positive factors, even if some doctors work in a shortage condition. This hierarchy CME pattern is only an intervention in the special time. After the intervention, we hope it can help patient give more trust to doctors in other level hospitals, balance the patient number in different level hospital, let doctors in all level hospital experience a number of cases and then improve them, hence relieve the public medical service issue in China.

References

1. Chinese Ministry of Health (2012) 2012 China health statistics. http://www.moh.gov.cn/publicfiles/business/htmlfiles/mohwsbwstjxxzx/s9092/201206/55044.htm
2. National Bureau of Statistics of the People's Republic of China (2011) China statistical yearbook. http://www.stats.gov.cn/tjsj/ndsj/2011/html/D0304e.htm
3. Zhou CF, Kolmos A, Nielsen JD (2012) A problem and project-based learning (pbl) approach to motivate group creativity in engineering education. Int J Eng Educ 28:3–16
4. Havet E, Duparc F, Peltier J, Tobenas-Dujardin AC, Freger P (2012) The article critique as a problem-based teaching method for medical students early in their training: a french example using anatomy. Surg Radiol Anat 34:81–84
5. Gingerich A, Mader H, Payne GW (2012) Problem-based learning tutors within medical curricula: An interprofessional analysis. J Interprof Care 26:69–70

Chapter 278
The Reverse Effects of Saikoside on Multidrug Resistance

Huiying Bai, Jing Li, Kun Jiang, Xuexin Liu, Chun Li and Xiaodong Gai

Abstract *Aim* To research the reverse effects of saikoside (SS) on the multidrug resistance (MDR) of human leukemic cell line K562/ADM and the related mechanism. *METHODS* K562 cells and K562/ADM cells in the culture were treated with SS at the concentrations of 1–100 mg/L. The inhibitory rate of the cell proliferation was measured by MTT assay. Non-cytotoxic dose of SS was determined. K562/ADM cells were treated with SS at non-cytotoxic doses of 1.25, 2.5 and 5.0 mg/L with different concentrations of adriamycin (ADM, 0.05–100 mg/L). The 50 % inhibitory concentration (IC_{50}) and the reversal index in all groups were determined. The cell morphology was observed after treated with SS + ADM. The effects of SS on ADM accumulation in K562/ADM cells, the cell cycle profile was examined by flow cytometry. *Results* The inhibitory rates were significantly increased in a dose-dependent manner when the cells were treated with different doses of SS(1–100 mg/L). The available reversal concentration of SS was 5.0 mg/L and the reversal index was 21.5 folds for K562/ADM cells. After treated with SS + ADM, the number of tumor cells was decreased and aoptotic cells were increased in a dose–response relationship. ADM accumulation in K562/ADM cells treated with SS was significantly higher than that in control cells ($P < 0.05$). K562/ADM cells treated with SS were blocked in the stage of G_0/G_1. *Conclusion* SS has effect on proliferation inhibition and MDR reversal in K562/ADM cell line. The reversal mechanisms of SS may be due to increasing the accumulation of chemotherapeutics in the cell, and arresting the cells in G_0/G_1 phase.

H. Bai · J. Li
The People's Hospital of Jilin, Jilin 132011, China

H. Bai · J. Li · K. Jiang · X. Liu · C. Li (✉) · X. Gai (✉)
Department of Pathology, Basic Medical College of Beihua University, Jilin 132013, China
e-mail: lichunjl@126.com

X. Gai
e-mail: bhdxgaixiaodong@126.com

Keywords Saikoside · Multidrug resistance · Reversal of drug resistance · K562/ADM cells

278.1 Introduction

Multidrug resistance (MDR) is the important cause of cancer chemotherapy failure and tumor recurrence. Up to now, there were at least 13 kinds of MDR-related ATP-binding cassette transporter. P-glycoprotein (P-gp) is one of the most important one [1]. Verapamil, cyclosporine and other resistance reversal agents were limited to clinical application because the drug concentration of normal blood could not achieve a therapeutic effect or the obvious adverse reactions were existed. Traditional Chinese medicines were widely used in clinical cancer treatment, One of its important objective is to improve the sensitivity of tumor cells to chemotherapeutic agents. There has been found that the traditional Chinese medicines have a better role of reversing MDR, its mechanism were related to inhibiting the activity of MDR proteins, affecting the expression of MDR gene and promoting the apoptosis of drug-resistant tumor cells [2, 3]. Bupleurum is one of traditional Chinese medicines, with the effect of solution table and inside, liver qi stagnation, its crude extract can reverse MDR [4]. In our preliminary experiments, we filtered components such as polysaccharides (Bupleurum chinese Polysaccharides, BCPS), saponins(Saikoside,SS) from Bupleurum. As a result, we found that SS has MDR reversal effect. Our objective is to explore the application value of SS in anti-human leukemia MDR by detecting the MDR reversal effect of SS on K562/ADM cells and its related mechanism.

278.2 Materials and Methods

278.2.1 Material

IMDM medium is Gibco product. MTT, DMSO are Sigma products. Vera Pammy (Ver) is Shanghai Hefeng pharmaceutical Limited by Share Ltd products. Adriamycin(ADM) is Zhejiang Hisun Pharmaceutical Co. product. Super newborn calf serum is Shanghai excell biology products Co. The North Chaihu (commercially available, were identified as genuine North Bupleurum). K562 cells and K562/ADM cells were provided by the Institute of Jilin University regeneration. Tecan Genios. Beckman.

278.2.2 Methods

278.2.2.1 Saikosaponin Extraction

Bupleurum was placed in 40–50 °C oven drying 7–8 h. It will be crushed into powder by the plant mill after sufficiently dried. 100 g Bupleurum powder were treated with 70 % ethanol 500 ml, 60° for 2 h and reflux extraction for 2 h, filtration, the filter residue and repeated 3 times of extraction, decompress, rotated, evaporation, solvent recovery and get extract. With appropriate amount of distilled water to dissolve it, it is added to the water-saturated n-butanol and extracted three times repeatedly. The extract was rotated through 55° under reduced pressure after the majority of the solvent was removed by evaporation, it is placed in a thoroughly dried in an oven at 80°, grated to obtain 2.8 g of total saponin of Radix Bupleuri powder, the yield was 2.8 %.

278.2.2.2 Toxic Effects of SS by MTT

K562 and K562/ADM cells (1×10^8/L) were seeded in 96-well plates. The experimental group were added different concentrations of SS(1–100 mg/L) and an equal volume of medium without drugs as control. Each well was added 15 µl of MTT after training in 5 % CO_2, 37 degrees for 48 h. After incubating for 4 h, each hole were add 150 µl DMSO, Enzyme immunoassay A570 values was detected.

278.2.2.3 Reversal Effect of SS by MTT

K562 and K562/ADM cells (1×10^8/L) were seeded in 96-well plates. The non-cytotoxic dose of SS 1.25, 2.5, 5.0 mg/L and positive control 5 mg/L VER respectively in K562 cells were combined with different concentrations of ADM (0.05–100 mg/L). A570 value was detected and 50 % inhibitory concentration of each group was calculated reversion index (RI), RI = Resistant cells reversed before IC50/Resistant cells after the reversal of IC50.

Computing two kinds of drugs A, B coefficient of Drug InterAction (CDI), CDI = AB/(A × B), A is A drug alone with the control group the ratio,B is B drug alone with the control group the ratio. CDI < 1, The two drugs have a significant synergistic effect [5, 6].

278.2.2.4 Intracellular ADM Concentration by Flow Cytometry

In order to detect intracellular concentration of ADM more effectively, we use 50 mg/L ADM on K562/ADM cells. K562/ADM cells (4×10^8/L) were seeded in 6-well plates. Experimental groups are as follows: (1) K562/ADM; (2) K562/

ADM + ADM 50 mg/L; (3) K562/ADM + ADM 50 mg/L + VER 5 mg/L; (4) K562/ADM + ADM 50 mg/L + SS 5 mg/L; (5) K562/ADM + ADM 50 mg/L + SS 2.5 mg/L; (6) K562/ADM + ADM 50 mg/L + SS 1.25 mg/L. Cells were collected after 4 h. Based on the fluorescence characteristics of the ADM itself, the fluorescence intensity was measured by flow cytometry (Laser wavelength of 488 nm, emission wavelength 575 nm).

278.2.2.5 Cell Cycle by Flow Cytometry

K562/ADM cells (4×10^8/L) were seeded in 6-well plates. Experimental groups are as follows: (1) K562/ADM; (2) K562/ADM + ADM (50 mg/L); (3) K562/ADM + ADM 50 mg/L + VER (5 mg/L); (4) K562/ADM + ADM 50 mg/L + SS (1.25, 2.5, 5 mg/L). Cells were collected after 4 h and 70 % Ethanol were treated at 4° overnight. Cell cycle were detected by Flow cytometry (Laser wavelength of 488 nm, emission wavelength 575 nm).

278.2.3 Statistical Processing

SPSS11.0 software were used. The data are expressed as mean ± standard deviation, Diversity Honma mean comparison by Single factor analysis of variance. There were statistically significant differences in $P < 0.05$.

278.3 Result

278.3.1 The Toxic Effects of SS on the K562 and K562/ADM Cells

After using six concentrations of SS (1–100 mg/L) for 48 h, with concentrations increasing, the proliferatory inhibition rate of K562 and K562/ADM cells were also corresponding increase. The dose-effect relationship were displayed, See Fig. 278.1. The non-cytotoxic dose of SS on K562/ADM cells is 5.0 mg/L, which is less than 10 % inhibitory rate.

278.3.2 Reversal Effect of SS on K562/ADM Cells

1.25, 2.5 and 5.0 mg/L SS with different concentrations of ADM (0.05–100 mg/L) were added to K562/ADM cells. As can be seen from Table 278.1, three concentrations of SS combined with different concentrations of ADM can be

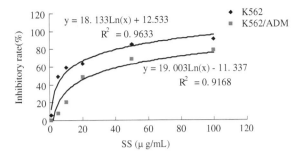

Fig. 278.1 Inhibitory rates of SS on proliferation of K562 and K562/ADM cells after treated with SS

significantly decreased IC50 of K562/ADM cells in a dose-dependent manner ($P < 0.01$).

278.3.3 Synergistic Effect of SS and ADM

By calculating, the CDI value of 1.25, 2.5 and 5.0 mg/L SS were 0.92, 0.89 and 0.82 mg/L. They were all <1 and showed a synergistic effect between SS and ADM. Cell morphology was observed under inverted microscope. After SS collaboratived ADM, the tumor cells were not only suppressed, but also showed a large number of apoptotic cells, expressed as cytoplasmic concentration, volume reduction, nuclear fragmentation as small pieces in a dose—response manner, Seen as Fig. 278.2.

278.3.4 The Change of ADM Concentration in K562/ADM Cells by SS

Non-cytotoxic dose of SS combined with ADM were added to K562/ADM cells for 4 h. With the increase of the SS concentration, the fluorescence intensity of ADM were increased accordingly. There was a significant difference compared to

Table 278.1 Reversal index (RI) of K562/ADM cells after treated with SS and ADM

Groups	Dose (μg/mL)	IC_{50}	Reversal index (RI)
ADM	0	49.53 ± 3.10	—
ADM + SS	1.25	5.93 ± 0.12*	8.4
	2.5	4.98 ± 0.13*	10.0
	5.0	2.31 ± 0.36*	21.5
ADM + VER	5.0	3.67 ± 0.33*	13.5

$P < 0.05$ versus ADM group

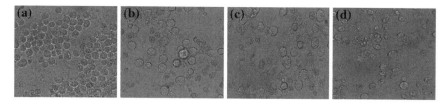

Fig. 278.2 The morphology of K562/ADM cells after treated with different concentrations of SS and ADM for 48 h. **a** K562/ADM, **b** SS1.25 μg/ml + ADM5 μg/ml, **c** SS2.5 μg/ml + ADM5 μg/ml, **d** SS5 μg/ml + ADM5 μg/ml

ADM in K562/ADM cells ($P < 0.05$). The fluorescence intensity of ADM were increased in positive control VER group ($P < 0.05$). Seen as Table 278.2.

278.3.5 The Phase Change of Cell Cycle Distribution by SS

When ADM were respectively treated with different concentrations of non-cytotoxic dose of SS on K562/ADM cells after 4 h, G0/G1 phase cells were increased and S-phase cells were reduced significantly in each SS group compared to ADM group alone ($P < 0.05$), Seen as Table 278.3.

Table 278.2 The change of ADM level in K562/ADM cells after treated with SS and ADM

Groups	MFI	
	K562/ADM	K562
ADM	22.80 ± 2.39	50.70 ± 2.67
ADM + SS 1.25 μg/mL	31.90 ± 2.04*	54.30 ± 2.12
2.5 μg/mL	35.20 ± 1.98*	53.10 ± 1.89
5.0 μg/mL	38.50 ± 2.56*	53.90 ± 2.92
ADM + VER	46.70 ± 2.24*	56.20 ± 3.89

$P < 0.05$ versus ADM group (K562/ADM)

Table 278.3 The change of cell cycle in K562/ADM after treated with SS and ADM (n = 3, ± S)

Groups	G_0/G_1(%)	S(%)
Control	24.80 ± 5.64	72.30 ± 2.98
ADM	32.90 ± 3.29*	61.50 ± 3.65*
ADM + SS 1.25 μg/mL	41.50 ± 3.94*#	52.10 ± 4.77*#
2.5 μg/mL	49.60 ± 4.67*#	46.60 ± 3.95*#
5.0 μg/mL	55.70 ± 5.28*#	34.20 ± 5.74*#
ADM + VER	49.60 ± 4.76*#	42.30 ± 4.21*#

$P < 0.05$ versus control group; # $P < 0.05$ versus ADM group

278.4 Discussion

Leukemia MDR is a major obstacle to leukemia chemotherapy. To overcome the leukemia MDR, enhancing the efficacy of anti-cancer drugs has become a key issue to be solved in leukemia treatment. It was confirmed to have many compounds or biological agents with reversal activity in vitro, Such as cyclosporine, verapamil and so on. But because of there are toxic to heart and kidney, its clinical application is limited. Looking for an effective and low toxicity reversal agents have been the hot point in leukemia MDR.

Since Tsuruo [7] reported that Verapamil has reversal effect on tumor drug resistance, several kinds of chemotherapy drugs reversal agents have been found, especially the calcium channel blocker (CCB). But because of its side effects, CCB was limited its clinical application. Radix Bupleurum has the effects of reconciliation and discharge heat, Xiere liver gas stagnation and anti-tumor, its crude extract has also played reversing MDR role in tumor cells [4]. SS is an effective active ingredient which extracted from Bupleurum. Non-toxic dose 1.25, 2.5 and 5 mg/L of SS were able to enhance the sensitivity of K562/ADM cells to ADM and make IC50 of ADM decreased. The reversal fold were 8.4 times, 10.0 times and 21.5 times and showed that SS may reverse MDR in K562/ADM cells. A synergistic effect between non-toxic dose of SS and ADM were confirmed in K562/ADM cells, CDI values were 0.92, 0.89 and 0.82. In addition to the proliferation of tumor cells were inhibited, a large number of apoptotic cells also have been observed by morphological observation.

Because ADM can emit fluorescence, the fluorescence intensity of ADM in cells and the intracellular ADM concentration was positively correlated, that means the fluorescence intensity and intracellular ADM concentration can be reflects [8]. The results of this study showed that the fluorescence intensity was significantly improved after SS combined with ADM in K562/ADM cells. The results suggested that SS may increase ADM accumulation in K562/ADM cells. The formation mechanism of MDR are intricate, including classic resistant marker proteins P-gp, cell cycle regulation abnormal apoptotic gene expression out of control and enhanced DNA repair capacity and other factors [9, 10].

The experimental results showed that G0/G1 phase cells were indicating, after SS treatment. G1 phase is the stage of cell differentiation and the sensitive period of drug action, indigating that SS may play a MDR role by arresting in G0/G1 phase.

In summary, SS could inhibit the proliferation and reversal effect on the K562/ADM cells. The reversal effect may be achieved by increasing intracellular drug accumulation, and arresting the cell in G0/G1 phase thus inhibiting the cell proliferation. Other related reversal mechanism need to be further studied.

Acknowledgments The work was funded by Science and Technology Department of Jilin Province (20110728), science and technology project of Jilin city (201262501) and department of education of Jilin Province (2013193).

References

1. Jabr-Milane LS, van Vlerken LE, Yadav S et al (2008) Multi-functional nancarriers to overcome tumor drug resistance. Cancer Treat Rev 34(7):592–602
2. Xu S, Xu C (2006) Multidrug resistance mechanism and chinese medicine reverse of progress. Chin J Cancer Biother 13(6):404–411
3. Leung MK, Shan B (2004) Chinese medicine research progress antagonize P-glycoprotein-mediated multidrug resistance mechanisms. Chin Herbal Med 35:466–469
4. Gai X, Zeng QC, Hong M (2005) Of Bupleurum reversing hepatocellular carcinoma multidrug resistance mechanisms. Chin J Chem 26(8):1446–1450
5. Li X, Hu Y et al (2010) PHII-7 reverse the resistance mechanisms of tumor cell K562/A02. Chin Pharmacol Bull 26(6):750–753
6. Xu S, Sun G, Wang H et al (2006) Synergistically suppressive effect of paeonol and cisplatin on the proliferation of human hepatoma cell line SMMC-7721. Acta Univer Med Anhui 41(1):63–65
7. Tsuruo T, Iiad H, Tsukagoshi S et al (1981) Overcoming of vincristine resistance in P388 leukemia in vivo and in vitro through enhanced cytotoxicity of vincristine and vinblastine by verapamil. Cancer Res 41(5):1967–1972
8. Gai X, Cheng P, Calendar Spring et al (2010) The novel polyamine the conjugate NMMB reversal multidrug resistance K562/ADM cells and its mechanism. J Jilin Univ 3(2):238–241
9. Admas JM, Cory S (2007) The Bcl-2 apoptotic switch in cancer development and therapy. Oncogene 26(9):1324–1337
10. Ghoshal K, Bai S (2007) DNA methyltransferases as targets for cancer therapy. Drugs Today (Barc) 43(6):395–422

Chapter 279
Research and Practice on "Three Steps of Bilingual Teaching" for Acupuncture and Moxibustion Science in Universities of TCM

Xiang Wen Meng, Dan Dan Li, Hua Peng Liu, Sheng Ai Piao, Cheng Hui Zhu and Karna Lokesh Kumar

Abstract Along with the development of acupuncture in different parts of the world, bilingual teaching of acupuncture and Traditional Chinese Medicine (TCM) is highly recommended in Universities of TCM in China. Although many new-type and integrated students of TCM have been cultivated, we still have some shortcomings. After analyzing the current situation of bilingual teaching methods of acupuncture and TCM, we had put forward a method of "Three Steps of Bilingual Teaching" including "disease study step, conversation step and writing step" which have got good result, in order to further improve the quality of bilingual teaching of acupuncture in universities of TCM and promote the spread and development of TCM around the world.

Keywords Universities of TCM · Acupuncture and moxibustion · Bilingual teaching

In 2001, the ministry of education had released a document (included several opinions to strengthen the teaching at universities and improve the quality of teaching) which asked a requirement that the foreign language teaching course of biomedical and other professionals should achieve a prescribed courses of 5–10 % within 3 years [1]. For internationalization and worldwide clinical practice of Acupuncture, bilingual teaching in the Universities of TCM is current trend of time. Through the training of both TCM and bilingual teaching knowledge,

---

Project source: 2012 Tianjin City undergraduate course of common colleges and universities teaching quality and teaching reform research project. NO: 20120204.

X. W. Meng (✉) · D. D. Li · H. P. Liu · S. A. Piao · C. H. Zhu
College of Acupuncture and Moxibustion, Tianjin University of TCM, Tianjin, China
e-mail: mengxiangwen116@hotmail.com

K. Lokesh Kumar
International Educational Center, Tianjin University of TCM, Tianjin, China

students can master the medical skills and be proficient in international language. This also helps to produce talents for international exchange programs in TCM. So it has become an inevitable trend in the teaching of TCM at present.

279.1 Existing Problems for the Bilingual Teaching

279.1.1 Lack of Rationality

University students enrolled in the learning process of TCM in bilingual specialized courses reflected a pattern of discontinuity due to curriculum schedule and can't complement each other. For example, the general acupuncture course takes three years to complete while the bilingual course takes one more extra year i.e. 4 years. This prolongation of the study period for same qualification appears to be burden for most of the students. So the students are unlikely to increase their learning burden.

279.1.2 Lack of Flexibility

Due to uneven English levels of different students, students in bilingual class show different learning abilities. High level students can be faster and better in grasping things, so their learning enthusiasm promotes the further clinical study. While low level students encounter difficulties that influence the enthusiasm of learning, thus forming a vicious cycle and eventually affect the clinical practice of acupuncture and Chinese medicine, resulting a polarization in the process of bilingual teaching.

279.1.3 Lack of Oral Practice

Although in the process of bilingual teaching, teachers can organize discussions or other forms of oral practice, the limited class hour and course arrangements make it tough.

279.1.4 Single Assessment Mode

The assessment for bilingual teaching is still a simple written test. So the students invest more energy dealing with the examination, and don't pay more attention in applied part of acupuncture and moxibustion in bilingual teaching and can't really improve the students' application level [2].

279.2 The Practice of "Three Steps of Bilingual Teaching"

Analyzing the problems in bilingual teaching and exploring the new ideas and combining with the characteristics of acupuncture and moxibustion, we summed up a method of "Three Steps of Bilingual Teaching" to further improve the quality of bilingual teaching of acupuncture which will help to promote and spread TCM in the world.

279.2.1 Disease Study Step

Students of TCM have the basis of ordinary English, but they lack professional knowledge of medical English. With the medical English, Chinese students can have international communication and master an indispensable tool in modern medicine. Paying attention to the basic theory of TCM, the formulas of Chinese medicine and treatment based on syndrome differentiation theory of TCM; the role of bilingual teaching should be highlighting the "syndromes" and common clinical symptoms of "disease". So to become a candidate of the international exchange program, one must master the common clinical symptoms of diseases in English language.

First of all, emphasize on how acupuncture helps to treat the disease such as Sciatica, lumbar pain, Lumbago, etc. Mastering the disease areas where acupuncture is really good is the premise of better treatment strategies, and understanding which diseases are more susceptible at abroad is the premise of good clinical reception and subsequent treatment. More focus should be given on the common diseases of European and American countries, such as Irritable Bowel Syndrome (Irritable Bowel Syndrome, IBS), amyotrophic lateral Sclerosis, Multiple Sclerosis, MS), etc. In specific learning process, we can enhance it through the specific cases in English according to the different branches of study. In spare time, through writing exercises or the students asking each other to do review in a timely manner could be beneficial for study.

279.2.2 Conversation Step

In the process of learning, students should be involved in oral conversation practice and listening exercises based on their curriculum. At the same time, the arrangement of our domestic students and foreign students together to participate in class discussion and English simulation trainings is beneficial [2]. The conversation trainings should incorporate following points.

Give full attention to the characteristic of TCM four diagnosis method, i.e. inspection (looking), auscultation and olfaction (listening and smelling), inquiry (asking) as well as pulse-taking and palpation. Among these, inquiry is one of the vital techniques which involve mainly listening to patient and asking questions. On the basis of the "Asked Ten Songs", a case of the full-scale inquiry involves listening to complaints of patient and asking purposeful questions according to the chief complaints of the patients.

Paying attention to cultural difference and communication taboos of east and west is most important. In clinical receptions, mastering in Chinese considerations and at the same time paying attention to the English communication habits and etiquette is very crucial. While communicating, euphemisms sentence patterns and very polite way should be used like "Could I help you…" or "Could you tell me…" etc. Since western countries' people are more concerned to their privacy, religion, age, weight and other problems, so when meeting such a sensitive topic; more attention should be paid to language appropriately and avoid causing unnecessary misunderstanding.

Students should be able to explain basic concepts of TCM and acupuncture treatment principle. As vigorously carried out international exchanges and clinical scientific research achievements, the curative effect of TCM is gradually accepted by more and more countries and regions. Unique theoretical system of TCM for people is becoming more and more interesting; so in the process of diagnosis, questions could be inevitably asked to the doctors. For example: what are the channels and collaterals? How acupuncture can relieve the pain? How doctors of TCM "cure" the disease? What's the meaning of "tongue observation"? And so on. In the process of explaining, students will use a brief and simple language to explain. So students are required to study systematically, summarize the ideas and practice properly.

279.2.3 Writing Step

This involves study and translation of English research papers and thesis. After a period of time of step I and II sessions, students should have significantly improved their vocabulary and listening and speaking skills. On this basis, students are required to consult some information, write paper in English, and have discussions on various topics [3]. When overseas students write papers, domestic students can assist them so that they could be familiar with English professional thesis writing [2].

Another important part is to be able to think and design clinical and scientific research tasks. So after they become familiar with the writing of professional papers in English, students are required to retrieve The American Journal of Chinese Medicine, The Journal of Clinical Acupuncture and Moxibustion or SCI journals in English. This will put them on forefront of clinical and scientific researches in TCM and they will be able to think and design a foundation for clinical research projects in the future.

279.3 Summary

After the 3 years of three steps bilingual teaching method practice, there are two hundred students in three grades accepting the method. In 2012, there was an experimental class which constituted by fifty students who choose the class of "bilingual teaching acupuncture", before given the "Three steps of Bilingual Teaching", an examination to inspect the ability of these students how do they good at the English names of TCM and basic knowledge, most of them got 40 average scores, after given the "Three steps of Bilingual Teaching", most of them got 90 average scores, having obvious improvement. The students showed improvement in Bilingual fundamentals and their consultation capabilities, especially the use of English explanation of TCM theory to patients. On the other hand, academic performance was excellent and good students in clinical teaching translation took part at various international conferences as translators. Last year, in a class of 20 TCM students, 10 had participated in clinical teaching and worked as a translator at international conferences and all of them had improved their English language ability while one of a classmate was admitted to the University of Melbourne, Australia for the master's study.

Nowadays, Bilingual teaching is a hot topic of education reform in our country and is in line with international standards, so it's now an inevitable trend of education reform [1]. Bilingual teaching in universities of TCM and Acupuncture has obtained great achievements and cultivated a large number of bilingual talents. The "Three steps of Bilingual Teaching" can promote the teaching content, the teaching method and a continuous reform. Such teaching model can stimulate students' bilingual learning abilities and at the same time improve their medical English level. It has really satisfied and met the needs of students learning and has achieved a better teaching effect. But still we need to further perfect the structure of this method to implement bilingual teaching method more effectively that will help to produce more qualified TCM bilingual talents for our country.

References

1. Xu YX (2006) The exploring of bilingual teaching of acupuncture and thinking. Chin Acupunct 26(9):673–675
2. Zhao L, Shen XY, Zhang HM (2007) The research of "bilingual teaching" about Meridians. J Shanghai Univ TCM 21(2):12–14
3. Wang Wei (2004) Acupuncture bilingual teaching experience. China's High Med Educ 3:16–17

Chapter 280
Current Status of Traditional Chinese Medicine Language System

Meng Cui, Lirong Jia, Tong Yu, Shuo Yang, Lihong liu. Ling Zhu, Jinghua Li, Bo Gao and Yan Dong

Abstract Traditional Chinese Medicine (TCM) is a complicated and huge knowledge system with a long history. As the information technology step forward, more and more problems about how to deal with plentiful TCM information come up. First of all, so we should normalize terminology in TCM, and use these terms to deal with TCM information. Then, the Traditional Chinese Medicine Language System (TCMLS) emerges as needed. Now, TCMLS has been the biggest ontology in the domain of TCM. It has been researched and developed for over ten years. And totally, more than 120,000 concepts and more than 600,000 terms have been added. Except this, other studies such as sematic research, system evaluation and application for TCMLS have been paid attention to. In short, the evolution of development and application for TCMLS will be briefly focused in this paper.

Keywords Traditional chinese medicine · Language system · Ontology

280.1 Introduction

With the rapid development of computer and networking technologies, there has been a huge change in the storage, processing, transmission, and application of information. How to organize and query the useful information has become an important problem. The emerging ontology technology gives a promising solution

M. Cui (✉) · L. Jia · T. Yu · S. Yang · L. liu. Ling Zhu · J. Li · B. Gao · Y. Dong
Institute of Information on Traditional Chinese Medicine, China Academy of Chinese Medicine Sciences, 100700 Beijing, China
e-mail: cui@mail.cintcm.ac.cn

to this problem. In 1986, the National Library of Medicine (NLM) built the Unified Medical Language System (UMLS), effectively integrating more than 100 controlled vocabularies. UMLS enables the interconnecting of 4,800 databases worldwide, and provides an information platform for the medical community.

Traditional Chinese Medicine (TCM) has been developing for thousands of years. Various factors, such as the evolution of language and the fusion of disciplines resulted into the richness of TCM language system, and the complexity of TCM knowledge representation, which caused the difficulty of understanding [1]. A unified TCM language system can resolve a series of complex problems such as Polysemy, Synonyms, and support various applications such as information retrieval and knowledge discovery.

In 2002, Institute of Information on Traditional Chinese Medicine (IITCM), China Academy of Chinese Medicine Sciences, collaborated with 13 organizations in China to devleop the Traditional Chinese Medicine Language System (TCMLS), which aims to utilize modern information techniques to achieve the normalization of the massive concepts and terms in TCM domain. Aining Yin et al. [2–4] conducted an in-depth study into the principles and methodology of TCMLS construction, and made a technical specification of TCMLS including the method and standard of collecting terms, semantic types, and semantic relations, which laid the foundation for the construction of TCMLS. TCMLS was initially developed by using Protégé, which is an open-source tool for ontology development. More than ten organizations in China participated in this project. They developed the modules of TCMLS is a distributed manner, and these modules were merged by IITCM. The distributed engineering of data, even under unified rules, resulted into the inconsistency and replication of data.

In 2006, a productive platform for constructing TCMLS was built using Web 2.0 technologies, such as the Spring Framework and Ajax [5]. This Web-based platform enabled collaborative editing online, and avoided the problem of data fusion. It provided flexible configuration and a rich set of functions such as computer-aided editing, reporting tool, and data import/export. This platform can support the concurrent editing of large-scale language system. This platform supported the concurrent and collaborative editing of large-scale language system by a distributive team with more than 100 experts from various domains. With the help of this system, there was a large increase in the efficiency and productivity of the TCMLS project, and the TCMLS system started to scale up.

Currently, TCMLS contains a classification system with 16 high-level classes and a semantic network with 58 semantic relations and 127 semantic classes. TCMLS also contains a thesaurus with 120,000 concepts, 600,000 terms, and 1,270,000 relations. TCMLS has been used in various applications such as terminological integration, translation, natural language processing.

280.2 The Organization of Traditional Chinese Medicine Language System

280.2.1 Thesaurus

As the core and fundamental component of TCMLS, *TCMLS Thesaurus* is a large scale repository created by analyzing, selecting, and organizing terms from various existing subject headings, classification schemes, databases, dictionaries. This thesaurus covers terms from TCM domain and related domains such as biology, chemistry and humanity [6]. The sources of this thesaurus include:

1. Controlled vocabularies from TCM and related domains, such as *"Chinese Traditional Medicine and materia medica subject headings"*, *"Medical Subject Headings (MeSH)"*, *"Chinese Library Classification ·Special Classification for Medicine (4th Edition)"*, and international controlled vocabularies.
2. Textbooks and authoritative dictionaries, including textbooks used by various universities and institutions, and TCM-related dictionaries such as *"Dictionary of Traditional Chinese Medicine"*, *"Prescription Dictionary of Traditional Chinese Medicine"*.
3. Various standards such as national standards, industry standards, and international standards.
4. TCM classics, modern literature, clinical cases, and clinical terms.
5. Terms form other related domains, such as medicine, biology, chemistry.

This thesaurus uses concepts as the basic unit for organizing terms, form a two-level structure of concepts and terms. Various terms representing the same concept are combined together. For example, *"lung"* and *"huagai"*, as well as *"心肾不交 (non-interaction between the heart and kidney)"* and *"水火不济"*, are two expressions of the same concept. On the other hand, a term can represent different concepts. For example, the term *"太阳(greater yang)"* refers to *"太阳穴(temple)"* and *"太阳经(greater yang meridian)"* in TCM domain. This kind of terms is classified into different concepts in this thesaurus.

280.2.2 Semantic Network

TCMLS Semantic Network (SN) provides a high-level ontology for TCMLS thesaurus. It is designed in reference to UMLS Semantic Network. The TCMLS SN conforms to the structural characteristics of TCM domain, and can satisfy the requirements of the digitization of TCM knowledge. The TCMLS SN contains two major parts:

TCMLS Semantic Type (ST): TCMLS SN defines 126 Semantic Types to cover the conceptual system of TCM domain (it also involves concepts from medicine, biology, and pharmaceutics). These STs are divided into two major categories: event and entity.

TCMLS Semantic Relations (ST): TCMLS SN imports the 54 semantic relations from UMLS, and add 4 TCM-specific semantic relations: correspond concepts to、inter_exterior and interior with、meridian tropism、similar concepts with [7].

280.3 Evaluation

In 2012, we conducted a systematic investigation of TCMLS, resulting into an evaluation of the soundness, capacity, and accuracy of this system [8]. The major conclusions are as follows:

The soundness of TCMLS: The disciplinary classification of TCMLS is reasonable, and conforms to the disciplinary system of TCM domain. The semantic classification of TCMLS is fairly reasonable, but some semantic classes need to be modified, and others need to be removed in that they are never used.

The capacity of TCMLS: The capacity of TCMLS is reflected in the completeness of terms. We survey the use of terms in clinical cases, data dictionary, and journal papers. The results show that the completeness of terms reaches 91.4 %, which is relatively good.

The accuracy of TCMLS: We search the literature repository for the co-occurrence of terms in papers and the usefulness and effectiveness of terms, in order to evaluate the accuracy of semantic relations. The results show that the accuracy of TCMLS is relatively low.

In summary, the soundness and capacity of TCMLS is qualified, but the accuracy of TCMLS is unsatisfactory. The major reason for the inaccuracy of TCMLS is that the knowledge expression is rather arbitrary, and is influenced by the knowledge structure and cognitive ability of editors.

280.4 Applications

TCMLS is applied in a platform for TCM literature retrieval. This platform utilizes the content of TCMLS to implement advanced functions such as synonymous search, and associative search, and provides more comprehensive and accurate results for users. This system also implements the same kind of search on Internet resources, increasing the accuracy and relevance of search results [9]. This platform includes two major functions:

1. *The presentation of TCMLS*

This system enables users to query the concepts in TCMLS, and provides the information about a concept, such as synonyms, definition, related concepts, and semantic types. This system also enables users to jump to a related concept for further investigation. This system provides two modes of navigation services:

Navigation through the concept hierarchy: the system use a tree-view to present the ISA relationships between concepts; when a user click a concept in the tree, the system will presents the detailed information of the concept.

Navigation through the semantic network: a user can first select a concept, and the system will present a semantic network around the concept and also present the detailed information of the concept.

2. *Literature retrieval service.*

The system utilizes the synonyms and concept relations in TCMLS to enhance literature retrieval. When a user search for documents about a concept, the system will find all the synonyms of the concept, and return all the related documents accordingly. For example, when a user searches for the concept "中风(stroke)", the system will consider all its synonyms, including "仆击","偏枯","卒中", "大厥","痱风","薄厥","脑卒中", and thus returns comprehensive searching results. In addition, the system will take the related concepts into consideration upon returning the results. For example, if a user input the concept "中风(stroke)", the system will find out that "牛黄清心丸(niuhuang qingxin pills)" can treat "中风(stroke)", and retrieve the documents that contains the two concepts. In addition, this platform enables users to search for the resources on the Internet, which improves the accuracy and relevance of searching results.

280.5 Conclusions

With more than ten years of development, TCMLS has achieved a considerable scale. Throughout this project, we conducted a series of studies on the methodology of system engineering, semantic relations, and TCM classics, which are significant for the construction and development for TCMLS. Currently, TCMLS has reached a new phase in which the emphasis is on how to apply TCM in practical applications. In addition, we will develop a technical specification for TCMLS in order to improve the data quality.

Acknowledgments This work is supported by "the Fundamental Research Funds for the Central public welfare research institutes (NO. ZZ070804, NO. ZZ070311, NO. ZZ070309)")", "the China Postdoctoral Science Foundation funded project (NO. 2012M520559)",

References

1. Zhu JP (2006) Standardization of terms of traditional Chinese medicine (TCM) and modernization internationalization of TCM. Chin J Traditi Chin Med Pharm 21:6–8
2. Yin AN, Zhang RE (2003) Traditional Chinese medicine language system technical standards. Chin J Inf Traditi Chin Med 10:92–94

3. Yin AN, Zhang RE (2003) Study of methodology about built traditional Chinese medicine language system. Chin J Inf Traditi Chin Med 10:90–92
4. Zhou XZ, Wu ZH, Yin AN et al (2004) Ontology development for unified traditional Chinese medical language system. J Artif Intell Med 32:15–27
5. Tang MY (2007) Ontology engineering and related application of traditional Chinese medicine language system. Zhejiang University
6. Fang Q (2004) Traditional Chinese medical language system based on ontology. Zhejiang University, Zhejiang
7. Jia LR (2005) A preliminary study about semantic relation of traditional Chinese medical language system. China academy of Chinese medical sciences, Beijing
8. Jia LR, Dong Y, Zhu L et al (2012) Study and establishment of appraisal system for traditional Chinese medical language system. Chin Digit Med 7:13–16
9. Jia LR, Liu LH (2012) Literature retrieval services platform based on traditional Chinese medical language system. J Med Inform 33:54–56

Chapter 281
The Selection Research of Security Elliptic Curve Cryptography in Packet Network Communication

Yuzhong Zhang

Abstract This paper studies the elliptic curve cryptography in a packet network communication security, the elliptic curve cryptosystem security elliptic curve select principles have been studied by several elliptic curve algorithm based on the analysis put forward the views of this article—that is, should be inclined to choose completely randomly generated by the ideal of security elliptic curve to construct the elliptic curve cryptosystem.

Keywords Packet network · Security · Elliptic curve

281.1 Introduction

With the rapid development of computer network, especially the Internet, and digital society has basically shaped. Due to the openness of the network, It makes the security problems of network communication activities are more prominent, particularly the various business activities and government affairs activities which are running on the grouping Internet. It could say that safety problem is the basis and prerequisite while the communication activities that all based on packet network performed normally. In order to better study the network information security problems; this paper analyzes the selection problem of security curve cryptography in packet network communication.

Y. Zhang (✉)
School of Information Technology and Engineering,
Yuxi Normal University, Yuxi, China
e-mail: zh1011@yxhu.net

281.2 Security Elliptic Curve Cryptography

Due to the elliptic curve cryptosystem is based on elliptic curve discrete logarithm problem in finite field, seeing from a security perspective, the more difficult the problem is, the better. In the same size of the elliptic curve discrete logarithm problems, if the discrete logarithm problem based on elliptic curve has a higher difficulty; It could say that the elliptic curve is more security [1].

In general, for a given elliptic curve E, if solving the discrete logarithm problem need index time, so it is called security elliptic curve. Seeing from the perspective of the application, security elliptic curve, namely that which can be chosen when people formulate the elliptic curve cryptosystem.

281.3 Elliptic Curve Algorithm Analysis

Now set elliptic curve E which is defined on finite field $GF(q)$, and $q = p^n$, p is a prime number. $\#E(GF(q))$ means the stair of Elliptic curve E rational subgroup $E(GF(q))$, setting L is the largest prime factor of $\#E(GF(q))$, about elliptic curve discrete logarithm problem $Q = mP$ which exist in the $E(GF(q))$, at present there has the best solving method [2]:

1. Pohlig-Hellman algorithm

The algorithm is applicable to the discrete logarithm problem of any limited Abel group. It utilized the ancient Chinese remainder theorem, which transformed the discrete logarithm problem of N stair finite group G into several discrete logarithm problems of prime factors cyclic subgroup, this algorithm is very effective when stair's factors of generating elements are all small primes factors.

2. Pollard-ρ algorithm.

The solution algorithm is effective to any discrete logarithm problems which are based on the limited Abel group. After the simplification of Pohlig-Hellmna algorithm, it can solve new elliptic curve discrete logarithm problem upon l prime number order subgroup. Aiming at the particularity of elliptic curve, the running time complexity of pollard-algorithm is $O(\sqrt{\frac{\pi l}{4}})$, and space complexity is negligible. After the Parallel processing, the running time complexity of distributed pollard-ρ algorithm can be dropped into $O(\frac{\sqrt{\pi l}}{2M})$. But the algorithm is still essentially index time algorithm.

3. MOV Method

Within polynomial time the minimum k to establish the $E[n] \subset E(GF(q^k))$ will simplified elliptic curve discrete logarithm problem into discrete logarithm problem on the finite field $GF(q^k)$ by MOV method. When k is not big, the DLP problems after simplification, using the Index algorithm, it can be solved in the Index time, and then can get the original ECDLP problem's result.

But the MOV method is only effective for the super odd heterotype elliptic curve and elliptic curve of Forbenius endomorphism trace $t = 2$[110]. For other types of elliptic curve, this method is invalid.

4. SSAS Method

For the elliptic curve of "deformity", the algorithm can solve its elliptic curve discrete logarithm problem within polynomial time. At this point, it has Forbenius endomorphism trace, namely $t = 1$ or $\#E(GF(q)) = q$.

Therefore, when Forbenius endomorphism trace $t = 0, 1, 2$ and P t of elliptic curve E, the attack methods mentioned above can solve problems of ECDLP within below the index time, the elliptic curve E cannot be used to construct cryptosystem.

281.4 Selection Principle of Secure Elliptic Curve

In terms of known attack methods aimed at the elliptic curve discrete logarithm, when selected the security elliptic curve $E(GF(q))$, we should follow the following two selection criteria's:

(1) The Forbenius endomorphism trace 0, 1, 2 and p of Elliptic curve $E(GF(q))$ cannot be divided exactly by t.
(2) The elliptic curve group's stair $\#E(GF(q))$ must contain a large prime number factor so as to avoid the attack of Pholig-Hellman algorithm, and increase the difficulty of the Pollard-ρ algorithm attack.

According to the above security elliptic curve selection criterion, when we judge the safety of chosen elliptic curve $E(GF(q))$ in practice, first calculate the elliptic curve group's stair $\#E(GF(q))$ and Forbenius endomorphism trace $t = q + 1 - \#E(GF(q))$, and then judge whether t satisfies the safety criterion (1); When meet the criteria, then make a decomposition to $\#E(GF(q))$, and judge whether it contains a large prime number factor greater than l, if has only one big prime number factor greater than l, so accept the elliptic curve as a secure elliptic curve.

Here is more complex to confirm the threshold value l. To ensure overall work performance of the system, it should make the l as small as possible under the premise of meeting certain security requirements.

281.5 Determine of the Security Elliptic Curve l Value

To determine the l value: the key factors of the minimum security requirements shall include the following respects:

(1) The importance of the protected information.
(2) The computing ability of existing computer.
(3) The prediction of improving future computing ability.
(4) The emerging situation estimates of new solution attack algorithm.

281.6 Type of Safety Elliptic Curve on Finite Field

Therefore, according to the rule of the selection of secure elliptic curve, safety elliptic curve can be subdivided on finite field type [4] as follows:

First species: The finite field characteristic is the elliptic curve of prime number p. This kind of curve can be subdivided into the following several kinds:

(1) $q = p$, $GF(q) = GF(p)$, at this point, the elliptic curve E define on prime field GF (P). Here, P is a big enough prime numbers so that the elliptic curve group E stair, $\#E(GF(q))$ contains a big prime number factor, it is better that $\#E(GF(q))$ is a prime number, then call the curve as the "ideal" security elliptic curve.
(2) $q = p$, $GF(q) = GF(p)$, p is a smaller prime numbers (e.g., $p = 3, 5, 7, 11$ etc.), to the elliptic curve E defined on the prime field $GF(p)$. At this moment, for a prime number n, considering E in extension field of $GF(p)$, $GF(p^n)$ on the elliptic curve rational subgroup. When $\#E(GF(p^n))$ contains a big prime number factor, $E(GF(p^n))$ can be used to construct the elliptic curve cryptosystem. At this moment, from improving operation performance of the system, the general requirements to p is a prime number whose size is close to handling the most characters length by using the system CPU.

For example, when using the password system CPU word length is 8 bits, select approach to 8 bits, namely prime numbers of 256, such as 257.

Second species: Elliptic curve whose finite field characteristic is 2.
This kind of curve can be subdivided into the following several:

(1) $q = 2^n$, Elliptic curve E defined on binary finite field $GF(q)$. To combat Weil descend algorithm, where n is a prime number, and 2^n should be large enough, so that $\#E(GF(2^n))$ contains a big prime number factor.
(2) $q = 2$, Elliptic curve E defined on finite field $GF(2)$, then the non-odd heterotype elliptic curve has only two:

$$E_1 : y^2 + xy = x^3 + x^2 + 1$$
$$E_2 : y^2 + xy = x^3 + 1$$
(281.1)

In terms of a prime number n, $E_i(GF(2^n))$, which E_i is on $GF(2)$ the extension field $GF(2^n)$. When $\#E_i(GF(2^n))$ contains a big prime number factor, it can construct cryptosystem by $E(GF(2^n))$. In general, this kind of curve is called as Koblitz curve.

(3) $q = 2^r$, Elliptic curve E defined on binary finite field GF (q). In order to improve the operation performance of the system, generally take the r and word length of the use of the system CPU's. For example, for a 32-bit CPU, take r = 32. And then to a prime number n, considering the rational subgroup $E(GF(q^n))$, which E is on the extension field of $GF(q)$, namely $GF(q^n)$. When $\#E(GF(q^n))$ contain a big prime number factor, $E(GF(q^n))$ can be used to construct the elliptic curve cryptosystem.

(4) $q = 2^n$, n = ed, e, d general are prime number, E defined on the binary finite field $GF(q) = GF(2^n)$, when $\#E(GF(q))$ contained the big prime number factor, $E(GF(q))$ can be used to construct cryptosystem.

281.7 Type Advantage Analysis of Secure Elliptic Curve Over Finite Field

In the various kinds of elliptic curves, The first type's first kind of curve and second type's second kind of curve are two of the most typical and the most basic security elliptic curve. Choosing the two curves to construct cryptosystem has the following several advantages:

(1) It can flexibly select the size of p or 2^n in basic field $GF(p)$ and $GF(2^2)$.
   For the prime number p, take p as the Fermat prime number, Mersenne prime number, etc. Such as p = $2^{196} - c$ is a small integer. But for 2^n in the $GF(2^n)$, take n as prime number which is close to 2 exponentiation of m. In this way, it can greatly improve the speed of the system.
(2) Curve selection space is big enough.
   For the fixed base domain $GF(p)$ and $GF(2^n)$, Due to p or 2^n is very big, So in finite field $GF(p)$ and $GF(2^n)$ have enough of the elliptic curves, which makes the selection space of secure elliptic curve is large enough and meet the needs of the various occasions application.
(3) Security is the best.
   At present it is generally believed that the elliptic curve cryptosystem based on the random selection of secure elliptic curve has the best security in all kinds of elliptic curve.

281.8 Type Defect Analysis of Safety Elliptic Curve on Finite Field

But on the other hand, using the two types of elliptic curves has two obvious weaknesses:

(1) It is difficult to select a right curve

When choosing the two types of elliptic curve, must first calculate the elliptic curve group's stair $\#E(GF(p))$ or $\#E(GF(2^n))$. Although in the present, the next chapter to discuss the SEA numbered algorithm, which is used to calculate the finite group stair of elliptic curve has reached the level of practical application, but the algorithm still is very complicated. and that, when using the SEA algorithm work out of the stair $\#E(GF(p))$ or $\#E(GF(2^n))$, It is necessary to make a decomposition to # E so as to ensure whether which contain a large prime number factor.

Experimental data show that, in the two kinds of curves which are randomly selected; roughly every 1,000 curves, only two curves can satisfy the security requirement. It is a very complex job to find out the work of security elliptic curve in the random generation two types of elliptic curves. When taken these two kinds of curve construction password security system, the selection of curve is a serious problem.

(2) Run slowly

The reason why these two kinds of curves implement at a slower speed is that:

There is generally a big coefficient in order to make a description of the elliptic curve Weiersrtass equation, and thus to a certain extent, it reduced its group operation speed; On the other hand, namely is multiplication operation to the two types of elliptic curves.

281.9 Packet Network Security Selection of Elliptic Curve cryptosystem

Besides two kinds of curves mentioned above, other various curves all have a common characteristic, Using finite field $GF(q)$ which is used to define the curve Weiersrtass equation is involved a child domain of finite field $GF(q^n)$ when using the curve. Therefore, generally referred them as "subdomain curve", also known as special curve [5]. For subdomain curve, the generally required n in the field $GF(q^n)$ is a prime number so as to enhance security.

Selecting subdomain curve to construct cryptosystem has the following two advantages:

(1) It is easily to calculate stair of elliptic curve finite group $E(GF(q^n))$ so that we can more easily to find suitable n, which makes $\#E(GF(q^n))$ contain a big prime number factor.
(2) This scalar multiplication number group operation is easily to proceed on the elliptic curve.

But, choosing this seed domain curve also has the following two shortcomings:

(1) This curve is too few.
Such for the Koblitz curveE_1, Just when taken n as 3, 5, 7, 11.17, 23, 101, 109, 163, 283, 311, 331, 359, $\#E_1(GF(2^n))$ is the product of 2 with a prime number. But for the Koblitz curveE_2, Just when take n as 5, 7, 13, 19, 23, 41, 97, 103.107, 131, 233, 239, 277, 283, 349, 409, $\#E_2(GF(2^n))$ is the product of 4 with a prime number.
(2) People's security concerns
Safety concerns that there are two main aspects:

On the one hand, people fear that the special structure of the curve is likely to become the breach of the attacker, so elliptic curve cryptosystem based on the curve has less security.

On the other hand, due to the amount of the curve are limited, which makes it possible that some special structures make a special attack to concreted every curves, and the repeated use of the same curve might also provides a large number of available data for the attacker.

Therefore, through the analysis of this article, in the packet network communication, we should tend to choose the ideal security elliptic curve that generated randomly, and construct the elliptic curve cryptosystem.

281.10 Conclusion

The innovation of the paper: after this paper summarised and concluded all kinds of solutions for safety elliptic curve algorithm problems, then given the two selection principles on the secure elliptic curve, On the basis of analyzing and comparing the several possible secure elliptic curves, identified the ideal secure elliptic curve, which is used to construct safe elliptic curve public key password system in packet network communication.

References

1. Chen L, Bian Z-Z, WeiLi G (2002) The applications of elliptic curve public key cryptosystem in the security e-commerce. Comput Eng 5
2. Shann CE (1949) Communication theory of secrecy systems. BellSystemTecnhiclaJournla 28(4):656–715

3. Li X-J, Jing Z-L, Dai G-Z (2002) Public key cryptography based on elliptic curve discrete logarithm problem. Comput Eng Appl 6:20–22
4. Wang J-M, Liu J-M (1999) Communication network security theory and technology. Xidian University press, Xi'an
5. Yu X (2007) Micro-processing structure research of special command block cipher. Microcomput Inf 9:84–86

Chapter 282
Improvement of Medical Imaging Course by Modeling of Positron Emission Tomography

Huiting Qiao, Libin Wang, Wenyong Liu, Yu Wang, Shuyu Li, Fang Pu and Deyu Li

Abstract With the development of nuclear medical imaging, the medical imaging course has been developed in Beihang University. As an important part of nuclear medical imaging, Positron Emission Tomography (PET) is introduced in the imaging course with the methods of modeling and simulation. Phamacokinetics model, Monte Carlo N-Particle Transport Code (MCNP) and Visible Human Project (VHP) datasets have been used to simulate the principle of PET imaging, which have made students understand the course more easily. The method that integrates imaging and modeling is potential and effective in the interdisciplinary teaching.

Keywords Imaging · Modeling · Simulation · Education

282.1 Introduction

As a discipline of interdisciplinary nature, Biomedical engineering (BME) aims to understand physiology and medicine, and to solve the problem by using engineering principles. Though the major course varies according to the education target of each university [1, 2], the biomedical imaging course is always of the core course [3]. With the development of nuclear medicine, positron emission tomography (PET) appears in the course of medical imaging as a new imaging mode. Unlike X-ray, CT and other traditional image methods, PET has a complicated imaging process and involves the random decay of radionuclide. Therefore the biomedical imaging course was developed in Beihang University.

H. Qiao · L. Wang · W. Liu · Y. Wang · S. Li · F. Pu · D. Li (✉)
School of Biological Science and Medical Engineering, Beihang University,
Beijing 100191, China
e-mail: deyuli@buaa.edu.cn

Besides imaging, modeling and simulation is also a major course of biomedical engineering education in Beihang University, aiming to describe physiological systems and biomedical process quantitatively. They are the important methods and widely used in research. In education of medicine, modeling and simulation play an role [4, 5], so do they in biomedical engineering. In Johns Hopkins University, simplified modeling experiments have been used to introduce the research fields of BME to freshmen [6]. For researches of medical imaging, models are also effective methods. Thus, we tried to use modeling and simulation to develop the biomedical imaging course. This study may enrich the education of BME.

282.2 The Application of Models in Nuclear Medical Imaging Education

As functional imaging, PET is an indispensable part of medical imaging education. The complex imaging process of PET includes: (1) the transport of radiation tracer in body, (2) the decay of the radiation tracer, (3) the transport of pairs of photon, (4) the detection of photon, and (5) the reconstruction of 3D image. To improve the understanding of the imaging process, modeling and simulation have been used as follow.

282.2.1 The Model for the Transport of Radiation Tracer

For imaging education, the foundation of imaging and the diagnosis criterion are significant. Simplified model could help students to understand. Positron Emission Tomography (PET) can realize the dynamic observation of metabolic process in vivo by using radionuclide as tracer. Injected into the body, the tracer could participate in some physiological metabolic process, and distribute in different part of the body. Since the tracer metabolism is the foundation of PET imaging [7], the pharmacokinetic model, known as compartment model [8], has been involved to medical imaging education. By using the model, the tracer metabolism in different tissue could be compared. For example, the tracer's time-concentration curve in cancer could be received by model simulation, and be contrasted with that of normal tissue. With the comparison of tracer's time-concentration curve, it is easy to understand when could be optimal imaging schedule.

282.2.2 The Simulation of the Tracer Decay and Photon Transmission

Before detected, the distributed tracer could emit positron, produce pairs of photon, pass through the tissue, and then reach the detector outside. The whole process is stochastic. Monte Carlo simulation is a better way to introduce the stochastic nuclear imaging process [9]. Monte Carlo N-Particle Transport Code (MCNP), developed by Los Alamos National Laboratory, is used to describe the transport of photon in complicated situation. As a tool to simulate nuclear processes, MCNP can also be used in nuclear medicine imaging course to depict the imaging process. In the simulation of MCNP, the complex structure of body is presented by simple geometric structure, the random decay and scattering is described by probability, and the transport character in different tissue is depicted according to photon-cross-section database. The complex process has been described by model with MCNP, and simulated with computer. Though the simulated results are rough, the simulation process can be understood more easily than before.

282.2.3 The Simulation of Reconstructed PET Images

Not only the process of imaging, but also the influence of imaging parameters should be included in medical imaging course. Reconstructed PET images have been simulated on the base of Visible Human Project (VHP) [10], a detailed anatomic model of human. The simulation help students recognize the difference of reconstructed PET images with varied imaging parameters. The tracer kinetic model and VHP datasets compose a simulation platform of PET images, on which the influence of radiation dose, imaging time, scan duration and resolution could be simulated. Firstly, we obtained a sequence of concentration of radiation tracer in each tissue with the tracer kinetic model. Secondly, the certain time concentration of tracer was translated into activity value in unit voxel. Then, the noise, according to the scan duration, was added to the activity value. At last the activity value with noise was assigned to form the simulated images. Finally, the volume rendering method was used to represent the assigned VHP data in 3D views. On the simulation platform, students could modify the imaging parameters, and observe the varieties of simulated images. It makes the teaching process easier to understand.

282.3 Teaching Methods and Assessment

The syllabus of medical imaging has been modified since 2011 in Beihang University. PET, as the example of nuclear medical imaging, has been included.

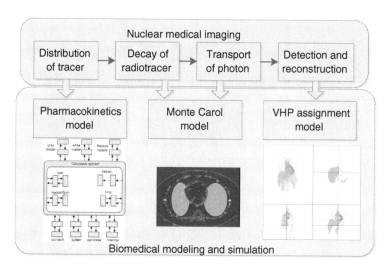

Fig. 282.1 The relation between two important BME courses

Some biomedical models and simulation form a demonstration platform of nuclear medical imaging, which come from the biomedical modeling and simulation courses.

The content of PET imaging highlights the principle and the imaging process. The imaging process is divided into four steps. For each step, there is a model to explain the principle, as shown in Fig. 282.1. It is not only the support for imaging course, but also the application of modeling and simulation that could be seen in this teaching study. The interdisciplinary teaching has integrated the techniques of imaging and modeling. In this way, students are likely to form an interdisciplinary view and a better understand of nuclear medical imaging.

282.4 Conclusion and Discussion

Since biomedical engineering is a fast developing discipline, the courses of BME should be improved constantly. The medical imaging course has been developed in the school of biological Science and medical Engineering at Beihang University. Nuclear medical imaging has become one of the contents in medical imaging course. To help the students understand, a simulation platform was established with three models, pharmacokinetic model, MCNP model and VHP data mapping model. The simulation platform has been used to demonstrate the principle of PET imaging and received good response.

The development of the imaging course not only strengthens students' understanding of the imaging principle, but also improves the comprehension of models' application. In traditional curriculum system, courses are usually taught independently, although there are so many interaction. This study is the experiments of combined teaching module in imaging course. The combined teaching module could spread out in other biomedical engineering courses. The combined teaching module focuses on one special problem including more than one technique. For example, to develop the comprehension of sphygmomanometer, some content of physiology, modeling, medical sensor, medical electronics and other courses may be united. This module may gives students an overall view of a special biomedical problem.

As shown in this study, modeling and simulation could be used to enhance the education of medical imaging. The association of multiple course education may benefit more to interdisciplinary education.

Acknowledgments This work was supported by the National Natural Science Foundation of China (No. 81101123, No. 61108084), Fundamental Research Funds for the Central Universities of China and Education development Project of Beihang University.

References

1. Kourennyi DE, Sankovic JM (2002) Interdisciplinary skills development in the biomedical engineering laboratory course. Montreal, Que., Canada, pp 1585–1592
2. Saterbak A, San K-Y, McIntire LV (2001) Development of a novel foundation course for biomedical engineering curriculum. Albuquerque, NM, United states, pp 3733–3738
3. Chan KL (2000) Biomedical engineering course at the City University of Hong Kong, in engineering in medicine and biology society 2000. In: Proceedings of the 22nd annual international conference of the IEEE, 2000, vol 1. pp 741–743
4. Demir SS Velipasaoglu EO (2003) Simulation-based education and training resource: iCell, in information technology applications in biomedicine, 2003. In: 4th international IEEE EMBS special topic conference on, 2003, pp 106–109
5. Demir SS (2004) An interactive electrophysiology training resource for simulation-based teaching and learning, in engineering in medicine and biology society, 2004. In: IEMBS '04. 26th annual international conference of the IEEE, 2004, pp 5169–5171
6. Wong WC, Haase EB (2010) A course guideline for biomedical engineering modeling and design for freshmen. College Park, MD, United states, pp 56–60
7. Townsend DW (2004) Physical principles and technology of clinical PET imaging, Annals of the Academy of Medicine. Singapore 33:133–145
8. Hays MT, Segall GM (1999) A mathematical model for the distribution of fluorodeoxyglucose in humans. J Nucl Med 40:1358–1366
9. Jan S, Collot J, Gallin-Martel ML, Martin P, Mayet F, Tournefier E (2005) GePEToS: a Geant4 Monte Carlo simulation package for positron emission tomography. IEEE Trans Nucl Sci 52:102–106
10. Bai J, Qiao H (2011) Dynamic simulation of FDG-PET image based on VHP datasets. In: 2011 5th IEEE/ICME international confererce on complex medical engineering, CME 2011, Harbin, China, 2011, 22–25 May 2011 pp 154–158

Chapter 283
The Research of Management System in Sports Anatomy Based on the Network Technology

Hong Liu, Dao-lin Zhang, Xiao-mei Zhan, Xiao-mei Zeng and Fei Yu

Abstract Using network technology, combined with the current problem of Sport Anatomy Experiment, the design of experiment management system which based on the structure of B/S, including students, teacher, educational administration and virtual simulation are proposed to improve the teaching quality of Sports Anatomy, enhance the practical ability of students and achieve the Network management of experimental class.

Keywords ASP · The database of SQL · Structure of B/S · Virtual experiment · Sports anatomy

283.1 Introduction

Sports Anatomy is one of the compulsory courses for students majoring in Physical Education, which includes two parts of the theoretical teaching and experimental teaching. Under the influence of traditional education idea, Sports Anatomy experimental teaching is often neglected, being the "tail" and "subsidiary" of the theoretic teaching [1]. Many sport professional institutions which lacked in experimental anatomy teachers, laboratory equipment scarce and the unreasonable circumstances for experimental class schedule, have serious impact on the overall teaching quality of the Sports Anatomy. For a long time, utilization rate of laboratory is low, due to using just in the experiment conditions.

H. Liu (✉) · D. Zhang · X. Zhan · X. Zeng · F. Yu
Institute of Physical Education, Jiangxi Normal University, No. 99 Ziyang Avenue,
Nanchang 330027 Jiangxi, China
e-mail: 15079046089@163.com

H. Liu · D. Zhang · X. Zhan · X. Zeng · F. Yu
Institute of Physical Education, East China Institute of Technology, Nanchang 330013
Jiangxi, China

meanwhile, the experimental class has so much people that they mainly observe and cannot play for their autonomy and innovation potential [2]. To solve the problem in the experimental teaching of anatomy and improve the quality of experiment teaching and students' innovation ability in practice, the study targeted to design a kind of network teaching management system, and make the use of modern information technology of anatomy open experiment teaching guidance.

283.2 Technologies on the Design of Experiment Education Management System on Sport Anatomy

283.2.1 B/S Three-Layer Architecture

Browser/Web Server (B/S) architecture is a Web technology-based system platform mode, which makes the server part of the traditional C/S mode be decomposition of a data server and one or more application servers (Web server), and then constitutes a three-layer structure of the client–server system. Web client make a first connect with the Web server via the HTTP protocol, and request the Web server by the browser, finally the Web server processes the results output to the browser. The advantages of B/S structure:

1. Simplified the client-side by installing generic browser software.
2. Cross-platform operating system based on B/S structure, users on a variety of platforms can access information through a browser, as the browser and the Web server software can support a variety of platforms, and unified communication protocol is used.
3. Uniform standards and simplified development and maintenance system. Using the B/S mode, development work can be concentrated to the server, and only the server-side application development and maintenance are needed, which greatly reduced the cost of software maintenance and upgrade.
4. B/S structure makes the user's operation simpler. the client have only a simple, easy-to-use browser software, while the browser provides a unified, friendly and easy-to-use interface and users can used directly without training [3].

B/S architecture closely integrated network technology, creating the experiment management system of the B/S structure in school LAN may make different staff from different locations with different access methods (such as LAN, WAN, Internet/Intranet, etc.) access and manipulate a common database, and effectively protect data platform, manage access rights and maintenance security of the database server.

283.2.2 ASP and SQL Server

ASP is a powerful web development tool. Based on DCOM (Distributed DCOM), which makes that framework program can be performed in a distributed manner on a local or network, combining with a dynamic, interactive Web server applications of HTML Web page, the script (Script) program, ActiveX establishment and implementation. The users through the ASP access the database, the Web server calls the ASP engine to establish the connection to the database, then the database will check the legality of the request and perform the appropriate SQL commands, and the result set is returned to the HTML page to the Web server in response to user requests. Because of its running in the server and the users' browser are receiving a standard HTML page, so it can support a variety of browsers. To achieve the workflow service and maintenance of various kinds of information with the Web server and take advantage of powerful data processing and security management functions of the relational database for data processing and user rights management and access through ODBC. In addition, the ActiveX component can extend its function by combination of ASP and ADO component, and access to the database can be easier.

Seen from Fig. 283.1, the entire system will combine the advantages of different platforms. ASP web programming and SQL Server database technology, which not only can complete document workflow, interactive communication, information sharing and query functions etc., the function of the SQL Server database can also be used to record laboratory data, equipment and experimental condition as well as users' access rights assignment [4].

283.2.3 Virtual Experiment System

As combination of described above ASP and SQL development system, a virtual laboratory platform client-side will be built, the different resources of the system by database technology be linked, and virtual experiment system with Flash animation software for sport anatomical experimental class be created. The collection and processing of the experimental material are made by sport anatomy teachers in accordance with all aspects of the experimental teaching requirements: the experimental specimens or map shoot by digital cameras and scanners and other

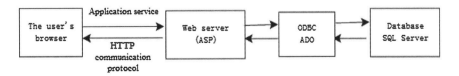

Fig. 283.1 ASP access database [7]

equipment from different angles (15° angle every turn) and scanning the movement image of the system, and then the image material are carried out after Photoshopes3 software batch processing, and classified and stored in the material library as the name and chapter, so that developers can create virtual three-dimensional simulation animation, finally released synthetic animated films to SWF file, which are named by the pre-established coding requirements, and combined SWF files together by database technology to form a complete virtual experiments [5, 6].

283.3 Design of Sports Anatomy Experimental Teaching Management System

To meet experiment management and teaching requirements of open network education system, The Sports Anatomy experimental class management system designed the management system that shown in Fig. 283.2. The system is divided into four parts, which are students' window, teachers' window, window for educational administration and virtual experiments. And public function of the system can be modified in the password including each account login. And the message, questions can be left and asked in the teacher-student interaction platform.

283.3.1 Students' Window

Students with their student number and password enter into the student window interface after successful authentication, which is made of several pages and each page is relatively independent. The left side of the page shows the personal information of Log in students and the function menu. In addition to the common functions, the students' window includes query and elective. That's to say, students can query the semester pilot projects in place of experimental (laboratory), as well as completion of the pilot of the experimental arrangement after the results of the query. If the experiment did not pass, the message will be displayed next to the experimental results and the student number will be locked before the start of the program. Then teachers will arrange the experiment according to the number. But students can transfer courses and changes prior to this. Students can see other student elective experimental period in a pilot project, and can also view the arrangements of the various experiments in the next two weeks, which includes the number of remaining optional of each projects at a time, while an experimental unit is selected fully or experiment with the unit teachers locked and cannot be elective, then the unit will display the number of course full. That means you cannot select any more. But if selection of the student has not been locked, which can be modified again. According to the published experimental projects arranged

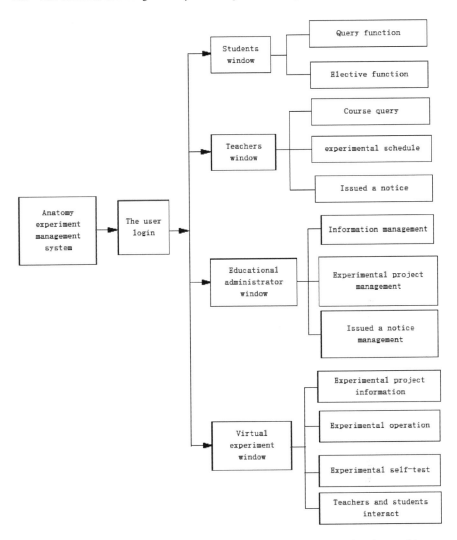

Fig. 283.2 Sports anatomy experimental course management system function architecture diagram

by the teachers, students can have several experimental projects appointment. After all the optional selections are submitted, elective course record is saved to the database.

283.3.2 Teacher Window

Teachers through a login screen, with their own job number and password log into the window. In addition to public functions, the arrangement of the experimental time course of query and issued notices included. According to the arrangement of educational administration at the scheduled weeks, teachers can make their own arrangements of specific experimental time, and the number of students accommodated each time period. To a certain extent, you can lock the time period of the full number. If the number of students during a certain time period not achieves the basic number of commencement of the experiment, the student election can be cancelled. Or else be locked in this time period. Teachers can also publish a notice and scores input of students, statistics and publication, and modify or delete the issued notices.

283.3.3 Educational Administration Windows

Educational administrators select the administrator access to the system management interface through the same interface, which can manage information for students, and being registered by the administrator can the student enter the experimental course, query, modify the password of students and help students to retrieve password. For the teacher Information Management, new experimental teachers can be added and register. Arrangement of experimental project as well as teachers account for providing the password to modify and restore be designed. arrangement of all open experiment teaching, the arrangement of the laboratory, the limited number of students each time, and the introduction to experiment project, experiment requirements and test report been submitted are conducted by the administrator on the per semester.

283.3.4 Virtual Experiment Windows

Both of Students and teachers can login the virtual experiment window through their account number and password, select virtual simulation of the corresponding experimental project. Login to the interface, several features choice of experimental projects can be seen, experimental project information including name of the experimental project, experimental requirements, and experimental appliances, etc.), experimental operation, self-test, teachers and students interact. According to their own requirements, students select the experimental project, a preliminary understanding of its requirements, objectives and experimental tools, and then perform the experiment, invoke Flash animation files, conduct virtual simulation, press, drag and move the mouse to the operation object, zoom, rotate, turn left and right and click "Play" to play the animation, so students can observe the specimens from different angles to identify the various parts and click "Stop" to stop the playback. Click on the "Names of parts" the animation specimens of the site name and a description can be watched until the experiment be familiar with, then click "Exit" to exit this experiment. After own experimental self-testing, exchange of consultation or message your questions can be done through an interactive platform online for teachers and students.

283.4 The Superiority of Sports Anatomy Experiment Network System Management

For students, Sports anatomy experiment network system management facilitate the query of experiment, make the students more freedom in time course arrangement, and make project selection and evaluation of experiments more flexible. Only simply login at ordinary times, the virtual simulation system can be carried out to the experimental operation and self test, the problems can be consulted online or leave a message to ask questions to teachers in teachers and students interact. For teachers and educational administrators, through platform management, the network of teaching plan, students basic information, experiment arrangements, experiment grade etc. can be done by manual into the computer management; and the workload of experimental teaching be reduced at maximum. Virtual simulation experiment also effectively relieves in school funding, sites, equipment apparatus and difficulty and pressure should be faced.

Based on B/S structure of design for the sports anatomy experimental teaching management system, which improves the quality of sports anatomy experiment teaching and the students' practice ability and realize the network management of the LABS, and deepen the teaching reform, the only way to solve the contradictions between learning and teaching, and have a good prospects to be widely used. However, virtual simulation experiment cannot be touched so that there is certain difference in tangible operation, therefore the combination of traditional anatomy virtual simulation experiment teaching and network teaching will be more beneficial to improve the teaching quality of sports anatomy.

References

1. Li H, Liang Y, Zhu Y et al (2012) Network open experiment booking management system based on B/S structure. Exp Sci Technol
2. Liu X, Chen H, Jiang S et al (2011) Constructing acoustics teaching experiment center under a new concept of open innovation. Exp Technol Manage
3. Qiao Y, Lu X, Zhang H et al (2008) Innovation and practice of sports anatomy experiment's curriculum system and teaching mode. Shanxi Normal University Institute of Physical Education

4. Sun W (2006) Design and implementation of B/S-based administration system of students' results. Anhui Institute of Education
5. Xu X, Han Z, Liu H et al (2012) Talk about in the anatomy experiment teaching of construction and application of the network virtual experiment system. Educ Explor
6. Zhang T, Chen X, Zhang Y et al (2007) Design and application of the virtual laboratory of the regional anatomy. Anatomy
7. Zhang Y (2006) Construction of open laboratory management system based on campus network. China Mod Educ Equip

Chapter 284
Innovation of Compiler Theory Course for CDIO

Wang Na and Wu YuePing

Abstract Compiler theory course is a very important compulsory basic course in professional computer education, and it is also an important branch in the computer system software. But the practice of this course is lack or immature especially in CDIO education. And the curriculum need be reformed since it is unreasonable for CDIO education. In our paper, we propose a new innovation of compiler theory course which combine theory and practice and divide compiler into two levels: compiler technology and compiler theory. The result showed that the using of new teaching method and curriculum are effective in compiler theory teaching.

Keywords Compiler · Innovation · CDIO · Practice · Curriculum

284.1 Introduction

CDIO engineering education is the latest achievement of international engineering education reform in recent years. CDIO represents Conceive, Design, Implement and Operate. If engineering colleges want to meet the CDIO engineering education model and improve the practice and innovation capability of engineering graduates, first and foremost task is to strengthen the practice of teaching.

With the rapid development of higher education in our country, there has been a complete and special education system. In fact, teaching could achieve a combination of theory and practice, book knowledge and practical application, and hands-brain combination [2].

W. Na (✉) · W. YuePing
Shanghai Second Polytechnic University, Shanghai, People's Republic of China
e-mail: wnoffice@126.com

W. YuePing
e-mail: ypwu@sspu.cn

284.2 Current Situation of Compiler Theory Course

Compiler technology course is a very important compulsory basic course in professional computer education, and it is also an important branch in the computer system software. The main teaching objective of compiler technology is making students re-understand algorithms and programs on the level of system to enhance the students' system capacity. It is the most difficult course in computer professional courses covering both formal language and abstract automata theory. It is also a comprehensive reflection of knowledge including data structure, programming languages, algorithms and software design.

In recent years, the comment of college graduates from employment sector is good, they think that the university graduates are active, full of passion, good at English and computer application, and know more about new developments in science and technology. However, there are also problems that some students who divorced from reality and just have high scores but less ability to solve practical problems. The same problem exists in the teaching process of complier theory.

284.3 Course Reform for CDIO

284.3.1 Teaching Method

Firstly, we start with the internal structure of the knowledge system to seize the internal relations and laws of the various functional stages of the compilation process, using meaningful questions to guide students' positive thinking. Disclose theoretical difficulties and abstract concepts in compiler theory by presenting problems to students. By answering questions from different perspectives, students can seek the principle and means to solve problems, thus guiding students to independently analysis and solve problem, deepening the understanding of compiler theory and technology.

Compiler theory is a strong theoretical course. In order to visualize abstract problems to facilitate students to understand and apply knowledge points, the use of multimedia tools can present principle knowledge in the form of animation, graphics to transform static to dynamic, teach through lively activities to stimulate students' interest in learning. The effect is as Fig. 284.1.

In order to provide large number of exercises for students to review, we also use Web-based Collaborative Teaching Model which is the process of utilizing the computer network and multimedia technology to let different learners to interact and cooperate on the same learning content in order to make the students have a deeper understanding and better command of the courses.

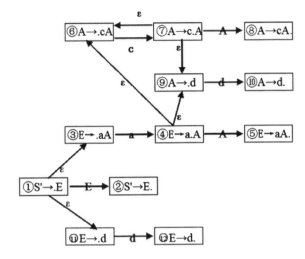

Fig. 284.1 The multimedia interface of compiler theory course

284.3.2 Course Curriculum

In consideration the character of CDIO, we must take practice into account when configure the content of compiler theory course. We divide compiler into two levels: compiler technology and compiler theory. Compiler theory is set as an optional course emphasis on deep content introducing formalized principle for students interesting in compiler. While compiler technology introduced the basic methods and techniques to meet basic application and requires, then achieving the purpose of language transfer.

In theory-based teaching part, we introduce knowledge about compiler theory including automata, regular expression and the conversion method between regular expression and automata. And we introduce technology through the whole compiler process such as lexical analysis, parse and the syntax-directed method of compiling. During the procedure, there may be some new concept, for example syntax tree, NFA, DFA etc.

In projects-based experiments part, the two types of projects are validation experiments and comprehensive experiments. The former is tied in with the content of classroom instruction that is compiled by teachers according to the original rationale taught order to sync certain confirmatory experimental subject, allowing students to complete related sub-module one by one by either coding or tool, and gradually expanding to improve the entire compiler. The step-by-step method not only increases the sense of accomplishment and self-confidence of the students, but also enables them to develop a solid basis. It can also stimulate students' interest and enthusiasm in learning.

Certain scale comprehensive design experiment is essential to ensure the effect of practice. We design projects about compiler technology programming carefully. Students will be divided into several groups according to students and their topics

Table 284.1 Score statics

Score segment	90–100 %	80–89 %	70–79 %	60–69 %	0–59 %	Excellent rate %	Pass rate %	Average score
Normal score	3/3.3	54/59.3	28/30.8	2/2.2	4/4.4	3.3 (3/91)	95.6 (87/91)	77.67
Terminal score	2/2.2	7/7.6	22/23.9	27/29.3	34/37	2.2 (2/92)	63 (58/92)	60.5
Overall score	1/1.1	12/13.2	28/30.8	36/39.6	14/15.4	1.1 (1/91)	84.6 (77/91)	66.47

of interest. Students selected the leader of each team. Each leader is equivalent to project manager, and is responsible for the entire software project organization and coordination. Each member should put forward their own ideas and views of other team members to evaluate by listening to special reports, documentation, inspection, such as aspect, and then by the team leader determine the group's research projects.

284.3.3 Development of Teachers' Ability

Practical ability of teachers is directly the effect of practice teaching. Therefore, in order to do a good job in the practice teaching, there must be excellent teachers with practical skills and strengthen the professional capacity of teachers. We must focus on doing the following things in developing teachers' practical ability:

First, let young teachers take turns to industrial and mining enterprises for some time to receive training and practice and improve their project quality. And select some large state owned enterprises to develop some bases for young teachers' training.

Second, build a team of teachers who are "Double Type"(teachers and engineers). Schools should encourage teachers to take part-time jobs in enterprises and support them to take part in educational conference, therefore they can improve their skills and learn new experiences from experts of famous university.

Third, if the number of teachers in current practice teaching is inadequate, schools could also create part-time teachers who come from enterprises with professional practical experience or skills.

Teachers also should insist on a combination of teaching and research, cite the latest scientific research and education reform into teaching and combine classical compiler theory with organically modern compiler technology. For example, we can introduce embedded compiler, timed automata, distributed parallel compilers, and multi-core compiler to enrich compiler theory courses. In addition, we can also introduce the specific applications of compiler technology in artificial intelligent, parallel computing, and natural language processing to foreshadow the subsequent courses.

284.4 Conclusions

With the application of new configure and method in compiler theory course, the effect of study improve a lot as shown in Table 284.1. The pass rate is up to 95.6 % and the excellent rate is 15.4 % which is a serious progress comparing with the score of last term.

Practice teaching is an important part of the process of personnel training and it is the key for higher education to achieve the objectives. Engineering colleges in

China must continuously deepen the CDIO engineering education model, target personnel training, increase funding for practice teaching, and strengthen the teacher team.

Web-based teaching method and project-based experiments has been put into practice to solve realistic problems like lack of practice in theory-based course. Teachers use flexible methods to induct content and lead students to think, discover and practice by themselves. Through several years' experience, students can not only master principle theories in compiler technology but also complement a compiler in groups.

References

1. Dongyong Y (2009) Return to engineering: education reform to foster applied innovative software talents. In: Proceedings of 2009 4th international conference on computer science and education, 2009
2. Qidi Wu (2007) Reform and development of China higher engineering education[J]. Chin High Educ Eval (Chin) 2007(4):3–7
3. Chengcheng Z, Shiying G (2011) A Survey on the outline of national long-term education reform and development plan. Paper presented at the IEEE 3rd international conference on communication coftware and networks (ICCSN), 2011
4. Hong D, ChuanYin Z (2011) Discussions on the reform of higher vocational education from training the IT students' occupational ability. Paper presented at the international conference on E-business and E-government (ICEE). 2011
5. Xiao M, Hu G (2010) Research on reform of computer elementary education in University. Paper presented at the Second International workshop on Education technology and computer science (ETCS). 2010

Chapter 285
The Design and Implementation of Web-Based E-Learning System

Chunjie Hou and Chuanmu Li

Abstract The Web-based E-learning System overcomes time and space limitations in traditional universities. Teachers and students are now accessing to large amounts of information and resources via the web. In this paper, we provide a learning model of Web-based system, which is based on the principles of constructivism, to provide motivation and collaborative learning for students in the Web environment. The practical results show that the system is mainly to complete the autonomous learning, including learning resource management, grading test, students' management, unit test, etc. and it is proved that the system is effective and useful.

Keywords Web-based · Learning · E-learning system

285.1 Introduction

In view of the Internet being able to overcome the space and time barriers of learning, people have started to think about the process of integrating this information technology with teaching and teaching materials, there by, the establishment of Web-based learning system as the basis of the educational environment is flourishing. With the assistance of software and hardware facilities, people are able to have a breakthrough in the various limitations of time, environment and distance, and adequately use abundant learning resources to extend the educational activities, create a "timely and appropriate" learning environment for the

---

C. Hou (✉)
School of Foreign Language, Jimei University, 361021 Xiamen, People's Republic of China
e-mail: cjhou@jmu.edu.cn

C. Li
College of Computer Engineer, Jimei University, 361021 Xiamen, People's Republic of China
e-mail: cm@jmu.edu.cn

"appropriate persons", and also allow Web-learning to become an integral part of a diverse education [1–5]. Internet technology has brought a new look of learning concepts and redesigning of learning strategies to educationists, and proceeds to develop a learning environment that verifies learning concepts and provides opportunities for learning strategies [6]. Internet technology can be used for teaching activities, and become the main form of teaching in the future.

285.2 System Architecture

The system covers the course teaching plan, scheduling, and outcome based teaching and learning objectives. It consists of the project assignment, review and tutorial questions, hands-on and E-learning exercises, and references etc. The Grade web page is to list out students' grades for each submitted assignment. The open forum is for students to communicate with each other and the lecturers for general discussion on the lecture. The system architecture is shown in Fig. 285.1.

In the E-learning system, every web page contains a header and a navigation bar; the consistency layout enables the user to easily browse the web site without getting lost. It is good for both search engine optimization and the accessibility of the users who use the screen readers.

In each course, lesson notes, written notes, references, review questions, tutorial questions, hands-on and E-learning exercises are all put into the web for students to review and comprehend.

For teachers, after logging on, they can view student information, release public notices, give assignments and answer questions. There are six functional modules, i.e. teaching materials management, pubic notice management, program content management, student information management, assignment management and answers to questions. Instead of uploading and downloading the files from the web site and local drive for each update, the system provides an easy way for teachers to change the content of the website so as to make the website more user-friendly. For students who will be the end users, they can download lesson notes, written notes, references, review questions and tutorial questions from the web site.

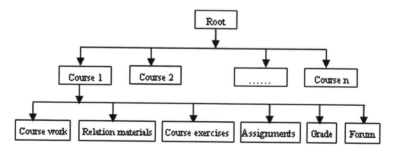

Fig. 285.1 The architecture of the Web-based system

For students, they can register, logon, test themselves, upload assignments, practice, and so on. In order to achieve different learning goals for different degrees of students, more levels of courses can be elaborately designed by teachers. Each level of courses contains several lectures and literature readings to train students' skills. Students can choose the appropriate lecture according to their own learning pace. Once a student accomplishes the objectives of a course, he can write a refection or an essay composition and turn it in online through an upload interface. Subsequently, the teacher can correct it or give feedbacks. Teacher can give a general plan whether for a certain teaching or learning period, while students can find the related web pages to learn and complete the assignments. All the learning process can be recorded by means of learning duration and submitted answers for teacher assessment.

For exercises, self-assessment tool in our system is designed to evaluate the learning efficiency of students. Several types of exercises, such as listening exercise, cloze exercise, and choice exercise, are designed as specific lecture material. The questions for different types of exercise are prepared beforehand by the teacher and stored in the Exercise pages. We provide a Web-based management interface to generate questions by teachers for different types of exercise. The functions in this management tool include the creation of a new question and re-editing an existing question.

If a student wants to do an exercise, he can choose the type of exercise and the number of questions for this exercise. The system will retrieve the questions randomly from exercise repository to generate the exercise. After he finishes the exercise and submits the answers, the answer to each question will be checked and the score will be shown to him. The exercise information, including the type of exercise, questions of exercise, student's answers to exercise, and score of exercise, will be recorded for the evaluation of the student's learning efficiency. Additionally, the statistics of answers to each question can be further analyzed and provide as a clue for teachers to determine the difficulty of each question.

For the test subsystem, a great number of students can access the system online concurrently with great stability and usability and teachers or researchers can easily diagnose the learning condition from those students. The system is divided into the client side and server side for different purposes. On the client side, a friendly User Interface is designed as a learning environment to collect students' answer texts. Students are asked to produce their ideas and answers to each question, and then fill them in divided answer cells. The test subsystem is designed to be more structured with explicit identification of divergent and convergent thinking so that the answers are easier to be processed by computers. When the test paper is designed, teacher can set the timer. When students begin taking the test, they have to finish it in limited time. And teacher can also choose to provide the correct answer right after students submitting theirs or a day or a week later. All the records of students' performance can be downloaded for teacher assessment.

In order to encourage peer-to-peer learning, a forum is put on the web site for students to discuss problems and solution among themselves. They can also ask teachers on the courses. The forum applies blogging system so that students are free to append their comments to each particular course that they are interested in. Security needs to be implemented to block non-students intruders who may erase the blog messages.

285.3 Conclusion and Future Work

The system has been implemented in our university to which all students in our university have access. In this system, we analyzed the current state of the e-learning system. Then we proposed a functional model of an e-learning environment. In developing and testing the system for its online use, the management tools are good for managing online courses and self-assessment questions, and it is easy to use. The assessment tool is also well-done to create exercise more conveniently and to evaluate their achievement of courses by self-assessment. The system has been a very helpful online tutor for different course teaching/learning.

Web Services provide a standard means of communication among different software applications, running on a variety of platforms and/or frameworks. We can use Web Services technology to implement the interoperability on different platforms. There are many challenges for implementing such an e-learning system because Web Services and E-learning standards are all newly-emerged technologies and are undergoing changes and developments. The security of Services, the encryption of messages, and the common taxonomies to describe Services and service access points in E-learning systems environments are all in need of consideration.

In next step, we will keep improving user interface of the management tools which are frequently used by teachers and students.

References

1. Yu Z-J, Lin X-T,Yuan X-M (2005) The famework of Web-based versatile brainstorming system. Paper presented at the global Chinese conference of computers in education (GCCCE), pp 502–510 2005
2. Na R (2008) A research into the online education interactive system. Mode Distance Edu Res 1:62–64
3. Ling X, Ma W (2009) The research of blending leading of web2.0 based College English. E-educ Res, vol 06
4. Botchy L, Cankering P (2010) On the impact of formal methods in the SOA. Electron Notes Theor Comput Sci 160:113–126
5. Erming L (2012) Basic principles and mode of multimedia network teaching design. Mod Distance Educ 2:47–50
6. Alva M (2008) Computer-mediated collaborative learning: an empirical evaluation. MIS Q 18:159–174

Chapter 286
Complex System Ensuring Outstanding Student Research Training in Private Universities

YueYu Xu

Abstract Improving the quality of education is always a key consideration in the universities. Especially for the private universities which focus more in the students, setting up a training system for outstanding students is a promising and interesting task. In this paper, an information technology based outstanding student training programme, which includes training objectives, organizational structure, core curriculum courses, teaching staff, support policies, learning and self-management and other aspects, are presented.

Keywords Information technology · Private universities · Outstanding students · Quality of education · Training programme

286.1 Introduction

According to "2011 the National Educational Development Statistics Bulletin" released by Ministry of Education the end of 2011. The enrolment of general undergraduate students reaches 23.0851 million, while private colleges and universities college now have 5.0507 million full time students. It is observed that the student in private colleges or universities are hosting 21.9 % students, which is a consideration part of students can not be ignored [1].

Compared with public universities, the lack of excellent students and teachers greatly impact the quality of education in the private colleges. However, improving the quality of education is of great importance for the enrolment of

---

Y. Xu (✉)
Department of Fundamental Education, Zhejiang Shuren University, Hangzhou, People's Republic of China
e-mail: xyy.zjsru@gmail.com

students and consequently, the income of tuition fee of the universities. The improvement of the quality of education is therefore a critical factor in the survival and development of private colleges.

286.2 Outline of the Programme

The target of this training programme is to develop the type of talent and its specifications as well as quality requirements. Based on the school's practice, the programme is designed for general education-oriented but high-level application-oriented talents within the overall goal of training excellent students of private universities.

The characteristic of this outstanding student-training programme lies in a general education instead of "professional" defects, which widely implemented in current private colleges. The goal in this outstanding student-training programme in private colleges and universities is to improve the quality of students in terms in general education.

286.3 Educational Resources

It is necessary to re-set and enhance the general education curriculum-based in private colleges and universities to support this outstanding student-training programme. Overall, the curriculum includes specialised courses and general education courses.

The organization of curriculum of this programme is also owned by the colleges or departments respectively. These courses are in accordance with professional standards organization outstanding graduates of the teaching. The most important characteristic or the difference of this training programme lies the general education. In this new general education curriculum, the education of science and art are both emphasized, which constantly improves the technological literacy of students in liberal arts and science and engineering students in the human spirit. It is necessary to set up "literature and art," "technological civilization", "moral philosophy" and "historical culture" and other courses, the formation of distinctive, value-based general education with curriculum. In the context of the era of information technology with special emphasis on the introduction of the world's elite network of curriculum resources, its integration into the curriculum, making it the new General Education courses in the subject. Given the current quality of private college students generally weak human status, general education "should be more emphasis on the humanities-oriented, focusing on training in the humanities and foster the coordinated development of human qualities" [2].

Traditional core curriculum courses tend to enhance the target bit-oriented curriculum reform. "College Language" to appreciate the special focus on improving student reading ability, verbal skills and writing skills; "College English" to enhance students' English listening and speaking skills training, to lay a solid foundation for students to graduate enrollment; "Higher Mathematics" curriculum reform, according to teaching standards aiming at national graduate entrance examination and professional requirements set content, the implementation of classified teaching for all students to lay the foundation for further studies; "college sports" should be to improve students' physical fitness as the goal, students exercise habits, improve their athletic ability, and sports and students will develop the quality of the combination. And so on.

From another aspect, the teaching staffs are critical in this training programme as well. Private colleges and universities to strengthen the teaching staff is the key to an outstanding student to achieve training objectives. It is important for the Management Committee to offer excellent teaching staff in this programme through attractive policies, measures to noble morality. "Teaching quality is the lifeblood of private colleges and universities, teaching staff of private universities is directly related to educational quality" [3].

Among all the measures taken in this programme, an important aspect is "double-mentoring." The so-called "double-mentoring", is the school management committee for each outstanding student with two teachers, that is general and professional mentor teacher, instructors need to have the title of professor or Ph.D degree. General Education's main functions of instructors teaching general education classes, college career planning, development and implementation of comprehensive, personalized guide the whole process, general mentor actually act as a finance teacher, counselor and teacher as a whole.

286.4 Policy Support

The outstanding student-training programme is a new system in nowadays private colleges, it is a new challenge. It is therefore necessary for the Management Committee to establish a series of new policy to support the training programme. Hence to integrate the educational resources from the University level, and finalize the running mechanism. Only by this means the policy support can effectively ensure the perfectly running of the outstanding student programme. The support from policy of the University lies in three important parts.

286.4.1 Policy of Students

First of all, a student recruiting system should be establish. Based on school yearly undergraduate students college entrance examination scores in terms of total score and single subject results such as English and mathematics. For this first round, there will be around 300 candidates be shortlisted. After that, a voluntary registration with the combination of comprehensive admission interview will be carried out. Finally, there will be about 80 students (two classes) recruited into Jia-Yang college every year. A triage system is also applied in this programme. That is, each end of the semester (to 3 end of the semester only), based on the subjective wishes of students, tutors and comprehensive views of performance, the students not suitable for continue learning will be send back to the college for professional learning. Secondly, there are two major research area for the students. Recruited students are divided into two categories after one year of fundamental education, namely, liberal arts (including business management, language and art) and engineering. College students after Year two may be relatively independent choice of profession. Students can choose the college admission profession completely independent.

286.4.2 Policy of Teachers

The Management Committee should work together with the personnel, academic, research and other departments to mobilize outstanding teachers in training outstanding student enthusiasm. In detail, some special policy which can improve the wiliness of excellent teaching staffs in joining this programme, for example, teaching assessment, research assessment, remuneration and job promotion are formulated to support this training programme.

286.4.3 Policy of Facilities

The committee is also work with should work together with logistics, academic and other departments, that the students create a good learning environment for the target, in classrooms, dormitories, websites, sports venues and other aspects of development policy tilt.

286.5 Creative Learning and Self-management

Innovative learning is the key characteristic of an outstanding student. In this training programe, it is carried out from the following three aspects.

Firstly, general education courses are work under the unified implementation of teaching plans, students no longer participate in related professional course of study enrollment; professional courses of study are established by the relevant professional training colleges, teaching implementation of the plan, an outstanding student teachers and classes are free to choose time; if general course of study is in conflict with the professional course of study, students need to choose a professional course of study, related to general education courses under the guidance of instructors to students primarily in the form of complete self-study.

Secondly, the original course credits remain unchanged under the conditions of general education classroom time to reduce the overall 1/2-1/3; through course work and other forms, greatly increasing the student's extracurricular self-study time, improve learning efficiency.

Finally, measures are taken to achieve the goal of teaching effectiveness of the reform of teaching methods. General education teachers to completely change the way output is characterized by the "one-way only" teaching methods. By introducing exploration and inquiry form, discussion, project-based, scenario-based and other two-way communication with students characterized by "participation" teaching methods, and strive for 1-2 years, so that the "participatory" teaching method to be teaching the basic teaching methods, as Klingberg said, the interactive dialogue are excellent nature of teaching as a logo [4].

Mentor the students should be able to fully understand the actual situation, according to their characteristics, to help and guide students to form a personalized self-study habits and abilities. Reform of teaching methods, teaching students to emphasize the subject, "Only the real implementation of the student's dominant position in order to mobilize the enthusiasm and creativity; only allow students to self in order to truly develop their personality, to promote the development of each student" [5].

Student Affairs and Development Center to highlight the "development" concept, highlighting the characteristics of students' self-management, to become a train and improve their overall quality of an important organizational platform. Student Affairs and Development Center by students form the backbone of the members, organizing students to participate in courses, seminars, student organizations, "second class", social practice and other activities, is responsible for students' daily life management. Student Affairs and Development center is located instructor appointed by the General Education part-time instructors, both counselor and teacher responsibilities.

286.6 Conclusion

In this paper, an outstanding student research training program in a Chinese private college, learning from the Fudan University, Xi'an Jiaotong University and other public universities to develop an outstanding student of the college system model concept and content related to [6], is presented. More importantly, this study is based on students of private universities and educational resources the actual.

The programme proposed here is not only an outstanding student to develop the implementation plan needs, but also enrich the school training model needs. Private colleges and universities to develop an outstanding student as the starting point, to promote the school's style of study, thus improving the overall quality of the training has an important practical significance.

References

1. Ministry of Education Ministry of Education (2011), National Educational Development Statistics Bulletin [N]. China Educ, -7-6 http://www.gov.cn/gzdt/2012-08/30/content_2213875.htm
2. Xu D (2003) Trial college school of disciplines to explore the quality of education system, a new model. China Educ Res (1):21
3. Tian J (2011) College culture on intensive development of private universities inspiration. Heilongjiang High Educ Res (6):79
4. Liu Q (2001) Beginning dialogue on teaching. Educ Res (11):66
5. Xiao Z (2006) The characteristics of today's university teaching college teaching reform. Jiangsu High Educ (3):78
6. Ming HH (2010) The college system and the residential college system management mode comparative study of college students. High Eng Educ Res (3):111

Chapter 287
The Influence of Short Chain Fatty Acids on Biosynthesis of Emodin by *Aspergillus ochraceus* LP-316

Xia Li and Lv Ping

Abstract Emodin or 1,3,8-trihydroxy-6-methyl-anthraquinone is a naturally occurring pigment found in many plants, molds and lichens. Our previous studies revealed that a strain of Aspergillus ochraceus LP-316 (from LP-118 isolated from Chinese potato) had produced emodin efficiently. In this article, the production of emodin in 5-L bioreactor and resting cells system was studied with adding short chain fatty acids as precursors in order to identified the biosynthesis pathway type of emodin. The result illustrated that acetic acid was propitious to enhance the content of emodin and provided valuable information for the further searching the biosynthesis mechanism of emodin.

Keywords Emodin · Short chain fatty acids · Biosynthesis

287.1 Introduction

Emodin or 1,3,8-trihydroxy-6-methyl-anthraquinone is a naturally occurring pigment found in many plants [1], molds and lichens, exhibiting diverse biological activities including anticancer functions [2–4] and anti-inflammatory functions [5]. Early studies on its therapeutic benefits were mainly focused on its laxative functions as it is abundant in traditional Chinese medicinal herbs used for laxative formulation, such as rhubarb, the root and rhizome of Rheum palmatum L [6]. The health benefit of emodin has been linked to its involvement in many cellular

---

X. Li · L. Ping (✉)
Department of Biotechnological and Environmental Engineering, Tianjin Professional College, Tianjin 300410, China
e-mail: bestman_0429@163.com

X. Li
e-mail: lixia6804@163.com

processes, such as the suppression of tumor-associated angiogenesis through the inhibition of extracellular signal-regulated kinases [7]. There was also a report that emodin can sensitize certain types of breast cancer cells to the treatment of paclitaxel [8]. Its inhibitory effect on tumorogenesis-associated cell signaling pathways has made emodin an interesting molecular entity for antineoplastic studies and formulations.

Recently, we reported our studies on a strain of Aspergillus ochraceus isolated from Chinese potato, which constantly produced emodin which were isolated using Silica gel column chromatography and purified by preparative high performance liquid chromatography [9]. It was very important that the induced mechanism of Emodin from *Aspergillus ochraceus* was studied for industrialization production of emdon based on high yield fermentation. At the same time, two polymorphic amplification segments about producing emodin were found by RAPD analysis. One was homologous with XM_002374227.1 and AY585205.1, which indicated the biosynthesis of emodin was related to SOD and oxygen free radicals (Data unpublished).In order to reveal the pathway of emodin biosynthesis, the identification of emodin biosynthesis-type was urgent and necessary with discovering the influence of short chain fatty acid on biosynthesis of emodin by *Aspergillus ochraceus*.

287.2 Materials and Methods

287.2.1 Fungal Strain

The strain LP_118 of *Aspergillus ochraceus* was isolated from Chinese potato, and the strain LP_316 and LP_276 of *Aspergillus ochraceus* were obtained by low energy ion implantation into LP_118. The content of emodin from LP_316 was high at 1.518 mg/L, however, LP_276 had almost lost its ability of producing emodin.

287.2.2 Fermentation in Shake Flasks

A. ochraceus strain lpzhequ188 was initially isolated and identified from Chinese potato. The *A. ochraceus* strain was first grown in flasks containing 150 ml of Czapek-Dox (CD) medium, which was adjusted to pH 6.8 before autoclaving. The flasks were inoculated with a conidial suspension obtained from a 3-day old culture. The fermentation process was carried out at 29–32 °C on a rotary shaker (220 rpm).

287.2.3 Emodin Biosynthesis Using 5-L Bioreactor

The cells of Aspergillus ochraceus LP_118 in flasks (150 mL) was aseptically poured into a 5-L bioreactor containing 3,500 mL culture medium, at 28−30 °C and 0.9 v/m (air only) at 150, 180 and 200 rpm. Cellular growth was monitored every hour by optical density determination (660 nm). After 72 h, 10, 30, 50 and 70 g/L of short chain fatty acids (acetic acid, propionic acid, Methylmalonic acid, propanedioic acid) and incubated in the same conditions for 88 h. The bioreactor broth kept pH during 5.5−5.8 with 1.0 M HCl and 1.0 M NaCl, and Soil -80 was as defoamer in fermentation. After this time, the emodin content in 5-L bioreactor was assayed by RP-HPLC.

287.2.4 Emodin Biosynthesis Using Resting Cells

Pre-culture a 250 mL flask containing 100 mL of sterile culture. A medium was inoculated from an agar plate (3 days old) and incubated at 28−30 °C on an orbital shaker (170 rpm) for 48 h. The cells were collected by centrifugation at 4,500 rpm for 15 min. Cells were washed twice with potassium phosphate buffer (0.1 mol L^{-1}, pH 7.0). The cells were incubated in 50 mL phosphates buffer, 0.1 mol L^{-1}, pH 7.0, for 30 min at 28−30 °C on an orbital shaker (170 rpm), then 20, 40, 60 and 80 g/L of the short chain fatty acids (acetic acid, propionic acid, Methylmalonic acid, propanedioic acid) were added to the whole cells, and shaked in the same conditions for 8 h, depending of short chain fatty acids. After this time, the emodin content in resting cell system was assayed by RP-HPLC.

287.2.5 Emodin Content Determination

An accurately weighed sample of 5 g centrifuged, filtered and dried from fermentation liquid and 20 mL chloroform were added to a flask, and extraction was conducted in anultrasonic bath for 30 min. The extraction process was repeated three times. The primary extracts were combined, filtered, evaporated under vacuum and diluted to volume with chloroform in a 25 mL methanol volumetric flask 2 mL of the solution was then filtered through a 0.23 μm membrane and applied to HPLC for analysis. Separation was achieved using a Nacalai Cosmosil C18-MS-II column (5 μm, 250 × 4.66 mm, San Diego, USA) at 20 °C on an Agilent 1,100 HPLC system (Ramsey, Minnesota, USA). The mobile phase consisted of organic phase A (methanol containing 0.05 % acetic acid) and aqueous phase B (water containing 0.05 % acetic acid) and operated at a flow rate of 1.0 mL min^{-1} with an organic phase A gradient from 30 to 90 % in 10 min. The injection volume was 5 μL. The chromatograms were recorded at 254 nm.

287.3 Results and Discussion

287.3.1 The Influence of Short Chain Fatty Acid on Biosynthesis of Emodin in 5-L Bioreactor

In most cases, the production of secondary metabolites can be enhanced by treating the undifferentiated cells with Precursors. Short chain fatty acid has been reported to have the ability to induce many secondary metabolic processes to enhance the in vitro production of many compounds of interest. In nature, the process of elicitation induces the synthesis of secondary metabolites to ensure their survival, persistence and competitiveness. Another successful strategy used in influencing the biosynthetic pathways to activate and increase the production of secondary metabolites is by feeding cell cultures with precursors [10]. Precursors such as amino acids have been successful used when they are cheaper than the desired end products [11]. In this study, we pointed out the individual effect of Short chain fatty acid as precursors on the biosynthesis of emodin in 5-L bioreactor.

The effect of short chain fatty acids on emodin biosynthesis in 5-L bioreactor was investigated by a set of experiments using four kinds of short chain fatty acids separately (including acetic acid, propionic acid, Methylmalonic acid, propanedioic acid) at the concentration of 0, 10, 30, 50 and 70 g/L, and the result was showed in Fig. 287.1. Acetic acid was the best precursor for emodin production. With the increase of acetic acid, the content of emodin also added in linear relationship, and the biggest content of emodin reached to 1.358 mg/L. However, other short chain fatty acids were not useful for improving the content of emodin in 5-L bioreactor. As a result, Acetic acid was selected as an excellent precursor to confirm pathway-type of emodin biosynthesis and industrial fermental optimization.

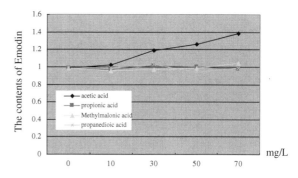

Fig. 287.1 Effects of short chain fatty acids on emodin biosynthesis in 5-L bioreactor

287.3.2 The Influence of Short Chain Fatty Acid on Biosynthesis of Emodin in Resting Cells System

Metabolically active resting (i.e., non-growing) bacterial cells have a high potential in cofactor-dependent emodin biotransformations. Where growing cells require carbon and energy for biomass production, resting cells can potentially exploit their metabolism more efficiently for biosynthesis of emodin allowing higher specific activities and product yields on energy source. Resting cells commonly showed higher specific activities as compared to growing cells in a similar setup. Emodin formation rates decreased steadily resulting in lower final product concentrations. That is say, emodin inhibition was identified as a limiting factor, in growing cells culture system, however, deactivation of enzyme system of emodin biosynthesis did not occur on the basis of the results in pre-experiments. The resting cell setup allowed high product yields of emodin, which makes the use of resting cells a promising approach for ecologically as well as economically sustainable whole-cell bioreactor for emodin.

Effects of short chain fatty acids on emodin biosynthesis in resting cell system were observed in Fig. 287.2, acetic acids enhanced the production of emodin better than the other short chain fatty acids. The content of emodin was increased to 1.358 mg/g at 70 mg/L of acetic acid, while the other short chain fatty acids were found to have insignificant influences on emodin production. The similar results have been observed in 5-L bioreactor. This stimulating effect of acetic acid was probably caused by acetic acid was one of unit-moculers in the biosynthesis pathway of emodin, so it should be chosen as precursor in the improved medium of cultivation and was helpful for later metabolite pathway analysis.

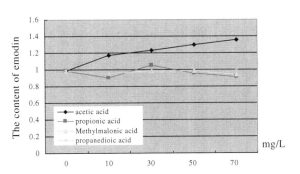

Fig. 287.2 Effects of short chain fatty acids on emodin biosynthesis in resting cell system

287.4 Conclusion

In short, our study illustrated that acetic acid was propitious to enhance the content of emodin from *Aspergillus ochraceus* LP-316 and provided valuable information for the further searching the biosynthesis mechanism of emodin.

Acknowledgments The financial support of Tianjin Natural Science Foundation (**A Study of Biosynthesis Pathway and Induced Mechanism from Reactive Oxygen Species of Emodin by Fermentation from Aspergillus ochraceus, No: 12JCYBJC19000**), is gratefully Acknowledged.

References

1. Izhaki I (2002) Emodin—a secondary metablosite with multiple ecological functions in higher plants. New Phytol 55:205–217
2. Lin SY, Lai WW, Ho CC et al (2009) Emodin induces apoptosis of human tongue squamous cancer SCC-4 cells through reactive oxygen species and mitochondria-dependent pathways. Anticancer Res 29:327–335
3. Muto A, Hori M, Sasaki Y et al (2007) Emodin has a cytotoxic activity against human multiple myeloma as a janus-activated kinase 2 inhibitor. Mol Cancer Ther 6:987–994
4. Srinivas G, Babykutty S, Sathiadevan PP et al (2007) Molecular mechanism of emodin action: transition from laxative ingredient to an antitumor agent. Med Res Rev. 591–608
5. Ding Y, Zhao L, Mei H et al (2008) Exploration of emodin to treat alpha-naphthylisothiocyanate-induced cholestatic hepatitis via anti-inflammatory pathway. Eur J Pharmacol. 590:377 − 386
6. Wang L, Li D, Bao C et al (2008) Ultrasonic extraction and separation of anthraquinones from rheum palmatum L. Ultrason Sonochem 15:738–746
7. Kaneshiro T, Morioka T, Inamine M et al (2006) Anthraquinone derivative emodin inhibits tumor-associated angiogenesis through inhibition of extracellular signal-regulated kinase 1/2 phosphorylation. Eur J Pharmacol 553:46–53
8. Zhang L, Lau YK, Xia W et al (1999) Tyrosine kinase inhibitor emodin suppresses growth of her-2/neu-overexpressing breast cancer cells in athymic mice and sensitizes these cells to the inhibitory effect of paclitaxel. Clin Cancer Res 5:343–353
9. Lu P, Zhao XM, Cui T (2010) Production of emodin from *Aspergillus ochraceus* at preparative scale. Afican J Biotechnol 9(4):512–517
10. Smetanska I (2008) Production of secondary metabolites using plant cell cultures. Adv Biochem Eng Biotechnol 111:187–228
11. Tumova L, Gallova K, Rimakova J (2004) Silybum marianum in vitro. Ceska Slov Farm 53(3):135–140

Chapter 288
Relationship Between Reactive Oxygen Species and Emodin Production in *Aspergillus ochraceus*

Ping Lv

Abstract Content of emodin, enzyme activity of SOD, enzyme activity of CAT and content of ROS were investigated simultaneously in fermentation process of Aspergillus ochraceus LP_318 and LP_276 in order to reveal relationship between Reactive Oxygen Species and emodin production for speculating the mechanism of high-yield emodin from Aspergillus ochraceus LP_318. The result showed that emodin was identified as an antioxidation in vivo and an explosion of ROS which was found from 36 to 84 h in LP_318 stimulated to produce emodin efficiently with deficiency in enzyme activity of SOD in LP_318.

Keywords Reactive · Oxygen · Species · Emodin · SOD · CAT

288.1 Introduction

Emodin or 1,3,8-trihydroxy-6-methyl-anthraquinone (Fig. 288.1) is a naturally occurring pigment found in many plants [8], molds and lichens, exhibiting diverse biological activities including anticancer functions [10, 12, 13] and anti-inflammatory functions [5]. Early studies on its therapeutic benefits were mainly focused on its laxative functions as it is abundant in traditional Chinese medicinal herbs used for laxative formulation, such as rhubarb, the root and rhizome of Rheum palmatum L [15]. The health benefit of emodin has been linked to its involvement in many cellular processes, such as the suppression of tumor-associated angiogenesis through the inhibition of extracellular signal-regulated kinases [9]. There was also a report that emodin can sensitize certain types of breast cancer cells to the treatment of paclitaxel [16]. Its inhibitory effect on tumorogenesis-associated

P. Lv (✉)
Department of Biotechnological and Environmental Engineering, Tianjin Professional College, Tianjin 300410, China
e-mail: bestman_0429@163.com

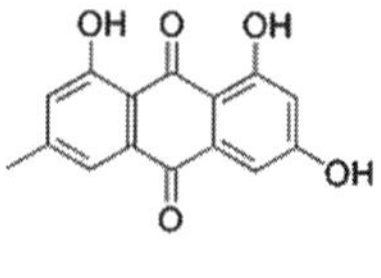

Fig. 288.1 Chemical structures of emodin

cell signaling pathways has made emodin an interesting molecular entity for antineoplastic studies and formulations.

Recently, we reported our studies on a strain of Aspergillus ochraceus isolated from Chinese potato, which constantly produced emodin which were isolated using Silica gel column chromatography and purified by preparative high performance liquid chromatography [11]. It was very important that the induced mechanism of Emodin from Aspergillus ochraceus was studied for Industrialization production of emdon based on high yield fermentation. At the same time, two polymorphic amplification segments about producing emodin were found by RAPD analysis. One was homologous with XM_002374227.1 and AY585205.1, which indicated the biosynthesis of emodin was related to SOD and oxygen free radicals. (Data unpublished).

It was well known that Emodin, a natural anthraquinone polyphenol, was reported to possess promising in vitro antioxidation [7, 14]. Franklin investigated the ability of emodin inhibit free radicals or reactive oxygen species generated in cell-free systems using isoluminol and luminol-enhanced chemiluminescence and electronic absorption spectra. The result showed emodin had an efficient and dose-dependent scavenging activity of reactive oxygen species [6]. We identified emodin function of scavenging oxygen free radical in vitro again. According to the results of above experiments, emodin was speculated to scavenge oxygen free radicals. So it was very necessary to research on relationship between Reactive Oxygen Species and emodin production with comparison of LP-318 and LP-276.

288.2 Materials and Methods

288.2.1 Materials

The strain LP_118 of Aspergillus ochraceus was isolated from Chinese potato, and the strain LP_318 and LP_276 of Aspergillus ochraceus were obtained by low energy ion implantation into LP_118. The content of emodin from LP_318 was high at 1.518 mg/L, however, LP_276 had almost lost its ability of producing emodin.

288.2.2 Fermentation in Shake Flasks

The strain LP_118 of Aspergillus ochraceus was initially isolated and identified from Chinese potato. The Aspergillus ochraceus strain was first grown in flasks containing 100 ml of Czapek-Dox (CD) medium, which was adjusted to pH 6.8 before autoclaving. The flasks were inoculated with a conidial suspension obtained from a 3-day old culture. The fermentation process was carried out at 29–32 °C on a rotary shaker (220 rpm).

288.2.3 Emodin Content Determination

An accurately weighed sample of 5 g centrifuged, filtered and dried from fermentation liquid and 20 mL chloroform were added to a flask, and extraction was conducted in an ultrasonic bath for 30 min. The extraction process was repeated three times. The primary extracts were combined, filtered, evaporated under vacuum and diluted to volume with chloroform in a 25 mL methanol volumetric flask. 2 mL of the solution was then filtered through a 0.23 μm membrane and applied to HPLC for analysis. Separation was achieved using a Nacalai Cosmosil C18-MS-II column (5 μm, 250 mm × 4.66 mm, San Diego, USA) at 20 °C on an Agilent 1100 HPLC system (Ramsey, Minnesota, USA). The mobile phase consisted of organic phase A (methanol containing 0.05 % acetic acid) and aqueous phase B (water containing 0.05 % acetic acid) and operated at a flow rate of 1.0 mL min-1 with an organic phase A gradient from 30 to 90 % in 10 min. The injection volume was 5 μL. The chromatograms were recorded at 254 nm.

288.2.4 Preparation of Enzyme Complex

A weighed sample of 10 g centrifuged, filtered from fermentation liquid and added to a flask, then rinsed with cold distilled water and homogenized in 100 mmol/L cold tris-HCl buffer (pH 6.5) and the homogenate was then centrifuged at 10,000 × g for 20 min. The preparation containing the enzyme complex was obtained from the supernatant by freeze-drying and was stored at −80 °C.

288.2.5 SOD Enzyme Activity

SOD (EC 1.15.1.1) activity was assayed by monitoring the inhibition of photochemical reduction of nitro blue tetrazolium (NBT), according to the method of Beyer and Fridovich (Beyer and Fridovich [3] with some modifications. For the total SOD assay, a 5 ml reaction mixture contained 50 mM HEPES (pH 7.6), 0.1 mM EDTA, 50 mM Na2CO3, 13 mM methionine, 0.025 % (w/v) Triton X-100, 75 μm NBT, 2 μm riboflavin and an appropriate aliquot of enzyme extract. The reaction mixture was illuminated for 15 min at a light intensity of 350 μmol m-2 s-1. One unit of SOD activity was defined as the amount of enzyme required to cause 50 % inhibition of the reduction of NBT as monitored at 560 nm.

288.2.6 Catalase Enzyme Activity

Catalase activity assay was performed by Aebi [1] method. 1.8 ml 0.05 M phosphate buffer (pH 7.0) and 40 mM H2O2 containing substrate buffer added to 0.2 ml extraction supernatant and spectrophotometric measurements were taken at 240 nm wavelength.

288.2.7 Electron Spin Resonance-Spin Trapping Determinations of ROS

A weighed sample of 2 g centrifuged, filtered from fermentation liquid and was immediately transferred to an ESR spectrometry cell, and the ESR measurement was started after 45 s. The measurement conditions of ESR (JES-FA-100, JEOL, Tokyo, Japan) were as follows: field sweep, 330.80–340.80 mT; field modulation frequency, 100 kHz; filed modulation width, 0.07 mT; amplitude, 400; sweep time, 1 min; time constant, 0.1 s; microwave frequency, 9.430 GHz; microwave power, 4–5 mW.

288.2.8 Statistical Analysis

All of assay results were expressed as relative data with computing standards of content of emodin at 60 h, enzyme activity of SOD at 48 h, enzyme activity of CAT at 48 h, content of ROS at 36 h, in order to all the curves of LP_0318 or LP_0276 on a figure for comparing each other and finding the characteristics. All the statistical analyses were done using SPSS v.11.5 for Windows.

288.3 Results and Discussion

288.3.1 Relationship Between Reactive Oxygen Species and Emodin Production in LP_318

To evaluate the mechanism of producing emodin in LP_318, relative content of emodin, relative enzyme activity of SOD, relative enzyme activity of CAT and relative content of ROS were investigated simultaneously in fermentation process. As shown in Fig. 288.2, relative content of emodin increased with fermentation time adding, especially a liner growth exhibited from 60 to 120 h. Content of ROS had almost no change at first phase (0–35 h). However, content of ROS increased rapidly from 36 to 60 h and added up to 7.12, but decreased sharply to former level at 84 h. It suggested that there was an explosion of ROS at 60 h. Relative enzyme activity of SOD was not changed obviously and only fluctuated within 1 ± 0.15. Relative enzyme activity of CAT increased slowly in the fermentation process. It was well known that SOD which catalyzed the dismutation of superoxide into oxygen and hydrogen peroxide was an important antioxidant defense in nearly all cells exposed to oxygen. In the process of removing superoxide free radicals, SOD rarely operated alone. It required CAT to remove hydrogen peroxide molecules which are by-products of the reactions created by SOD. Nevertheless, the enzyme activity of SOD in LP_318 was not enhanced when explosion of ROS was appeared, at the same time, the content of emodin had a huge increase. It hinted that emodin probably acted as an antioxidant to convert superoxide anion radicals to H_2O_2, and then H_2O_2 was converted to O_2 by CAT, so the enzyme activity of CAT was a synchronous increase with the content of emodin. That was to say emodin (not SOD) and CAT realized the process of removing superoxide free radicals in LP-318.

288.3.2 Relationship Between Reactive Oxygen Species and Emodin Production in LP_276

Figure 288.3 showed changes of the relative content of emodin, relative enzyme activity of SOD, relative enzyme activity of CAT and relative content of ROS in LP_276 fermentation process. The relative content of emodin was near zero, which exhibited LP_276 lost its ability to produce emodin. An explosion of ROS did not appeared but a little increase about 45 % from 36 to 84 h, at the same time, relative enzyme activity of SOD added steadily. The relative enzyme activity of SOD at 120 h almost increased three times as well as at 48 h. It suggested that SOD emerged normally and scavenged ROS, but had a delay about 12 h. Relative enzyme activity of CAT increased in the process of fermentation and exhibited the same variation trend of that of LP_318.

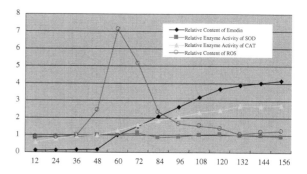

Fig. 288.2 Change of relative content of emodin, relative enzyme activity of SOD, relative enzyme activity of CAT and relative content of ROS in LP_318

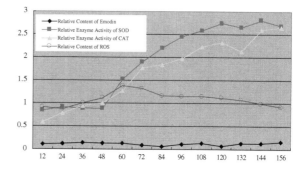

Fig. 288.3 Change of relative content of emodin, relative enzyme activity of SOD, relative enzyme activity of CAT and relative content of ROS in LP_276

288.4 Conclusion

In short, our study hinted emodin was also an antioxidation in vivo and an explosion of ROS was a trigger of high-yield emodin production on the base of deficiency in enzyme activity of SOD in LP_318.

Acknowledgments The financial support of Tianjin Natural Science Foundation (A Study of Biosynthesis Pathway and Induced Mechanism from Reactive Oxygen Species of Emodin by Fermentation from Aspergillus ochraceus, No: 12JCYBJC19000), is gratefully Acknowledged.

References

1. Aebi H (1984) Catalase in vitro. Methods Enzymol 105:121–126
2. Brook J, Barry O (2005) The source of abnormal returns from strategic alliance announcements. Pac Basin Financ J 13(2):145–161
3. Beyer WF, Fridovich I (1987) Assaying for superoxide dismutase ctivity: some large consequences of minor changes in conditions. Anal Biochem 161:559–566
4. Curch TR, Vikram N (2003) Divisional diversity and the conglomerate discount: evidence from spinoffs. J Financ Econ 70(1):69–98

5. Ding Y, Zhao L, Mei H, Zhang SL, Huang ZH, Duan YY, Ye P (2008) Exploration of emodin to treat alpha-naphthylisothiocyanate-induced cholestatic hepatitis via anti-inflammatory pathway. Euro J Pharmaco 590:377–386
6. Vargas FR, Díaz YH, Carbonell KM (2004) Antioxidant and Scavenging Activity of Emodin, Aloe-Emodin and Rhein on Free-Radical and Reactive Oxygen Species. Pharm Biol 42(4–5):342–348
7. Huang SS, Yeh SF, Hong CY (1995) Effect of anthraquinone derivatives on lipid peroxidation in rat heart mitochondria: structure-activity relationship. J Nat Prod 58:1365–1371
8. Izhaki I (2002) Emodin—a secondary metablosite with multiple ecological functions in higher plants. New Phytol 55:205–217
9. Kaneshiro T, Morioka T, Inamine M, Kinjo T, Arakaki J, Chiba I, Sunagawa N, Suzui M, Yoshimi N (2006) Anthraquinone derivative emodin inhibits tumor-associated angiogenesis through inhibition of extracellular signal-regulated kinase 1/2 phosphorylation. Euro J Pharmacoy 553:46–53
10. Lin SY, Lai WW, Ho CC, Yu FS, Chen GW, Yang JS, Liu KC, Lin ML, Wu PP, Fan MJ, Chung JG (2009) Emodin induces apoptosis of human tongue squamous cancer SCC-4 cells through reactive oxygen species and mitochondria-dependent pathways. Antican Res 29:327–335
11. Lu P, Zhao XM, Cui T (2010) Production of emodin from Aspergillus ochraceus at preparative scale. Afr J Biotechnol 9(4):512–517
12. Muto A, Hori M, Sasaki Y, Saitoh A, Yasuda I, Maekawa T, Uchida T, Asakura K, Nakazato T, Kaneda T, Kizaki M, Ikeda Y, Yoshida T (2007) Emodin has a cytotoxic activity against human multiple myeloma as a Janus-activated kinase 2 inhibitor. Molecul Can Therap 6:987–994
13. Srinivas G, Babykutty S, Sathiadevan PP, Srinivas P (2007) Molecular mechanism of emodin action: transition from laxative ingredient to an antitumor agent. Med Res Rev 27:591–608
14. Vargas F, Dı'az Y, Carbonell K (2004) Antioxidant and scavenging activity of emodin, aloe-emodin, and rhein on free-radical and reactive oxygen species. Pharm Biol 42:342–348
15. Wang L, Li D, Bao C, You J, Wang Z, Shi Y, Zhang H (2008) Ultrasonic extraction and separation of anthraquinones from Rheum palmatum L. Ultrasons Sonochem 15:738–746
16. Zhang L, Lau YK, Xia W, Hortobagyi GN, Hung MC (1999) Tyrosine kinase inhibitor emodin suppresses growth of HER-2/neu-overexpressing breast cancer cells in athymic mice and sensitizes these cells to the inhibitory effect of paclitaxel. Clin Canr Res 5:343–353

Chapter 289
A Studies of the Early Intervention to the Diabetic Patients with Hearing Loss by Hypoglycemic Anti-deaf Party

Kaoshan Guo, Ruiyu Li, Meng Li, Jianqiao Li, Liping Wu, Junli Yan, Jianmei Jing, Weiya Guo, Yang Liu, Weihua Han, Yanfu Sun and Qing Gu

Abstract Objective to discuss the effect of the early intervention to the patients with hearing loss by the hypoglycemic anti-deaf party. Methods 44 (56 ears) patients with diabetes and deafness treat by the hypoglycemic anti-deaf party, control group of 40 healthy persons Refuses to accept any drug and observe the same number of days with the treatment group. All patients were given the control diet, diabetes knowledge, education, sports and other treatment. Measured the two groups fasting blood glucose (FBG), 2 h postprandial blood glucose (2 hPBG), glycosylated hemoglobin (HbAIc), FINS, insulin (2 hINS), TCM syndromes and compared the before and the after. Results After treatment, FBG, 2 hPBG HbAIc decreased significantly than before treatment ($P < 0.05$), and control group after treatment in addition to 2 hPBG was decreased ($P < 0.05$), FBG, HbAIc despite changes, but not statistically significant ($P > 0.05$). After treatment FINS, 2 hINS than before treatment decreased significantly ($P < 0.05$), with the control group, representing a drop of gap significantly ($P < 0.05$), control group after treatment compared with before treatment FINS, 2 hINS, BMI, despite changes, butno statistically significant ($P > 0.05$) the two groups' BMI before and after treatment had no statistically significant ($P > 0.05$) Before and after treatment syndromes

---

K. Guo · R. Li (✉) · J. Jing · W. Guo · Y. Liu · W. Han · Y. Sun · Q. Gu
Second Affiliated Hospital of Xing Tai Medical College, No. 618 Gangtiebei Road, Xingtai, Hebei, China
e-mail: liruiyu651021@163.com

M. Li
Health Team of Hotan Prefecture Detachment of Chinese Armed Police Force,
Xinjiang, China

J. Li
Chinese Medicine Hospital, Luquan, Hebei, China

L. Wu
Xingtai People's Hospital, Xingtai, Hebei, China

J. Yan
Renxian County Hospital, Xingtai, Hebei, China

treatment group than the control group. Conclusion Hypoglycemic anti-deaf glue combined to control diet, diabetes knowledge, education, sports, and other patients with hearing loss early treatment of diabetes was significantly lower FBG, 2 hPBG, HbAIc, improve insulin secretion, control diabetes and development.

Keywords Hypoglycemic anti-deaf party · Early stage of diabetes · Deaf

289.1 Introduction

At home and abroad diabetes induced sensorineural deafness for its mechanism is not yet clear, so no definite therapy, we have to hypoglycemic developed anti-deaf Treatment of diabetes and deafness to achieve a certain effect, and found the syndrome and is closely related to concurrent deafness proposed "control card" development ideas and methods [1–4].Therefore, this paper carried out on diabetic hearing loss in patients with early application hypoglycemic anti-deaf party intervention, are as follows.

289.2 Materials and Methods

289.2.1 General Information

The group of 44 patients (56 ears) with type II diabetes mellitus (NIDDM) with deaf patients, were 18 males and 26 females, aged 36–73 years, mean 54.6 years, duration of 1–11 years, an average of 4.8 years. Deafness level published by the International Organization for Standardization (ISO) 1954 standard, is a mild hearing loss in 12 ears, moderate hearing loss in 16 ears, severe hearing loss in 17 ears, Severe deaf in 8 ears, depth deaf in 2 ears; Unilateral deafness 34 ears, 20 ears bilateral deafness. Sudden deafness 12 ears, gradually 42 ear, BMI (23 ± 2) kg/M2, IFG 10 cases, IGT 16 cases, both in 5 patients; according to the Chinese dialectical is yinxuzaore. Control group for the normal 40, including 26 males and 14 females, aged 34–69 years, mean 59.4 years, BMI (22 ± 3) kg/m2, IFG 16, IGT in 17 cases, two by both 4 cases. Two sets of general information, not statistically significant ($P > 0.05$).

289.2.2 Pre-diabetes Diagnostic Criteria

This group of patients with pre-diabetes diagnostic criteria for diabetes according to a 1999 World Health Organization (WHO) Expert Committee Report and the 2007 version of "Chinese type 2 diabetes Guide" [5] published diagnostic criteria to develop.

(1) impaired glucose tolerance (IGT): fasting blood glucose (FBG) < 7.0 mmol/L and 2 h plasma glucose glucose tolerance test (2 h PBG) ≥ 7.8 mmol/L;
(2) impaired fasting glucose (IFG): 6.1 mmol/L ≤ fasting blood glucose < 7.0 mmol/L glucose tolerance test 2 h PBG < 8 mmol/L;
(3) At the same time meet the above conditions.

289.2.3 Yinxuresheng Syndrome Diagnostic Criteria

Refer to the *Chinese medicine clinical research guiding principles* [5].

Where the main symptoms of essential, both secondary symptoms two or more than two, combined with tongue and pulse can be dialectical.

289.2.4 Inclusion Criteria

(1) comply with pre-diabetes diagnosis, that is in line with IFG and (or) IGT diagnostic criteria;
(2) comply with deficiency heat syndrome Diagnostic Criteria;
(3) dyslipidemia or in an abnormal edge;
(4) age 34–69 years;
(5) systolic blood pressure <140 mmHg, diastolic blood pressure <90 mmHg are taking antihypertensive drugs or not taking would be free;
(6) not taking other hypoglycemic, lipid-lowering drugs;
(7) signed informed consent.

289.2.5 Exclusion Criteria

In the near future cardiovascular events; Glucocorticoids, beta blockers, thiazide diuretics, nicotinic acid drug use within the past 3 months; Serum creatinine ≥ 130 μmol · L^{-1}; elevated liver transaminases to more than two times the upper limit of the normal range; Moderate or severe hypertension, endocrine diseases uncorrected; Fasting plasma triglyceride levels > 5.7 mmol · L^{-1}; Thyroid-stimulating hormone (TSH), more than 1.5 times the upper limit of the normal range or below the lower limit of normal; TCM two and see no primary or secondary or other syndromes and witness-type complex.

289.2.6 Clinical Criteria

Diabetes syndromes in TCM syndromes standard (Reference 2002 Chinese new drug clinical research guidelines criteria [6]) recovered: TCM symptoms and signs disappeared after treatment, symptom score was reduced by ≥ 95 %.

Markedly: TCM clinical symptoms and signs of significant improvement in symptom scores decreased $\geq 70\ \%$.

Effective: the TCM clinical symptoms and signs were improved symptom scores decreased $\geq 30\ \%$.

Invalid: the TCM clinical symptoms, signs were not significantly improved, or even increase, symptom scores decreased to less than 30 %.

Nimodipine: efficacy index = (Points before treatment score—points after treatment)/treatment $\times$ 100 %.

289.2.7 Determination of Indicators

FBG and 2 h PBG before and after the detection of two groups of patients with drug and non-drug interventions, insulin (FINS and 2 h INS).

289.2.8 Treatment

The two groups were given control diet, diabetes knowledge, education, sports and other treatment. Diabetes and deafness group (treatment group): oral hypoglycemic anti-deaf side "gegen (Radix Puerariae), danshen (Radix Salviae Miltiorrhizae), chuanxiong (Rhizorna Chuanxiong), shudihuang (Radix Rehmanniae), huaishanyao (Rhizoma Dioseoreae), fuling (poria), danpi (Cortex Moutan), zexie (Rhizoma Alismatis), shanzhuyu (Fruetus Comi), cishi (Magnetite)" is made according to the above formula 0.5 g capsules, five times a day orally, three times a day. Yinxuzaore plus capsules one (made by shigao (Gypsum Fibrosum), zihmu (Rhizoma Anemarrhenae), huanglian (RhiZoma Coptidis), xuanshen (Radix Scrophulariae)); each piece 0.5 g, 3–5 tablets each time, three times a day. Before treatment was measured by the above method, measured after 48 days of treatment compared with before treatment, during treatment by these drugs. The control group refused to accept any medication, observe the number of days with the treatment group.

289.2.9 Security Outcome Measures

(1) laboratory tests blood, urine, liver function, renal function (once each before and after treatment).
(2) adverse reaction: any possible adverse reactions.

289.2.10 Statistical Methods

SPSS11.0 statistical software analysis and processing of the test results, the measurement data are expressed as mean ± standard deviation ($\bar{x} \pm S$) between the two groups were compared using the t test.

289.3 Results

289.3.1 Before and After Treatment TCM Syndromes are Shown in Table 289.1

Table 289.1.

289.3.2 Before and After Treatment FBG, 2 hPBG, HbAIc Comparison

After treatment, FBG, 2 hPBG The glycosylated hemoglobin level than before treatment decreased significantly ($P < 0.05$), the control group after treatment in addition to 2 hPBG decreased outside ($P < 0.05$), FBG, The glycosylated hemoglobin level Notwithstanding changes, but not statistically significant ($P > 0.05$) (Table 289.2).

Table 289.1 Before and after treatment syndromes compare (%)

Grouping	The number	Be cured	Markedly	Effective	Invalid	Total efficiency
Treatment Group	44	26	8	6	4	90.9✕
Control Group	40	15	9	6	10	75

Note Compared with the group before treatment ✕ $P < 0.05$

Table 289.2 Two groups before and after treatment FBG 2 hPBG The glycosylated hemoglobin level comparison ($\bar{x} \pm S$)

Groups		The number	FBG (mm01/L)	2 h PBG (mm01/L)	HbAIc (%)
Treatment group	Before treatment	44	6.38 ± 0.54	8.61 ± 2.55	6.41 ± 0.65
	After treatment		5.67 ± 0.40✕	7.23 ± 1.87✕	5.84 ± 0.59✕
Control group	Before treatment	40	6.42 ± 0.53	8.71 ± 2.71	6.42 ± 0.62
	After treatment		5.96 ± 0.63	7.72 ± 2.75✕	6.36 ± 0.65

Note Compared with the group before treatment ✕ $P < 0.05$

Table 289.3 Before and after treatment by FINS, 2 hINS and BMI (x ± s)

Groups		The number	FINS (mIU/L)	2 hINS (mIU/L)	BMI (Kg/m2)
Treatment group	Before treatment	44	13.25 ± 8.82	49.22 ± 9.48	25.28 ± 1.58
	After treatment		8.90 ± 5.04*△	36.50 ± 8.99*△	24.51 ± 0.87
Control group	Before treatment	40	13.50 ± 7.15	50.15 ± 9.88	25.59 ± 1.66
	After treatment		12.64 ± 6.96	47.59 ± 9.65	24.89 ± 1.78

Note Compared with the same group before treatment * $P < 0.05$; compared with the control group over the same period △ $P < 0.05$

289.3.3 Before and After Treatment by FINS, 2hINS and BMI Comparison

After treatment, FINS, 2 hINS than before treatment decreased significantly ($P < 0.05$), with the control group, representing a drop of the gap significantly ($P < 0.05$) in the control group with before treatment the FINS, 2 hINS, BMI, despite changes, but not statistically significant ($P > 0.05$). The BMI the two groups before and after treatment had no statistically significant ($P > 0.05$) (Table 289.3).

289.4 Discussion

Sensorineural deafness caused by diabetes, at home and abroad for its mechanism is not yet clear, therefore, extremely limited efficacy for the treatment of diabetes, there is no clear treatment, Western medicine hypoglycemic drugs in the treatment of diabetic sure, but long-term use varying degrees of adverse reactions, can not effectively control complications. Chinese medicine treatment of diabetes, efficacy, adverse reactions, which can effectively prevent complications [7, 8]. Columbia University is closely related to research diabetes and osteocalcin, experimental study found that osteocalcin by play to fat and pancreatic send signals to the secretion and regulation of insulin action. Diabetes is closely related to the kidney, Chinese herbal medicine which invigorate the kidney to promote the proliferation and differentiation of bone cells to secrete osteocalcin [9–13]. According to the theory of renal bone, through Drug card and found that kidney deficiency rat model of nerve-endocrine-immune and nerve-endocrine-route of two gene regulation of bone metabolism disorders, kidney can correct the network function. We asked the diabetes-kidney-bone-ear is one of scientific hypothesis, in accordance with the hypothesis of the occurrence and development of prevention and treatment of diabetes, diabetes early intervention.

"Disease prevention, not disease prevention", is the essence of the theory of Chinese medicine prevention. Diabetes is a traditional Chinese medicine,

"Diabetes" category, and kidney-oriented machine, hot flashes as the standard, therefore, kidney-based treatment of dry standard, Based on the principle of treating the symptoms, focusing on the relationship between whole and part, hypoglycemic anti-deaf side arrowroot, Salvia root, Rehmannia, Chinese yam, Poria, Alisma, Dan, dogwood, magnet, Fang Chuan Xiong and Salvia are the blood circulation of power, Kudzu has the role of thirst, Rehmannia sweet soft blood ney fill fine yam spleen to help transport, Poria to infiltration Lee spleen wet, the Alisma short vent kidney turbidity, Dan Qing diarrhea anger, dogwood liver and kidney tonic, magnet Kennedy yin and ears and eyesight role All parties have nourishing yin, promoting blood circulation-based effect. In the light of TCM Syndrome Types of diabetes in patients with early performance Yin hot patients increased of gypsum, Anemarrhena, berberine, Scrophulariaceae, the heat Runzao palliative, prevention and treatment philosophy of the whole party reflect the overall concept of diagnosis and treatment.

By the early application of hypoglycemic diabetic patients with deafness anti-deaf party to control diet, diabetes knowledge, education, sports and other treatment. 40 and normal control after treatment, FBG, 2 hPBG The glycosylated hemoglobin level than before treatment decreased significantly ($P < 0.05$), except 2 hPBG control group after treatment was decreased ($P < 0.05$), FBG, The glycosylated hemoglobin level, despite changes in but not statistically significant ($P > 0.05$).After treatment FINS, 2 hINS than before treatment decreased significantly ($P < 0.05$), with the control group, representing a drop of gap significantly ($P < 0.05$), control group after treatment compared with before treatment FINS, 2 hINS, BMI, despite changes, butno statistically significant ($P > 0.05$). BMI the two groups before and after treatment had no statistically significant ($P > 0.05$) before and after treatment syndromes treatment group than the control group. The results showed that hypoglycemic anti-deaf rubber combination to significantly reduce FBG to control diet, diabetes knowledge, education, sports and other treatment of diabetic patients with deafness early 2 hPBG The glycosylated hemoglobin level, improve insulin secretion, control diabetes and development.

References

1. Li RY, Li M, Wang R et al (2008) Jiang Tang Fang Long Jiao Nang in treating non-insulin dependent diabetes mellitus with hearing loss. J Otol 3(1):45–50
2. Li RY, Li B, Guo YJ (2009) The effect of blood insulin C peptide and glucagon by Jiangtang Fanglong capsule on different syndromes diabetes patients with deafness. J Liaoning Tradit Chin Med 36(4):510–511
3. Li RY, Guo YL, Liu JW et al (2011) The influence of prescription of tonifying kidney to diabetes with deafness. J Mod Tradit Chin West Med 20(6):654–656
4. Li RY, Li M, Li B (2008) Control syndromes development thinking of prevention and treatment of diabetes accompanied with deafness. J Mod Tradit Chin West Med 17(3):5237–5238
5. Diabetology branch of Chinese medical association (2008) Chinese type 2 diabetes prevention guidelines. Chin Med J 88(18):1227–1245

6. Zheng XY (2002) Guiding principle of clinical research on new drugs of traditional Chinese medicine trial. Beijing China Press of Traditional Medical Science and Technology, Beijing, pp 233–237
7. Chen JS, Zheng C (2011) Application of traditional Chinese medicine in the treatment of diabetes and complications. J China Exp Pharmacol 17(23):276
8. Zhang YP, Liu J, Li YM (2011) Research survey of treating diabetes by Chinese medicine clinical medicine. J Chin Clin Exp Pathol 17(22):277
9. Shen ZY, Chen Y, Huang JH et al (2006) Two gene network regulation route map by drug test certificate to rendering kidney. J Tradit Chin Med 26(6):521
10. Zhang H, Ni Q, Ren Y et al (2010) The correlation of Yaoxisuanruan and diabetic kidney deficiency symptom. J Tradit Chin Med 51(5):409
11. Zhang H, Wang JR, Tan CG et al (2010) Quantitative study of diabetes and kidney deficiency syndrome. J Liaoning Tradit Chin Med 37(6):1023
12. Tan CG, Wang MQ, Ni Q et al (2010) The relationship between characteristics of diabetes family genetic and kidney deficiency. J Liaoning Tradit Chin Med 37(7):1197
13. Yuan J, Lin YP (2006) The progress of experimental study on osteoblast proliferation and differentiation by TCM serum. J Fujian Univ Tradit Chin Med 16(4):70

Chapter 290
Effect of T Lymphocytes PD-1/B7-H1 Path Expression in Patients with Severe Hepatitis Depression from Promoting Liver Cell Growth Hormone Combinations from Gongying Yinchen Soup

Zhang Junhui, Gao Junfeng, Zhao Xinguo, Li Meng, Ma Limin, Hou Jinjie, Sun Yanfu, Gu Qing and Li Ruiyu

Abstract *Objective* To investigate the effect of T lymphocytes PD-1/B7-H1 path expression in patients with severe hepatitis depression from promoting liver cell growth hormone combinations from Gongying Yinchen soup. *Methods* With reference to the American psychiatric association's diagnostic statistical manual of mental disorders, fourth edition (dsm-iv) criteria, 88 cases of fulminant hepatitis in patients with depression were collected as treatment group, which consist of acute severe hepatitis (n = 31), chronic severe hepatitis (n = 28) and subacute severe hepatitis (n = 29),120 mg promoting liver cell growth hormone to join within 250 ml of 10 % glucose injection, intravenous drip, 1 times a day, 15 d for a period of treatment, At the same time to add with the Gongying Yinchen soup (dandelion, radix et rhizoma rhei, radix bupleuri, herba artemisiae capillaris, glabrous greenbrier rhizome, radix isatidis, grifola, bitter arguments). Three period of treatment. Thirty healthy persons of control group come from blood donor of

Z. Junhui · H. Jinjie
Xingtai Medical College, No. 618 Gangtiebei Road, Xingtai, Hebei Province, China

G. Junfeng · S. Yanfu · G. Qing
Second affiliated hospital, Xingtai Medical College, No. 618 Gangtiebei Road, Xingtai, Hebei Province, China

Z. Xinguo · M. Limin
Chinese Medicine Hospital of Lincheng County, Hebei Province, China

L. Meng
Health Team of Hotan Prefecture Detachment of Chinese Armed Police Force, Xinjiang, China

L. Ruiyu (✉)
Institute of Integrated Traditional and Western Medicine, second affiliated hospital, Xingtai Medical College, No. 618 Gangtiebei Road, Xingtai, Hebei, China
e-mail: Liruiyu651021@163.com

central blood stations. The expressions of PD-1/B7-H1 of T lymphocytes and T lymphocyte subsets of two groups were determined by flow cytometry. *Results* The positive expression of PD1 and B7—H1of T lymphocytes in patients of the treatment group was significant higher than that in healthy control group ($P < 0.05$); The positive expression of PD1and B7—H1of T lymphocytes significantly decreased after treatment in the treatment group ($P < 0.05$). The amount of $CD4^+$, $CD8^+$ cells of the treatment group was significantly lower than that of control group ($P < 0.05$). The amount of $CD4^+/CD8^+$ cells of the treatment group was higher than that of control group ($P < 0.05$), significantly decreased after treatment ($P < 0.05$). *Conclusion* Promoting liver cell growth hormone combination from the Gongying Yinchen soup can influence expression of T lymphocytes PD-1/B7-H1 path in patients with severe hepatitis depression, enhance the body's immune response.

Keywords Hepatocyte growth-promoting factors · Gongying yinchen soup · Severe hepatitis · T lymphocyte PD-1/B7-H1

290.1 Introduction

The body's immune response demand positive and negative signals to work together to maintain the balance of the signal, the negative signals which generated by the PD-1/B7-H1 is now considered one of the most factors of chronic viral infection [1], and become one of the targeted is of great application prospect. PD-1 and its ligand binding, can block positive signal molecules CD28, thereby activating PI3K pathway, as well as inhibiting T cell proliferation and differentiation [2]. PD-1 show a high level of expression in virus specific $CD8^+$ T cells, and PD-1/B7-H1 pathway plays a key role in regulating T cell function failure [3]. This paper discusses effect of T lymphocytes PD-1/B7-H1 path expression in patients with severe hepatitis depression from promoting liver cell growth hormone combinations from Gongying Yinchen soup, early report as below.

290.2 Materials and Methods

290.2.1 General Data

The treatment group of 88 cases (57 male and 31 female, ages 26 to 75 years old) came from Department of Integrated Traditional and Western Medicine from November 2003–August 2007, including 31 cases of acute severe hepatitis (21 male and 10 female, ages 18 to 52 years old, average 29.7 years old); 29 cases of subacute severe hepatitis(17 male and 12 female, ages 19 to 50 years old, average 30.4 years old); 28 cases of chronic severe hepatitis (19 male and 9 female age 28 to 58 years old, average 38.6 years). The control group of 30 cases(21 male and 9 female, ages 24–72 years old, average 40.7 years old) are healthy blood donor of xingtai blood donation center.

290.2.2 Criteria of Diagnosis

Severe hepatitis diagnostic criteria: refer to the Chinese medical association infectious diseases and parasitic epidemiology branch, liver disease, viral hepatitis prevention scheme [4]. The diagnosis of depression (western medicine diagnostic criteria): refer to the Chinese classification and diagnosis standard of mental illness, third edition (CCMD-3) [5]. Diagnostic criteria of traditional Chinese medicine of depression: reference about depression in literature of traditional Chinese medicine [6].

290.2.3 Classification Standards of Depression Severity

With reference to the American psychiatric association, the diagnostic statistical manual of mental disorders criteria, fourth edition (dsm-iv).

290.2.4 Inclusion Criteria

(1) Conform to the diagnosis of depression of patients with mild and moderate depression. (2) Stable vital signs, conscious, have certain skills.

290.2.5 Exclusion Criteria

(1) Belong to major depression. (2) There are some disruptive symptoms, or belong to depression after schizophrenia. (3) Clinical doctors psychosis diagnosed as depressed. (4) Those were not included in the standard of inclusion, or the data is not complete. Conforming to the item 1 above will be ruled out.

290.2.6 Treatment Method

In treatment group, promoting liver cell auxin 120 mg add in 250 ml of 10 % glucose solution, intravenous drip 1 times a day, 15 d as a course of treatment. At the same time to add with the Gongying Yinchen soup. Its composition was: dandelion, radix et rhizoma rhei, radix bupleuri, herba artemisiae capillaris, glabrous greenbrier rhizome, radix isatidis, grifola, bitter ginseng, daily 1 agent, water decoction, 15 d for a period of treatment, shared 3 period of treatment.

290.2.7 Main Reagents and Instruments

CD3-FITC/CD8-PE/CD45-PreCP/CD4-APC, hemolysin FITC-CD3 antibody, PE-rat anti CD279 (PD-1), PE-rat anti CD274 (B7-H1) and FACS Calibur flow cytometry instrument were purchased from BD company, the United States.

290.2.8 Sample Collection

Using EDTA-K2 Anticoagulation vacuum blood collection tube, we pick vascular venous blood 2 mL, SH, CHB patients with Fasting venous blood after 2 day morning to the time of be hospitalized, healthy physical examines with Fasting venous blood, blood specimens was saved at 4 °C.

290.2.9 PD-1/B7-H1 Detection

3 flow cytometry analysis tube respectively to join anti CD3, CD3 + CD274, CD3 + CD279 antibody 3 uL, and 25 uL venous blood specimen, 15 min at room temperature away from light, each tube plus 1 mL of hemolysin in 10 times diluted, let stand for 10 min, 300 × g centrifuge for 5 min, abandon supernatant, PBS washing cells 2 times, 300 × g centrifuge for 5 min, abandon supernatant. Add PBS 0.5 mL, detection were carried out by FACS Calibur flow cytometry instrument.

290.2.10 T Cells Subgroup Detection

Take 1 flow cytometry analysis tube, add single anti CD3-FITC labeled/CD8-PE/CD45-PreCP/CD4- APC 20uL, and venous blood samples of 100 uL, incubation

15 min at room temperature away from light, puls hemolysin 2 mL by 10 times dilution, let stand for 10 min, 300 × g centrifuge for 5 min, abandon supernatant. PBS washing cells 2 times, 300 × g centrifuge for 5 min, abandon the supernatant, add 1 % paraformaldehyde 0.5 mL, detection were carried out by FACS Calibur flow cytometry instrument.

290.2.11 Statistical Methods

SPSS11.0 statistical software was used to analyze the above inspection result processing, data of measurement were presented as $\bar{x} \pm S$, t test was used to compare the difference between control group and treatment group.

290.3 Results

290.3.1 The Expression of PD-1/B7-H1 in T Lymphocytes of Severe Hepatitis Patients and Normal Person Blood (see Table 290.1)

Table 290.1 The expression of PD-1/B7-H1 in T lymphocytes of severe hepatitis patients and normal person blood ($\bar{x} \pm s$ %)

Group	n		PD-1	B7-H1
Acute severe hepatitis	31	Prior treatment	5.18 ± 0.74	7.75 ± 0.90
		Posttreatment	3.20 ± 0.50*△	4.79 ± 0.69*△
Chronic severe hepatitis	28	Prior treatment	10.29 ± 1.26	16.85 ± 10.89
		Posttreatment	8.30 ± 1.11*△	13.89 ± 2.10*△
Subacute severe hepatitis	29	Prior treatment	6.38 ± 1.48	4.95 ± 0.74
		Posttreatment	4.25 ± 1.32*△	3.10 ± 0.32*△
Normal			1.74 ± 0.26	1.98 ± 0.32

Note Compared with control group*$P < 0.05$; Comparison of before and after treatment △$P < 0.05$

290.3.2 Test Results of T Lymphocyte Subgroup (see Table 290.2)

Table 290.2 Test results of T lymphocyte subgroup ($\bar{x} \pm s$ %)

Group	n		$CD3^+$	$CD4^+$	$CD8^+$	$CD4^+/CD8^+$
Acute severe hepatitis	31	Prior treatment	55 ± 11.4	44 ± 8.5	12 ± 5.6	3.69 ± 0.28
		Posttreatment	60 ± 10.1*△	49 ± 6.9*△	19 ± 6.2*△	2.99 ± 0.16*△
Chronic severe hepatitis	28	Prior treatment	60 ± 12.1	47 ± 7.7	18 ± 7.5	3.12 ± 0.12
		Posttreatment	62 ± 10.3*△	49 ± 8.2*△	20 ± 7.9*△	2.94 ± 0.15*△
Subacute severe hepatitis	29	Prior treatment	63 ± 10.3	48 ± 10.7	18 ± 7.4	2.96 ± 0.14
		Posttreatment	70 ± 11.1*△	53 ± 10.3*△	20 ± 7.0*△	2.41 ± 0.13
Normal			73 ± 12.4	55 ± 11.4	25 ± 8.4	2.19 ± 0.19

Note Compared with control group*$P < 0.05$; Comparison of before and after treatment △$P < 0.05$

290.4 Discussions

Apoptosis factor 1 (programmed death 1, PD-1) is a new CD28 family members, and its ligand B7-H1 (B7 homolog 1) are the total stimulus molecule [7]. Virus infection can induce T cells expressing PD-1/B7-H1, resulting in a loss of specific T lymphocyte immune function. Blocking the PD-1/B7-H1 signaling pathways, can enhance specific T lymphocyte function [8]. The immunity of the liver is closely related to the expression of B7-H1 in intrahepatic non parenchymal cells, including endothelial cells and hepatic clearance macrophages, B7-H1 inhibits the proliferation and differentiation of T cells in the liver [1, 3]. This study suggests that the expression of PD-1, B7-H1 of T lymphocytes in patients with severe hepatitis is significantly higher than that of control group, expression of PD-1 and B7-H1 of T lymphocyte in chronic severe hepatitis group is significantly higher than patients with severe hepatitis, account for lymphoid cells as antigen, it can antigen-presenting cell and express PD-1/B7-H1 pathways, involve in total stimulus way induced by HBV infection to activate T lymphocytes, but cellular level of induced expression are not completely the same. The expression of PD-1/B7-H1 of T lymphocytes in severe hepatitis group is less than the group of patients with subsevere hepatitis in this study, whether this phenomenon was correlated with the pathogenesis of severe hepatitis need further discussion.

T lymphocytes play an important role in cellular immunity and T lymphocyte subsets CD3, CD4 and CD8 is important surface antigen of the logo, as the immune effector cells play important roles in immune regulation, have been widely as a standard of assessment of cellular immune function change [9]. CD3 of T lymphocytes continues to reduce showed that cellular immune suppression; CD4 (helper T lymphocytes) and CD8 (weak T lymphocytes) are two kinds of important subgroup of T lymphocytes, the fall of CD4 lymphatic factor lead to assist the B lymphocytes to produce antibodies and other auxiliary lymphocyte function abate, CD4/CD8 ratio descend shows that the body reduce the balance between T lymphocyte subsets, more can reflect the immune state [10]. In the pathogenesis of severe hepatitis, cell immune-mediated liver injury plays a key role. Studies suggest that peripheral blood lymphocyte reduced in early severe hepatitis patients [11]. This study suggested $CD4^+$ and $CD8^+$ in severe hepatitis group and the control group were decreased ($P < 0.05$), showed that patients with severe hepatitis have obvious cell function disorder phenomenon in the body. Causes of this phenomenon is likely to be consumption of a large number of lymphocytes by severe hepatitis acute immune reaction [12]. Most severe hepatitis were harmed by immune of $CD4^+$, $CD8^+$ cells inducing, what to consume most, so $CD4^+$, $CD8^+$ cells consumed most, also reduced obviously.

Promoting liver cell auxin (Hepatocyte growth promot—ing factor, pHGF) is low molecular peptide substances extracted from fresh pig liver, can promote regeneration liver of rats DNA synthesis, eliminate endotoxin, and can reduce mortality of the D-galactose amine induced rat experimental liver failure [13, 14]. In the self-made Gongying Yinchen Decoction,the dandelion has the function of heat-clearing and detoxifying, eliminating carbuncle and dissipating, removing dampness and treating ssoupuria; The capillary artemisia has the function of clearing heat and removing dampness, curing jaundice by normalizing function of the gallbladder. Radix bupleuri has the function of dispersing the stagnated liver-qi and uplift yang-qi to raise sinking.Rhei could remove stagnation by purgation, clear away heat and purge fire, remove toxin and promote blood circulation to remove blood stasis. Smilax glabra and grifola has the function of clearing damp and promoting diuresis. Radix isatidis could clear away heat and remove toxin, cool the blood and relieve sore throat, in latest Pharmacological research, when it combined with other herbs to treat oxyhepatitis, it can alleviate the symptoms, promote the improvement of liver function [15]. Radix sophorae flavescentis is good at heat-clearing and damp-drying, diuresis and insecticidal action. The study suggested the positive expression rate of T lymphocytes PD-1, B7-H1 in patients of the treatment group was higher than that of healthy control group, statistical significance were significant ($P < 0.05$); PD-1, B7-H1 positive expression rate of T lymphocytes in patients of the treatment group significantly decreased after treatment, compared with before treatment ($P < 0.05$). $CD4^+$, $CD8^+$ cells of the treatment group patients were significantly lower than that of normal group ($P < 0.05$). The $CD4^+/CD8^+$ cells of the treatment group patients was higher than that of normal group ($P < 0.05$), significantly decreased after treatment ($P < 0.05$). Confirmed to promoting liver cell growth hormone combination from the Gongying Yinchen soup can influence expression of T lymphocytes PD-1/B7-H1 path in patients with severe hepatitis depression, can enhance the body's immune response.

References

1. Xu XF, Ye JS, Jiang LH et al (2011) The expression and significance of PD-1/B7-H1 pathways of T lymphocytes in patients with fulminant hepatitis. J Clin Exam 29(9):670–671
2. Han JM, Li HR (2010) Factors of influencing the prognosis of severe hepatitis. Chin J Exp Clin Infect Dis Electron 4(3):44
3. Zhou YX, Ceng YX (2010) Detection and its clinical value of plasma endotoxin, tumor necrosis factor alpha in patients with severe hepatitis. Lab Med Clin 7(6):528–529
4. Chinese Medical Association Infectious Diseases and Parasitic Epidemiology Branch (2001) Liver disease, viral hepatitis prevention scheme. Chin J Infect Dis 12 (1):56–62
5. Psychiatric Branch of Chinese Medical Association (2001) The diagnosis of depression with western medicine diagnostic criteria: refer to the Chinese classification and diagnosis standard of mental illness, third edition (CCMD-3). Jinan: Shandong Science And Technology Press, 87–89
6. Chen ZJ, Hu SY, Zhang HN et al (2005) Research of depression common syndrome standard. J Tradit Chin Med 46–48(1):47–49
7. Okazakj T, Honjo T (2006) The PD-1-PD-L pathway in immunological tolerance. Trevds Immunol 27(4):195–201
8. Barber DL, Wherry EJ, Masopust D et al (2006) Restoring function in ex-hausted CD8 T cells during chronic viral infection. Nature 439(7077):682–687
9. Pellegrini JD, DeAK KodysK et al (2000) Relationship between lymphocyte apoptosis and energy following trauma. J SurgRes 88(2):200–206
10. Cai WQ, Wang BR (1994) Practical immunocytochemistry and nucleicacid hybridization technology. Sichuan Science and Technology Publishing House, Chengdu, pp 241–243
11. Xie ZB, Li NF (2010) Detection and significance of $CD4^+$ and $CD8^+$ lymphocytes subgroup in severe hepatitis. J Cell Mol Immunol 26(6):587–588
12. Wu CX, Chen L (2007) Clinical analysis of T cell subgroup detection of viral severe hepatitis. J Qiqihar Med Coll 28(22):2711–2712
13. Kong XP, Zheng GC, Zhang YJ et al (1991) Liver cell stimulating factor treatment of experimental liver failure in rats and its mechanism of experimental research. Chin J Dig 11(1):23
14. Zheng GC, Kong XP, Zhang YJ et al (1990) The protection research of promoting hepatocyte growth factor in CCl_4 hepatic injury in the rat. Tianjin Med J 18(9):539
15. Sun JN (2007) Chinese medicine pharmacology version 2. China's Traditional Chinese Medicine Press, p 95

Chapter 291
The Influence of Hepatocyte Growth-Promoting Factors Combined with Gongying Yinchen Soup for Depression in Patients with Fulminant Hepatitis Peripheral Blood T Lymphocyte Subsets and Liver Function

Liping Wu, Junfeng Gao, Xinguo Zhao, Huilong Li, Jianqiao Li, Limin Ma, Meng Li, Weihua Han, Qing Gu and Ruiyu Li

Abstract *Objective* To investigate the effect of the influence of hepatocyte growth-promoting factors combined with Gongying Yinchen soup for depression in patients with fulminant hepatitis peripheral blood T lymphocyte subsets and liver function. *Methods* Choose 61 cases of fulminant hepatitis patients with depression, With reference to the American psychiatric association *Mental disorders diagnostic and statistical manual* (DSM-IV) Classification standard, 31 cases patients were randomly divided into treatment group, which was given intravenous drip of 10 % glucose injection 250 ml containing Hepatocyte growth-promoting factors 120 rag, once daily, 15 days for a course of treatment and 30 in the control group, Application of above methods at the same time to add with the

L. Wu
Xingtai People's Hospital, Xingtai, Hebei Province, China

J. Gao · H. Li · W. Han · Q. Gu
Second Affiliated Hospital of Xingtai Medical College, No. 618 Gangtiebei Road, Xingtai, Hebei Province, China

X. Zhao · L. Ma
Chinese Medicine Hospital of Lincheng County, Xingtai, Hebei Province, China

J. Li
Chinese Medicine Hospital, Luquan, Hebei Province, China

M. Li
Health Team of Hotan Prefecture Detachment of Chinese Armed Police Force, Xinjiang, China

R. Li (✉)
Institute of Integrated Traditional and Western Medicine, Second Affiliated Hospital, Xingtai Medical College, No. 618 Gangtiebei Road, Xingtai, Hebei Province, China
e-mail: Liruiyu651021@163.com

Gongying Yinchen soup, etc. (Dandelion, radix et rhizoma rhei, radix bupleuri, herba artemisiae capillaris, glabrous greenbrier rhizome, radix isatidis, grifola, bitter ginseng). After the treatment for three courses, the peripheral blood T lymphocyte subsets (by FACSCalibur flow cytometry) and liver function were detected. *Results* After the treatments the level of $CD3^+$ $CD4^+$ $CD4^+/CD8^+$ increased in two groups with more marked elevation in control group ($P < 0.01$); The level of $CD8^+$ counts decreased. Compared with the treatment group, the change of control group was more significant ($P < 0.05$); The level of ALT AST and GGT in two groups decreased, But the control group decreased obviously ($P < 0.05$, $P < 0.01$). *Conclusions* Hepatocyte growth-promoting factors combined with Gongying Yinchen soup in patients with fulminant hepatitis depression can affect the peripheral blood T lymphocyte subsets, can enhance the body's immune response ability.

Keywords Hepatocyte growth-promoting factors · Gongying Yinchen soup · Fulminant hepatitis · T lymphocyte subsets · Liver function

291.1 Introduction

Chronic fulminate hepatitis was induced by the interaction of a variety of complications, which includes chronic liver dysfunction and disorder of the immune mechanism. T lymphocyte subsets play an important role in liver cells immunopathological damage of chronic fulminate hepatitis [1]. To further explore the effect of immunization of hepatocyte growth-promoting factors associated with self-production gongying yinchen soup against patients with chronic fulminate hepatitis-mediated depression, the thesis observed the changes of peripheral blood T lymphocyte subsets and liver function of hepatocyte growth-promoting factors associated with self-production Gongying Yinchen soup against patients with chronic fulminate hepatitis-mediated depression, preliminary report are as follows.

291.2 Materials and Methods

291.2.1 General Information

From November 2003 to August 2007, 61 patients in Department of Integrated Chinese and Western Medicine were treated, 61 cases were divided into two groups. The treatment group 31 cases, 21 males, 10 females, age 26–75 years, an average of 49.2 years; Hepatitis A 12 cases, Hepatitis B 10 cases, The overlap of hepatitis A and hepatitis B 2 cases, Undifferentiated hepatitis 4 cases, Alcoholic hepatitis 3 cases; Control group 30 cases, 21 males, 9 females, age 24–72 years, an average of 47.7 year; Hepatitis A 9 cases, Hepatitis B 15 cases, The overlap of hepatitis A and hepatitis B 1 cases, Undifferentiated hepatitis 3 cases, Alcoholic hepatitis 2 cases.

291.2.2 Criteria of Diagnosis

Fulminant hepatitis diagnostic criteria with reference to the Chinese medical association of infectious diseases and parasitic epidemiology branch-hepatology branch Viral hepatitis prevention and treatment programmes [2]. The criteria of depression with western medicine diagnostic criteria: *According to the Chinese Classification and Diagnosis of Mental Diseases*-3rd edition (CCMD-3) [3], certainty what exactly depression is for patients. TCM diagnostic criteria: Referring to the relevant TCM literature [4].

291.2.3 Classification Standards of Depression Severity

Reference to the *American Psychiatric Association's Diagnostic and Statistical Manual-IV* (DSM-IV).

291.2.4 Inclusion Criteria

① Conforms to the diagnosis of depression in patients with slight or midrange depression. ② Stable vital signs, conscious, Have certain language ability.

291.2.5 Exclusion Criteria

① Belong to major depressive disorder. ② There is some form of schizophrenia,or belong to the symptom of post-schizophrenia depression. ③ Clinical diagnosis was Non depression psychosis. ④ Does not accord with the inclusive criteria; or data not congruent effect observation of patients. Comply with the above one of the patients, and to exclude.

291.2.6 Therapeutic Method

Treatment group application on hepatocyte growth-promoting factors 120 mg, add in 250 ml of 10 % glucose, Intravenous fluids,once daily, 15 days for a course of treatment. Control group applied this method at the same time to add with the gongying yinchen soup decoction created by ourselves. Gongying yinchen soup decoction create by ourselves, its composition is: dandelion, Herba artemisiae capillaris, radix bupleuri, herba artemisiae capillaris, prepared rhubarb,glabrous greenbrier rhizome, radix isatidis, grifola, bitter ginseng, daily one agent, water decoction, 15 days for a period of treatment, Shared 3 period of treatment, merger gastrointestinal cold should be used with caution.

291.2.7 Observational Index

The detection of peripheral blood T lymphocyte subsets: extraction of peripheral venous blood 2 ml, heparin anticoagulation. Use the FAC—SCalibur flow cytometry instrument produced by BD company in United States and detection of peripheral blood $CD3^+$, $CD4^+$ and $CD8^+$ T cells by indirect immunofluorescence (monoclonal antibody) (fluorescein labeled goat anti mouse antibody produced by Beijing biological product institute).

291.2.8 Statistical Methods

The data of the results were analysed by SPSS11.0, Measurement data with mean standard deviation ($\bar{x} \pm S$), T test was adopted in group measurement data.

291.3 Results

291.3.1 Comparison of the Changes in T Cell Subsets Before and After the Treatment of Treatment Group and Control Group (Table 291.1)

Table 291.1 Comparison of the changes in T cell subsets ($\bar{x} \pm s$ %) before and after the treatment of treatment group and control group

Group		ALT	AST	GGT
Treatment group (44 cases)	Before treatment	94.69 ± 28.64	53.72 ± 21.726	69.77 ± 31.93
	After treatment	51.76 ± 19.68②	37.23 ± 14.74①	43.90 ± 26.11②
Control group (40 cases)	Before treatment	96.95 ± 29.70	52.34 ± 19.72	74.51 ± 28.41
	After treatment	39.52 ± 16.20②④	29.12 ± 12.68②③	42.66 ± 27.15①

Note compared with before treatment, ①$P < 0.05$, ②$P < 0.01$; compared with control group, ③$P < 0.05$, ④$P < 0.01$

291.3.2 The Changes of the Liver Function Before and After the Treatment of Treatment Group and Control Group (Table 291.2)

Table 291.2 Comparison of the changes in T cell subsets ($\bar{x} \pm s$ %) before and after the treatment of treatment group and control group

Group		$CD3^+$	$CD4^+$	$CD8^+$	$CD4^+/CD8^+$
Treatment group (44 cases)	Before treatment	55.62 ± 8.96	32.33 ± 7.60	33.93 ± 5.43	0.92 ± 0.26
	After treatment	59.33 ± 9.70①	35.73 ± 8.62①	31.33 ± 6.12①	1.11 ± 0.33①
Control group (40 cases)	Before treatment	55.13 ± 8.22	37.75 ± 7.19	34.12 ± 6.48	0.90 ± 0.27
	After treatment	69.66 ± 9.96②③	38.96 ± 8.67②③	28.62 ± 5.61②③	1.33 ± 0.36②③

Note compared with before treatment, ①$P < 0.05$, ②$P < 0.01$; compared with control group, ③$P < 0.05$, ④$P < 0.01$

291.4 Discussions

For effect of T lymphocyte subgroup and function, in theory after practice have effect. It depends on the co-synergy or co-restricting effects among a variety of immune cells, especially the T-lymphocyte subsets, to maintain the normal balance of the immune system and to produce moderate immune response, witch can protect the self-tissue from damaging and clear up the foreign antigen [5]. According to the phenotypes, the mature T cells can be divided into $CD3^+$ $CD4^+$ $CD8^-$ and $CD3^+$ CD4–CD8(+) types, which are also known as $CD4^+$ T cells and $CD8^+$ T cells. According to the different functions, it can also be divided into helper T cells (Th), cytotoxic T cells (Tc), T cells mediated delayed-type hypersensitivity reaction (TDTH) and suppressor T cells (Ts). Because most $CD4^+$ T cells is Th cells and $CD8^+$ T cells is mainly Tc cells, the $CD4^+/CD8^+$ ratio is often used as the assessment indicator of the immune status [6].

Insufficient of $CD4^+$ quantity in peripheral blood of chronic fulminate hepatitis, reactive T cells (mainly is the hepatitis B virus specific $CD8^+$ cells) excessive proliferating, and continuously attacking the hepatitis B virus infected target cells, results a large number of target cells necrosis. In addition, there is some positive correlation between the percentage of $CD4^+$ regulatory T cells in peripheral blood and the HBV DNA load [7], Hepatocyte growth promoting factor (pHGF) is a low molecular peptide which extracted from fresh liver of pig, with the promotion of regenerating rat liver DNA synthesis, eliminating endotoxin, that can reduce the death rate in D-galactosamine induced rats experimental hepatic failure [8, 9]. In the self-made Gongying Yinchen Decoction, the dandelion has the function of heat-clearing and detoxifying, eliminating carbuncle and dissipating, removing dampness and treating ssoupuria; The capillary artemisia has the function of clearing heat and removing dampness, curing jaundice by normalizing function of the gallbladder. Radix bupleuri has the function of dispersing the stagnated liver-qi and uplift yang-qi to raise sinking. Rhei could remove stagnation by purgation, clear away heat and purge fire, remove toxin and promote blood circulation to remove blood stasis, smilax glabra and grifola has the function of clearing damp and promoting diuresis radix isatidis could clear away heat and remove toxin, cool the blood and relieve sore throat, in latest Pharmacological research, when it combined with other herbs to treat oxyhepatitis, it can alleviate the symptoms, promote the improvement of liver function [10]. Radix sophorae flavescentis is good at heat-clearing and damp-drying, diuresis and insecticidal action.

Here we used Gongying Yinchen soup combining with the hepatocyte growth-promoting factors to treat fulminant hepatitis patients with depression and finally proved that this therapeutic regimen can improve the immune response ability by affecting T lymphocyte subsets and liver function.

References

1. Ding QY, Yu HY, Sun WW et al (2010) Peripheral blood T lymphocyte subsets changes fulminant hepatitis. Jiangsu Med J 36(19):2336–2337
2. Chinese medical association infectious diseases and parasitic epidemiology branch (2001) Liver disease, viral hepatitis prevention scheme. Chin J Infect Dis 12(1):56–62
3. Psychiatric branch of Chinese medical association (2001) The diagnosis of depression with western medicine diagnostic criteria: refer to the Chinese classification and diagnosis standard of mental illness, 3rd edn (CCMD-3). Shandong science and technology press, Jinan, pp 87–89
4. Chen ZQ, Hu SY, Zhang HN et al (2005) Studying on common TCM syndromes of depression. J Tradit Chin Med 46(1):47–49
5. Gong FL (2000) Medical immunology. Science press, Beijing, p 160
6. Jin BQ, Li ES, Xu H et al (1999) Cellular and molecular immunology. World Publishing Corporation, Beijing, pp 259–285
7. Zhang LL, Zhou ZS (2007) $CD4^+$ $CD25^+$ regulatory T cells in the role of fulminant hepatitis B disease. Liver Mag 10(12):371–373
8. Kong XP, Zheng GC, Zhang YZ et al (1991) Hepatocyte stimulating factor of rat experimental liver failure factors and the experimental mechanism research. Chin J Dig 11(1):23
9. Zheng GC, Kong XP, Zhang YJ et al (1990) Promoting liver cell toxicity of auxin in CCl_4 rat liver injury research. Tianjin Med J 18(9):539
10. Sun JN (2007) Chinese medicine pharmacology, Version 2. China's Traditional Chinese Medicine Press, Beijing, p 95

Chapter 292
The Impact of Hepatocyte Growth-Promoting Factors Combined with Gongying Yinchen Soup on Peripheral Blood SIL-2R of Depression in Fulminant Hepatitis Patients

Guo Kaoshan, Gao Junfeng, Li Jianqiao, Zhao Xinguo, Li Huilong, Ma Limin, Li Meng, Sun Yanfu, Gu Qing, Han Weihua and Li Ruiyu

Abstract *Objective* Discuss the effect of Hepatocyte growth-promoting factors combined with Gongying Yinchen soup on peripheral blood SIL-2R of depression in fulminant hepatitis patients. *Methods* Choose 88 cases of fulminant hepatitis patients with depression,With reference to the American psychiatric association *Mental disorders diagnostic and statistical manual* (DSM-IV) Classification standard, The treatment group 88 cases, which was given GongYing Yinchen soup and intravenous drip of 10 % glucose injection 250 ml containing Hepatocyte growth-promoting factors 120 rag, once daily, 15 days for a course of treatment, Application of above methods at the same time to add with the Gongying Yinchen soup, etc. (Dandelion, radix et rhizoma rhei, radix bupleuri, herba artemisiae capillaris, glabrous greenbrier rhizome, radix isatidis, grifola, bitter ginseng). After the treatment for three courses, Peripheral blood levels of SIL-2R in all patients with severe hepatitis depression were detected,and 30 healthy blood donors were used as controls. Methods Adopt the method of ELISA for levels of SIL-2R in all patients of two groups were detected pre and post-treatment. *Results* Compare the

---

G. Kaoshan · L. Ruiyu (✉)
Second Affiliated Hospital of Xing Tai Medical College, No. 618 Gangtiebei Road, Xingtai, Hebei Province, China
e-mail: liruiyu651021@163.com

G. Junfeng · L. Huilong · S. Yanfu · G. Qing · H. Weihua
Second Affiliated Hospital of Xingtai Medical College, Xingtai City, Hebei Province, China

L. Jianqiao
Chinese Medicine Hospital, Luquan, Hebei Pronvince, China

Z. Xinguo · M. Limin
Chinese Medicine Hospital, Lincheng, Hebei Province, China

L. Meng
Health Team of Hotan Prefecture Detachment of Chinese Armed Police Force, Xinjiang, China

blood level of SIL-2R of Each group patients with severe hepatitis and health adults, there is significant statistical significance ($P < 0.05$, $P < 0.05$). Treatment group after treatment level of serum SIL-2R significantly decreased, There was a significant difference in comparison with the pretreatment ($P < 0.01$). *Conclusions* Hepatocyte growth-promoting factors combined with Gongying Yinchen soup can influence peripheral blood SIL-2R of depression in fulminant hepatitis patients, efficacy significantly on severe hepatitis, Can enhance the body's immune response.

Keywords Hepatocyte growth-promoting factors · Gongying yinchen soup · Fulminant hepatitis · SIL-2R

292.1 Introduction

SIL-2R is from activated lymphocyte membrane IL-2 receptor α chain parts, It combines with low affinity interleukin-2, Thus has immune adjustment and immune inhibition. Since Rubin's etc. found in 1985, Has confirmed that it is involved in the pathogenesis of autoimmune diseases. Serum soluble interleukin 2 receptor (SIL-2R) mainly released by activated T cells. In the hepatitis, The pathological mechanism of hepatic damage is directly related to T lymphocyte function [1]. This article explores the impact of Hepatocyte growth-promoting factors combined with Gongying Yinchen soup on peripheral blood SIL-2R of depression in fulminant hepatitis patients. A preliminary report as follows:

292.2 Materials and Methods

292.2.1 General Information

From November 2003–August 2007, 88 patients in Department of Integrated Chinese and Western Medicine were treated, 88 cases(treatment group), 57 males and 31 females, 26–75 years old, Among them acute sever hepatitis 31 cases, 21 males and 10 females, 18–52 years old, an average of 29.7 years; subacute severe viral hepatitis 29 cases, 17 males and 12 females, 19–50 years old, an average of 30.4 years;chronic severe hepatitis 28 cases, 19 males and 9 females, 28–58 years old, an average of 38.6 years.The control group 30 cases, 21 males and 9 females, 24–72 years old, an average of 40.7 years, They are from blood banks in Xingtai City of healthy blood donors.

292.2.2 Diagnostic Criteria

Fulminant hepatitis diagnostic criteria with reference to the Chinese medical association of infectious diseases and parasitic epidemiology branch—hepatology branch Viral hepatitis prevention and treatment programmes [2]. The criteria of depression with western medicine diagnostic criteria: According to the *Chinese Classification and Diagnosis of Mental Diseases* -3rd edition (CCMD-3) [3], certainty what exactly depression is for patients. TCM diagnostic criteria: Referring to the relevant tcm literature [4].

292.2.3 The Severity of the Depression Classification Standard

Reference to the American Psychiatric Association's *Diagnostic and Statistical Manual-IV* (DSM-IV).

292.2.4 The Inclusion Criteria

①Conforms to the diagnosis of depression in patients with slight or midrange depression. ②Stable vital signs, conscious, Have certain language ability.

292.2.5 Exclusion Criteria

①Belong to major depressive disorder; ②There is some form of schizophrenia, or belong to the symptom of post-schizophrenia depression; ③Clinical diagnosis was Non depression psychosis; ④Does not accord with the inclusive criteria; or Data not congruent effect observation of patients; Comply with the above one of the patients, and to exclude.

292.2.6 Treatment

Treatment group application on hepatocyte growth-promoting factors 120 mg, add in 250 ml of 10 % glucose, Intravenous fluids, once daily, 15 days for a course of treatment.Treatment group applied this method at the same time to add with the gongying yinchen soup decoction Create by ourselves. The self-made gongying yinchen soup, which made up of Pugongying Yinchen CHaihu ZHidahuang

Tufuling Banlangen ZHuling Kushen, one dose each day, Make into decoction and use as tea,10 doses constituting one course;altogether used 3 period of treatments, deficiency-cold of spleen and stomach persons used with caution.Control group applied this method at the same time added nutgrass galingale rhizome, radix curcumae, radix angelicae sinensis, radix paeoniae alba, radix aucklandiae and other drugs.

292.2.7 Observational Index

Detection of peripheral blood SIL-2R: Peripheral blood levels of soluble interleukin 2 receptor (SIL-2R) in all patients of two groups were detected pre and post-treatment, Methods Adopt the method of ELISA for levels of SIL-2R. Kit: They are supplied by the Department of Immunology of Hebei medical university,In strict accordance with the instructions.

292.2.8 Statistical Methods

The data of the results were analysised by SPSS11.0, Measurement data with mean standard deviation ($\bar{\chi} \pm S$), T test was adopted in group measurement data.

292.3 Results

292.3.1 Severe Hepatitis Patients Compared with Normal Serum SIL-2R Levels (Table 292.1)

Table 292.1 Severe hepatitis patients compared with normal serum SIL-2R levels ($\bar{x} \pm s$)

Group	case	SIL-2R(u/ul)
Normal group	30	131.0 ± 34.1*
Acute sever hepatitis group	31	521.2 ± 97.7△*
Subacute severe viral hepatitis group	29	571.4 ± 97.2△*#
Chronic severe hepatitis group	28	520.3 ± 95.6△*★

Note Compared with normal group *$P < 0.01$; Compared withchronic severe hepatitis group △$P < 0.01$; Compared with acute sever hepatitis group #$P < 0.01$; Compared with subacute severe viral hepatitis group ★$P < 0.01$

Table 292.2 The changes of serum levels of SIL-2R pre and post-treatment in Treatment group

Group	case	prior treatment	post treatment
Acute sever hepatitis group	31	516.7 ± 97.2	196.5 ± 37.4△
Subacute severe viral hepatitis group	29	577.1 ± 95.1	290.6 ± 42.7△
Chronic severe hepatitis group	28	525.2 ± 94.4	282. ± 60.2△

Note Before and after treatment comparison △$P < 0.01$

292.3.2 Compare the Changes of Serum Levels of SIL-2R Pre and Post-treatment in Treatment Group(Table 292.2)

292.4 Discussion

Interleukin-2 (IL-2) 1976 Morgan [5] etc. in induce to foster peripheral blood mononuclear cells found in the first place, At that time was named the T cell growth factor (TCGF). Since found, International and domestic academics for its structure, biological characteristics, action mechanism, purification, identification, genetic analysis and clinical application and so on have done a lot of research. Unified named IL-2 in 1979, Because of IL-2 has a wide range of biological activities and potential prospect of clinical application, and has been widely concerned. Interleukin 2 receptor (IL-2r) was founded in 1985 by Rubin [6] a protein found in the first place,It can exist in two forms,A located on the cell membrane that is membrane IL-2R (mIL-2R), Another appear in blood and in the bacterium spent culture supernatant that is soluble IL-2R(SIL-2R), The increasing of SIL-2R is associated with many diseases, and detect eaSILy,Thus cause the attention of clinical workers.

SIL-2R is by the activation of T cells surface of IL-2r extracellular structure zone formed under part fall off. (1) HBV replication invivo can stimulate T cells release a large number of SIL-2R, It and MIL-2R can be combined with IL-2, neutralization and activated the IL-2 of T cells surrounding, Can be used as an immunosuppressive factor, so the elevated levels of IL-12 can reduce patient's antiviral immune activity, Compound the immune dysfunction; (2) Remove SIL-2R's ability are reduce after Liver damage. Also SIL-2R in blood circulation does not effectively rule out in vitro. Sometimes the elevated levels of IL-12 associated with the degree of liver disease and liver function decline [7–9]. Wan Wei [10] etc. study found that various types of hepatitis in pediatric patients with serum IL-2 and SIL-2R were significantly higher than the control group ($P < 0.05$), The IL-2 increased most obviously in the acute hepatitis, SIL-2R most significantly elevated in chronic severe hepatitis ($P < 0.05$), IL-2 and SIL-2R in infantile viral hepatitis damage degrees there is a certain value. It has directing significance in prognostics of chronic severe hepatitis.

Hepatocyte growth promot-ing factor (pHGF) is a low molecular peptide which extracted from fresh liver of pig, with the promotion of regenerating rat liver DNA synthesis, eliminating endotoxin, that can reduce the death rate in D- galactos-amine induced rats experimental hepatic failure [11, 12]. In the self-made Gongying Yinchen Decoction, the dandelion has the function of heat-clearing and detoxifying, eliminating carbuncle and dissipating, removing dampness and treating ssoupuria. The capillary artemisia has the function of clearing heat and removing dampness, curing jaundice by normalizing function of the gallbladder. Radix bupleuri has the function of dispersing the stagnated liver-qi and uplift yang-qi to raise sinking. Rhei could remove stagnation by purgation, clear away heat and purge fire, remove toxin and promote blood circulation to remove blood stasis. Smilax glabra and grifola has the function of clearing damp and promoting diuresis. Radix isatidis could clear away heat and remove toxin, cool the blood and relieve sore throat, in latest Pharmacological research, when it combined with other herbs to treat oxyhepatitis, it can alleviate the symptoms, promote the improvement of liver function [13]. Radix sophorae flavescentis is good at heat-clearing and damp-drying, diuresis and insecticidal action.

This article through to each group in severe hepatitis and normal serum SIL-2R level detection, There is significant statistical significance ($P < 0.05$, $P < 0.05$); Treatment group after treatment level of serum SIL-2R significantly decreased, There was a significant difference in comparison with the pretreatment ($P < 0.01$). Suggests that hepatocyte growth-promoting factors combined with Gongying Yinchen soup can influence peripheral blood SIL-2R of depression in fulminant hepatitis patients, efficacy significantly on severe hepatitis, Can enhance the body's immune response.

References

1. Li K, Liu JX, Nan YM (1997) Serum soluble interleukin 2 receptor and T lymphocyte subsets of the significance of combined detection of hepatitis c[J]. Chin J Clin Hepatol 13(2):151–155
2. Branch Association of Infectious diseases and parasitic epidemiology, Branch Association of Hepatology. Chinese Medical Association (2001) Virus hepatitis integrated control measure. Chin J Infect Dis 19(1): 56–62
3. . Branch of the Chinese Medical Association of psychiatry. (2001) The Chinese Classification and Diagnosis of Mental Diseases 3rd edition (CCMD-3). Jinan: Shandong Science & Technology press, 87–89
4. Chen ZQ, Hu SY, Zhang HN et al (2005) Studying on common TCM syndromes of depression [J]. J Tradit Chin Med 46(1):47–49
5. Morgam DA, Rusceff FW, Gallo R (1976) Selectibe vitrogrouth of Lymphocytes from normal human bome marrows. Science 193:1007–1009
6. Rubin LA, Kurman CC, Fritz ME et al (1985) Soluble interleukin-2 receptors are released from activated human lymphoid cells in vitro. J Immunol 135(5):3172–3177
7. Jing RL, Lu QS, Guo YB et al (2000) Th1/Th2 cells in the role of chronic hepatitis b virus infection. Acad J First Mil Med Univ 20(2):103–105

8. Jia HY, Du J, Zhu SH et al (2003) Clinical observation of serum IL-18, IL-10 and SIL-2R levels in patients withchronic hepatitis C pre and post antiviral treatment[J]. Chin Med J 116(4):605–608
9. Tangkijvanich P, Vimolket T, Theamboonlers A et al (2000) Serum interkeukin-6 and interferon-gamma levels in patientswith hepatitis-associated chronic liver disease [J]. Asian Pac J Allergy Immunol 18(2):109–114
10. Jiang W, Lederman MM, Salkowitz JR et al (2005) Impaired monocytematuration in response to CpG oligodeoxynucleotide is related to viralRNA levels in human immunodeficiency virus disease and is at leastpartially mediated by deficiencies in alpha/beta interferon responsivenessand production. J Virol 79(7):4109–4119
11. Kong XP, Zheng GC, Zhang YZ et al (1991) Hepatocyte stimulating factor of rat experimental liver failure factors and the experimental mechanism research. Chin J Digestion 11(1):23
12. Zheng GC, Kong XP, Zhang YZ et al (1990) Promoting liver cell toxicity of auxin in CCl4 rat liver injury research [J]. Tianjin Med J 18(9):539
13. Sun JN (2011) Pharmacology of Chinese materia medica (Version 2). Chinese Medicine Press, p 95

Chapter 293
Design and Development of Learning-Based Game for Acupuncture Education

Youliang Huang, Renquan Liu, Mingquan Zhou and Xingguang Ma

Abstract Traditional teaching-and-learning environments often do not address the learning needs of students who prefer experiential activities and the use of new technology. In this paper, it is provided a new method to create a game platform that includes the acupuncture knowledge. When students use this platform, they will find learning is an interesting thing. This is the so-called Serious Games. It is rising in a wide range of fields like education, training and simulation, etc. We develop a game for acupuncture education and use a different platform, Unity3D, as our game engine. 3D models and other scenes are designed with 3ds Max 2012, then converted to *.fbx format to load in the Unity 3D. When students log in the game, the game presents a series of scenes include some questions and asks students to make decisions about the acupuncture knowledge. It is also discussed some details of the game for acupuncture learning and provided some references for the development of the Serious Games.

Keywords Acupuncture education · Serious games · Unity 3D

293.1 Introduction

With the further development of acupuncturology's modernization and internationalization [1], the combination of acupuncturology and modern science and technology has become one of trends for acupuncturology. It is of great

---

Y. Huang · R. Liu (✉) · X. Ma
Information Center, Beijing University of Chinese Medicine, Beijing 100029, China
e-mail: liurq@bucm.edu.cn

Y. Huang · M. Zhou
College of Information Science and Technology, Beijing Normal University,
Beijing 100875, China

significance and application value to train acupuncture learners with modern information technology. The use of 'serious games' is rapidly growing part of educational technology. Serious Games research has shown that learning through games has positive effects, since the users can abstract themselves from the learning process itself, and learn while playing. For this reason, we decided to create a serious game for education of acupuncture. This paper describes a project that will see the design and development serious game to facilitate learning of the concepts related to acupuncture. It can help medical students to focus on and develop an understanding of the acupuncture knowledge.

293.1.1 Acupuncture

Acupuncture was originated from ancient China with the typical Chinese thinking and special philosophy, and recently has been accepted as a useful curing method, attracting quite much interest and being studied by many medical institutions worldwide [2]. It is one of the key components of traditional Chinese medicine. It is a collection of procedures which involves the stimulation of points on the body using a variety of techniques.

293.1.2 Serious Game in Education

Serious games are (digital) games used for purposes other than mere entertainment. Serious games are a new educational approach, extremely attractive for professional and adult education, since they allow the participants to assume the roles of decision-makers in simulated situations that recreate reality [3]. It also can save cost and time. Many graduate courses (like, business administration, medicine) and post-graduate programs have computerized simulations and serious games deeply integrated into their curricula [4].

The rest of this paper is organized as follows. Section 293.2 presents the architecture of our system. Section 293.3 describes the implementation details. Results are discussed in Sect. 293.4. Conclusion and future work will be shown in Sect. 293.5.

293.2 Architecture

The purpose of all the work is to generate an acupuncture game. For the development of our game, the workflow was followed: (i) Data collection and assessment of the educational needs of the students, (ii) Game planning and design, (iii) Integrate game module, (iv) Game test and optimize.

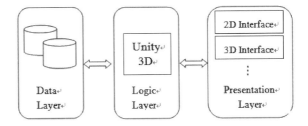

Fig. 293.1 The architecture of our framework

We designed a framework for brower-based single-player online game. This framework includes three layers: data layer, logical layer and presentation layer. The architecture of our system is shown in Fig. 293.1.

293.3 Design and Development

It is made up by five function modules such as: underlying principle, choosing a game engine, 3D modeling and scene, game design, game play.

293.3.1 Underlying Principle

The developed game serves three major goals:

- Create a game that would teach medical students the basic functioning of the acupuncture knowledge.
- Improve the traditional teaching methods to stimulate students' enthusiasm for learning.
- Allow students to experience situations that would be unreason able in real life due to safety reasons, excessive cost, etc.

293.3.2 Choosing a Game Engine

Game engine is a platform to process underlying technologies, through which game developers need not pay more attention to technologies related to system structure and graphic process. Serious Games call engine supported API directly. Game engine provides API, some core class libraries and assist toolkit, which greatly improves efficiency and reduce development cost [5]. In this paper, we selected Unity 3D as game engine. Unity 3D is one of the most famous virtual reality tools, user-friendly interface, and lots of target platforms (mobiles, web, PC/MacOS, etc. are supported). Unity3D supports three scripting languages:

JavaScript, C# and a dialect of Python called Boo. These three languages in game development projects can also be mixed-use. Unity3d also supports the Windows platform, C#, VB.net, VB6, Delphi and other programming languages [6].

293.3.3 3D Modeling and Scene

3D modeling is an important piece of the acupuncture game. 3D models and scenes can be generated using a number of different tools such as 3D Studio Max, Maya, and Blender among others. The choice of modeling system dictates what type of geometry will appear in the game. In this paper, the main tools for modeling are 3ds Max 2012. The game models and scenes consist of human body, drugstore, study, buildings and so on. The snapshot of the model in the game is shown in Fig. 293.2.

293.3.4 Game Design

The acupuncture point of the body contains a vast amount of acupuncture point, but in order to adapt the process to the level of young students, we had to simplify it. According to the story-line, we design three levels. In the first level, we select Chinese culture as the background. The task is to understand and learning culture of the traditional Chinese medicine. In the second level, the task is to learn acupuncture knowledge in the study scene. In the third level, we select drugstore as the main scene, the task is acupuncture training and testing. The game allowed students interaction (via dialog, exam) and students can reach a higher level after they complete a task in the game.

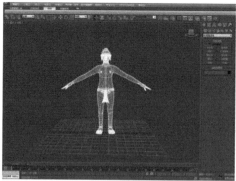 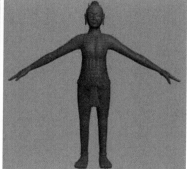

Fig. 293.2 The snapshot of the model in the game

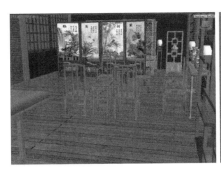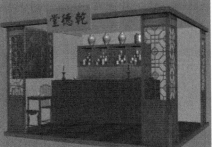

Fig. 293.3 The picture of the game

293.3.5 Game Play

Students view the environment through their avatar in a first-person perspective. In the game, this view mode is flexible and easy to use, good operability, making the students browsing scenes easily, greatly enhancing students' sense of reality. Students can move and rotate the "camera" using the mouse in a first-person manner thus allowing them to move within the scene. A cursor appears on the screen and students can use this cursor to point at specific objects and locations in the scene. The task of the students is to answer the question following the appropriate steps and choosing the correct tools for each step.

293.4 Result

According to the above method, we designed the acupuncture game. We conducted a similar set of experiments to test the performance of the system. The tests were carried out using an Intel Core2 Quad CPU Q6600, 4 GB of RAM, a GeForce 8800GT and Windows 7 SP1 32 bits. The result shows that the acupuncture game is feasible and practicable. After a series of the tests, the students will also be asked to fill out a short satisfaction questionnaire. We want to improve the playability of the game, based on the results before a final release. The picture of the game was shown in Fig. 293.3.

293.5 Conclusion and Future Work

Serious Games are proving to be valuable assets for teaching and training in various different outlets. In this paper, we described a new method that using game platform for solving the problems in acupuncture education. It can help teachers achieve an innovative and more effective way of teaching or training. However, the game has some shortcomings as well. We also want to improve the knowledge base in our game in our following work. Finally, we believe that our game will be a useful, educationally adequate tool for education of acupuncture learning, with the additional advantage of being more fun and attractive to students.

Acknowledgments This paper was supported in part by the Beijing University of Chinese Medicine Educational Research Fund (XJY12015).

References

1. Wang X (2004) Internationalization and modernization of acupuncture. Chin Acupunct Moxibustion 24(2):75–77 (in Chinese)
2. Shirota F (2002) Acu-points quick cure. Kodansha Sophia Books (in Japanese)
3. Aldrich C (2009) The complete guide to simulations and serious games: how the most valuable content will be created in the age beyond Gutenberg to Google. Pfeiffer, San Francisco
4. Shute V, Ventura M, Bauer M, Zapata-Rivera D (2009) "Melding the power of serious games and embedded assessment to monitor and foster learning," in Serious Games. In: Ritterfeld U, Cody M, Vorderer P (eds) Mechanisms and effects. Routledge Publishers, New York, pp 97–122
5. Cheng-yong X, Wei-ming X (2010) Constructing 3D game engine based on XNA. Comput Knowl Technol 6:3401–3402. doi: CNKI:SUN:DNZS.0.2010-13-042
6. Wang S, Mao Z, Zeng C, Gong H, Li S, Chen B (2010). A new method of virtual reality based on unity3D. In: 18th IEEE international conference on geoinformatics, Peking University, Beijing

Chapter 294
Clinical Research on Using Hepatocyte Growth-Promoting Factors Combined with Gongying Yinchen Soup to Cure Depression in Patients with Fulminant Hepatitis

Guo Kaoshan, Hou Shuying, Gao Junfeng, Zhao Xinguo, Li Jianqiao, Li Huilong, Hou Jinjie, Ma Limin, Li Meng, Sun Yanfu, Gu Qing and Li Ruiyu

Abstract *Objective* Discuss the effect of using Hepatocyte growth-promoting factors combined with Gongying Yinchen soup to cure depression in patients with fulminant hepatitis. *Methods* Choose 61 cases of fulminant hepatitis patients with depression, With reference to the American psychiatric association *Mental disorders diagnostic and statistical manual* (DSM-IV) Classification standard, 31 cases patients were randomly divided into treatment group, which was given Gongying Yinchen soup and intravenous drip of 10 % glucose injection 250 ml containing Hepatocyte growth-promoting factors 120 rag, once daily, 15 days for a course of treatment and 30 in the control group, application of this method at the same time added nutgrass galingale rhizome, radix curcumae, radix angelicae

---

G. Kaoshan · G. Junfeng · L. Huilong · S. Yanfu · G. Qing
Second Affiliated Hospital of Xing Tai Medical College, Xingtai, Hebei, China

H. Shuying
Qianjiudian Primary School of Guangzong County, Xingtai, Hebei, China

Z. Xinguo · M. Limin
Chinese Medicine Hospital of Lincheng County, Hebei, China

L. Jianqiao
Chinese Medicine Hospital of Luquan, Hebei, China

H. Jinjie
Xingtai Medical College, No. 618 Gangtiebei Road, Xingtai, Hebei, China

L. Meng
Health Team of Hotan Prefecture Detachment of Chinese Armed Police Force, Xinjiang, China

L. Ruiyu (✉)
Second Affiliated Hospital of Xing Tai Medical College, No. 618 Gangtiebei Road, Xingtai, Hebei, China
e-mail: liruiyu651021@163.com

sinensis, radix paeoniae alba, radix aucklandiae and other drugs. After three courses of treatment, HAMD rating scale, scores of TCM symptoms. Determine the efficacy. *Results* Use Gongying Yinchen soup combined with promoting liver cell growth hormone treatment of severe hepatitis patients with depression after treatment, pretherapy and post-treatment in the two groups of HAMD scale total score, treatment group before treatment 45.23 ± 17.29, after the treatment 44.25 ± 18.14; the control group before treatment 43.25 ± 18.30, after the treatment 28.46 ± 14.08, the therapeutic effect of control group patients was much better than that of treatment group cases ($P < 0.05$); Chinese medicine symptom curative effect as a whole,Treatment group total effectiveness 80.6 %, control group 93.3 %, had significant statistical differences were compared ($P < 0.05$). *Conclusions* Promoting liver cell growth to combination the Gongying Yinchen soup curative effect in patients with severe hepatitis depression significantly.

Keywords Hepatocyte growth-promoting factors · Gongying Yinchen soup · Fulminant hepatitis · Depression

294.1 Introduction

Severe hepatitis is caused due to various reasons extensive necrosis of liver cells that a group of liver disease, according to the disease process can be divided into acute, subacute, and chronic severe hepatitis. One similar to the pathogenesis of the acute and subacute severe hepatitis, mainly due to the host for invading virus produces strong immune reaction, cause liver cells large necrosis, occurrence liver failure. In addition and tumor necrosis factor (TNF) secretion, expression of histocompatibility locus antigens (HLA), interleukin-1 (IL-1) and interleukin-6 (IL-6) and other cytokines activity enhancement, enterogenous endotoxin levels, as well as the relevant mechanisms such as apoptosis [1]. And chronic severe hepatitis is a chronic, hypohepatia, liver detoxification, defensive ability to drop, the body's immune system disorder, caused by various complications, interaction, mutual influence. This disease not only physical pain to the patient, and change a spirit, on the impact of depression in patients with fulminant hepatitis is still rare, this chapter discusses promoting liver cell growth hormone combinations from Gongying Yinchen soup changes of depression in patients with severe hepatitis, a preliminary report as follows.

294.2 Materials and Methods

294.2.1 General Information

From November 2003 to August 2007, 61 patients in Department of Integrated Chinese and Western Medicine were treated, 61 cases were divided into two groups. The treatment group 31 cases, 21 males and 10 females, 26–75 years old, an average of 49.2 years; hepatitis A 12 cases, hepatitis B 10 cases, co-infection of HAV-HBV 2 cases, Undifferentiated type 4 cases, AlcoholicHepatitis 3 cases; The control group 30 cases, 21 males and 9 females, 24–72 years old, an average of 47.7 years; hepatitis A 9 cases, hepatitis B 15 cases, co-infection of HAV-HBV 1 cases, Undifferentiated type 3 cases, AlcoholicHepatitis 2 cases.

294.2.2 Diagnostic Criteria

Fulminant hepatitis diagnostic criteria with reference to the Chinese medical association of infectious diseases and parasitic epidemiology branch-hepatology branch Viral hepatitis prevention and treatment programmes [2]. The criteria of depression with western medicine diagnostic criteria: According to the *Chinese Classification and Diagnosis of Mental Diseases*-3rd edition (CCMD-3) [3], certainty what exactly depression is for patients. TCM diagnostic criteria: Referring to the relevant TCM literature [4].

294.2.3 The Severity of the Depression Classification Standard

Reference to the American Psychiatric Association's *Diagnostic and Statistical Manual-IV* (DSM-IV).

294.2.4 The Inclusion Criteria

1. Conforms to the diagnosis of depression in patients with slight or midrange depression.
2. Stable vital signs, conscious, have certain language ability.

294.2.5 Exclusion Criteria

1. Belong to major depressive disorder;
2. There is some form of schizophrenia, or belong to the symptom of post-schizophrenia depression;
3. Clinical diagnosis was non depression psychosis;
4. Does not accord with the inclusive criteria; or data not congruent effect observation of patients; Comply with the above one of the patients, and to exclude.

294.2.6 Treatment

Treatment group application on hepatocyte growth-promoting factors 120 mg, add in 250 ml of 10 % glucose, Intravenous fluids, once daily, 15 days for a course of treatment. The self-made Gongying Yinchen soup, which made up of Pugongying Yinchen CHaihu ZHidahuang Tufuling Banlangen ZHuling Kushen, one dose each day, make into decoction and use as tea, 10 doses constituting one course; altogether used 3 period of treatments, deficiency-cold of spleen and stomach persons used with caution. Control group applied this method at the same time added nutgrass galingale rhizome, radix curcumae, radix angelicae sinensis, radix paeoniae alba, radix aucklandiae and other drugs.

294.2.7 Observational Index

HAMD scale and chinese medicine symptom were used for assessing treatment effects before treatment and after treatment 45 days. Reference to Chinese Medicine Clinical Research of N new Drugs Guiding Principles [5], TCM symptoms curative effect evaluation standard for grade 4 (A zero as no symptoms; two points as Mild; 4 points as Moderate; 6 points as Severe).

294.2.8 Statistical Methods

The data of the results were analysed by SPSS11.0, measurement data with mean standard deviation ($\bar{x} \pm S$), T-test was adopted in group measurement data.

294.3 Results

294.3.1 Effect Judgment Standard

Clinical recovery: After treatment symptoms and signs disappeared, $N \geq 95\%$; Excellent: Most of the signs and symptoms disappeared after treatment, $70\% < N < 95\%$; Invalid: After treatment symptoms and signs not disappear or exacerbation, $N < 30\%$. $N =$ (Symptom integral before treatment-symptom score after treatment)/Symptom integral before treatment $\times 100\%$.

294.3.2 Before and After Treatment in the Two Groups of HAMD Scale Total Score Comparison

HAMD scale score to process after statistics ($P < 0.05$), has the significant difference, the control group obviously group surpasses the treatment, control information of fulminant hepatitis depression has obvious treatment effect (Table 294.1).

294.3.3 Chinese Medicine Symptom Overall Curative Effect

Refer (Table 294.2).

294.4 Discussion

Labrecque begin from just 1975 weanling rats liver extract liver cell stimulus material [6], subsequently found in other animals (including dogs, pigs, fetal liver) also have a similar material [7], the molecular weight of 10–17 kda heat-resistant of short peptide, named as hepatocyte growth-promoting factors (PHGF). The experiment found that PHGF can stimulate monolayer hepatocytes DNA synthesis

Table 294.1 HAMD scores were compared before and after treatment ($\bar{x} \pm s$, ms)

Group	HAMD total score	
	Prior treatment	Post treatment
Treatment group	45.23 ± 17.29	44.25 ± 18.14[a]
Control group	43.25 ± 18.30	28.46 ± 14.08

[a] After treatment in treatment group is obviously better than the control group, there was significantly statistical difference ($P < 0.05$)

Table 294.2 In the two groups pretherapy and post-treatment efficacy comparison (n) (%)

Grouping	Case number	Recovery	Excellent	Effective	Ineffectiveness	Total effective rate
Treatment group	31	2	10	13	6	80.6[a]
Control group	30	4	12	12	2	93.3

[a] Compared with the group before treatment ($P < 0.05$)

in active substances, with D-galactosamine induced rat experimental hepatic failure can reduce the mortality rate [8], can reduce the animal models of acute liver failure of lipid peroxidase level, can stabilize cell membrane, promotes mitochondrial repair and proliferation. PHGF has got satisfactory effect in the clinical treatment [9], but the current lack of ideal therapy in patients with hepatitis gravis patients with depression. Reports of hepatitis gravis and chronic liver disease patients psychological burden and appear typical symptoms, depression, anxiety, moderate depression are 61.129 % [10, 11]. Most studies have confirmed, hepatitis patients psychological problems serious, depression disorders are more prominent. Depression may induced or contributed to physical disease [12], and physical diseases may increase psychological burden, serious hepatitis affect the cathartic of liver function, TCM believes liver controlling dispersion, Liver governs discharging in function, including freeing qi activity, harmonizing emotion, soothing spleen and stomach, and regulating blood. So soothing the liver and relieving depression is its therapeutic principles, above-mentioned rhizoma cyperi with the effect of qi Jieyu, radix curcumae with adjustable air JieYu, white Paeony Root with nourishing blood and liver, costustoot with soothe the liver and regulate the Qi. In this paper, by using Gongying Yinchen soup combined with hepatocyte growth-promoting factors hormone treatment of fulminant hepatitis patients with depression after treatment, HAMD scores were compared before and after treatment: Treatment group before treatment 45.23 ± 17.29, posttreatment 44.25 ± 18.14; the control group before treatment 43.25 ± 18.30, posttreatment 28.46 ± 14.08, treatment group was much better than the control group, there was significantly statistical differences ($P < 0.05$); chinese medicine symptom overall curative effect: The validity rate in treatment group was 80.6 %, and the control group was 93.3 %, there was notable diversity ($P < 0.05$), Suggests that hepatocyte growth-promoting factors combinations from the Gongying Yinchen soup curative effect significantly in patients with fulminant hepatitis depression.

References

1. Wang Q (2011) 42 cases of fulminant hepatitis risk factor of prognosis analysis. Jilin Med J 32(2):233–234
2. Branch association of infectious diseases and parasitic epidemiology (2001) Branch association of Hepatology, Chinese medical association. Virus hepatitis integrated control measure. Chin J Infect Dis 19(1):56–62

3. Branch of the Chinese medical association of psychiatry (2001) The Chinese classification and diagnosis of Mental Diseases, 3rd edn (CCMD-3). Shandong Science & Technology Press, Jinan, pp 87–89
4. Chen ZQ, Hu SY, Zhang HN et al (2005) Studying on common TCM syndromes of depression. J Tradit Chin Med 46(1):47–49
5. SFDA (2002) Refer to directions of new drugs clinical research (try out). China Press of Traditional Chinese Medicine, Beijing, p 105
6. Labrecque DR (1975) Rogeneration stimulator substance (HSS) from preparation and partial characterization of hepatic rat liver. J Physiol 248(5):273
7. Michalopoulos GK, Zarnegar R (1992) Hepatocyte growth factor. Hepatology 15(1):149–155
8. Kong XP, Zheng GC, Zhang YZ et al (1991) Hepatocyte stimulating factor of rat experimental liver failure factors and the experimental mechanism research. Chin J Digestion 11(1):23
9. Zhang YZ, Zheng GC, Kong XP et al (1991) J Clin Hepatol 7(1):15
10. Shi SM, Zhang X (2000) Blood transfusion or blood products infected with hepatitis c patient's mental nursing. J Heze Med Coll 12(3):140
11. Xu B, Wang XD, Liu SL (2000) Psychosomatic medicine. China Science and Technology Press, pp 248–250
12. Sui ZQ, Xu ZG, Wang Y (2012) Depressive disorders and study on the relationship between the physical diseases. J Psychiatry 25(2):153–156

Chapter 295
The Development of Information System in General Hospitals: A Case Study of Peking University Third Hospital

Jiang Xue and Jin Changxiao

Abstract Healthcare Information system (HIS) building is an important way to improve hospital efficiency and health care quality. This article describes the process of HIS development in general hospitals in china as the Peking University Third Hospital (PUTH) for example. By expanding wirelesses AP and digital system in PUTH, the hospital has made great achievements in the building of electronic medical record system, public reservation registration platform, personal digital assistant, treatment before settlement and the DRGs. According to the previous experiences, it also gives some suggestions for further HIS development in general hospitals. The suggestions include reasonable planning, efficiency and effectiveness, data processing, information standardization, staff participation and updating information system.

Keywords Healthcare information system · General hospital · Peking university third hospital

295.1 Introduction

Healthcare Information System (HIS) is an important component of informationization of the whole society. Among the Chinese medical system reform, known well by the public, a more efficient medical and health service system is to be established, which requires a strengthened hospital information system, so as to increasingly improve the level of hospital management and modernization, to effectively deal with the issue of difficult access to medical service and high price for the public. Based on the previous experiences, the China Ministry of Health

---

J. Xue (✉) · J. Changxiao
Peking University Third Hospital, North Garden Road 49, Beijing 100191, China
e-mail: pkujiangxuer@yahoo.com

and local governments regulate and guidance on the HIS development. In 2002, the Ministry of Health issued Regulation on Hospital Information System, stating that the regulation is not only a criteria towards the evaluation to developers, but a guidance paper on the information technology development of hospitals and basic evaluation criteria of HIS. In 2001, Beijing Municipal government issued the 12th Five-year Plan of Beijing Health Development, stating that electronic medical records, health files and reservation registration will be promoted in the future 5 years. These policies provide an important regulation and guidance to the HIS development. This study will employ the HIS of Peking University Third Hospital (PUTH) as a case, discuss the process of information system in China's general hospitals, and propose some valuable suggestions on how healthcare information system will go further.

295.2 Information System in PUTH

295.2.1 Basic Information of PUTH

Peking University Third Hospital (PUTH) was founded in 1958 under the supervision of the Ministry of Health. It is a modernized and comprehensive upper first-class hospital with integration of medical services, medical education/teaching, research and prevention as well as health care. At present, the Hospital has a staff of 2,331 and 1,284 clinic beds, 34 clinical departments, 10 medical technique departments.

In recent decades, PUTH has been improving greatly on its operation and medical services quality level. In 2012, the hospital accepted more than 3.8 million outpatient and emergency visits, about 13,000 per day. The annual discharged patients were over 70,000. The annual operation quantity was over 40,000 cases. The average length of stay was 6.6 days. The overall management indexes have achieved advanced level that won praises and honors from the Ministry of Health and Beijing Municipal Health Bureau.

295.2.2 HIS in PUTH

Through the years' efforts, the healthcare information system of PUTH has passed the period of PAC period. An E-hospital featured by a whole coverage of information technology has been established, developing to be a hospital with regional medical health information system. A platform of dealing with multimedia information like digitals, words, waveforms and pictures has been established. The patients-oriented management model has been forming, transformed from the original financial focused model. Information technology is now becoming an indispensible platform for the hospital management and patients acquiring medical services. The objectives of hospital information system are to improve efficiency, reduce mistakes, control cost and better services.

295.2.3 Information System Development

The PUTH initiated a computer room in 1984, and the information management center in 1991. From 2002 to 2005, the hospital continues to expand the use of information technology, developing case management and digital system, medicine e-purchasing management system, digestive endoscopy, pharmacy intravenous admixture service (PIVA). From the year of 2007, the hospital initiated outpatient computer-based prescription record, outpatient calling and queuing system, clinic anesthesia information system (CAIS), and all-in-one card.

In the following 3 years, the hospital gradually achieved bar code management system for hospital test specimens,promoted electronic medical record system (EMR), infectious disease monitoring, patient self-service system, outpatient medical insurance card real time settlement, hospital medical supplies management information system, inpatient electronic medical record, initiated the management function of clinical path (CP) and established the remote diagnostic system. From 2011, the hospital started the trial of diagnosis related groups (DRGs) and pathology information system (PIS). In 2012, the hospital started transfusion outpatients management system, upgraded the laboratory information system (LIS), ultrasonic image management and teaching management system.

At present, the hospital information system and picture archiving communication system have reached a high level. HIS is covering administrative information system, such as portal site, coordinate office system, teaching management system, scientific research system and employees ID card, clinic information system, such as LIS, doctor working station, EMR, medicine monitoring, antibacterial monitoring, CP management, medical files system; management information system, such as medical cards management system, reservation registration platform, calling and queuing system for outpatient triage, outpatient charges, inpatient charges, medical insurance charges, settlement system of charges, pharmacy administration system, device and consumable material management system, material supply system, patient self-service system.

PACS developing covers radiology department, ultrasound department, gastroenterology department, pathology department, and gastroenterology department. The PACS could be applied in clinic anesthesia information system (CAIS), infectious disease monitoring system and remote diagnostic system.

295.2.4 Achievements of Information System

295.2.4.1 Infrastructure

There are 17,559 information points, 14 computer rooms including central and candidate computer rooms, 80 distribute rooms, 3 central units, 23 aggregations, 3-level gigabit Ethernet of 272 network as core redundancy. Wireless internet is working in the hospital with 795 wirelesses AP.

295.2.4.2 Reservation Registration

Public reservation registration platform is established for the hospital to meet the patients' needs. The patients could reserve their registration through telephone, internet, doctors working station, consulting room and ward. Till now, the total number of patients from reservation registration is 1.6 million, among which 52 % are further consultation patients.

Moreover, PUTH sets up comprehensive reservation system covering diagnosis and treatment, and puts examination reservation in this system, such as radiology department, ultrasonography department, electrocardiographic room, digestive endoscopy room, etc.

295.2.4.3 Expand the Usage of Treatment Before Settlement

As the medical card used in the reservation system, the fees will not be confirmed when the patients go consulting or get examination. By the end of 2012, the number of patients using the treatment before settlement has reached 677,066. This method has improved the medical experience of patients.

295.2.4.4 Make Achievements in DRGs

PUTH has built 455 clinical pathways, which covered 108 category diseases using DRGs ways to settle, and this way will firmly ensure the quality of medical treatment. Through the building of case management system, doctors may get the diagnosis coding quickly, and achieve the clinical message of the patients. This will ensure the patients settle accounts following the DRGs in a short period.

295.2.4.5 Building of Electronic Medical Record System

In November of 2008, the building of electronic medical record system (EMRS) was started. In September of 2010, EMRS had covered 53 wards of PUTH. Now,

PUTH has 430 resident doctor workstations, and has built 3,623 EMR formworks, 2,274 surgery record formworks. The total number of EMR is 183,642, and the number of outpatients records reached 72,445. The system has combined the data and information of doctor's advice, electric application form, electric examination report and structured medical documents.

295.2.4.6 Application of Mobile Nursing

Based on the WIFI, personal digital assistant (PDA) can be used with the mobile devices. This will supply mobile nursing, changing the traditional medical model to prescribed closed-loop management model. And the mobile nursing system with its coordination system, such as NIS, EMR, LIS and PACS will be settled together.

295.3 Challenges in General Hospitals

295.3.1 General Situation

Studies have reported evidence of the positive impact of hospital information technology on healthcare quality, including lower mortality rates, higher vaccination rates, and patient safety indicators. And there are also some findings that greater automation of hospital information is associated with improving the efficiency of hospitals, reduced complications, costs and length of stay [1–3]. When evaluating the health care quality, the following six aspects may be concerned, which are hospital quality improvement practices and strategies, adherence to process of care measures, risk-adjusted inpatient mortality, patient satisfaction, assessment of patient care quality by hospital quality managers and front-line clinicians [4].

But not all hospitals pushing the HIS construction get what they want. One research in Brazil revealed that there were still weaknesses and problems relative to planning, selection, implementation and use of the management technology and tools at the researched hospitals. So it is possible for us to identify the hospitals which better use and take better advantage of resources and easiness of information technology so as to facilitate the routine and work processes from their doctors, patients and directors [5].

As the adoption of information technology in hospitals concerned, the hospital size, located in urban or rural, stand-alone or affiliated, profit or non-profit, will influence the adoption of HIS. Neset's investigations find that hospital size appears to be less relevant for administrative hospital information technology, where its effect is compensated by those of system membership and tax status [6]. Another studies also give us some useful information. Ning's find that organizational factors appear to be more influential than market factors when it comes to information technology adoption in hospitals [7].

295.3.2 Reasonable Planning of HIS

Healthcare information system development is a gradual process. The various characteristics of different hospitals decide that there is no repeat, and no possibility that technologies and equipments applied at the same period. For example, the application of EMR could not always lead to the high efficiency in hospital management, while the features of hospital should be considered [8]. Some researches show that more attention should be focused on the scientific and effective procedures of decision-making and the administration in its process.

Meanwhile, information system development should be reviewed from the perspectives of integrity, which falls into two aspects. On one hand, some projects cannot be isolated from the integrated planning. Otherwise, the mismatch of new and old systems will lead to the phenomenon of Information Island. On the other hand, information system development is not the responsibilities of one single department or several departments of a hospital, but needs coordination of different departments, especially at the premium stage of system running, so that the whole system could start to work well as soon as possible [9].

295.3.3 Efficiency and Effectiveness of HIS

295.3.3.1 Data Processing

At present, most of HIS application in Chinese hospitals is limited in the operation level, such as simplify procedures, improve efficiencies of human operating and storage, while cloud processing of data is usually neglected. We can see the trend of using E-files, CP management and other electronic statistics, but generally speaking, they are still quite weak. So if we can strengthen the analysis and application on the basic data and processed data in the information system development, we will more effectively improve the efficiencies and benefits of hospital management.

295.3.3.2 Information Standardization

Information Standardization is always regarded as the issue planned by governments and Health Departments. But generally speaking, there is some flexibility for the information system development, so that various types of medical institutions in different regions with differences of economic development degrees could select their information technology path based on their own situations. It's a complicate procedure to regulate a standard clinic data and apply it as well. Some terminologies vary with the continuous development of health care. So information standardization of hospitals should be planned as an integrated part from the long term, and this will help the quantitative management of clinic data and complete maintaining of original E-files, so as to reduce the unnecessary and repeated work of establishing information platforms.

295.3.3.3 Staff Participation

The users of healthcare information technology are the medical working staff. Whether information technology could play its role or not depends on how medical working staff use it. According to some reports, the attitudes of medical staff towards the information technology decide if it can succeed in hospitals [10]. So in the process of information system development, medical staff needs to improve their ability to manipulate IT, and be mobilized to participate in the information technology innovation. In this way, the information system in the hospitals could function better.

295.3.3.4 Updating Information System

The information technology is changing very fast with the times. The capital investment in the hardware and software updating of information technology is large, which is the basic guarantee of the information system development. However, according to some studies, the advancement and high technological performance of hospital information system is lagging behind far compared with other industries, such as bank, post and transportations [11]. This is largely decided by the goal of health information system. Under such circumstances, updating information system should be considered from the macro perspectives, with no blind capital investment, especially when deciding to renew those equipments of high technologies. Meanwhile, we should take more energy to promote the information technologies which have profound impact on the quality of healthcare. On the other hand, fundraising for healthcare information system updating should be diversified, such as government support and corporate sponsor.

295.4 Conclusion

As decades' use of information technology in hospital, such as the HIS and PACS, the health care in PUTH has been more efficient and diversified with little mistakes. And the information technology is now dramatically becoming an indispensible platform for the PUTH management and patients. But when developing the information technology in the general hospital, we still have something more to do. Strengthening the analysis and application on the basic data and processed data in the information system is an important way to effectively improve the efficiencies and benefits of hospital management. And when planning the information standardization in hospital, long-term sight should be not neglected. Medical staffs are the main bodies of hospital who use the information technology, so it needs to improve their mobility to participate in the information technology innovation. The last suggestion is that hospitals should take more energy to promote the information technologies, and the fundraising for healthcare information system updating should be diversified, such as government support and corporate sponsor.

References

1. Amarasingham R, Plantinga L, Diener M et al (2009) Clinical information technologies and inpatient outcomes: a multiple hospital study. Arch Intern Med 169(2):108–114
2. Aron S, Dutta R, Janakiram PS et al (2010) The impact of automation of systems on medical errors: evidence from field research. In: Working paper. Johns Hopkins University, Baltimore
3. Dexter F, Perkins SM, Maharry KS et al (2004) Inpatient computer-based standing orders versus physician reminders to increase influenza and pneumococcal vaccination rates: a randomized trial. J Am Med Assoc 292(19):2366–2371
4. Joseph DR, Alan BC, Jedediah NH et al (2012) Hospital implementation of health information technology and quality of care: are they related? BMC Med Inform Decis Mak 12(109):online
5. Saulo BO, Antonio JB, Favio AT (2011) The use of information technology in public hospitals in the city of Rio de Janeiro. Commun Comput Inf Sci 221:347–360
6. Neset H, Anol B, Nir M et al (2008) The role of organizational factors in the adoption of healthcare information technology in Florida hospitals. Healthc Manag Sci 1(11):1–9
7. Ning JZ, Binyam S, Thomas W et al (2013) Health information technology adoption in U.S. acute care hospitals. J Med Syst 37:9907
8. Natalia AZ, Mark LD, Look I (2012) U.S. hospital efficiency and adoption of health information technology. Healthc Manag Sci 1(15):37–47
9. FU Z (2008) Thoughts on hospital information status and measurement. Chin Hosp 12(1):4–7
10. Pouyan E, Murali S, Naresh Kr et al (2011) Adoption of technology applications in healthcare: the influence of attitude toward knowledge sharing on technology acceptance in a hospital. Commun Comput Inf Sci (264):17–30
11. Mirou J, Marcia MW, Guy P et al (2005) Clinical information technology in hospitals: a comparison between the state of Iowa and two provinces in Canada. Int J Med Inf (74):719–731

Chapter 296
Several Reflections on the Design of Educational Computer Games in China

Nie Yun and L. V. Ping

Abstract With the development and application of computer technology and Internet in China, educational computer Games come into schools as a new education technology and have profound influences on the Chinese education system. For the purpose of promoting the joyful function and education value, a good design of educational computer games is essential. This paper describes some of the considerations that must be taken into account in creating effective interactive games, such as a well-designed educational computer game itself can become an effective learning environment; design tactics of excellent educational computer games ought to be on base of theory of multiple intelligences; the match between children's psychology and game characters design should be implemented in a well-designed educational computer game and analysis of education objectives and contents is the first step for the design of educational computer Games.

Keywords Design educational computer games China

296.1 Introduction

Educational computer games are types of serious computer games. Serious computer games are those computer games designed for a strong purpose other than pure entertainment. Although serious computer games can be entertaining, their main purpose is to train, investigate, or advertise. Educational computer

N. Yun · L. V. Ping (✉)
Department of Biotechnological and Environmental Engineering, Tianjin Professional College, Tianjin 300410, China
e-mail: bestman_0429@163.com

N. Yun
e-mail: nieyun57@yahoo.com.cn

games are those games that have been specially designed to teach people about a certain subject, expand concepts, reinforce development, understand a historical event or culture, or assist them in learning a skill as they play.

Educational computer games in the last decade is the remarkable development, and its development can be attributed to the game to become a new knowledge carrier and achieve enlightenment effect; educational computer games have a broad range of players, strong game development team as a backup, and rich cultural heritage to become the subject of inexhaustible game library. The combination of computer games and education is not only entertaining way to learn, but also a very good computer game development [1]. More and more of the education sectors and students have gradually accepted these new digital learning games, educational computer games have penetrated into our daily lives. In some developed countries, educational computer games are being there for some years. And the research has obtained so much. The computer game combines with education; it has some fans who like it very much [2]. Compared with this, in our country, the research on educational computer game just begins, the theory and the technology are not enough, the current games cannot balance the education and entertainment, so it cannot attract the students to play and like the games. In some products of educational computer games education is epidemically at variance with game itself which radically reflects conceptual and designable warp in educational computer games. Many education experts, concerning about the educational value of games, always regard games as teaching media. Under the influence of such thinking, some designers one-sidedly regard games as tools for knowledge transfer. While for the lack of reasonable and feasible guidance in design models and strategies, they can only imaginatively take the game elements and knowledge graft together. At this time, the most important work is to find the strongpoint of the successful computer games, then combine with education, hoping this will help to develop the good and successful educational computer games. So it is very important to research on design tactics of educational computer games for development and application of educational computer games in Chinese education.

296.2 Educational Computer Games Become Effective Learning Environments

A well-designed educational computer game itself can become an effective learning environment on the basis of consulting a number of relevant materials both at home and abroad about the close relationship between educational computer games and motivation theory, flow experience (immersion experience) theory, effective learning environment. It's inevitable to produce flow experience while being immersing in an effective learning environment. And it's nature to stimulate learning motivation in the circumstances of flow experience. Therefore, educational computer games can be regarded as games based learning environments to design [3]. To create an effective learning environment as orientation, we can try to use the methods and techniques of game design to express the prerequisites of effective learning environment, so as to stimulate learners' flow experience and learning motivation, and eventually realize the perfect fusion of education effect and game effect. Thus, an EFM model for educational computer game design was constructed and some design strategies and a design process were propound based on the model. Besides, "Hope Summer", with the content of "Law on Protection of Minors", had been designed and developed as a case to detail the production process of an educational computer game based on the EFM model.

296.3 Design Tactics on Base of Theory of Multiple Intelligences

Since Gardner theory of multiple intelligences put in the world, the education field has resulted in a strong response. In the United States, theory of multiple intelligences brings new theoretical guiding ideology and the education practice of theory of multiple intelligences for countries opens a new field. This theory reveals a theme of global concern, especially to all students' intelligent development. Students are the future of all countries, so development of children intelligence also reflects the diversity of the world culture. Hence, it is beneficial to seek out the new estimated standard of the kinds of games by reaching out a new visual angle to evaluate and judge the intelligent type and to find strong intelligent type of the students according to their intelligent behavioral expression in the game. It is helpful to make more scientific the results by taking the educational computer games as a learning environment, discussing the behavioral research of simulation game-teaching method. It is favorable to heighten the acceptability of educational computer games for teachers and students, on the basis of having investigation about the influence of the different types of games on the learners. Then modern design tactics of educational computer game should be in the light of theory of multiple intelligences, combining modern instructional design theory, constructivism theory, situated cognition, flow theory and gaming theory, talked the overview flowchart and the basic framework of educational computer games; Taking the "Teaching Media Function" as a bridge, the author does a research on building the educational gaming systematic design method by integrating the "Teaching Design" and "Gaming Design" general approach to educational computer games software.

296.4 Emphasis on Match Children's Psychology with Game Characters Design

There are some problems in education computer Game characters design strategy, including of without the use of good character, no definition of characters, and the accuracy of different age stages without considering the psychological characteristics of different students, no effective incentive mechanism, the game without balance between education function and entertainment function in the design of education computer Game [4]. To solve these problems, education role of game design process, must notice psychoanalytic theory, hierarchy theory of needs, cognitive theory of design concept. In order to make the characters to create more plentiful and full consideration to the role of psychological and physiological characteristics, role conflict between the consistency of the role, and the role of language and characters, grow factor perspective. At the same time, In order to develop more and better education computer Games to guarantee children's happy and healthy lives, more and more people should truly understand and concern with the need of children's psychology and get involved in the design and exploitation of education computer Games. The study of cognitive and emotional characteristics of students in the field of education computer Games can give an inspiration to the design of education computer Games. Emotional experience factors in education computer Games are identified and analyze, and then based on this, a set of design strategy and related emotional engineering technology of emotional experience summed up in education computer Games.

296.5 Notice Analysis of Education Objective and Content

To ensure that the education function of education computer game, analysis of education activity is the first step, including of analysis of education objective and analysis of education content. Study on any key factors in the education computer Game around game assignment is a very important foundation for Design procedure of education computer Game [5]. In the education computer Games, players are both learners and the players. Meanwhile, education computer Games need to realize certain teaching objectives, so analysis of knowledge which players must be learn and skills which must be master is first of all. Then analysis of gap between the current study state and the target of education, and determine whether study content can be realized in the form of education computer Game, in order to convert teaching goals into the game tasks. Analysis of study content contains definition of study topics, classification of types of study contents and establishment relationship of study contents. According to study topics, types of study contents and relationship of study contents, design factors of education computer Games melt organically into education computer Games to create a pleasant learning environment in which they immersed them to experience the fun of learning for students in the form of games, which can really achieve the goal of "learning in fun".

296.6 Conclusion

It was confined that excellent education computer Games have a lot of important uses in many education aspects, they can enlighten students' thoughts, cultivate students' ability of finding questions and problem solving, promote the information literacy of students, cultivate students' innovation and cooperation capability. The motivational and immersive traits of game-based learning have been studied in chinese education, but the systematic design and implementation of education computer Games remain an elusive situation in Chinese education systems. Some important relevant requirements for the design of education computer Games are analyzed and a general game design principle and method that includes adaptation and assessment features is proposed. Because of the restriction of many objective conditions, however, the study of the case in this paper was not perfect, and was in need of further improvement.

Acknowledgments This research was supported by grants from the Tianjin education scientific planning projects (Teaching resources construction and practice of the modern biotechnology curriculum in vocational college, No. 2007AA021506) and Twelfth Five Years scientific planning projects of Higher education from Higher Education Academy of Tianjin (Teaching resources construction and practice of biotechnology major in vocational college, No. 125q202).

References

1. Squire K (2003) Video games in education. Int J Intell Simul Gaming 2(1):49–62
2. Van Eck R (2006) Digital game-based learning: it's not just the digital natives who are restless. Educ Rev 41(2):16–30
3. Squire K (2005) Game-based learning: an X-learn perspective paper. MASIE center: e-learning consortium.http://www.masieweb.com/research-and-articles/research/game-based-learning.html
4. Michael D, Chen S (2006) Serious games: games that educate, train, and inform. Thomson, Boston
5. Jonassen DH (1994) Thinking technology: toward a constructivist design model. Educ Technol 34(4):34–47
6. Vogten HMH et al (2006) Coppercore service integration integrating IMS learning design and IMS question and test interoperability. In: 6th IEEE international conference on advanced learning technologies, Kerkrade. IEEE Computer Society Press, The Netherland

Chapter 297
A Rural Medical and Health Collaborative Working Platform

Jiang Yanfeng, Yin Ling, Wang Siyang, Lei Mingtao, Zheng Shuo and Wang Cong

Abstract Medical and health care is underserved in rural areas in China. To solve this problem, a collaborative medical and health working platform is proposed, which combines Information Processing System and Computer Aided Diagnosis System. It provides eight key technologies, which are Statistics Survey, Information Collection, Case Analysis, Professor Team, Project Management, Telemedicine Module, Medical Image Processing and Real Disease Analysis. With this platform, efficiency, safety and other aspects are promoted substantially.

Keywords Computer aided diagnosis · Telemedicine · Medical image processing

297.1 Introduction

With the advent of the information age, the rapid development of science and technology, especially the innovation of computer artificial intelligence technology and pharmaceutical biotechnology, contributes a lot to the integration of medical and computer technology. Computer aided diagnosis (CAD) means an auxiliary diagnosis that medical workers using computer technology and equipment to diagnose patients [1]. Combined with imaging, medical image processing, as well as physiological, biochemical, and other means, CAD makes use of the

J. Yanfeng (✉)
School of Public Health, Lanzhou University, Donggangxi Lu. 199, Lanzhou 730000, China
e-mail: yfyf518@163.com

Y. Ling
Telemedicine Center, Chinese PLA General Hospital, Fuxing Lu. 28, Beijing 100853, China

W. Siyang · L. Mingtao · Z. Shuo · W. Cong
Beijing University of Posts and Telecommunications, Xitucheng Road. 10, Beijing 100876, China

computer analysis to help physicians to find the nidus, thus improving the accuracy of the diagnosis [2].

For a long time, high quality medical and health resources are over concentrated on cities or developed areas, while in rural areas and communities, the development of medical service is lagging behind. To help rural doctors and researchers to carry out the basic rural medical and health work and research, guarantee the efficiency of operations, improve the basic rural medical and health services, a rural medical and health collaborative working platform is designed. The platform could be able to store large amounts of information, which provides platform service for medical data collection, case analysis, medical project management and collaborative working chance between urban and rural medical workers, thus improving the hospital's capabilities in transaction processing, the result of which makes more patients could receive high level medical treatment.

This paper is organized as follows. Section 297.2 introduces the related work about CAD technology and medical image processing. Section 297.3 describes the platform structure. Conclusion and future work are written in Sect. 297.4.

297.2 Related Work

A rural medical and health collaborative working platform is actually a system using CAD technology, and medical image processing technology provides indispensable quantitative data for the computer-aided diagnosis. Therefore, to get familiar with our platform, it is necessary to understand the concept of CAD, collaborative working platform and medical image processing.

297.2.1 Computer Aided Diagnosis

With the proposal of the concept of CAD [3–6], research in CAD becomes more and more popular in abroad. Data acquisition, processing and visualization applied to CAD have a great influent on medical imaging in recent years. However, specific expression of medical knowledge meanings of medical image is still done by professional physicians. The development of artificial intelligence and image processing shows that CAD still has a huge development potential [7].

Computer-aided diagnosis process, including the collection of general data and checking data of patients, quantitative processing of medical information, statistical analysis, until finally arrive at the diagnosis. In the 1990s, the application of CAD based on mathematical approach to mimic working principle of human brain, this led to the rapid development of Artificial Neural Network (ANN). Artificial Neural Network has the ability to self-learning, memory and prediction development of events, etc. Compared with traditional probability statistics and mathematical model, ANN has better performance and it represents the most advanced artificial intelligence technology at that time [8]. In twenty-first century, CAD expands research in various clinical disease. Up to now, CAD breast cancer based on the X-ray imaging has been the most widely used and successfully applied to clinical diagnosis [9].

297.2.2 Collaborative Working System

Beyerlein et al. [10] defines collaboration as the collective work of two or more individuals where the work is undertaken with a sense of shared purpose and direction, which is attentive and responsive to the environment. Collaborative working system break the barrier of distant collaboration and electronic communication [11] and let more people join in the collaborative working. This system support distant communication and CAD process bringing advanced technic and professional medical aid towards rural area.

Kondylakis et al. [12] proposes a collaborative platform which will empower patient with knowledge about his/her health condition and at the same time it will assist the physician to have a better understanding about the patient's unique psychological profile. This is collaboration between patient and physician.

Chen [13] presents a collaborative decision-making method which develops a multi-person, multi-attribute model for patient-centered decision-making.

297.2.3 Medical Image Processing

Medical image processing technology is divided into image segmentation, medical image registration and three-dimensional image visualization [14]. Image segmentation is proposed by Pham DL etc. in 2000 [15], it is to split the different regions of the image that have special meanings. These regions makes each mutually disjoint region meet the consistency of a particular region. Image segmentation has been further developed on the basis of gray threshold segmentation method and edge detection segmentation method, it could help doctors to qualitative and quantitative analysis of diseased tissue, thus providing an accurate diagnosis. Medical image registration proposed by Zitova B etc. [16] makes many times and many kinds of equipment fully use of imaging information. The two corresponding points of the image achieve consistency in spatial location with anatomy, at least matches point with diagnostic significance and surgical area. Now there are two types of image registration, namely the image registration based on external characteristics and the image registration based on internal characteristics. Three-dimensional medical image visualization refers to two-dimensional tomographic images are acquired from CT/MR, through computer processing, 3D image reconstruction is obtained [17].

297.3 Platform Structure

The rural medical and health collaborative working platform (RMC platform) combines the technology of computer aided diagnose, medical image processing and collaborative working platform providing the function of remote collaborative treatment for primary hospitals and patients.

The RMC platform has two main systems, the Information Processing System and CAD System. In the RMC platform, all the information is stored on case database through the internet. In this way, the burden of data management could be reduced and the efficiency of data storage and retrieval would be improved. Figure 297.1 shows the structure of RMC platform.

With the basic modules above, RMC platform has the following benefits.

1. Avoid single point of failure. Each module work independently. If one stop working, another module won't be influenced.
2. Balance different work loads. This way could save a lot of resources and reduce the fault rate of devices. So availability will be guaranteed.
3. Guarantee security. Each module works on a virtual machine, which is isolated with each other. And different access rights are provided.

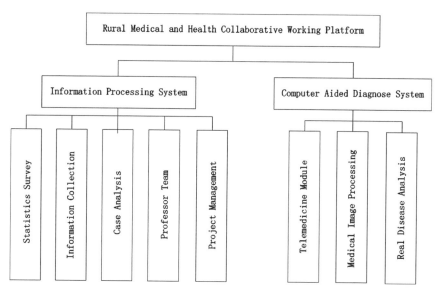

Fig. 297.1 Platform structure

297.3.1 Information Processing System

The Information Processing System consists of five modules, which are statistics survey, information collection, case analysis, professor team and project management. The statistics survey module realizes the disease investigation survey of different regions, such as the morbidity, distributing situation and occurrence regularity. The information collection module collects and stores medical information about patients and respondents. The case analysis module collects diagnose opinion based on patient information from authorized professors, which is the important part of case database. In professor team module, users can obtain information about professors and researchers. As many primary hospitals participate in some medical projects, the project management module in RMC platform helps them manage their project information and funds.

The Information Processing System provides simple entry function which could guarantee the completeness and accuracy of data. The entry staff use private user information with different access rights to get access to the system. In this way, data secure could be protected. The Information Processing System also support different kinds of databases and entry modes, which would be convenient for users. Also, this distributing platform could improve the efficiency of data entry for being deployed case database.

297.3.2 Computer Aided Diagnosis System

The CAD System is divided into three modules. Telemedicine module provides the service of remote consultation, training, education, guidance and teaching rounds. Medical image processing module uses computer to deal with the processing and analysis of medical images. Intelligent diagnosis and normalized treatment reference, as the most crucial function of RMC platform, are offered in real disease analysis module.

In the part of platform, important diagnosis analysis function is provided. Based on the data gathered by the Information Processing System, the CAD System is responsible for data analysis and statistics and generating data analysis report of certain disease. Also, diagnosis can be offered by CAD System in real analysis module using data analysis technology. Since medical data analysis and remote visualization service are supported, CAD System provides telemedicine, intelligent analysis of cases treatment advice and guidance for primary healthcare workers.

297.3.3 Important Module

297.3.3.1 Real Case Analysis Module

Among all the modules in RMC platform, real case analysis module (RCA module) in CAD system is the most important one. RCA module uses statistical information and case data to provide intelligent diagnosis and normalized treatment reference. The RCA module is supported by cloud storage technology and data retrieval technology. Figure 297.2 shows the working process of RCA module. The real case analysis method is as follows:

1. Primary healthcare workers collect medical information from patients and entry this new case into the RCA module.
2. The RCA module generates standardized new case and inquiries from index database.
3. The index database forms index and inquiries from case database.
4. The case database provides similar historical cases and reuses them to inquiries to get diagnosis and treatment of similar historical cases.
5. Based on diagnosis and treatment of similar historical cases and real situation of patient, doctor correct historical diagnosis opinion and provides confirmed diagnosis and treatment method.
6. The standardized new case and confirmed diagnosis and treatment method are sent into the case database.

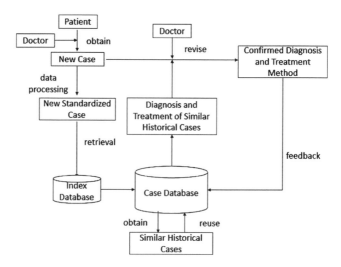

Fig. 297.2 Real case analysis method

297.3.3.2 Medical Image Processing Module

Medical image processing module uses the technology of medical image processing and data analysis to offer medical service. This module could support not only primary healthcare workers with medical technology and skill training, but patients with high quality telemedicine as well. In the medial image processing module, remote video consultation, medical training, remote mentoring and remote medical image processing are included. These remote support methods makes professors get involved in the treatment in primary hospitals which would be helpful for both patients and primary medical workers. Remote medical image processing uses image segmentation, medical image registration and three dimensional image visualization to support telemedicine.

297.3.3.3 Project Management Module

The project management module helps users manage their project information and funds. This module has the following functions to help primary hospitals participate in medical projects managing.

1. Task progress management. The project management module in RMC platform monitors task progress and shows user task list and measures project accomplishments with task completion. Authorized users can login in and see task completion percentage (the percentage of the tasks that are finished) indicated by progress bar.
2. Message management. Users of RMC platform can communicate with each other in project management module. Also, this module support message notification to specified user and attachments can be added.
3. Web mail management. Web mail is supported by project management module. A user can send web mail to any other members in the same project with him/her. And if users did not check their tasks in time, project management module will remind him/her with a web mail.
4. Fund management. To meet the requirement of Ministry of Science and Technology (MOST), our project information module provides fund management function. In this module, detailed management of fund usage is offered, fund subjects and spending. Those authorized users can see the fund situation of the sub-project of the project that they are participating. And financial statement can be uploaded and shared among authorized users.
5. Integration management. In some complex projects, numbers of research reports, thesis, books, patents and equipment are involved. It is a time-consuming effort to manage them. However, in project management module, those thesis, books and patents are numbered and stored with reference number in this module. Physical equipment and resources are also numbered and related information is saved. In this way, integration management efficiency is increased.

297.4 Conclusion and Future Work

The rural medical and health collaborative working platform makes the collaborative working of professors and primary medical workers come true and provides valuable opportunity for improving the rural medical service. The built of case database needs support of a wide range of data. Many research institutions and hospitals have a wealth of data resources, but lack the database interface with our case database. The interface section would be improved to connect more data resources. Also, primary health care institution, rural medical and scientific research institutes lack coordination office module. Adding this module would help carry out the business and research work of the rural medical and health service. In the future, the interface section and coordination office module will be improved.

Acknowledgments This work is supported by the National Key Technology R&D Program of the Ministry of Science and Technology of China (2012BAJ18B07, 2012BAJ18B08). This work relies on rural key crowd nutrition and health key technology integration and application demonstration research (2012BAJ18B07-05, 2012BAJ18B07-08) and the rural three-level health service comprehensive demonstration research.

References

1. Song F, Wang J (2011) Computer aided diagnosis system application in clinical practice. J Inf Technol 3:34–36
2. Zhang Z (2009) Conception of medical image processing technology. J Changzhi Univ 26(3):26–28
3. Taylor P, Champness J, Given-Wilson R, Johnston K, Potts H (2005) Impact of computer-aided detection prompts on the sensitivity and specificity of screening mammography. Health Technol Assess 9(6):1–70
4. Montani S, Portinale L, Leonardi G et al (2006) Case-based retrieval to support the treatment of end stage renal failure patients. J Artif Intell Med 37:31–42
5. Xu N (2007) The applied research of medical diagnose based on case- based reasoning. M Comput Knowl Technol 1:18–19
6. Xin L, Wang L (2011) The design for the clinic diagnosis support system based on CBR. M Comput Knowl Technol 7(13):3195–3196
7. Teng W, Chang P (2012) Identifying regions of interest in medical images using self-organizing maps. J Med Syst 36(5):2761–2768
8. Brem RF, Baum J, Lechner M et al (2003) Improvement in sentsitivity of screening mammography with computer-aided detection:a multinational trial. Am J Roentgenol 181:687–693
9. Dio K (2005) Current status and future potential of computer-aided diagnosis in medical imaging. British J Radiol 78(1):3–19
10. Beyerlein M, Freedman S, McGee G, Moran L (2002) Beyond teams: building the collaborative organization. The collaborative work systems series. Wiley
11. Collaborative working system. Wikipedia. http://en.wikipedia.org/wiki/Collaborative_working_system#cite_ref-Beyerlein2002_1-1
12. Kondylakis H, Koumakis L, Genitsaridi E et al (2012) IEmS: a collaborative environment for patent empowerment the 2012. In: 12th IEEE international conference on bioinformatics and bioengineering (BIBE), Larnaca 535–540

13. Chen T (2012) J collaborative decision-making method for patient-centered care based on interval type-2 fuzzy sets. J Chin Inst Ind Eng 29(7):494–513
14. Tian J, Bao SL, Zhou MQ (2003) Medical image process and analysis. Publishing House of Electronics Industry, Beijing
15. Pham DL, Xu C, Prince JL (2008) A survey of current methods in medical image segmentation. J Ann Rev Biomed Eng 2(8):315–337
16. Zitova B, Flusser J (2003) Image registration methods: a survey. J Imag Vis Comput 21(11):977–1000
17. Kaufman AE (1996) Volume visualization. J ACM Comput Surv 28(1):165–167

Chapter 298
Application of Internet in Pharmacological Teaching

Chen Jianguang, Li He, Wang Chunmei, Sun Jinghui, Sun Hongxia, Zhang Chengyi and Fan Xintian

Abstract The demand of the rapid development of internet and the information construction of the education industry has prompted the research of educators on the combination of the internet resource with the science of education. In this paper, from the view of point of teaching preparation and practice, combining with the actual situation of pharmacology teaching, some specific ideas and practices are discussed and introduced. The use of the internet for teaching has become a new method for education, a new model, a trend of medical teaching, and the only way which must be passed for the education to face the mass and the modern time. Although it is still in the exploratory stage, a training system for the medical professional personnel can be established through the continuous exploration and the further accumulation of experience on it since the medical education is a very practical science and the higher education reform is a long-term and systematic project.

Keywords Internet · Pharmacology · Education

298.1 Introduction

Pharmacology is a required course in medical education. Because of a wide coverage of pharmacology, divergent knowledge points, and a wide range of disciplines involved in it, it is difficult for students to understand it. Due to the dramatic development in the modern science and technology, and the rapid update of medical knowledge, how medical students can improve their learning efficiencies within the limited time has become an important subject that a teacher in a

---

C. Jianguang (✉) · L. He · W. Chunmei · S. Jinghui · S. Hongxia · Z. Chengyi · F. Xintian
Pharmaceutical College of Beihua University, Jilin 132013, China
e-mail: chenjg118@sohu.Com

medical college or university has to face. The internet as a modern information exchange platform has been widely used in every field of social life to promote the progress of human society, and also brought a great revolution in medicinal education, certainly including the mode of pharmacology teaching. The transition from the traditional mode, teaching with chalk and blackboard, to the mode of multimedia teaching has improved the quality of teaching, and the application of internet in the medical teaching has attracted more attention of teachers in colleges and universities. In this paper, the application of internet in the pharmacology teaching was focused in the undergraduate students based on our practical teaching experience [1, 2].

298.2 Fully Utilization of Advantages of the Internet

298.2.1 Facilitation to Mobilize the Enthusiasm of Students

Pharmacology is involved in an extensive and abundant knowledge on many disciplines of basic medicine and pharmacy so that the students generally reflect that it is difficult for them to learn and memorize it, thus they are not so enthusiastic about the learning of it. Due to this reason, how to mobilize the enthusiasm of students in the study of pharmacology and make them more deeply understand it is a problem that should be further discussed and studied. In our teaching practice, the students universally accepted the form of the network with entertainment. Moreover, the diverse teaching form, the illustrated method with figures and tables, the synchronization of display with both audio and video, the close and friendly feelings from a computer interface, and the transfer of a large amount of information to the students all could facilitate the mobilizing of their enthusiasms to learn their courses, especially for pharmacology due to the characteristics of pharmacology itself described above. This advantage made the classroom teaching more lively, and some abstract, difficult, and boring pharmacological knowledge more vivid and intuitive. After school, students were also happy to take advantage of online resources to conduct the review. It can be believed that it should be easy for the students to enhance their enthusiasm and initiative in their learning pharmacology to understand it better.

298.2.2 Facilitation for Students' Self-Study

In contrast to the past, the content of pharmacology is more, and the teaching hours are limited today because so many subjects have been established. The teaching content by teachers in the classroom is also limited so that more contents of pharmacology are learned by the students relying on their self-learning. How to enhance the enthusiasm of the students' self-learning and facilitate the students' self-study is one of the problems we have to solve. The internet is one of common ways in which students learn and entertain after class. Some pharmacology websites have provided pharmacology syllabus, teaching content, lesson plans, background knowledge, and review questions for students. In our practice, the students could visit the websites provided by us for self-study at any time after school, so as to get rid of the learning mode of "holding a book", indicating that they could both improve their learning interests, but also broaden their horizons to deepen their understanding of the knowledge in the textbook, thus enhancing their independence in learning pharmacology. It may be considered that in the teaching process, the main role of the students could be embodied, and the teaching method might be focused on improving the students 'interests, mobilizing the students' self-learning initiative, inspiring the students' thinking, and developing the students' intelligence.

298.2.3 Facilitation to Reduce Teachers' Burden

Writing teaching plans or making electronic teaching plans is an important preparatory work for teachers before class. In the past, teachers had to spend a lot time and effort to look up the related contents by referring to textbooks and literatures. The internet is a carrier with the mass of information and has a large number of pharmacological resources. Teachers can utilize the search engines to easily get the picture, animation and other materials, and refer to lesson plans from other fellow teachers, which can save a lot of duplication for teachers.

298.3 Application of Internet in Pharmacology Teaching

One of the main functions of the internet is to provide vast amounts of information resources, and a lot of information can be gotten by an appropriate search for a topic of interest through it. If it is properly used, it can be more effective [3–5].

298.3.1 Application of Courseware

Computer-aided multimedia teaching need is required for the support of the related courseware and PPT slides file is still commonly used. If the corresponding courseware materials used for a teaching preparation can be achieved, it is most desirable. Through some large search engines such as Baidu or Google, as long as we add the keyword "PPT", a large number of slides courseware, especially courseware in foreign language can be found, which should often be illustrated, informative, full and new. Both Google and Baidu make a direct search of images and audio and video files available. In addition, a large amount of information can be obtained from PDF documents.

298.3.2 Application of the Medical Literature

In order to make students adapt to the development of modern medicine, the forefront disciplinary information should be timely introduced to them. In this regard, the massive medical research literature plays an irreplaceable role. Although many teaching and research institutes have bought all kinds of good foreign language and Chinese literature database, this kind of situation is not common and it is impossible for the database to cover all the literature comprehensively. In fact, a lot of free literature with full text can be found, which can make up for the lack of the database. In addition to the direct use of free literature provided by some websites, the full-text documents that one wants to have can be obtained through PDF search based on titles, abstracts, search terms of the documents.

298.3.3 Application of Teaching Website

The emergence of the internet has provided an open teaching environment and greatly enriched the traditional pharmacology classroom teaching. With the gradual popularization of E-Learning and distance education in colleges and universities, the construction of online teaching resources has been put a more and more important position. Various institutions have constructed their own teaching websites and set up network courses. These websites have provided very rich contents closely related to the teaching of pharmacology (Table 298.1). There have been lesson plans, teaching papers, courseware, question bank, chemical

Table 298.1 Websites of excellent course of pharmacology

Courses	Websites
Pharmacology, Xian Jiaotong university	http://pharmacology.xjtu.edu.cn/jp/web/index.asp
Pharmacology, China medical sciences university	http://www.cmu.edu.cn/course/viewpage.aspx?cid=1&pageid=86
Pharmacology, Beijing university	http://jpkcsb.b-jmu.cn/yaoli06/index.asp
Pharmacology, Guangdong college of medicine	http://branch.gdpu.cn/jpkc/ylx/ylxjxzy/index.asp
Pharmacology, Central south university	http://www.xysm.net/yaoli/
Pharmacology, Zhongshan university	http://202.116.64.61/jpkc/2005/yaolixue/
Pharmacology, The Fourth Military Medical University	http://course.xlb.fmmu.edu.cn:8080/

software, as well as a lot of teaching material, including pictures, text, video, animation and audio, in our websites. The teachers can make full use of them to eliminate the need for a lot of duplication of effort to improve the work efficiency now. On the other hand, students can deepen the understanding of the pharmacology knowledge by browsing network pharmacology courses [2–5].

In summary, the use of the internet for teaching has become a new method for education, a new model, a trend of medical teaching, and a way which must be passed for the education to face the mass and the modern time. Although it is still in the exploratory stage, a training system for the medical professional personnel can be established through the continuous exploration and the further accumulation of experience on it since the medical education is a very practical science and the higher education reform is a long-term and systematic project.

References

1. Xiaoli Z (2012) Talking about pharmacology teaching. Mod Read 10(222):120
2. Enping J, Yundong W, Chunmei W et al (2011) Characteristics and advantages of application of multimedia technology in pharmacological teaching. J Beihua Univ 12:495–496
3. Wen W, Yuexiu W, Houxi A et al (2012) Use of network resources to build medical pharmacology teaching platform. Chin J ICT Educ 19:39–40
4. Zhipeng W, Qibing M (2007) Make full use of the internet resources, and improve the effect of pharmacology teaching. J shanxi med univ 9:585–588
5. Yandong L, Jiachun L, Yixiong L et al (2005) The application of internet in preventive medicine education practical. Prev Med 12:961–962

Chapter 299
Assessing Information Literacy Development of Undergraduates

Fei Li, Bao Xi and Hua Jiang

Abstract Assessing information literacy development (ILD) of undergraduates becomes more important for universities to confirm their efforts in helping students to cope with challenges in information age. We suggest ILD construct concept of behavior of using IT in academic activities, perception on institution emphasis on using IT, and proficiency of using IT. The concept was tested using survey data from college students. Results from reliability and construct validity suggest that the ILD construct is rational.

Keywords Assessing · Information literacy development · Undergraduates

299.1 Introduction

The information technology is changing the face of the world in the 21th century, where exists the paradox between the proliferation and unending resources, and the citizens all over the world must possess the ability to process information [1]. Undergoing primary and secondary educations, undergraduates have grasped basic knowledge about computer and information technology. So it's important for higher education to foster students' information literacy to cope with challenges in information society, and to help students develop the information skills that will enable them to be successful in both their academic programs and their professional lives [2].

Under the commitment to educate students to be information competent ones, assessing the outcomes of the efforts has become more important. Some universities have their standardized assessments, such as Kent State University's Project

F. Li (✉) · B. Xi · H. Jiang
School of Management, Harbin Institute of Technology, 150001 Harbin, China
e-mail: thanksall@hit.edu.cn

SAILS, and James Madison University's Information Literacy Test, and so on. The assessments are focusing on curriculum [3, 4], strategy [5], and distance education [6] Then it's vital to assess information literacy of students. Few studies pay attention to assessing undergraduates' information literacy development. We try to develop some indicators to assess it.

The rest of the paper is organized as follows. In the next section, we confirm the concept of information literacy development. Subsequent section to describe the construct operationalization and data collection, present the data analysis procedure and the results of the concept testing.

299.2 Information Literacy Development

Information literacy in this paper refers to capacity to processing information using information technologies. College students situate a special period, during which they not only use information technologies in academic work, but also need developing their information capacity for working socially. As a result, the information literacy is developed. The development of information literacy (DIL) depends mainly on three factors.

The first one is student' behavior of using IT in academic activities (BU), refers to some initiative behavior. College students are required to acquire new study habits as they adapt to new instruction, assessment, and learning styles. They should consciously use IT during their autonomous learning so that they can exchange information more effectively and conveniently through those media. In general, there is in general base for using IT with universities' fine IT infrastructure and students' computer for life, entertainment and study. Here we focus on BU for it showing to some extent special academic information ability which indicates professional competence.

The second one is students' perception on institution emphasis on IT (CIE). College atmosphere can affect students' thinking and behavior. Now the internet becomes the primary research information source, a body of academic information is in virtual form in every industry. So the universities have responsibility to educate students to use them and in turn to show themselves outcomes in virtual forms for more efficient communicate. If students accept the institution emphasis on information technology, they should attempt to use IT. Reliance on a particular source of information does not predict greater perceived credibility of the information available through the source [7]. And Universities are obliged to prepare students to be successful and productive in processing information. Then DIL may be come true.

The third one is proficiency of using IT (PU). Although high school students' information literacy skills prepare them for academic work in digital age, students entering the university often lack the IL skills necessary to effectively and efficiently locate, assess and use information [7]. Transition from secondary school to University means more kinds of information resources, and skills occupied seemed limited. And IL policies and practices in university have been tested effective in improving the proficiency [8]. PU reflects the effectiveness of universities' decisions on IL.

299.3 Research Design and Data Analyses

299.3.1 Research Design

We used the survey method to measure the construct concept of information literacy development. The survey tool is China-Nsse. The target students are undergraduates of one university in China. The concept construct come from three questions about information dismissed in different parts, we suggests those questions reflect students' information development in university. The survey was administered to undergraduates from 1–4 grades. For the useful three questions, 1,020 questionaires were effective, and enough for the study.

We test the construct from reliability and construct validity and use respectively the methods of Cronbach α and exploratory factor analysis.

299.3.2 Data Analyses

We test the reliability of data. As shown in Table 299.1, the Cronbach's Alpha of three items is 0.520, which is over the lowest critical value and lies. While three Cronbach's Alpha if item deleted are in turn 0.478, 0.378 and 0.407, all less than 0.52. The results indicate that the data has acceptable consistence and is reliable. Then we tested the construct validity from feasibility of factor analysis and factor analysis if the feasibility is acceptable. As shown in Table 299.2, the KMO value is 0.610, and indicates that there exit some common factors among three items, and the Bartlett x^2 (205.625) is significant at the 0.001 level. So factor analysis is feasibility. Table 299.3 shows that one component is extracted, the initial eigenvalues is 1.541 (over 1), and the extraction sum of squared loadings is 51.345 %. We can see it clearly in Fig 299.1 scree plot. The component matrix is shown as Table 299.4, the factor loadings are 0.673,745 and 730, they are all over the low bound 0.3. So the results are acceptable.

299.4 Conclusion and Discussion

Our interest in assessing ILD of undergraduates was triggered by efforts for college students' ILD. IT from computer to internet requires citizens more proficient in IL. Universities need to foster students preparing for their professional work in

Table 299.1 Cronbach's alpha comparison

LDU items	Scale mean if item deleted	Scale variance if item deleted	Corrected item-total correlation	Cronbach's alpha if item deleted
BU	4.12	1.669	0.305	0.478
CIE	4.53	1.735	0.359	0.378
PU	4.44	1.929	0.346	0.407
Cronbach's alpha of 3 items				0.520

Table 299.2 KMO and bartlett test

Kaiser–Meyer–Olkin measure of sampling adequacy		0.610
Bartlett's test of sphericity	Approx. chi square	205.625
	df	3
	Sig.	0.000

Table 299.3 Total variance explained

Component	Initial eigenvalues			Extraction sums of squared loadings		
	Total	% of variance	Cumulative %	Total	% of variance	cumulative %
1	1.541	51.354	51.354	1.541	51.354	51.354
2	0.776	25.874	77.228			
3	0.683	22.772	100.000			

Extraction method: Principal component analysis

Fig. 299.1 Scree plot of component

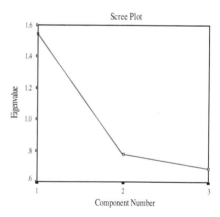

digital society. So assessing DIL become more important. It's provided rational that the ILD construct concept consists of behavior of using IT in academic activities, perception on institution emphasis, and proficiency of using IT.

Table 299.4 Component matrix (a)

	Component 1
UI	0.673
IE	0.745
IA	0.730

Extraction method: Principal component analysis
a 1 components extracted

While we believe we have a rational construct concept of ILD. There exit also some limits in research, the reliability and KMO value are meet the low bound of statistics significance. We consider that may be caused by fewer number of three items. So in the future research we will extend items of ILD to improve reliability and community.

Acknowledgments Sponsored by Teaching and Learning Research Program of HIT ([2010]548–098)

References

1. O'Sullivan C (2002) Is information literacy relevant in the real world? Ref Serv Rev 30(1):7–15
2. Fain Margaret (2011) Assessing information literacy skills development in first tear students: a multi-year study. J Acad Librarianship 37(2):109–119
3. Kong SC (2008) A curriculum framework for implementing information technology in school education to foster information literacy. Comput Educ 51(1):129–141
4. Dunn Kathleen (2002) Assessing information literacy skills in the California State University: a progress report. J Acad Librarianship 28(1):26–35
5. Jennifer L, CoxT, van der Pol Slifka D (2005). Promoting information literacy: a strategic approach. Res Strat 20:69–76
6. van de Vord R (2010) Distance students and online research: promoting information literacy through media literacy. Internet High Educ 13:170–175
7. Hong T (2006) Contributing factors to the use of health-related websites. J Health Commun 11:149–165
8. Gross M, Latham D (2012) What's skill got to do with it?: information literacy skills and self-views of ability among first-year college students. J Am Soc Inform Sci Technol 63:574–583
9. Smith JK, Given LM, Julien H, Ouellette D, DeLong K (2013). Information literacy proficiency: assessing the gap in high school students' readiness for undergraduate academic work. Library and Inf Sci Res 35:88–96

Chapter 300
Improved Access Control Model Under Cloud Computing Environment

Yongsheng Zhang, Jiashun Zou, Yan Gao and Bo Li

Abstract With the development of cloud computing, cloud security problem has become a hot topic. Some scholars put forward the role access control based on mapping, which is used to solve the leakage problem of data storing in the cloud. This paper briefly describes the cloud computing and traditional access control model based on the latest research. Then the paper sums up the work and puts forward a new kind of access control model based on the hop named HBAC. It is based on the role access control that based on mapping. It is used to control the length of path to access the data in outer domain. At last, the paper gives the concrete steps to describe the principle of its operation in detail. And this paper makes a comparison with other related researches. Then this paper summarizes the advantages and disadvantages of HBAC.

Keywords Cloud security · Access control · RBAC · HBAC

Y. Zhang · J. Zou (✉) · Y. Gao
School of Information Science and Engineering, Shandong Normal University, Shandong Provincial Key Laboratory for Novel Distributed Computer Software Technology, Jinan 250014, China
e-mail: 1010336028@qq.com

Y. Zhang
e-mail: zhangys@sdnu.edu.cn

Y. Gao
e-mail: 15553109740@163.com

B. Li
Academic Affairs Office, Shandong Polytechnic, Jinan 250104, China
e-mail: 24874890@qq.com

300.1 Cloud Computing

300.1.1 Concept of Cloud Computing

The cloud computing has not been clearly defined up to now. Although the exact meaning of cloud computing has not yet been fully understood, everywhere is various related service. The understanding of this paper is: Cloud computing is a kind of service used for data storage and applications through the Internet and remote service center [1].

300.1.2 Cloud Security Issues

Under the cloud computing environment, users will not store their information data in their hard drives, but in the remote server data center [2]. Because of the change of data center from the client to the server, the data security of the server is very important. Therefore trusted cloud security technology is also developing rapidly. Many scholars have done research on the aspects of destruction and protection of data, such as the proposed Dissolver system [3].

300.2 Traditional Access Control Model

ISO, the international organization for standard proposed the hierarchical security architecture in the design standard of the security of network system (ISO7498-2), and defined five security services: authentication service, access control, data confidentiality, data integrity, non-repudiation service. As one of the five services, access control service plays an irreplaceable role in network security system [4]. Traditional access control models mainly include four types: access control matrix, Discretionary Access Control (DAC), Mandatory Access Control (MAC) and Role Based Access Control (RBAC) [5].

1. DAC increases the characteristic of "independent" based on access control matrix. Authorized subjects can give authority to other subjects. So it has strong flexibility.
2. MAC is mainly used in military application of multi-level security level. It defines the trust level as user proposed a request or access to the system. The system carries out the comparison, to determine if the access is legitimate.
3. RBAC introduces the concept of the role between subject and object [6]. A user associates with one or more roles, and the role associates with one or more permissions. The users can activate the corresponding role by logging on system to get the corresponding permissions.

At present, RBAC has been widely studied, the experts have put forward some models. For example, the RBAC96 and ARBAC97 put forward by George Mason university of America [7].

300.3 Improved Access Control Model

300.3.1 Division of Logical Domain

Under the environment of cloud computing, users' information are stored in the cloud server, including some private and confidential data. Therefore under multi-tenant environment, data security issues are very important. Here, the paper divides data center under computing environment into different security domains. Resource belongs to different companies or enterprise will be divided into different security domains, which we call the logical domain [8].

300.3.2 Hop-Based Role Access Control

In each logic domain, we use role-based access control model. But to establish the role, this paper adopts a Hop-Based Access Control (HBAC), to make the access in different logical domain a fine-grained limit. It will be described in detail below. For the roles in the logical domain, we record them as three byte R = {(Role, Domain, Hop)}.

300.3.3 The Mapping of Role Between Domains

Under the multi-domain environment, a subject of a security domain has no access to another security domain unless it can pass the permission check of the resource-requested domain. Only when it is cognized by the access control system and it has appropriate permission, the subject can have access to the resource in the foreign domain [9]. We use the role access control based on the mapping as the strategy to visit from one domain to another. The example is Fig. 300.1.

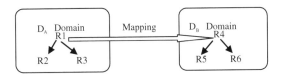

Fig. 300.1 Mapping diagram

300.4 The Defects and Improvements of Role Mapping

300.4.1 A Brief Introduction to the HBAC

To solve the problem of permeation of authority, the paper puts forward a kind of access control based on hop count (HBAC). Assuming the existence of A, B, C, D four security domain, four domain resources are expressed as O = {(Object, Domain)}.The roles are denoted as R = {(Role, Domain, Hop)}. And all the initial value of hop in four domains is set by 0. If B assuming that there is role mapping relation between B and C. Then there is role mapping relationship between C and D. When we want to establish mapping relationship between A and B, we can have fine-grained access control through the 'Hop' fields. Each value of hop should minus 1 if the role wants to visit resources in foreign domains. If its hop = 0, the access is rejected. Else, the value of hop will minus 1, and the visit will be permitted. So, it can prevent problem of penetration of authority.

300.4.2 The Disadvantages and Solution in the HBAC

Although the HBAC mechanism has fine-grained access control, there is also such a situation that when the value for the hop field of the role in A is assigned, we assuming it equals 2, the user have two choices at the moment. One is to continue visiting domain C which has mapping relationship with ask B domain. The other choice is that the user may withdraw from the B domain, and then visit B domain again. In all the situations, the Hop's value will minus 2. But users in the second case (we call it the inverse domain access) cannot visit the resources in C, which is contrary to our original intention. In addition, if different users need different hop value, the same role not be authorized to different users. Therefore, the HBAC mechanism requires strict restrictions on these problems. The solution is as follows:

1. All the initial values of hop are set by 0.
2. Establish a Mapping Hop (MH), table. The table only records the information of the roles which have mapping relationship. Common role won't be recorded into the table.
3. In the process of mapping of role (the role is visiting the resources in foreign domain), the access control system will check the hop's value in the MH table. If the user doesn't exist or the hop's value of the role is 0, then the visit will be turn down, and error will be returned. Otherwise the corresponding hop's value will minus 1, allowing the role mapping.
4. The users' information will be automatically deleted when the access is over. Users should be reauthorized if they want to visit again. We will cancel the users' information in the MH table once the user finishes his visit to the resource in foreign domain and return his own domain.

5. MH table needs to be established by the reliable system which is safe. It is effective only when the identity-authentications of both the cooperation units are given. And once the MH table is set up, it cannot be modified by the provider of cloud service himself.

300.4.3 The Process of HBAC

Access process:

Step 1: As the users in secure domain D_A, P and S want to obtain the authorization of RB_2 in D_B. We need to make restrictions that the user P can only visit the resources in D_A and D_B but not in D_C. The user S can visit the resources in D_B and D_C. When the P and S are authorized with role, we should modify the MH table. Create Row $S(S, RA_1, 2)$; Create Row $P(P, RA, 1)$;

Step 2: When S or P want to visit the resources in D_B, the access system will check them: if $(S \wedge S \rightarrow hop!=0)\{S \rightarrow hop--;visit();\}else\{return\ ERROR;\}$

Step 3: After having visited the resources in the D_B, the result in MH table is as follows: Row $S(S, RA_1, 1)$; Row $P(P, RA_1, 0)$;

Step 4: If P and S want more visits to the resources in D_C, then the S will have the access, the result being Row $S(S, RA_1, 0)$ while the P will be turn down.

300.4.4 Advantages of HBAC Mechanism

The advantages of HBAC mechanism include fine-grained restrictions in access, avoidance of penetration of authority, saving more space compared with establishing the mirror role mapping to prevent penetration of authority, because the MH only records the information of users who has mapping relationship. So the needed space is very small. Secondly, the MH table is updated at dynamic runtime, which reduces the consumption.

300.5 Conclusions

Cloud computing can provide us with reliable and custom service and maximum utilization of resources. Cloud computing service will become popular in the future with its On-demand concept of service. The paper puts forward an improved mechanism based on the analysis about access control model. We believe that the cloud computing service will improve step by step. In the end, it will become a kind of service without any menace from the "rear".

Acknowledgments This research was supported by Natural Science Foundation of Shandong Province of China under Grant No. ZR2011FM019 and Postgraduate Education Innovation Projects of Shandong Province of China under Grant No. SDYY11117. It was also supported by the Project of Shandong Province Higher Educational Science and Technology Program under Grant No. J12LN61. In addition, the authors would like to thank the reviewers for their valuable comments and suggestions.

References

1. Fauzi AAC, Noraziah A, Herawan T, Zin NM (2012) On cloud computing security issues. In: Pan J-S, Chen S-M, Nguyen NT (eds.) Paper presented at the 4th asian conference on intelligent information and database systems. Berlin, Heidelberg
2. Zou J-S (2012) Security problems and its countermeasures in the cloud computing environment. CD Comp Softw Applicat 35–37
3. Zhang F-J, Chen J, Chen H-B, Zang B-Y (2011) Data privacy protection and self destruct in cloud computing. Compute Res Develop, 1155–1167
4. Li H, Li H (2010) Trusted cloud security key technologies and realization. People's Posts and Telecommunications Press, Beijing
5. Han D-J, Gao J, Huo H-L, Li L (2010) Progress of access control model research. Compute Sci, 29–33
6. Sandhu R, Coyne EJ (1996) Role based access control models. IEEE Compute, 38–47
7. Zou X (2006) Analysis and implementation of role-based access control model. Info Microcompute 108–111
8. Tan X (2011) Cloud computing environment access control model. Beijing Jiaotong University, Beijing
9. Zhang D-Y, Liu L-Z (2008) Multi-domain access control model. Compute Applicat, 633–637

Chapter 301
Research on Regional Health Information Platform Construction Based on Cloud Computing

Zhimei Zhang, Xinping Hu, Jiancheng Dong, Jian Yang and Tianmin Jiang

Abstract This paper proposes a service-oriented hierarchical architecture of regional health information service platform with five layers based on concept of cloud computing, and points out the key indicators of platform service level agreement. From views of system security and health information privacy preserving, it also puts forward a security model of the platform and a health information sharing model based on individual permission.

Keywords Cloud computing · Regional health information system

301.1 Introduction

In recent years, in order to promote the modernization of medical and health services, many countries have carried out the projects of regional medical information sharing. UK launched the national medical IT project and United States launched a national health information network project. Canada initiated Health-Infoway project of electronic health system. However, high information construction cost and lacking technical personnel lead to achieve a little progress of these projects. Cloud computing is changing the application mode of traditional computing resources. Information construction through purchasing the computing power from the service provider of cloud computing, medical and health institutions can focus on their own business and innovation. It will promote the developments of health information too. A series of surveys from TripleTree Institute and some investment banks show that cloud computing will eventually repair and improve a medical care system, and solve the inefficient and backward of the health care system over the past ten years in IT.

Z. Zhang · X. Hu (✉) · J. Dong · J. Yang · T. Jiang
Institute of Digital Medicine, Nantong University, Nantong 226001, China
e-mail: xphu@ntu.edu.cn

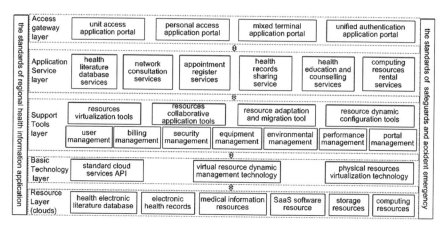

Fig. 301.1 Architecture of regional health information service platform

301.2 Architecture of Regional Health Information Service Platform

Regional health information platform ought to provide a secure medical and health information service including information collection, storage, access, processing, analysis, application, communication and sharing for all authorized users in a certain range with computer and network equipment supporting. Therefore, the goals of regional health information service platform should provide a new people-oriented environment of information service based on computation and communication. The important features of cloud computing are flexible scalability, with the Internet as the center, virtualization and user transparency. The architecture of regional health information service platform based on the cloud computing technology is shown in Fig. 301.1. Guided by the standards of regional health information application and the standards of security safeguards and accident emergency, it is a service-oriented hierarchical architecture and consist of the access gateway layer, application service layer, support layer, technology layer, tool based resource clouds.

301.3 Design of Platform Service Level

Service level agreement (SLA) is an agreement or a contract between service providers and customers on the quality, level, performance and other aspects of services. SLA can improve the development quality of platform, reduce the risk of project failure and strengthen relationships with customers. SLA can ensure the platform service functions meet the demands of all of users though regional health information platform providing a variety of complex application services to multi-class users. The methods of SLA construct are mainly based on services and on users. The key indicators of SLA include:

① security. Service providers must specify the access control policy, encryption algorithm, isolation mode of multi-tenant dada, data retention rules and deletion strategy in SLA.

② transparency. Providers must specify platform sharing architecture, system redundancy mode, the punishment of violation of the agreements and publish regular quality report to clients.

③ auditable. Platform service provider is responsible for lack of availability of any processing. Therefore, consumers should be able to audit systems and procedures of platform services providers. SLA should be clearly define how and when to audit. Consumers can also point third party organization as their proxy to detect performance of cloud service providing. At the same time, cloud service providers should produce evidences to prove their operations correctness.

④ automated on-demand service: SLA should clearly define what kinds of services can be on-demand, the standards of service charges and effective dates.

⑤ metrics definition: response speed, reliability, load balance, the possibility of data loss, flexibility, agility, automation request processing percentage and maximum system downtime must be defined objectively and clearly.

301.4 Design of Security Model

The security model of health information platform based on the cloud computing consists of three parts: cloud-edges, cloud terminal and the transport layer. It is shown in Fig. 301.2.

The services of regional health information platform providing are continuous, sustainable, migrating. In order to ensure high availability, high reliability and

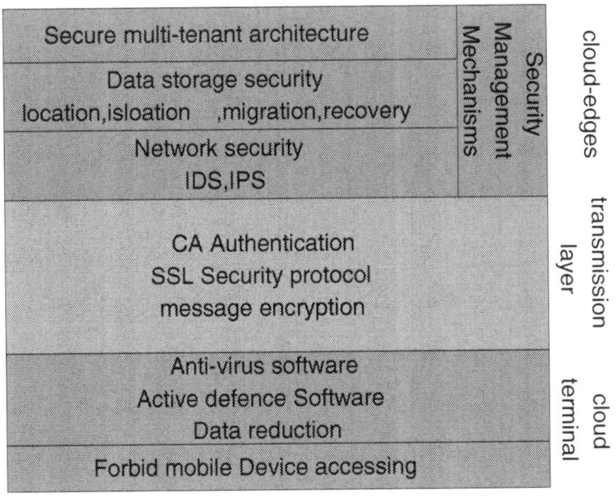

Fig. 301.2 Security model of health information platform

economy, service platform can adopt redundant storage and multi-tenant data isolation to guarantee the data availability and security. In addition, fault-tolerant management mechanism, fault rapid detection, advance fault solution strategies and task migration technology are important to improve platform reliability and security. Intrusion detection system (IDS) and intrusion prevention system (IPS) are two important technologies to solve the problems of network attacks. To the security of transmission layer, CA Authentication, SSL Security protocol and message encryption can prevent health information being abused and filched. In the aspect of cloud terminal, malicious attackers often obtain legal entrance to access system through controlling the cloud terminal and intercept and monitor information. Installing anti-virus software and active defence software can prevent cloud terminal being used by malicious attacker in a certain extent. The better scheme is to make terminal return to original state security using hardware reduction software. However, for the security of mobile devices, there is not a preferable management, so it is necessary to limit the mobile devices freely access to platform.

The focus of health information technologies are security, privacy preserving and data interoperability nowadays. Regional health information sharing model is based on individual independent permission as shown in Fig. 301.3.

Firstly, health authorities establish preliminary data access rules according to the health data using statute in order to regulate what kind of users or organizations how to access health data. Users must obtain CA identity from Certificate Authority and their query operations are record to the access logs to prevent abuse of medical data.

Secondly, patients make data access rules according to their medical data and privacy protection attitude. The rules can specify different access rights of row, column and field to restrict access of different users (Institutions).

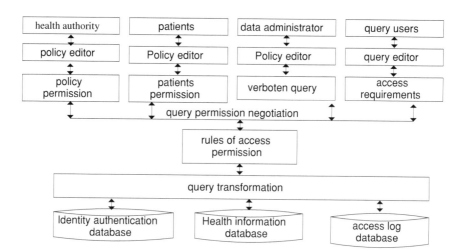

Fig. 301.3 Medical data sharing model based on individual permission

Finally, the data manager can make some access rules from a professional view to protect patient privacy and data security.

When users establish a health information query through query editor, system automatic parses the query and compares with policy access rules, patients' access rules and the data manager's access rules, then convert the users' query into a new query. For examples, a user wants to query all the information for all patients suffering from "hypertension", and the query sentence as following: Select * from patients where diagnosis = 'hypertension'. System automatic converts the users' query as: Select age, sex, occupation, diagnosis from patients where diagnosis = 'hypertension'. The query results which are prohibited to access will be deleted or instead of the null value in order to protect patient privacy and utilize health information availably and effectually.

301.5 Conclusion and Acknowledgments

Health informationization degree is lagged behind other fields, and cloud computing is contributed to promoting health information rapid development. The architecture and models based on cloud computing concept put forward in this article can expand the health information sharing and utilizing and enhance grassroots unit health informationization level. The research is supported by the National Natural Science Foundation of China (No. 81271668), Nantong Science and Technology Bureau (No. BK2011065, No. BK2013024) and Nantong University One-hundred Talent Programme of Humanities and Social Sciences.

References

1. NPfIT: The NHS National Programme for Information Technology (2013) http://www.bcs.org/upload/pdf/sociotechnical-041208.pdf. Accessed 15 Jan 2013
2. Nationwide Health Information Network(NHIN):Background and Scope (2013). http://healthit.hhs.gov/portal/server.pt?open=512&mode=2&cached=true&objID=1142. Accessed 15 Jan 2013
3. Infoway's EHRS Blueprint (2013). http://www.infoway-inforoute.ca/working-with-ehr/solution-providers. Accessed 15 Jan 2013
4. CanadaHealthInfoway. http://en.wikipedia.org/wiki/Canada_Health_Infoway. Accessed 15 Jan 2013
5. Chang HH, Chou PB, Ramakrishnan S (2009) An ecosystem approach for healthcare services cloud. In: IEEE International Conference on e-Business Engineering, pp 608–612
6. Cusumano M (2010) Cloud computing and SaaS as new computing Platforms. Commun ACM 53(4):27–29
7. Li B, Chai X, Hou B et al (2009) Networked modeling and simulation platform Based on concept of cloud computing. J Syst Simul 21(17):5292–5299

Chapter 302
Detection of Fasciculation Potentials in Amyotrophic Lateral Sclerosis Using Surface EMG

Boling Chen and Ping Zhou

Abstract Wide presence of fasciculation potentials is an important indicator for supporting diagnosis of amyotrophic lateral sclerosis (ALS). This study describes the use of surface electromyography (EMG) techniques for examination of fasciculation potentials in ALS patients. Multi-channel surface electrode arrays were used for fasciculation potential recording, while template matching techniques were used to discriminate whether the recorded fasciculation potentials were from the same or different motor unit origins. The results were assessed using independent processing of selected channels of electrode array surface EMG signals.

Keywords: Fasciculation potentials · Surface EMG · Amyotrophic lateral sclerosis

302.1 Introduction

Amyotrophic lateral sclerosis (ALS) is a fatal motor neuron degenerative disease, involving both upper and lower motor neurons. Electromyography (EMG) is one of the routinely used techniques for supporting diagnosis of ALS. Current clinical EMG diagnosis relies on invasive needle electrodes. The wide presence of fibrillation potentials or positive sharp waves is an important diagnostic indicator of ALS, according to E1 Escorial Criteria [1] published by World Federation of Neurology in 1994 [2, 3]. In 2008, new AWAJI criteria [4] emphasize the

---

B. Chen (✉) · P. Zhou
Institute of Biomedical Engineering, University of Science and Technology of China, Hefei, People's Republic of China
e-mail: boling@mail.ustc.edu.cn

P. Zhou
Sensory Motor Performance Program, Rehabilitation Institute of Chicago, Chicago, USA
e-mail: pzhou@ustc.edu.cn

importance of detection of fasciculation potentials in supporting the diagnosis of the disease [5]. It is believed that fibrillation potentials only can be detected by needle EMG. Because of the relative large amplitude, fasciculation potentials can be recorded by both needle and surface electrodes [6]. Recently developed surface electrode arrays, consisting of a number of probes, have provided a powerful approach for detection of fasciculation potentials from skin surface because of the large contact area and small inter-electrode distances [7–10]. In this paper, we present a method of detecting fasciculation potentials using surface EMG from ALS patients. We will study whether fasciculation potentials can be detected in surface EMG.

302.2 Methods

302.2.1 Experiments

Three ALS patients (2 males and 1 female, 48, 66 and 75 years old, respectively) participated in this study. All the subjects met the El Escorial criteria for "Probable" or "Definite" ALS [2]. Each subject was supine comfortably on an examination table. After placing the surface electrode array, the subject was asked to be relaxed completely. Three muscles were examined. For the first dorsal interosseous (FDI) and abductor pollicis brevis (APB) muscles, the hand was typically in semi-pronation. A flexible surface electrode array, arranged in an 8*8 rectangular matrix with a 4-mm interelectrode distance in both directions, was used. Each spontaneous muscle activity recording lasted for at least 100 s. The surface EMG signals were sampled at 2 kHz per channel, with a band pass filter setting of 20–500 Hz [11].

302.2.2 Data Processing

All data were processed using Matlab 2010b (MathWorks, Natick, MA). Every time a signal with duration of 5–10 s was selected for processing. This was performed independently for each channel. Wavelet (sym4 mother wavelet) thresholding based denosing was first used to preprocess the signal. Then, fasciculation potentials were detected using a template-matching technique, generating different classes of fasciculation potential waveforms and their discharge timing or inter peak interval (IPI). Specifically, there steps were involved.

(1) Active segment detection. This was realized by zero filtering. By threshold determination, the whole signal was segmented to individual motor unit potentials;

(2) Clustering. K-means is a typical classification algorithm based on distance. The study used it to cluster similar action potential spikes, resulting in a set of fasciculation potential templates representing different motor unit origins;
(3) Separation of superposition. The superposition waveforms were decomposed by template matching. The EMGLAB was used to help this process [12–14]. To align the set of templates with a given waveform to minimize the euclidean distance between them, the algorithm used a recursive approach to search all possible discrete-time alignments, starting with the most likely ones and stopping once it could be verified that the optimal alignment had been found.

302.3 Results

To show the results, here we demonstrate a 5-s portion in one channel of the surface EMG signal recorded with the 8*8 electrode array from the FDI muscle. This signal was segmented to be 147 individual potentials by threshold determination. For K-means, we used the initial clustering centers algorithm based on minimax distance, so 5 clusters were formed (Fig. 302.1).

We found that 48 of 147 action potential waveforms were not classified to any cluster. Then template matching was used to assess the motor unit components of these waveforms. Firstly, peak detection by nonlinear energy operator (NLEO) was used to retrieve the possible templates of the given waveform (Fig. 302.2). One peak was judged as individual MUAP, and multi-peak as superposition. Then correlation coefficients between superposition and one or two most possible

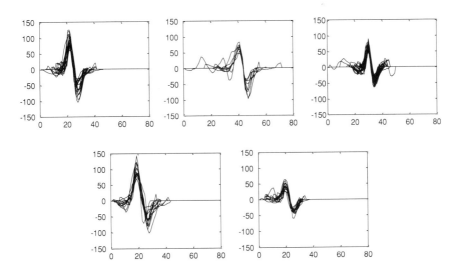

Fig. 302.1 147 potentials of a 5-s signal were classified into 5 clusters

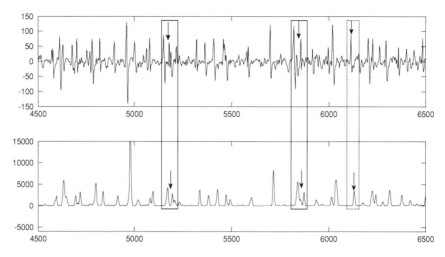

Fig. 302.2 Original signal and its NLEO. *Solid boxes* represent superimposed waveforms and the number of constituent MUAPs, while the *dashed one* represents individual MUAP waveform

templates were computed to find the optimal alignment. These steps were repeated until we got a comfortable firing pattern and relatively small residual signal. Eventual result was shown in Fig. 302.3.

Two-source method was used to verify the results. Traditional 2-source method used needle EMG to verify surface EMG, in this report, we compared IPI from adjacent channels of the arrar recording. Accuracies of the three subjects are shown in Table 302.1.

302.4 Discussion

We detected the fasciculation potentials in ALS patients using surface EMG. Classic pattern recognition method was used to cluster fasciculation potentials using their waveform information. The use of surface EMG is noninvasive and convenient, compared to intramuscular needle EMG, which has been routinely used in clinical neurophysiology for examination of neuromuscular diseases. This study suggests that it is feasible to detect fasciculation potentials using surface EMG. The diagnostic value of fasciculation detection has been emphasized by the Awaji criteria [5]. On the other hand, it is generally believed that other type of spontaneous activity such as fibrillation potentials and positive spikes (these are the important criteria for diagnose of ALS) cannot be detected by surface electrodes, due to the greater distance between the surface electrode and the muscle fibers.

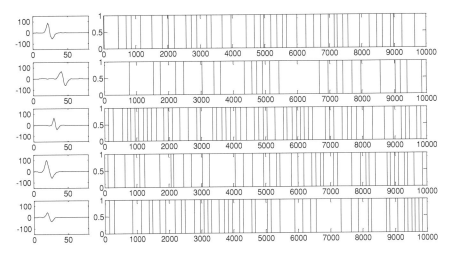

Fig. 302.3 The motor unit template waveforms and their respective firing patterns

Table 302.1 Individual decomposing accuracies by 2-source

Recording	FDI(%)	APB(%)
Subject 1	85.05	87.26
Subject 2	78.43	80.17
Subject 3	82.58	83.69

It is noted that the spatial information provided by multiple channel recording can offer additional useful motor unit information [15] (e.g. location of motor unit innervations zone, conduction velocity, etc.). Such information may not be obtained invasive needle electrodes. Our future work will involve extraction of additional useful information by taking advantage of the spatial information provided by the electrode array.

Acknowledgment This study was supported by National Nature Science Foundation of China (NFSC) under Grant 81271658.

References

1. Subcommittee on Motor Neuron Diseases of World Federation of Neurology Research Group on Neuromuscular Diseases, El Escorial "Clinical Limits of ALS" Workshop Contributors. El Escorial World Federation of Neurology criteria for the diagnosis of amyotrophic lateral sclerosis. J Neurol Sci 1994 124:96–107
2. Brooks BR, Miller RG, Swash M et al (2000) World Federation of Neurology Group on Motor Neuron Diseases: El Escorial revisited: revised criteria for the diagnosis of amyotrophic lateral sclerosis. Amyotroph Lateral Scler Other Motor Neuron Disord 1:293–299

3. Nandedkar SD, Barkhaus PE, Sanders DB et al (2000) Some observations on fibrillations and positive sharp waves. Muscle Nerve 23:888–894
4. de Carvalho M, Dengler R, Eisen A, England JD, Kaji R, Kimura K et al (2008) Electrodiagnostic criteria for diagnosis of ALS. Clin Neurophysiol 119:497–503
5. Benatar M, Tandan R (2011) The Awaji criteria for the diagnosis of amyotrophic lateral sclerosis: have we put the cart before the horse? Muscle Nerve 43:461–463
6. Howard RS, Murray NM (1992) Surface EMG in the recording of fasciculations. Muscle Nerve 15:1240–1245
7. Blok JH, van Dijk P, Dros G, Zwarts MJ, Stegeman DF (2002) A high-density multichannel surface electromyography system for the characterization of single motor units. Rev Sci Instr 73:1887–1897
8. Lapatki BG, van Dijk JP, Jonas IE, Zwarts MJ, Stegeman DF (2004) A thin, flexible multielectrode grid for high-density surface EMG. J Appl Physiol 96:327–336
9. Pozzo M, Bottin A, Ferrabone R, Merletti R (2004) Sixty-four channel wearable acquisition system for long-term surface electromyogram recording with electrode arrays. Med Biol Eng Comput 42:455–466
10. Merletti R, Botter A, Troiano A, Merlo E, Minetto MA (2009) Technology and instrumentation for detection and conditioning of the surface electromyographic signal: State of the art. Clin Biomech (Bristol, Avon) 24(2):122–134
11. Zhou P (2012) Duration of observation required in detecting fasciculation potentials in amyotrophic lateral sclerosis using high-density surface EMG. J NeuroEng Rehabil 9:78. doi:10.1186/1743-0003-9-78
12. McGill KC (2002) Optimal resolution of superimposed action potentials. IEEE Trans Biomed Eng 49:640–650
13. McGill KC, Dorfman LJ (1984) High-resolution alignment of sampled wave-forms. IEEE Trans Biomed Eng 31:462–468
14. McGill KC, Lateva ZC, Marateb HR (2005) EMGLAB:an interactive EMG decomposition program. J Neurosci Methods 149(2):121–133
15. Kleine Bert U, van Dijk Johannes P (2007) Using two-dimensional spatial information in decomposition of surface EMG signals. J Electromyogr Kinesiol 17:535–548
16. Drost Gea, Kleine Bert U (2007) Fasciculation potentials in high-density surface EMG. J Clin Neurophysiol 24:301–307
17. Kleine Bert U, Stegeman Dick F (2008) Firing pattern of fasciculations in ALS: evidence for axonal and neuronal origin. Neurology 70:353
18. Zhou P, Suresh NL, Rymer WZ (2011) Surface electromyogram analysis of the direction of isometric torque generation by the first dorsal interosseous muscle. J Neural Eng 8(3):036028. Epub 13 May 2011
19. Rosenfeld J (2000) Fasciculations without fibrillations: the dilemma of early diagnosis. Amyotroph Lateral Scler Other Motor Neuron Disord 1(Suppl 1):S53–S56
20. De Carvalho M, Swash M (1998) Fasciculation potentials: a study of amyotrophic lateral sclerosis and other neurogenic disorders. Muscle Nerve 21(3):336–344
21. Noto YI, Misawa S, Kanai K, Shibuya K, Isose S, Nasu S, Sekiguchi Y, Fujimaki Y, Nakagawa M, Kuwabara S (2011) Awaji ALS criteria increase the diagnostic sensitivity in patients with bulbar onset. Clin Neurophysiol.122 (12) Epub ahead of print
22. Mills KR (2010) Characteristics of fasciculations in amyotrophic lateral sclerosis and the benign fasciculation syndrome. Brain 133(11):3458–3469. Epub Oct 2010

Chapter 303
Biological Performance Evaluation of the PRP/nHA/CoI Composite Material

Ning Ma, Li Zhang, Di Ying, Pan He, Ming-guang Jin, He Liu and Chun-yu Chen

Abstract *Objective* Analyse the biological performance of the PRP/nHA/CoI composite biofilm. *Methods* Prepared nHA(nHA, *Nanosized hydroxyapatit*) by Chemical precipitation; Co- I (Co- I, Collagen I) was extracted by acid dissolution and protease digestion; Got platelet rich plasma (PRP, Platelet-Rich Plasma) by centrifugation. And crosslinked the composite material. Use the scanning electron microscopy, ELISA immunohistochemistry, 16-slice msct (msct, Multislice Spiral Computed Tomography) to observe composite material and analysis by computer software. *Results* PRP/nHA/CoI has a higher porosity in line with the tissue engineering material.

Keywords Tissue engineered · Platelet-rich plasma · Collagen · Nanosized hydroxyapatit · 16-slice msct · Computer software

Periodontal disease is a popular disease [1], periodontal tissue repair include periodontal ligament repair, cementum repair and alveolar bone repair. Tissue engineering technology opens up new therapeutic way for the reconstruction of periodontal tissues, There are three influential factors: seed cells, biodegradable scaffolds materials and regulating factors in cell growth. In bone tissue engineering, use suitable scaffold carried exogenous growth factors to promote the regeneration of bone tissue is the research focus [2–5].

nHA is the major inorganic component of vertebrate bone and teeth. nHA has osteoinductive function offer available a good environment for bone cell to adhere and grow, its porous structure, tissue regeneration, and vascular conditions is similar with natural bone, is good scaffold material [6, 7]. Co is a fibrini in human body, it has important biological functions can be composited with other synthetic materials, inorganic materials, organic materials, and bio-composite which make it a important scaffold materials in the field of tissue engineering [8–11]. PRP come

---

N. Ma · L. Zhang (✉) · D. Ying · P. He · M. Jin · H. Liu · C. Chen
Periodontics Specialty, School of Stomatology JiLin University, Changchun, China
e-mail: zlamy1009@sina.com

from the platelet concentrates, rich in platelet growth factor, PDGF (PDGF, platelet-derived growth factor), slowly release and promote the regeneration of bone tissue [12, 13].

The experiment we will mix PRP/nHA/CoI composite material together, and then text the complex's biological activity material bioactivities through a series of experimental.

303.1 Experiment Research

303.1.1 Preparation of Composites

303.1.1.1 Type I Collagen Extracted

Take fresh adult cattle Achilles tendon, remove muscle and fascia, wash, cut into thick 0.1 mm sheet and weigh it. Put it into 0.05 mol L-1 acid solution (pH3.2), and add pepsin digestive (100 mg pepsin/1 g tendon pieces) filtered, centrifuged, and discard the pellet in the supernatant, NaCl was added for salting out, see white flocculent precipitate, and then centrifuged, the precipitate collagen dissolved in acetic acid solution, and into a dialysis bag with 0.01 mol L-1 pH7.4PBS for 96 h, and finally dialyzed with distilled water. Dehydration by polyethylene glycol (PEG), after dialysis of the collagen add dropwise glutaraldehyde to the collagen to crosslink.

303.1.1.2 Preparation of nHA

Get nHA by precipitation synthesis. $Ca(OH)_2$ and H_3PO_4 stoichiometry by a Ca/P ratio of 1.67, respectively paired to a certain concentration of the solution, at room temperature, stirring H_3PO_4 solution was slowly added dropwise to the ethylene glycol solution with $Ca(OH)_2$ for 2 h, filtration, drying, then respectively calcined in 300, 600, 800° C at muffle furnace for 2 h.

303.1.1.3 nHA/CoI Composite Membrane

Take 0.5 g nHA to ultrasonic oscillation for 10 min, add 225 mL collagen I protein into it. dilute the solution to 800 mL with distilled water, at room temperature add in 0.025 mol L-1 NaOH (pH = 12.5) until pH rise to 6.2, keep pH at 7.2 for 10 min. Low speed centrifugation and remove the supernatant.

303.1.1.4 PRP/nHA/Co Composite Membrane

Get 10 mL blood from the center of the rabbit ear artery using 10 mL injector with 1 mL 10 % EDTA-Na$_2$. Centrifuged extract twice (1000 rpm × 15 min; 3000 rpm × 8 min), to obtain PRP. The PRP/of NHA/Co. composite membrane preparation: the obtained PRP mixed (10 % CaC$_{12}$, thrombin) 6:1, add to the composite film nHA/Co.

303.1.2 Determination of Biological Properties

303.1.2.1 Extract Osteoblasts and Culture with the nHA/Co Composite

Select 4 week-old white rabbits, weighing 2.5–3.5 kg, aseptic conditions suction total 3 mL bone marrow from bilateral femur, put into the DMEM with 15 % fetal bovine serum, made single cell suspension. 3 × 106 mL-1 cells were inoculated into 50 mL culture flasks, set to 37° C, 5 % CO$_2$ incubator culture. 5d later change half of the medium, after 2–3d change full. Vitro after three generations, and digestion with trypsin, replace the liquid sodium with containing dexamethasone (DEX), ascorbic acid and B-glycerol phosphate DMEM medium induce induced 2l, stain cell with Von Kossa.

Irradiation disinfection nHA/Co composite film with Co60, BMSCs cells were seeded with composite film by 5 × 106 mL-1. The composite membrane, remove culture diaphragm rinsed with PBS, 4 % glutaraldehyde, HE staining, light microscopy; the conventional production scanning electron microscopy (SEM) samples to observe cell adhesion and morphological characteristics.

303.1.2.2 The Rabbit Mandibular Experiment Repairing Composite Membrane

Take 20 healthy adult New Zealand rabbits, make the 1.0 cm × 0.5 cm rectangular bone defect in the middle of the lower edge of bilateral mandibular defect. The right side for the experimental group with composite membrane covering; the left was the control group. Postoperative 28d, 56d installments killed animals, take the bilateral mandibular line of soft X-ray radiography; doing routine HE staining, seen by light microscopy.

303.1.2.3 Composite Membrane Guide the Dog Periodontal Tissue Regeneration

Eight healthy adult male Miscellaneous dogs with 32 teeth. Surgical dissection gingival, exposed bone wall, drilling and grinding the "U" bone defects, bone wall under 5 mm of the cemento-enamel junction, mesiodistal width was 4 mm. Scrape the exposed root surface periodontal ligament and cementum, and make root planing. The right side of the experimental group with the composite membrane materials; The left is the control group put nothing. After 4 and 8 weeks, respectively killed 4 animals, cut bilateral the mandible specimens, shot 16-slice CT slices observed alveolar bone regeneration.

303.2 Results and Discussion

303.2.1 PRP/nHA/CoI Material Physical Performance Tests

Extracting collagen-polyacrylamide gel electrophoresis (SDS-PAGE) results appear a band (molecular weight of about 98KD), proving that the extraction was the CoI, CoI was three-dimensional mesh structure scanned by electron microscope (Fig. 303.1). It has the same size with the natural bone,and relatively uniform pore size distribution of the surface of the composite material, the nHA are evenly distributed in the collagen matrix, and a good combination with collagen interface (Figs. 303.2 and 303.3).

303.2.2 Using Composite Membrane Repairing Rabbit Mandibular Experiment

This experiment successfully isolated and cultured rabbit BMSCs [14], serial subcultivation cells to spindle cells, the polygonal cell transformation and some extend pseudopodia, with a number of projections, rabbit BMSCs, after dexamethasone (DEX), ascorbic acid and β-glycerophosphate induced a significant positive reaction. After Von Kossa staining after 2ld, the black nodules showed up, turned out that the transformation BMSCs to the osteoblast-like cells was successfully.

Scanning by electron microscopy (SEM) materials having larger pores develop early cells scattered in that the surface of the material, was a plurality of projections of the spindle or polygonal, loosely connected cells. With the incubation time, cell proliferation, connected with a single-layer or growth attached to the larger pore surface, tightly packed cells. The membrane surface visible to a large number of BMSCs adhered cell growth, attached close, the partial region of the formation of extracellular matrix. Biocompatible composite material developed in this experiment, negative stimulus to the cells, cytotoxic materials (see Figs. 303.4 and 303.5).

Above experiment the rabbit BMSCs was the characteristics of bone tissue engineering seed cells. The rabbit BMSCs the nHA/Co composite culture together

Fig. 303.1 The result of SDS-PAGE

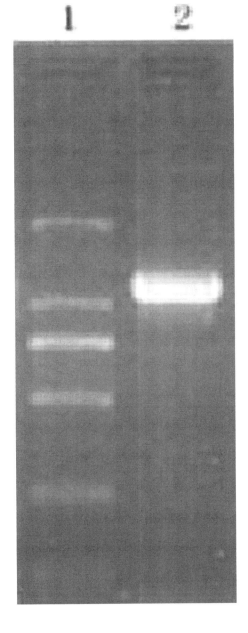

proved this composite material was biocompatible, non-cytotoxic cells without adverse stimulus. In this study, the development of the material was a fine bone substitute material [18–22].

Fig. 303.2 Microscopy of natural bone

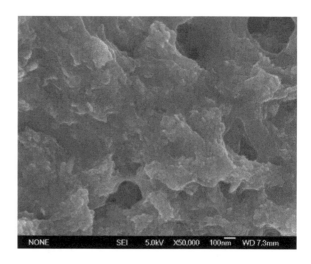

Fig. 303.3 Microscopy of synthesis

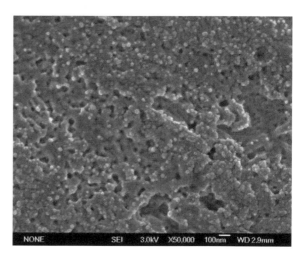

303.2.3 PRP/nHA/CoI Composite Membrane Repair Mandible Experiment

56d later, Soft X-ray: the control group, almost no new bone still the previous the mandibular defects notch (Fig. 303.6); the experimental group bone density increase, complete healing bone defect, the defect area of new bone and the original bone edge healing well, between bone healing line can be seen (Fig. 303.7).

Fig. 303.4 Von Kossa Staining of BMSCs cultured for 21 days with DMEM × 40

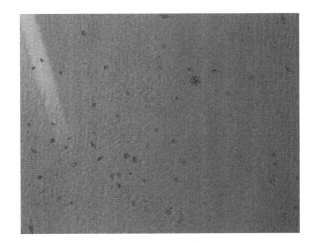

Fig. 303.5 SEM result of Co-Culture of BMSCs and material × 2000

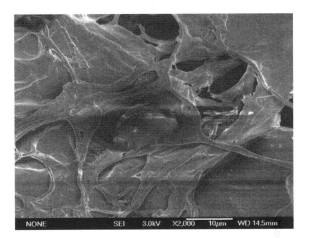

Fig. 303.6 The notch was still seen 56 days

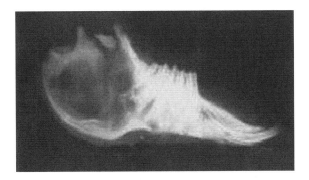

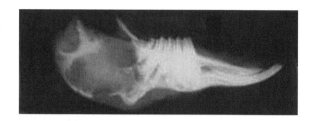

Fig. 303.7 Bone density increased and the defect area healed completely 56 days

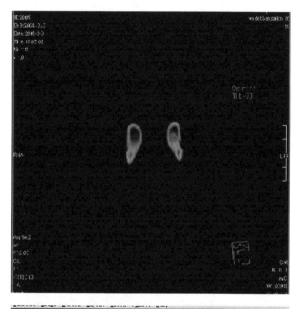

Fig. 303.8 The alveolar bone has not healed to its original height 8 weeks of the control group

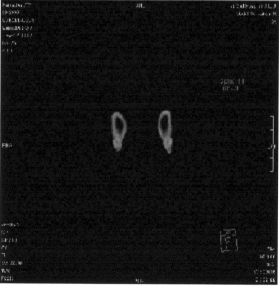

Fig. 303.9 The alveolar bone height healed to normal 8 weeks of the experimental group

303.2.4 16-Slice CT Observed Dog Periodontal Tissue Regeneration

The alveolar bone has not healed to its original height 8 weeks of the control group. The alveolar bone height healed to normal 8 weeks of the experimental group. Prove that PRP/nHA/CoI composite membrane can repair the periodontal tissue.

303.3 Conclusion

By using the advanced technology to evaluate the biological performance PRP/nHA/CoI composite has good biocompatibility, can repair defect tissue. Confirm that the composite material is a new type of the biological activity material replacement material in bone tissue engineering (Figs. 303.8 and 303.9).

References

1. Liu K, Meng H, Hou J (2012) Activity of 25-hydroxylase in human gingival fibroblasts and periodontal ligament cells. PLoS ONE 7(12):e52053
2. Woo KM, Chen VJ, Jung HM, Kim TI, Shin HI, Baek JH et al (2009) Tissue Eng Part A 15(8):2155e62
3. Seyedjafari E, Soleimani M, Ghaemi N, Shabani I (2010) Biomacromolecules 11(11):3118e25
4. Bohner M (2010) Design of ceramic-based cements and putties for bone graft substitution. Eur Cells Mater 20:1–12
5. Johnson AJW, Herschler BA (2011) Acta Biomater 7:16–30
6. Gałkowska E, Kiernicka M, Owczarek B (2003) The use of HA-Biocer in the complex treatment of aggressive periodontal diseases. Ann Univ Mariae Curie Sklodowska Med. 58(1):231–235
7. Zietek M, Gedrange T, Mikulewicz M (2008) Long term evaluation of biomaterial application in surgical treatment of periodontosis. J Physiol Pharmacol 59(5):81–86
8. Koutouzis T, Haber D, Shaddox L, Aukhil I, Wallet SM (2009) Autoreactivity of serum immunoglobulin to periodontal tissue components: a pilot study. J Periodontol 80(4):625–633
9. Hendler A, Mulli TK, Hughes FJ (2010) Involvement of autoimmunity in the pathogenesis of aggressive periodontitis. J Dent Res 89(12):1389–1394
10. Marelli B, Ghezzi CE, Barralet JE, Boccaccini AR, Nazhat SN (2010) Biomacromolecules 11:1470e9
11. Chen R, Hunt JA (2007) Biomimetic materials processing for tissue-engineering processes. J Mater Chem 17:3974e9
12. Kang J, Sha YQ, Ou-yang XY (2010) Combination therapy of periodontal intrabony defects with demineralized freeze-dried bone powder and platelet-rich plasma. Beijing Da Xue Xue Bao (Chinese) 42(1):24–27
13. Pepelassi EA, Markopoulou CE, Dereka XE (2009) Platelet-rich plasma effect on periodontally affected human gingival fibroblasts: an in vitro study. J Int Acad Periodontol 11(1):160–8

14. Chen K, Ng KS, Ravi S, Goh JC, Toh SL (2013) In vitro generation of whole osteochondral constructs using rabbit bone marrow stromal cells, employing a two-chambered co-culture well design. J Tissue Eng Regen Med
15. Roostaeian J, Carlsen B, Simhaee D (2006) Characterization of growth and osteogenic differentiation of rabbit bone marrow stromal cells. J Surg Res 133(2):76–83
16. Jiang XQ, Chen JG, Gittens S (2005) The ectopic study of tissue-engineered bone with hBMP-4 gene modified bone marrow stromal cells in rabbits. Chin Med J (Engl) 118(4):281–288
17. Zhang C, Ma Q, Qiang H (2010) Study on effect of recombinant adeno-associated virus vector co-expressing human vascular endothelial growth factor 165 and human bone morphogenetic protein 7 genes on bone regeneration and angiopoiesis in vivo. Zhongguo Xiu Fu Chong Jian Wai Ke Za Zhi (Chinese) 24(12):1449–1454
18. Tamaki Y, Nakahara T, Ishikawa H, Sato S (2012) In vitro analysis of mesenchymal stem cells derived from human teeth and bone marrow. Odontology
19. JulKim SH, Kim YS, Lee SY (2011) Gene expression profile in mesenchymal stem cells derived from dental tissues and bone marrow. J Periodontal Implant Sci 41(4):192–200
20. Kim SH, Kim KH, Seo BM (2009) Alveolar bone regeneration by transplantation of periodontal ligament stem cells and bone marrow stem cells in a canine peri-implant defect model: a pilot study. J Periodontol 80(11):1815–1823
21. Li H, Yan F, Lei L, Li Y, Xiao Y (2009) Application of autologous cryopreserved bone marrow mesenchymal stem cells for periodontal regeneration in dogs. Cells Tissues Organs 190(2):94–101
22. Ueno T, Kagawa T, Ishida N (2001) Prefabricated bone graft induced from grafted periosteum for the repair of jaw defects: an experimental study in rabbits. J Craniomaxillofac Surg 29(4):219–223
23. Matsumoto G, Hoshino J, Kinoshita Y (2012) Evaluation of guided bone regeneration with poly(lactic acid-co-glycolic acid-co-ε-caprolactone) porous membrane in lateral bone defects of the canine mandible. Int J Oral Maxillofac Implants 27(3):587–594
24. Martinez LA, Gioso MA, Lobos CM, Pinto AC.Localization of the mandibular canal in brachycephalic dogs using computed tomography.J Vet Dent. 2009 Fall;26(3):156-163
25. Soukup JW, Lawrence JA, Pinkerton ME, Schwarz T (2009) Computed tomography-assisted management of a mandibular dentigerous cyst in a dog with a nasal carcinoma. J Am Vet Med Assoc 235(6):710–714

Chapter 304
An Integrated Service Model: Linking Digital Libraries with VLEs

Deng Xiaozhao and Ruan Jianhai

Abstract Digital libraries and virtual learning environments (VLEs) have been designed, developed and maintained separately in China, so it is essential to explore a possible innovative service model that could add value to VLE communities and facilitate greater liaison between libraries and VLEs. This paper aims to bring a theoretical and conceptual framework to the practices of an integrated service of digital libraries and VLEs from the library community perspective. The integrated service model conceived could focus on two types of library service, the course-centered service and the discipline-centered service and supply users with following resources and services: course repository, reading list, subject resource list, disciplinary repository, one-stop access and subject librarian service.

Keywords Digital libraries · Virtual learning environments · Integration · E-learning

304.1 Introduction

Virtual learning environments (VLEs) are complementary virtual community support tools aimed at supporting the needs of teachers and learners. It is designed to act as a focus for students' learning activities and their management and facilitation, along with the provision of content and resources required to help make the activities successful [1]. Meanwhile, digital libraries are also information

D. Xiaozhao (✉)
School of Computer and Information Science, Southwest University, Chongqing 400715, China
e-mail: dxz@swu.edu.cn

R. Jianhai
Library Southwest University, Chongqing 400715, China
e-mail: rjh@swu.edu.cn

environments which include abundant excellent learning resources and services. Therefore, in virtual learning environments, digital libraries are likely to be considered as a federation of services and collections that function together to create a digital learning community.

The literature shows that a lot of institutional VLE implementations featured some form of integration to allow a library service presence, typically including a resource list tool, inside the virtual classroom in developed countries [2]. The JISC programme of VLE projects was shown to be a significant positive influence facilitating the development of learning resources and pedagogical understanding [3]. In China, however, digital libraries and VLEs have been designed, developed and maintained separately. Therefore, it is essential to explore a possible innovative service model that could add value to VLE communities and facilitate greater liaison between libraries and VLEs.

304.2 Fundamental Issues for Integrating Digital Libraries and VLEs

304.2.1 Reasons to Integrate Digital Libraries and VLEs

The benefits to users with respect to effective VLE library integrations have been identified as:

- Positioning library services within the virtual classroom environment;
- Promoting greater awareness and increasing utilization of electronic resources of library;
- Delivering online instruction through information literacy courses, tutorials, videos, worksheets and quizzes;
- Providing students with a one-stop access to all relevant services; and
- Improving faculty-librarian liaison and better matching between resources and their availability.

304.2.2 Resources that Could Be Integrated

Usually, the integrated course resources could be grouped as:

- Structured resources in libraries or VLEs, such as textbooks, reference books, glossaries, E-journals, databases, reading list or E-reserves, which are standardized, bibliographic controlled and peer reviewed;
- Less structured resources, including syllabus, courseware, handouts, course notes, teaching cases, teaching video, information literacy instruction from librarians and such like which may poorly structured and not subject to bibliographic controls;

- Unstructured resources, which might emerge from discussion forums in VLEs, virtual reference service of libraries, announcements or e-mail lists and which is changing dynamically and being amended.

304.2.3 Approaches to Integrate Digital Libraries and VLEs

A variety of approaches to integrate digital libraries and VLEs have being implemented in some developed countries, which can be divided into three types. Firstly, an approach is resources-oriented, which regards the library as information resources provider and embed the content in VLEs. Secondly, there is a way for integrating both resources and services, including digital collection, OPAC and virtual reference service, online library instruction, etc. Thirdly, the view of organizational restructuring exists, which includes the library as a whole organization merged with VLE communities and its activities.

Compared with the third one, the first two are more practicable and have been adopted by many universities abroad. This gave us great enlightenment for our study.

304.3 Framework for an Integrated Service Model

Learning from the practices of universities abroad, an integrated service model could be discussed here. In this model, every course in a VLE is guided to the "library" link, as shown in Fig. 304.1. When users click the linkage, the system would first help them to seeking for the page directly related to the course. If the page of specific course cannot be found, the system will navigate its users to a broader level of resources and service—the page of the specific discipline. If none of them exists, the library homepage will be delivered to the users. Anyway, the integrated service model provides users with relevant information more or less and ensures they can acquire pertinent resources and services from libraries as far as possible.

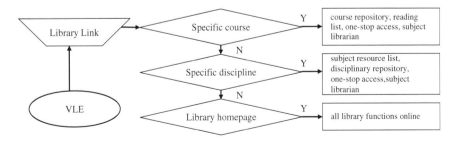

Fig. 304.1 Application flow of an integrated service model

For simplicity's sake, the proposal below will focus on two types of library service, the course-centered service and the discipline-centered service.

304.3.1 Course-Centered Service

Based on specific course resources, the course-centered service model integrates the library resources and services and assists users in seeking course-centered resources.

For this type of service, librarians are supposed to gather resources in response to the information needs of faculty and students and then filter, classify and integrate them into the resources page related to the course. Meanwhile librarians are obliged to participate in developing and maintaining the course website, in order to provide point-to-point services.

Such kind of service model could supply users with following information.

304.3.1.1 Course Repository

A course repository contains course atlas and course description. It covers offerings from one or more education providers and thus allows user to search and find comparable courses exploring the implications of learning objectives, syllabus, courseware, handouts, method of instruction, text books, faculty level, pre-requisites, credits, evaluation methods, study abroad programs, curriculum alignment initiatives and so on.

304.3.1.2 Reading List Service

Reading list service is designed to improve communication between VLEs and materials held in the library to improve user satisfaction in terms of resource availability and accessibility. The reading list will typically be closely embedded in the virtual learning environments. It gives the users a 'course/module' view on library resources. Links will be made from the reading list citation to the full text of book references, E-journal articles and digitized chapters/articles which have been accurately described by librarians. Thus it provides easy access to relevant materials for users who can then subscribe the resources as they like.

304.3.1.3 One-Stop Access

The integration of library facilities and the VLE allows for the integration of course modules from the point of view of users and of the course designers. One-stop access is built in the integrated service model that guides users through a simple interface to search all the resource in the fully integrated learning environment in which users do not perceive the joins between systems.

304.3.1.4 Subject Librarian

Subject librarians are the glue and intermediary between digital libraries and VLEs. In supporting E-learning, subject librarians often customize resources or services for particular subject fields, match information to users' need and answers or pathways to users' questions. Particularly, subject librarians can use the reference transaction not only to answer questions but also to improve the information retrieval skills and information literacy of their patrons.

To help users find the subject librarian in time, librarian's contact information is published online, including that of personal profile, job responsibility and co-operation of academic faculty.

304.3.2 Discipline-Centered Service

The discipline-centered service model caters to users' need of discipline-related resources or services, which covers disciplinary repository, subject resource list, one-stop access and subject librarian service.

This kind of service will be recommended to users when users fail to find relevant information from the course-centered service, as shown in Fig. 304.1. In particular, subject resource list and disciplinary repository are two special components in this service model.

304.3.2.1 Subject Resource List

A subject resource list means a digital collection gathering and providing access to the literature of a particular subject area or a set of related subjects. It may include a wide range of content for users. Typically it contains credible scholarly books, articles, or data associated with these works of scholars, research groups, institutions, organizations. Moreover, disciplinary repositories often have no limitations on the types of publications or types of data that can be held, so these can range from peer-reviewed journal articles to grey literature, data sets, theses and teaching materials and subject-based gateways.

304.3.2.2 Disciplinary Repository

A disciplinary repository is a knowledge base that encompasses all of the relevant information of a particular disciplinary, major, or cutting-edge knowledge on service delivery for the purposes of upscaling of learning initiatives.

Unlike a subject resource list, the disciplinary repository focus on capturing, processing and then supplying both of explicit knowledge and tacit knowledge based on knowledge service level objectives and requirements, rather than simply navigating users to literature/document service. For this purpose, besides traditional approaches in the filed of information management, domain ontology would be exploited to offers a direction towards solving the interoperability problems brought about by semantic obstacles, in order to allows automatic reasoning for problems resolution.

304.4 Conclusion

Undoubtedly, it is essential for us to harness the potentials of integration of digital libraries and VLEs for achieving educational goals. But at the meantime, there are various issues of integration in the following categories: human and organizational, technical, expenditure and so on. For instance, we must ensure that our task is not simply to put effort into computer programming and software development, important though that is. Significantly, our traditional libraries must be towards full and active liaison and collaboration with teaching branches and librarians should seek to understand their role in the information management chain to their academic colleagues and to improve their learning support skills. Only then can we harvest an interoperable and harmonious integrated service of digital libraries and virtual learning environments.

References

1. Stiles MJ (2000) Effective learning and the virtual learning environment. http://www.staffs.ac.uk/COSE/cose10/posnan.html
2. Virkus S et al (2009) Integration of digital libraries and virtual learning environments: a literature review. New Libr World 110(3/4):136–150
3. Corrall S, Keates J (2011) The subject librarian and the virtual learning environment: a study of UK universities. Program Electron Libr Inf Syst 45(1):29–49
4. Bewick L, Corrall S (2010) Developing librarians as teachers: a study of their pedagogical knowledge. J Librarianship Inf Sci 42(2):97–110
5. Fleck J (2012) Blended learning and learning communities: opportunities and challenges. J Manag Dev 31(4):398–411
6. Garland P, Garland I (2012) A participative research for learning methodology on education doctoral training programmes. Int J Res Dev 3(1):7–25
7. Johnson AM et al (2011) Library instruction and information literacy 2010. Ref Serv Rev 39(4):551–627
8. Osorio NL (2011) New approaches to E-reserve: linking, sharing and streaming. Collect Build 30(4):185–186
9. Sánchez RA (2012) E-learning and the University of Huelva: a study of WebCT and the technological acceptance model. CampusWide Inf Syst 30(2):135–160

10. Saumure K, Shiri A (2006) Integrating digital libraries and virtual learning environments. Libr Rev 55(8):474–488
11. Stagg A, Kimmins L (2012) Research skills development through collaborative virtual learning environments. Ref Serv Rev 40(1):61–74
12. Vasileiou M et al (2012) Choosing e-books: a perspective from academic libraries. Online Inf Rev 36(1):21–39

Chapter 305
The Research and Application of Process Evaluation Method on Prosthodontics Web-Based Course Learning

Min Tian, Zhao-hua Ji, Guo-feng WU, Ming Fang and Shao-feng Zhang

Abstract *Aim* To explore and apply a comprehensive evaluation method for web-based prosthodontics course learning. *Methods* A set of evaluation index system of prosthodontics web-based course learning process was preliminarily constructed through analyzing the influencing factors of web-based course learning effect. Expert consulting method and analytic hierarchy process were applied for the determination of the quality model of web-based course and the weights of each indicator. Delphi technique was used for the evaluation of the rationality of every index weight. A standard evaluation system was finally formed. The evaluation system combined with topsis method was applied in the evaluation of the web-based course learning effect of the five-year system dental students. *Results* Through multiple screening and weighting, a multistage model of web-based courses' evaluation was established, including 4 primary indexes, 7 secondary ones and 19 third ones. The general scores and ranks of the students were obtained from the comprehensive evaluation method and combined with topsis method. *Conclusion* This evaluation method includes the learning process and outcome, integrates the qualitative analysis and quantitative analysis, which assures the evaluation results to be objective and just.

Keywords Prosthodontics · Web-based course · Analytic hierarchy process · Delphi technique · Topsis method

---

M. Tian (✉) · G. WU · M. Fang (✉) · S. Zhang
Department of Prosthodontics School of Stomatology, The Fourth Military Medical University, 145 Changle Xi Road, Xi'an 710032, China
e-mail: tianminno@163.com

M. Fang
e-mail: fmfmyouyou@qq.com

Z. Ji
Department of Epidemiology School of Public Health, The Fourth Military Medical University, 145 Changle Xi Road, Xi'an 710032, China

Web-based course learning assessment is a very important part in the learning process, but the evaluation of web-based courses is mostly concentrated on the network curriculum assessment or just a simple transplant of traditional classroom learning evaluation techniques, the evaluations pay too much attention to the learning outcomes, ignoring the evaluators in various stages of progress, effort and learning process. The excessive objective tests make the assessment unscientific, incomplete and not comprehensive. The web-based learning assessment should not just be a simple summary judgment, and should be run through the whole learning process, not only quantitative factors and non-quantifiable factors. The completeness and accuracy of evaluation plays a very important role in improving teaching quality. Our research departments established a web-based course evaluation index system to track students' learning process and combined with Topsis method to comprehensively evaluate the web-based learning activities of students.

305.1 Establishment of the Evaluation Index System

305.1.1 Preliminary Establishment of the Web-Based Course Evaluation Index System

Through analyzing the factors that affect the effectiveness of learners and the existing evaluation index case, the results showed that the web-based learning should be evaluated from the knowledge acquisition, cooperation and exchange, learning attitude and ultimately works. On the basis of the learners' needs analysis, literature reading and trial investigation, according to the definitions and principles of web-based courses, as well as network accredited index system frame model, we propose of prosthodontics network learning results certification indicators, including four aspects of a total of 20 indicators.

305.1.2 Using Delphi Method to Filter the Network Course Evaluation Index System

The Delphi method is a preparation of educational evaluation system in order to obtain certain indicators or some of the indicators of the degree of importance of a consistent understanding of expert consultation. Experts do not meet each other in the process, the opinion of senior officers or judgment of the indicators of the degree of importance was acquired in the form of a questionnaire, so that the unanimous opinions were obtain [1–3] In this way, the opinions of different authorities can be taken into account.

In order to make the consultants of this study higher authority and representation, 18 experts were selected from the Department of Prosthodontics,

Department of Oral Anatomy and Physiology who are experienced in web-based course teaching, oral medicine teaching management to consult. Among them there are 14 experts engaged in clinical teaching and 2 in the medical education management, including 4 professors, 5 associate professors, 5 lecturers, 4 teaching management. Issued a total of 18 copies of the consultation table, 18 were returned, recovery rate was 100 %. The results show that 2 experts thought the indicators were very reasonable, 12 experts thought they were basic reasonable and 4 experts thought that they needed appropriate adjustments.

The first web-based course evaluation system was formed according to the specific adjustments opinion of the experts index content (Table 305.1).

305.1.3 Applying AHP to Determine Index Weight

The AHP is a multi-attribute decision tool that allows financial and non-financial, quantitative and qualitative measures to be considered and trade-offs among them to be addressed. The AHP aimed at integrating different measures into a single overall score for ranking decision alternatives. Its main characteristic is that it is based on pair-wise comparison judgments [4].

Table 305.1 After the first adjustment network course evaluation index system

First-class indicators	Second-class indicators	Third-class indicators	
Knowledge acquisition	The degree of knowledge acquisition	x1:	Homework average scores
		x2:	Self-test average scores
		x3:	Online exam average scores
Cooperation and exchange	Interactive enthusiasm	x4:	BBS Browse total time
		x5:	BBS post numbers
		x6:	Numbers of question
	The quality of interaction	x7:	Times of post browsing
		x8:	BBS Reply
		x9:	The number of BBS essence post
		x10:	Times of participate in the Q & Views
	Punctuality	x11:	Homework submission on time
		x12:	Login on time
	Participation	x13:	Self-test frequency
		x14:	Submit homework frequency
		x15:	The number of online exam
	Resource utilization	x16:	The total time of browsing course
		x17:	The total number of browsing course
		x18:	The number of paper of browsing course
Final works	Case design capabilities	x19:	Case design results
		x20	Case design new ideas, new methods

The basic idea of Analytic Hierarchy Process is that firstly identify the main factors of the target issues, constitutes a hierarchical model according to the association and affiliation of these factors, and then compare the relative importance at each level to establish a judgment matrix, obtained the layer elements of the weights for the criteria through calculating the maximum eigenvalue of the judgment matrix and the corresponding orthogonal eigenvectors. Finally, on the basis of the above the combination weights of overall goal of all elements were calculated.

Specific method as previously described 18 experts issuing expert advice inquiry form, the indicators were divided into "very important", "important", "general", "less important" and "unimportant". Five grades were given 9, 7, 5, 3, 1 scores, experts scoring according to the degree of importance of the indicators. The arithmetic mean of the scores obtained to represent expert opinions concentration for the indicators, and the coefficient of variation of the scores represented the coordination degree of the expert opinions, the smaller the coefficient of variation of expert advice, the higher the degree of co-ordination.

Suppose X_{ij} represented expert i, j indicator scoring. There were n experts and m indicators.

$$M_j = \frac{1}{n}\sum_{i=1}^{n} X_{ij} \qquad (305.1)$$

$$S_j = \sqrt{\frac{1}{n-1}\sum_{i=1}^{n}(X_{ij} - M_j)} \qquad (305.2)$$

The coefficient of variation of the formula: $V_j = S_j/M_j$; V_j represents the coefficient of variation of index j; S_j represents the standard deviation of index j; M_j represents the arithmetic mean of index j; the smaller of V_j, the higher of index j expert advice coordination.

The expert advisory statistics suggested that the coefficient of variation for each index values show a high degree of coordination between 0–0.35. The "opinions concentration greater than 6.5 (means that arithmetic mean is greater than 6.5) indicators" were kept in the evaluation index system which composed of 19 indicators and the indicator "Login on time" was removed.

305.2 Using Topsis Method for Evaluation

The TOPSIS method is a multiple criteria assessment method developed by Hwang and Yoon in 1981 [5]. It has been widely applied in the selection of different types of decision-making problems [6].

TOPSIS method is the ideal solution for a similar order selection technology, which can be used to benefit evaluation, health decision-making and health services management and other field. The basic idea of the TOPSIS method was based on normalized raw data matrix to identify a limited program in the optimal solution and the worst solution, and then the distance between the evaluation object with the optimal solution and the worst solution were calculated, which obtained the evaluation object and the relative closeness of the optimal solution, as the basis for evaluation.

Using topsis method and self-developed SAS programs in SAS 9.1 platform to analyze the selected evaluation indicators, in order to obtain the general scores and ranks of the students. Taking the web-based course learning effect of 10 five-year system students of grade 2005 in the Fourth Military Medical University for example, the original simulated data in Table 305.2 and the optimal value of the relative closeness and sort results in Table 305.3.

According to the results of Topsis method, the C_i test distribution is the normal distribution consistent with the students' actual learning (i.e. learning, especially with particularly inferior students account for a minority, the majority of students in the middle level). Therefore, we consider the evaluation of the course learning activities of students' learning network score conversion into percentile (formula 3), in order to facilitate comparison.

$$S_i = 100 \times C_i \qquad (305.3)$$

In this comprehensive evaluation of the 5-year system students learning, number 05 student was closest to the learning of the optimal level of 0.74. The scores of 9 indicators were not the best for number 05 student, however, it was closest combination compared with the optimal matrix. All the 19 indicators played important role for the comprehensive web-based course evaluation. The proportion of the final score value greater than 0.60 students accounted for 80 % and 20 % of the students failed in this course, which was acceptable for the final result of course evaluation.

Table 305.2 The original simulated data of 19 indicators for 10 five-year system students

ID	x1	x2	x3	x4	x5	x6	x7	x8	x9	x10	x11	x13	x14	x15	x16	x17	x18	x19	x20
01	5	78	85	154	7	29	16	6	6	9	6	0	3	3	4	3	2	85	65
02	4	93	85	161	6	17	22	8	5	11	7	1	4	3	5	3	2	80	80
03	4	75	85	168	7	20	24	4	4	12	3	1	4	3	2	3	2	80	85
04	4	78	100	182	6	16	9	4	1	10	10	1	2	3	2	3	2	75	80
05	5	90	90	189	8	40	24	8	5	9	8	1	5	3	1	3	2	75	80
06	4.5	78	85	148	9	24	17	7	4	9	7	1	4	3	4	3	2	85	75
07	4	88	85	220	3	15	21	5	4	11	7	1	4	3	5	3	2	80	80
08	4	85	85	288	7	26	23	7	4	9	9	0	5	3	3	3	2	75	75
09	4	68	80	169	8	16	23	10	5	9	9	1	4	3	2	3	2	80	75
10	4	87	90	198	8	21	22	9	5	12	11	0	3	3	4	3	2	75	85

Table 305.3 The optimal value of the relative closeness and sort results of 10 five-year system students of grade 2005 learning web-based course

ID	D^+	D^-	C_i	Sort results	The final score
01	0.33	0.48	0.60	9	59.70
02	0.22	0.56	0.72	2	71.56
03	0.30	0.50	0.63	8	62.60
04	0.35	0.46	0.57	10	57.13
05	0.21	0.60	0.74	1	74.13
06	0.22	0.54	0.71	3	71.03
07	0.27	0.53	0.67	5	66.80
08	0.30	0.52	0.63	7	63.14
09	0.25	0.55	0.69	4	68.51
10	0.30	0.54	0.64	6	64.13

Note D^+ represents the distance between the evaluation of the object with the optimal solution; D^- refers to the distance between the evaluation object and the worst program; C_i refers to the evaluation of the object and the closeness of the optimal solution and the worst solution, $C_i \in [0,1]$, C_i is more close to 1, which means that the ith evaluation object is closer to the optimal level; Conversely, C_i is more close to 0, which means the ith evaluation object is closer to the most inferior level. The greater the C value, the more excellent evaluation results

305.3 Conclusion

The web-based teaching has many incomparable advantages compare to traditional teaching methods. It can make up for the deficiencies of the traditional teaching model. So they attract widespread attention of the institutions of higher learning. The Prosthodontics web-based course of School of Stomatology in the Fourth Military Medical University has played a good role in promoting undergraduate teaching.

Evaluation and feedback was an integral part of teaching. However, behind the web-based teaching growing prosperity, the corresponding evaluation system still had some shortcomings on the evaluation methods in China, which had led to the reduction of the utilization of network courses in some degree. In this study, through a comprehensive tracking the learning process, learner motivation, learning process and the results were evaluated to avoid focus only on the evaluation of learning outcomes, ignore the occurrence of learning methods and learning ability evaluation, and ensure effective evaluation and provide personalized guidance to promote the all-round development of the learners' ability. Teachers and education authorities can also reproduce the thought process of the learner through these evaluation information, get a comprehensive understanding of the learning process, find the problems of the learner in the learning process and its personalized guidance.

As the evaluation of the content and information was descriptive, so the fuzzy evaluation strategy and quantitative methods were adopted as the key to the design of network curriculum assessment. In this study, the analytic hierarchy process can change the complex qualitative issues into a hierarchy on the lower relations of domination, resolve the problem for quantitative questions through each level pairwise comparison and make the comprehensive evaluation problem easier, which was consistent with network curriculum evaluation. Therefore, the analytic hierarchy process to carry out the evaluation of network courses, increased the combined efforts of the qualitative evaluation and quantitative evaluation can be more objective, scientific results. TOPSIS method for evaluation not only avoided the complexity of heterogeneous data conversion, but also took into account the process and results of the learning activities to ensure that the evaluation results are objective and fair. Through the practical applications, the result was good, which might provide reference for the evaluation of other network courses.

References

1. Barrios M, Villarroya A, Borrego Á et al (2011) Response rates and data quality in web and mail surveys administered to Ph.D. holders. Soc Sci Comput Rev 29(2):208–220
2. Chang A, Gardner G, Duffield C et al (2010) A Delphi study to validate an advanced practice nursing tool. J Adv Nurs 66(10):2320–2330
3. Joinson AN, Reips U-D (2007) Personalized salutation, power of sender and response rates to web-based surveys. Comput Hum Behav 23(3):1372–1383
4. Rangone A (1996) An analytical hierarchy process framework for comparing the overall performance of manufacturing departments. Int J Oper Prod Manag 16(8):104
5. Hwang CL, Yoon K (1981) Multiple attribute decision making: methods and application. Springer-Verlag, Berlin
6. Kuo RJ, Wu YH, Hsu TS (2012) Integration of fuzzy set theory and TOPSIS into HFMEA to improve outpatient service for elderly patients in Taiwan. J Chin Med Assoc 75(7):341–348

Chapter 306
Application of Multimedia in the Teaching of Pharmacological Experiment Course

Wang Chunmei, Li He, Sun Jinghui, Sun Hongxia, Zhang Chengyi, Fan Xintian and Chen Jianguang

Abstract Pharmacology is a bridge course connecting the basic medicine to the clinical medicine and the pharmacology experiment course is an important part of it because pharmacology is an experimental science and all facts written in the pharmacology textbook have already verified by so many pharmacological experiments. Since the beginning of the new century, the computer-assisted teaching has been widely applied in class. With the development of multimedia technology, multimedia classroom teaching has been injected a fresh vitality, but its shortcomings are revealed with its wide use. In this study, the experience on the pharmacological experiment teaching during the past years is summarized to discuss the optimized application of multimedia in the pharmacological experiment teaching and the cognition on it.

Keywords Multimedia · Pharmacology · Experiment course

306.1 Introduction

With the development of modern science and technology, teaching methods have been transited from the traditional method to various modernized modes. The teaching with multimedia has been accepted by the majority of teachers and students due to its illustrated explanation and vivid presentation. The utilization of the multimedia technology can enrich the teaching method used in the pharmacological experiment teaching, greatly enhance the students' understanding of the teaching contents, leading to the synchronous improvement of the teaching effect in both the theoretical teaching and the experimental teaching [1–3].

W. Chunmei · L. He · S. Jinghui · S. Hongxia · Z. Chengyi · F. Xintian · C. Jianguang (✉)
Pharmaceutical College of Beihua University, Jilin 132013, China
e-mail: chenjg118@sohu.Com

306.2 The Superiority of the Multimedia Application in the Pharmacological Experiment Teaching

306.2.1 Convenience for Understanding and Remembering of the Knowledge

Multimedia is a modern teaching method, characterized by vividness and visualization. It can help students understand the knowledge well, and stimulate students' interest and improve students' emotion in learning. Combining with the specific experiment courses, drug actions, mechanisms of drug actions and adverse reactions learned by the students during the theoretical study were displayed in different ways in which video display was combined with the experimental performance. The results showed that the use of multimedia as a teaching tool could make a complex abstract theoretical problem simplified and specific, suggesting that through the advantage of multimedia in the information technology, it could display the development process of things and reveal the nature of them by changing a static state to a dynamic state, and an abstract concept to an intuitive thing.

306.2.2 Increase in the Amount of Information in Class

In general, the teachers often introduced the background knowledge to the students first, including the basic medical and clinical information, but the students had not learned the clinical course before they began to learn pharmacology. Therefore, the knowledge to be introduced in the classroom was so much that it could not be fully received by the students with the traditional teaching method. Our practice demonstrated that the teaching with multimedia in the experimental courses could meet this requirement, which might make the amount of information learned by the students extended, break the restriction with the traditional teaching method, thereby realizing the combination of the basic medical knowledge with the clinical medical knowledge.

306.2.3 Facilitation to Grasp the Experimental Operation Skills

Experimental animals are often used as the research objects in pharmacological experiments so that how to make the students quickly skilled in basic procedures related to the experimental animal is very important in the pharmacological experiment course. The teaching with multimedia played a key role in the improvement of the students' skills in our teaching practice. For example, in the administration experiment of commonly used in laboratory, the video was used to show the procedure to the students so that the students could understand the basic performance of the animal experiment, and then a specific operating point slide animation demo similar to the real operation was showed to them so that the students could have a certain degree of perceptual knowledge for each method before the experiment. In this way, the students could handle with the operating process with high proficiency.

306.2.4 Reduction of the Error Rate and Improvement of the Success rate in the Experiment

There are a variety of factors to affect the success of experiment. Before the experiment, under the guidance of teachers, the experimental purposes, experimental methods, experimental procedures and experimental precautions should be first cleared by the students. In our practice, for some more complex experimental procedures, the students were asked to watch the audio-visual film in which the whole process of the experiment was displayed, then the related flow charts or diagrams that were made by the teachers and could show the specific experimental procedures were repeatedly played, in which the key points worthy to be notice and easily leading to the experimental failure were emphasized, and finally the students were asked to perform the experiment themselves. As a result, students could perform correctly and have no overwhelmed feeling during the operating process.

306.2.5 Simplification of Data Processing and Statistics

During the observation on effects of drugs acting on the peripheral nervous system on the blood pressure and heart rate in dogs, to make the whole experimental process took a lot of time, the students often failed to grasp the main points, the experiment data processing was not convenient, and it was difficult to obtain accurate data due to some objective factors. However, it was easy for the students to understand the process, conduct the procedure, collect and analyze the data by using the multimedia teaching method, in which the animation or video could be used to explain the process and performance in a way of the static and dynamic combination, and the biological multimedia computer signal record systems were used the medical function experiment.

306.3 Measures to Improvement the Teaching Effect with Multi-media in the Course of Pharmacological Experiments

306.3.1 To Strive to Improve the Quality of Teachers

In addition to the essential pharmacological knowledge and skills, the teachers responsible for the experimental teaching should be required for striving to improve their own quality. They should pay attention not only to the lecture of the experiment itself, but also more the recognizing understanding of the inner world of students. Thus, the teachers should put themselves to share the joy of success, especially the anguish of failure in the experiment with the students to make their students enable to understand that the teachers' teaching is to contribute to the progress of their own and take the initiative to accept guidance from teachers with a positive attitude.

306.3.2 To Utilize the Update Multimedia Technology

The teaching method and content of experiment should keep up with the technological change. We have tried our best to introduce the latest technology into the classroom, which has promoted the improvement of the quality of the faculty, given the students a fresh sense of vision, broaden the students' knowledge and utilize the multimedia technology efficiently to promote its further development.

306.3.3 To Improve the Overall Quality of Students

In order to train the student's practical ability, the coordination and distribution of responsibilities were implemented the experimental teaching to make each student fuse himself into the experiment and develop a good teamwork spirit of coordination and distribution of responsibilities. The students are encouraged to take the initiative to think and ask a question with the purpose, which can stimulate the students' desire for knowledge, develop their observation ability to analyze problems, and fully enhance their overall quality in the experimental teaching. The use of multimedia tools should start from the teaching content and combine with the traditional teaching method. The multimedia technology used in the classroom should be taken as a teaching tool for the complement, supplement and perfection of the traditional teaching method, but it can not completely replace the writing on the blackboard and the other methods. We should pay attention to the multimedia tools organically combined with the traditional style of teaching to realize the purpose of the penetration of each other, learning from each other and improvement of teaching effectiveness. As a teacher in pharmacology should strive to make high-quality multimedia to meet the requirement of aesthetic, cognitive science, psychology and pedagogy law, and to be suitable for the teaching content, which may arouse students actively to learn and stimulate their creative thinking. It is believed that to master the rules of teaching, flexibly use teaching methods, and optimize the combination of multimedia teaching may be the only way to improve the efficiency and quality of teaching [4].

References

1. Yuming L, Miao Y, Lin L et al (2009) A positive reform of pharmacological experiment teaching in consistency with the personnel training objectives contemporary medicine. 15:162–163
2. Xiaoli Z (2012) Talking about pharmacology teaching. Mod Reading 10(222):120
3. Enping J, Yundong W, Chunmei W et al (2011) Characteristics and Advantages of Application of Multimedia Technology in Pharmacological Teaching. J Beihua Univ 12:495–496
4. Wen W, Yuexiu W, Houxi A et al (2012) Use of network resources to build medical pharmacology teaching platform. Chinese J ICT Educ 19:39–40

Chapter 307
THz Imaging Technology and its Medical Usage

Yao Yao, Guanghong Pei, Houzhao Sun, Rennan Yao, Xiaoqin Zeng,
Ling Chen, Genlin Zhu, Weian Fu, Bin Cong, Aijun Li, Fang Wang,
Xiangshan Meng, Qiang Wu, Lingbo Pei, Yiwu Geng, Jun Meng,
Juan Zhang, Yang Gao, Qun Wang, Min Yang, Xiaoli Chong,
Yongxia Duan, Bei Liu, Shujing Wang, Bo Chen and Yubin Wang

Abstract Compared with X ray, THz has a very strong complementary characteristic, its photon energy is extremely low, and has no ionization property as that of x ray, therefore, its testing effect is more accurate. The unmarked working method of genetic analysis in biochip technology has already been realized. As THz radiation is sensitive to water molecules, by testing water content through the THz test of the calf thymus, the healthy tissue and sick tissue can be distinguished. Therefore, THz imaging has a very vast medical applying prospect.

Keywords THz · THz Imaging · Laser Optics

Y. Yao · G. Pei · H. Sun · G. Zhu · W. Fu · B. Cong · A. Li · F. Wang · X. Meng · Q. Wu ·
L. Pei · Y. Geng · J. Meng · J. Zhang · Y. Gao · Q. Wang · M. Yang · B. Liu · S. Wang ·
B. Chen · Y. Wang
Engineer Academy of PLA, 376 Tongshan Road, XuZhou 221004, China

R. Yao (✉) · L. Chen
97th Hospital of PLA, 226 Tongshan Road, XuZhou 221004, China
e-mail: walkman_yao@sina.com

X. Zeng
School of Computer and Information Engineering, Hohai University,
NanJing 210098, China

X. Chong
8007# Building, Hongli West Road, Futian District, ShenZhen 518040, China

Y. Duan
Armored Force Institute of PLA, BengBu 233050, China

307.1 Brief Introduction of THz Wave

307.1.1 Discovery

Traditionally, electromagnetic waves are divided into radio wave, infrared ray, visible light, ultraviolet ray, α ray, γ ray, etc. With the development research done on the electromagnetic waves, people discovered an additional special position in the electromagnetic spectrum, as shown in Fig. 307.1 [1].

This is the THz wave, or THz ray, and before 1980s', scientists called it far infrared ray. Over the passed 100 years, the far infrared technology had become industrialized. However, the researching results and data referred to THz band were few, mainly limited by effective THz source and sensitive detector, hence this band was also called THz gap. With the development of a series of new technology and materials in 1980s', THz technology had developed rapidly.

307.1.2 The Characteristics of THz Wave

At present, a common understanding has been reached internationally on THz radiation is, THz is a new radiation resource with many special advantages, and a very important cross forward field. Following are the characteristics of THz wave:

1. The vibrating and rotating frequencies of many biological macromolecules, such as organic molecules are all in THz band, so they show very strong absorption and resonance in THz wave band.
2. THz radiation can run through objects such as ceramics, fat, carbon plate, etc. with very small attenuation, so it can be used to probe low density polarization gas, and is suitable for pollution control. It also runs through wall and cloth without being damaged, and this enables it to function in some special fields.
3. The signal-to-noise ratio of THz's time domain spectrum is very high, and this enables THz to be adaptable to imaging using.
4. Very short as THz pulse is, it has a wide band and some special characteristics that are different from others.

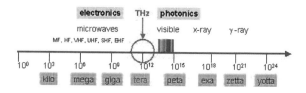

Fig. 307.1 The position of THz wave in the spectrum

307.2 THz Imaging Technology

The principle of THz imaging: THz wave with known wave form is used as light source to irradiate the surface of the sample, people analyze and deal with the amplitude information and other relevant information included by transmission or reflection spectrum that ran through the sample to get the image of the sample.

The absorption for THz ray of many non-metallic non-polar materials is very limited, so combined with relevant technology, to detect the materials' inner information is made possible. Polar material strongly absorbs the THz electromagnetic radiation, especially water. In THz spectrum technology, measures should be taken to avoid the influence of water, but this character can be used in THz imaging technology to distinguish different states of biologic tissue.

307.3 Biomedical Application of THz Imaging Technology

307.3.1 Dental Application

It's difficult to diagnose an early decayed tooth through radiography. But as a more sensitive imaging method, THz technology can. It not only accurately tests the position and degree of the its damage, but also differentiates the dentin and the enamel, and gets the stereo image of a tooth [2]. See Fig. 307.2 (left: a human being's tooth; right: transmission image absorbed by THz radiation, the red is the inner hollow of the tooth). Foreign scientists Crawley et al. did extracorporeal research by using THz ray, and discovered that the different contraction value between a decayed tooth and a normal tooth for absorbing THz wave is 1:2, which is more accurate than the result of X ray. And it avoids additional damage to human body got by taking X ray. Therefore, THz fills the important gap between X ray and the doctors' eyes (visible light) and is hopeful to become a substitute for dental X ray.

307.3.2 Cancer Research and Application

THz wave is hopeful to become an important tool to evaluate the boundary and infiltration depth of skin cancer. Scientists Woodward et al. carried out detailed research on basal cell carcinoma patients with TPI technology. Results show that

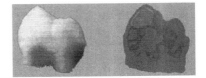

Fig. 307.2 THz pulse image of a decayed tooth

Fig. 307.3 THz pulse image for cancer cell

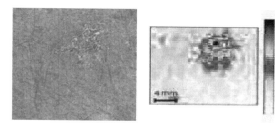

through THz wave imaging, the cancerous tissue, inflammation tissue, and healthy tissue can be distinguished. So far, in medical area, THz ray still stays in tissue near the skin [3]. But adult cancers include skin cancer, breast cancer, esophageal cancer, colon cancer, bladder cancer and prostate cancer, etc. all appear in skin tissue, so researchers believe that THz wave can examine these cancers.

The figure on the right (Fig. 307.3) shows basal cell carcinoma. Clinical photo TPI shows that when the depth of the cancer is 100, the red color is conspicuous, and that is the result of matching with the absorption of high energy THz.

THz wave technology is also hopeful to replace x ray to be applied in transmission examine and CT examine. THz's low power produces only a little damage to human body, so it effectively protects the patients' health and safety.

For cancer patients, the radiation therapy by using ion beam to cure cancer is called particle treatment, or more accurately, hadron therapy. Its working principle is to irradiate the cancer cells by high-energy hadron beam, such as proton or ion, to kill the cancer cells [4]. The main advantage of ion beam is its different absorbing characteristics. The iron beam can only be absorbed by the deep part inside the tissue of human body, so the tissues of other parts will not be affected. While γ ray has more effects on superficial cells because of the index attenuation law, which often does harm to the healthy tissue on the outer space of the tumour.

307.3.3 Directly Test Genetic Materials with THz Radiation

Experiments show that the more differences the DNA sequence have, the smaller the THz transmission and frequency of resonance will be. Therefore, THz spectrum can distinguish the free chain from the hybridization chain of DNA.

Biochip technology is another original part of present-day research. To directly test the combining state of genetic materials (such as DNA and RNA) by THz radiation, the unmarked working mode of genetic analysis is realized [5]. Besides, as THz radiation is very sensitive to water molecules, and is possible to distinguish bound water molecules from free water molecules, through testing water content we can distinguish healthy tissue from sick tissue. Figure 307.4 shows the THz absorption spectrum of calf thymus' DNA under different environmental humidity, and that of normal beef serum albumin (BSA) sample under different relative humidity, as well as the contrast with degenerated BSA (r.h. <5 %) [6].

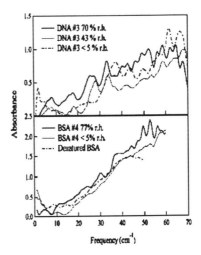

Fig. 307.4 Contrasting pictures between the THz absorption spectrum of calf thymus' DNA (*above*) and absorption spectrum of normal BSA sample in different relative humidity under different environmental humidity and degenerated BSA (r. h. <5) (*below*)

In 2012, Arun Arora et al. adopted the THz time-domain spectroscopy technology for the first time to do unmarked quantitative detection for amplified DNA under PCR polymerase chain reaction. Research showed that the absorption coefficient of the two DNA samples were in inverse proportion of their density. So THz technology has the prospect to become the new method of unmarked detection.

307.4 Conclusion

THz scientific technology has not developed for 30 years until now, hence some key technological problems such as THz radiation source and THz testing technology are still not mature. However, the applications of THz radiation have already carried out vigorously, as mentioned above, in dental and cancer applications. Directly testing genetic materials has also achieved a lot of achievements in biomedicine. With the rapid development of THz scientific technology and application, we can foresee that THz technology will bring further influence to human being like other bands of electromagnetic spectrum.

References

1. Zhang M, Ruan SS, Liu J et al (2007) Designing the Controlling Software of THz Imaging System. Micro Comput Inform 23(11):25–27 (in Chinese)
2. Zhang CH, Wang YY, B G et al (2007) THz Imaging Based on Far Infrared Laser Source. Superconduction Technol 35(3):245–247 (in Chinese)

3. Liu SG, Zhong RB (2009) The New Development of THz Scientific Technology and its Application. J China Electron Sci Res Acad 3:221–230 (in Chinese)
4. Xu JZ (2007) THz scientific technology and application. Beijing University Press, Beijing (in Chinese)
5. Fischer BM, Walther M et al (2002) Far-infrared vibrational modes of DNA components studied by terahertz time-domain pectroscopy. Phys Mel Biol 47:3807–3814
6. Samnel P, Mickan Addellah, Menikh et al (2002) Label-free bioaffinity detection using terahertz technology. Phys Med Biol 147:3789–3795

Chapter 308
Effects of Project-Based Learning in Improving Scientific Research and Practice Capacity of Nursing Undergraduates

Ruiling Li, Dongmei Dou and Yuanyuan Wang

Abstract *Objectives* To investigate the effect of project-based learning on scientific research and practice capacity. *Materials and methods* A total of 35 students from 244 sophomores were included in this study. Tests were done in three different stages: before training, after training and after implementation by a teacher who was blind to the project. The test included 4 items: skills of design questionnaires, methods of health education, abilities of communication and skills of data analysis. The total scores of each item were 25 points. In three different stages (before training, after training and after implementation), the mean scores were calculated for each item and analyzed using ANOVA. *Results* The mean scores of each item were significantly higher in the students after training compared to the scores before training ($p < 0.01$). After implementation the mean scores were also higher than those in students after training ($p < 0.01$). In comparison with the mean scores of each item before training, those were significantly higher in the students after implementation ($p < 0.01$). *Conclusion* Project-based learning can improve nursing students' scientific research and practice capacity.

Keywords Nursing · Students · Nursing research capacity

308.1 Introduction

Research capacity is an important way to measure advanced nursing professionals [1]. Undergraduate education's aim is not only to tell students ready-made knowledge, but more important is to guide students' exploration of unknown territory, to create more opportunities for research, to improve the awareness and

R. Li (✉) · D. Dou · Y. Wang
Nursing College, Henan University, Kaifeng, Henan Province, China
e-mail: lrl@henu.edu.cn

ability of students' research [2]. To early explore the practice of research projects and to plan systematically research training for nursing undergraduates, the project was carried out in 2007–2008 relying on the implementation of the Global Fund for AIDS projects.

308.2 Materials and Methods

308.2.1 Study Population

The Ethics Committee at Henan University, China approved this study. All subjects signed informed consent. Approved advertisement about the study's purpose, main contents and intended objectives in the nursing school, message boards, classes were used to recruit study students. A total of 35 sophomores voluntarily attended this project, these students had completed Nursing Research and Preventive Medicine—the two nursing courses—which were directly related to nursing research capacity.

308.2.2 Procedures

The project was performed between June 2007 and Oct 2008. From June 2007 to 10 days after summer holidays, about 1 month, in these days special skills training were undertaken by 5 teachers who undertook sixth China Global Fund AIDS Program to students, special skills training included skills of design questionnaires, methods of health education, abilities of communication and skills of data analysis. After training, students participated in "publicity messenger- youth out of school" AIDS intervention project, using weekends and holidays to design questionnaire about AIDS-related KAP (knowledge, attitude and practice towards) of youth out of school, information dissemination satisfaction questionnaire. Released pre-survey questionnaires and repeated revised the questionnaire; did health education plan and 3 on -site health education and investigated. After the implementation, students reorganized and analyzed the data based on the project information. In the whole process, teachers observed and guided.

Before training, after training and after implementation we did three independent tests to evaluate the students' scientific research and practice capacity. The test included four items, each item scores were 25 points. (1) skills of design questionnaires, questionnaire questions achieved the plan calls for 10 points, problem design reasonable 5 points, alternative answers comprehensive 5 points, the skills in title sequence, difficulty, privacy circumvent call for 5 points. (2) Health education and intervention implementation skills: Health education and intervention diagnosis call for 10 points, content design 10 points, education and the form of intervention 5 points. (3) Abilities of communication: Explain the purpose of the survey call for 10 points, the dialect or investigation object language adaptation 10 points, collect data completely 5 points. (4) Skills of data analysis: establish a database 10 points, handle data correctly 10 points, explain the data results reasonably 5 points.

308.2.3 Data Analysis

Testing scores were entered into a statistical software program for analysis by an operator blind to this study. The statistical analysis was performed with a statistical software package (IBM SPSS statistics standard 11.5 software package for PC, IBM Corp, NY, USA). The scores of each item were calculated for the different three stages ($\bar{X} \pm S$). The comparison between three different stages was analyzed by use of ANOVA. A $p < 0.01$ was considered to be statistically significant.

308.3 Result

Three independent tests had been carried out on three different stages—before training, after training and after implementation, neither of the three was same as each other. Before training each item scores were the lowest. After training the mean scores were higher than those of before training. After implementation the mean scores were the highest. The differences were statistically significant ($p < 0.01$), as shown in Table 308.1.

Table 308.1 Comparison of the scores of undergraduate students' research and practical abilities at different stages (points, $\bar{X} \pm S$)

Stages	n	Questionnaire skills	Health education	Communication skills	Data dialysis capacity
Before training	35	12.18 ± 2.63^{①}	13.88 ± 6.40^{①}	13.00 ± 0.87^{①}	12.71 ± 6.50^{①}
After training	35	13.94 ± 2.82^{②}	14.00 ± 8.53^{②}	21.28 ± 2.89^{②}	20.60 ± 6.45^{②}
After implementation	35	20.34 ± 3.25^{③}	20.56 ± 5.33^{③}	23.21 ± 3.12^{③}	23.33 ± 8.76^{③}
F		10.663	25.839	20.181	40.102
P		0.000	0.000	0.000	0.000

① Scores compared with the implementation, $P < 0.01$
② Scores compared with before training, $P < 0.01$
③ Scores compared with after training, $P < 0.01$

308.4 Discussion

308.4.1 Advantages of Project-Based Learning in Improving Scientific Research and Practice Capacity of Nursing Undergraduates

308.4.1.1 Project-Based Learning Stimulate Students' Interest in Scientific Research

In daily teaching, teachers often focused on research and survey instances, so when teachers public the project to students, students felt that they had the opportunity to personally participate in the project, so 35 nursing students attended this study voluntarily. Teachers used weekends to do theoretical training for the students who were voluntarily attended. As a result their research capacity had improved after participating in the implementation of the project. As shown in Table 308.1, after implementation, the scores of research and practical ability were higher than those of before, the difference was statistically significant ($p < 0.01$). It also played a further positive effect on other students. Many undergraduates who were interested in scientific research but not participated in this project paid more attention to the practice of nursing research. Interest is the best teacher. The research interest caused by the implementation of the project is conductive to the nursing undergraduate and it is good to further research and practice to carry out. So that it can truly promote the changes from simple classroom teaching to practice teaching and can improve undergraduates' research capacity.

308.4.1.2 In Process of this Project the Students Found their Deficiencies and Improved Capacity Gradually

To cultivate scientific research ability of undergraduate nursing students, we should not only expand corresponding curriculums, but also pay more attention to teaching and practice of relevant courses and practical teaching play an important role in the training of students abilities [3]. The students who attended in the project had already learned Nursing Research and related courses, but in the course of project implementation, many students found their own design questionnaires lacked of some important questions. Their health education and intervention could not operated very well. They still needed to improve communication skills and so on. With the increase of the implementation of on-site project, the students improved their own research's feasibility and improved their on-site implementation skills gradually. Simply theory teaching cannot achieve this objective.

308.4.1.3 Teachers can Clearly Affirm Research and Teaching Target when Guide Students in the Project

Through leading students involved in on-site implementation and record notes, observing students enthusiasm, skills of communication and on-site implementation, teachers could found lacks of daily teaching and theoretical training. Teachers benefit from these as well as students. Teachers accumulate experiences and these are good for teaching and guiding students in future research and teaching. The teachers can be more pertinency and practical; this can provide the basis for teachers to make a good decision.

308.4.2 The Problems Should be Noted

We achieved the desired results through practicing of project-based learning in improving scientific research and practice capacity of nursing undergraduates. At the same time, there are some issues that need our attention: ① Before every on-site implementation, teachers should organize students to fully understand the aim of the project, familiar with contents, pay attention to issues that need attention, reduce unnecessary errors and improve the implementation efficiency. ② After implementation, sum up experiences positively, check the data, discover faults, gain new knowledge by reviewing old, in order to improve the students ability effectively.

308.4.3 Inspiration

During teaching, teachers should do well in guiding and leading, pay full attention to students' automony and initiative, create a good learning environment, provide a rich learning resources [4]. Create the conditions for undergraduates and encourage them to connect the practice with scientific research. He training of the students' research quality extend from classroom to extra-curricular. Teachers should through various forms to encourage students to participate in research projects. He teacher research direction was combined with the students' interest, only in this way, it can achieve better teaching results.

308.5 Conclusion

In conclusion, project-based learning is effective in improving scientific research and practice capacity of nursing undergraduates.

Acknowledgments The authors would like to acknowledge the financial support from Global Fund for AIDS projects and the Educational Reform Fund at Henan University, Henan Province, China.

References

1. Cao BH, Chu J, Zhang YL et al (2009) Comparison between different levels of education in "Nursing Research". Nurs J Chin People's Lib Army 26:68–69
2. Liu C (2008) Characteristics and Implications of the American research university undergraduate research training activities. J Changsha Railw Univ (Soc Sci) 9:279–280
3. You LM, Zhang MF, Luo ZM et al (2009) A model for baccalaureate nursing education: emphasizing the formation of high quality and practice competence. Chine J Nurs Educ 6:65–67
4. Yao WJ, Chen JX, Zheng GH et al (2009) Application of self-inquiry educational model in the teaching of nursing research course. Chin J Nurs Educ 6:396–397

Chapter 309
Research on an Individualized Pathology Instructional System

Kai Hu and Zhiqian Ye

Abstract Due to the Internet, computers have been widely used in the educational field. In this paper, the current development of the pathology instructional system and the shortages of the system are presented. In order to improve the system, the concept of an individualized pathology instructional system is put forward. Next, the structure of the whole system is designed. Finally, the method to realize the individualized learning function is analysed and the development environment is recommended.

Keywords Pathology · Learning · Individualized · Instructional system

309.1 Introduction

With the development of technology, pathology teaching is in constant evolution. Here has been a qualitative leap from the microscopic teaching method to digital teaching method. The department of computer science at the University of Maryland, and department of pathology at the Johns Hopkins put forward the concept of "virtual microscope" for the first time in 1997.

In China, Zhejiang University introduced the Virtual Slice Scanning System during 2008 and built a digital slice library earlier than the other medical schools nationwide [1]. Currently, most medical schools through cooperation and various manufacturers have set up instructing system for pathology and related subjects.

K. Hu · Z. Ye (✉)
Colledge of Biomedical Engineering and Instrument Science, Zhejiang University, No. 38 of Zhejiang University Road, Zhejiang Province 310027 Hangzhou City, China
e-mail: yezq@greenlander.com.cn

K. Hu
e-mail: hukai666@126.com

For example, Guangxi Medical University have built the Web Instructing System based on digital slices [2]. South China Agricultural University has set up the "Microscopic Digital Slice Instructing System", based on the MOTIC Slice Scanning System [3].

In this paper, we focus on designing an individualized pathology instructional system to overcome the inherent deficiencies found in normal pathology instructional system. The second part of this paper will introduce the advantages of the individualized system. In the third part, the system structure will be shown. And the forth part will present the design.

309.2 The Improvements of the Individualized Pathology Instructional System

By research, it is found most existing instructional systems have the following features:

1. Concise style, convenient for user to log in and use.
2. Browser/Server structure. The browser is used as the client-side, and no software needs to be installed.
3. The slices are the only main material. They are classified by different human tissues.
4. Different students use the same materials. There is no way to extend further learning.
5. No individualized learning materials for students in accordance with their learning level.

Figure 309.1 briefly shows the procedural flow of the existing systems.

However, different students won't be satisfied with the same learning materials. In order to overcome the shortage of existing systems above, designing a new system, namely an Individualized Pathology Instructional System, is needed. This pathology instructional system can provide more materials for extended learning according to each student's learning events. Thus, the key function of this system is to realize individualized way of learning. Compared with the normal system, individualized system has these advantages below:

1. Student-centered. Teach students in accordance of their learning stage.
2. Help broadening the scope of knowledge.
3. Save time of searching learning materials.

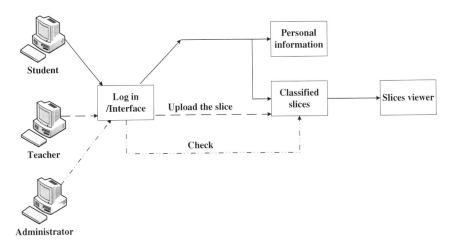

Fig. 309.1 Procedural flow of the existing system

309.3 Structure of the Individualized Pathology Instructional System

To make the system easily operated, the B/S architecture is adopted. The system is designed as a three-layer structure—browser layer, business logic layer and database layer. Thus it is more convenient for update and maintenance.

Furthermore, the users are divided into three groups—student, teacher and administrator. Each group has different requirements. The modules of the different users are listed in Fig. 309.2.

Figure 309.2 shows there are four basic modules— "Personal information", "Videos and digital slices", "Question & answer board", "Individualized learning". The module "individualized learning" is the key to realize the individualized learning function.

309.4 Design of the Individualized Function

Unlike other modules, the content of the "Individualized learning" can be updated by the change of student's learning level. The individual learning materials contains two parts designed below, recommendation of extended websites and slices. This key module needs to cost more operating time than others, so it is run on the backend server.

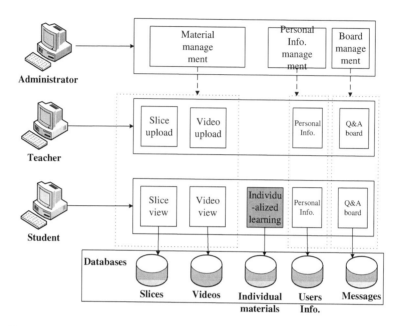

Fig. 309.2 Structure of the individualized instructional system

309.4.1 Recording Students' Learning Events

Recording of learning events is necessary to analyse a student's key words about learning events. When a student opens a slice or started a topic on the "Question & answer board", his action will be recorded in the "Learning Events" database with a unified format. Figure 309.3 gives the relationship and format of the data.

309.4.2 Mining Learning Events Data

During every set time interval, the data mining program will be run on the backend server. First, the backend server queries the "Learning events" database for the records. Then the backend server will do Chinese word segmentations on the text contents of the useful parts, "content" and "remark". After that, the important notional words will be picked out. The system computes the User Interest Degree of each word. Below, a simple formula is put forward to define the User Interest Degree. It is assumed that the time interval influences the Interest Degree linearly over the past 10 days.

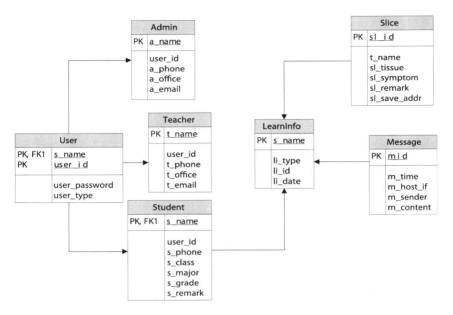

Fig. 309.3 Relationship of the data

$$UID = F \cdot \left(1 - \frac{\sum_{i=1}^{n} X_i}{10n}\right) \quad (309.1)$$

UID is User Interestingness. *X* equals the difference value between the present date and the recorded date. *F* is defined as the frequency of a word among all the words. The number of occurrence times of a word is represented by *n*. The expression in the brackets means the average time interval influence of a word and it can never be greater than one.

After the calculation, the results are placed in descending order.

309.4.3 Searching for the Recommended Learning Materials

The backend server chooses the top 5 words as the key words in that order. Then the search engine will search the related words on the Internet or in the digital slices library which is linked to this system. Here, an open source search engine is used. Hibernate Search, Compass, Nutch and Lucene are the common open source search engine based on the Java environment.

The hyperlinks of search results which include websites and slices will be stored in an "Individualized materials database". This database will be refreshed during a period chosen by the student user.

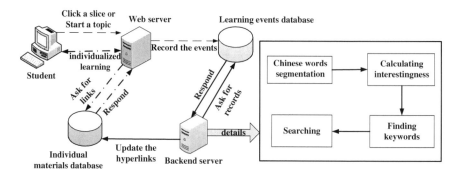

Fig. 309.4 Flow of the individualized learning function

When a student logs into the system and clicks the "Individual learning" button, the browser sends a command to the Web server. The Web server asks the "Individualized materials database" for hyperlinks and responds back to the browser. Figure 309.4 shows the flow of the whole path of the individualized learning function.

309.5 The System Development Environment

This system is based on following the environment:

1. Operating system: Windows XP.
2. Web server: Tomcat 7.0.
3. Database software: SQL server 2005.
4. Language: JSP, Servlet and JavaBean

The ICTCLAS is used as the Chinese words segmentation System. ICTCLAS has achieved a great effect for Chinese words segmentation in the 973 national specialists' assessment and the 2003 1st international competition of words segmentation. It is one of the best Chinese words segmentation systems [4].

309.6 Conclusions

This paper presented the development of an individualized pathology instructional system and analysed the shortages of present instructional systems. The concept of improved system based on individualized learning was proposed.

This new system is helpful to enhance pathology teaching and improve the students' clinical diagnosis ability.

However, the system still needs improvement. For examples, it is still required to set up the instructional system's connection to a regional pathology information network. Also, an intelligent analysis of ROI (region-of-interest) has not been yet implemented.

References

1. Dongmei LI, Genyou YAO, Lingling WANG, Xiaoli WEI, Jicheng LI (2010) Building the Medical Digital Slices Library on Web. J Anatomy 33(2):268–269
2. [2013-3-1]. http://www.myhistology.com/
3. [2013-3-1]. http://www.xwlab.com/dssweb/
4. Qun LIU, HuaPing ZHANG, HongKui YU, XueQi CHENG (2004) Chinese Lexical Analysis Using Cascaded Hidden Markov Mode. J Comput Res Devel 41(8):1421–1429
5. Yu TAO, Haoyuan LI, Yiming TAO (2004) The Teaching of Telepathology and Application of Technology. Chin Med Edu Tech 18(6):349–351

Chapter 310
Security Problems and Strategies of Digital Education Resource Management in Cloud Computing Environment

Li Bo

Abstract Cloud computing technology has an important influence on the development of digital education resource management, but also brings a lot of security problems to the digital education resource storage and sharing. This paper analyses the security problems of digital education resource storage and sharing in cloud computing environment, finally aimed at these problems, give the concrete security strategies.

Keywords Cloud computing · Digital education resources management · Security problems · Security strategies

310.1 Changes of Digital Education Resource Management Brought by Cloud Computing

Cloud computing could provide powerful compute capacity and storage capacity, simple interface, good scalability, good cross-platform service [1]. Using cloud computing as the underlying architecture to store the digital education resources, cloud computing is responsible for storage, management, allocation, load balancing, deployment, migration, cross-platform integration and security control of the education resources, while users don't need to care about where and how the resources are stored. That's the optimal solution with low price, high reliability and expansibility at present. But the storage and sharing of digital education resources also have many problems; we must carefully study and solve the possible challenges.

L. Bo (✉)
Shandong Polytechnic, No.23000 East Jingshi Road, Jinan, Shandong, China
e-mail: 24874890@qq.com

310.2 Security Problems of Digital Education Resource Management Based on Cloud Computing

As the digital education resources are all stored in the cloud, not in the managers' local servers, security, confidentiality, integrity and availability of the resources become uncertain [2].

310.2.1 Security and Confidentiality Problems of the Digital Education Resources

Storage security of digital education resources is the core problem should be considered in cloud computing environment. Compared with the traditional resource management model, open interfaces provided by cloud computing make illegal access to be possible [3].

First of all, the storage of cloud computing doesn't have clear boundary, it is very difficult to isolate from each other while customers' data sharing the same storage space.

Secondly, when the data disaster occurred, all data and applications will appear problems, so capacity and efficiency of cloud computing service providers to restore lost data determines the service reliability.

Third, cloud computing only provides data encryption service when transmitting; protection issues on data processing and storing remain unresolved, so the key or privacy information may be lost, stolen or destroyed.

Fourth, illegal users may access the digital education resources using super user identity which will avoid security protection systems. That will imperil the integrity and security of the education resources.

At last, how to avoid the cloud computing service providers unauthorized accessing to the resources, protect the intellectual property rights of the digital education resources, are also an important issues.

310.2.2 Reliability and Sustainability Problems of Cloud Computing Services

Cloud computing platform is integrated by various software modules and Web Services. Users rely more on the service reliability of the cloud computing platform, so software security events have more significant impacts. Therefore, the reliable and sustainable cloud computing software and services must have stronger ability to resist risks, prevent the cloud computing services, highly centralized digital education resources and software vulnerabilities from being exploited by hackers. In addition, robustness and ability of fast recovery are also important.

310.2.3 Problems of User Privilege Management and Access Control

Digital education resource management platform in cloud computing environment is a huge, complex, multi-user platform. Cloud computing service providers only support for safety, high efficiency and stability of the cloud computing platform, they don't pay attention to the resource management. Therefore, cloud computing platform should provide reasonable authority division and management for ordinary users, resource managers and cloud computing service providers, in order to ensure the data security and prevent the user information from being stolen or destroyed. At the same time, efficiently access control strategies are needed in cloud computing environment to ensure the effectiveness of security audit, ensure the monitoring of data operating, and protect the key or privacy information.

310.3 Security Strategies of Digital Education Resource Management Based on Cloud Computing

Considering the characteristics of the digital education resource management and the security threats in cloud computing environment, unique and comprehensive security policies and security technologies should be established in addition to traditional IT protection technology, to improve the security of education resources.

310.3.1 Secure Storage and Management Strategies of Digital Education Resources

First of all, virtual storage technology should be used. Data availability and access performance could be improved while multiple copies are created on each of the virtual disks.

Secondly, resource managers should timely backup the digital education resources and save the backup files reliably for a long time.

Third, core confidential data or important information should be encrypted and maintained in private cloud to prevent malicious users from illegal obtaining.

Fourth, when the cloud computing service provider is changed, storage spaces should be erased completely to avoid illegal recovery, which will make the files, directories or database records been revealed [2].

Fifth, a third party could be employed to review applications and strengthen the security of applications.

310.3.2 Confidentiality and Integrity Strategies of Digital Education Resources

Public Key Infrastructure (PKI) is the core of the security infrastructure in cloud computing environment which provides users encryption, certification and digital signature services [4]. Using PKI technology, encryption and digital signature technology could be widely used in the process of digital education resource storage and transmission, to ensure that the resources stored in the cloud cannot be maliciously downloaded, falsified or denied while storing and transmitting, so as to enhance the confidentiality and integrity of the resources.

310.3.3 Authorization Management Strategies of Digital Education Resources

In cloud computing environment, resources users are divided into several levels according to different needs and accessing to resources are strictly controlled by the platform. At present, the more mature authority management and control technology is the Privilege Management Infrastructure (PMI) [5]. PMI could provide authorization and authentication services to all users and create a secure communication between users and resource management platform. Ordinary users of the platform could only query, read, download data according to assigned roles; while resource managers can complete the specific data maintenance work according to assigned roles.

310.3.4 Access Control Strategies of Digital Education Resources

User authentication in cloud computing environment is vital important to data security, only certified users can access to the corresponding digital education resources. Cloud computing has heterogeneous, dynamic, cross-organizational characteristics [6], so in order to improve the management efficiency of resource users, single sign-on, unified authentication and interface could be used. Authorized users could visit all authorized resources while only need to login once. Through single sign-on authentication combined with the PMI access control technology, education resource management platform could set different access authority according to different user needs and user levels.

310.4 Conclusion

The emergence of cloud computing provides an opportunity for the application and development of digital education resources under the network environment but it still exist many problems. Security problems are the biggest obstacle mainly relate to both data security and cloud computing platform security and reliability. But on the whole, cloud computing will play a greater role in digital education resource management in the near future.

Acknowledgments This paper was supported by the Project of Shandong Province Higher Educational Science and Technology Program under Grant No. J13LN64. It was also supported by the Project of Shandong Province Higher Educational Science and Technology Program under Grant No. J12LN61. In addition, the author would like to thank the reviewers for their valuable comments and suggestions.

References

1. Changquan W, Fen A, Jianwen Y (2010) Research on information security strategy of digital library under the cloud computing environment. J intell 29(3):183–186 (in Chinese with English abstract)
2. Yandong Z, Yongsheng Z (2012) Cloud computing and cloud security challenges. In: Proceedings of 2012 international symposiumon on ITME, no I, pp 1084–1088
3. Lori MK (2009) Data security in the world of cloud computing, IEEE secur priv, vol 7, no 4
4. Darren P, Oleksandr O (2005) Privilege management infrastructure, Encyclopedia of multimedia technology and networking, Vol 1. DOI: 10.4018/978-1-59140-561-0.ch120
5. Tan W, Xie Y, Li D, Liu M (2011) A modified securities model based on public key infrastructure. Comm Comput Info Sci 226:252–259
6. Hong C, Zhang M, Feng DG (2011) AB-ACCS: A cryptographic access control scheme for cloud storage. J Comput Res Develop 47(I):259–265 (in Chinese with English abstract)

Chapter 311
Vocabulary Learning Strategies in Computer-Assisted Language Learning Environment

Liming Sun and Ni Wang

Abstract This paper attempts to explore the overall pattern of Vocabulary Learning Strategies adopted by English majors in the computer-assisted language learning (CALL) environment. It also tends to find out what strategies are correlated with students' performance in English proficiency test. In addition, a comparison study on beliefs and VLS in CALL environment adopted by High-achievers and Low-achievers is conducted via Independent-Sample *T* Test.

Keywords Vocabulary learning strategy · CALL environment · English majors · Adoption

311.1 Introduction

Research related to language learning strategies has prospered since the 1980s. Gradually, the importance of vocabulary acquisition in language learning has been proved and emphasized world widely. With the widespread of the use of computers among students, researchers are attracted to study the effects of computer-assisted language learning (CALL) on students' language development, such as learning beliefs, management strategies and language learning strategies in CALL environment. However, although the importance of vocabulary acquisition has

---

L. Sun (✉) · N. Wang
College of Foreign Language, Shijiazhuang University of Economics, Huaian Road 136, Shijiazhuang 050031, China
e-mail: sunlm1976@yahoo.com.cn

N. Wang
e-mail: wangni2005@yahoo.com.cn

been realized by most language learners and researchers, little work has been carried out on vocabulary learning strategies (VLS) especially on current occasion that CALL is widely applied, and little research has been conducted in finding out the change and the corresponding consequence. Therefore, the development of CALL has created the need and opportunity for investigating the effects of the computer and Internet on vocabulary acquisition.

This paper attempts to explore the overall pattern of VLS adopted by English majors in the CALL environment. It also tends to find out what strategies are correlated with students' performance in English proficiency test. In addition, a comparison study on beliefs and VLS in CALL environment adopted by High-achievers and Low-achievers (In order to deal with this question, participants are grouped into high achievers and low achievers, which will be explicitly explained in Chap. 4 is conducted via Independent-Sample T Test. The questionnaire adopted in the present study, refers to those of Stoffer (1995), Schmitt (1997), Nation (2001), Gu and Johnson (1996) respectively and Vocabulary Level Test is adopted from that of Nation (1990) in the college level, which are delivered to 114 English majors from Shijiazhuang University of Economics. The reason why these English majors are chosen is that CALL environment is generally available for them, they are greatly motivated to employ different kinds of VLS to help their vocabulary learning and, they are future English teachers so that their learning characteristics are implicational and of guiding significance. In order to find answers to these proposed research questions, both quantitative and qualitative research methods are adopted in this thesis to get the following findings.

311.2 Research Methodology

311.2.1 Research Questions

In an attempt to explore the overall pattern of VLS adopted by Chinese English majors in CALL environment and to find out what effects VLS in CALL environment might have on their vocabulary learning, a questionnaire is conducted among the third-year english majors in shijiazhuang university of Economics.

To achieve these ends, the current study will endeavor to answer the following research questions:

1. What are the English majors' beliefs towards computer-assisted vocabulary learning? What types of strategies are preferred by subjects in CALL?
2. Is there any correlation between VLS in CALL and their vocabulary achievements? If there are, what are they?
3. What are the major problems in utilizing computers in autonomous vocabulary learning?

311.2.2 Subjects

The study was conducted in the autumn semester in 2012. It involves about 114 junior English majors in Shijiazhuang University of Economics. They are all Chinese learners of English and have learned English in middle school for six years and more than two years in Shijiazhuang University of Economics. Their age ranges from 20 to 23 with the mean age being 21.5. Since all of them are in the English department, we do not take sex as a variable. As for the CALL environment, based on the data from the pilot survey, it is suggested that most of juniors have a personal computer and these students without a personal computer are provided enough opportunities to use computers because there is a autonomous language learning center in English department and there are many net-bars in the university. In addition, after more than two years of specific English learning, most juniors have sort out their own effective ways to acquire English vocabulary. Thus, they are most suitable for the investigation of the VLS adopted in CALL environment.

311.3 Findings

This paper reported an exploratory study on the beliefs and strategies of third-year English majors in Shijiazhuang University of Economics for EFL vocabulary learning in CALL environment, including the vocabulary learning beliefs and strategies adopted by some Chinese English majors, the relationship between their use of VLS and their vocabulary learning achievement, and the similarities and differences between the high-achievers and low-achievers of the test. Through the quantitative and qualitative analysis of the questionnaire and interviews, the following findings were obtained.

First, the present study has pronied the overall pattern of strategy used by Chinese English majors. Generally speaking, the students involved in this study hold the belief that the computer and the Internet are contributory to vocabulary learning, and do not think that words should be memorized mechanically. At the meantime, the majority of them hold positive beliefs towards the computer assisted vocabulary learning in the learning activities, especially reading and listening. In their vocabulary learning processes in CALL environment, the great majority of learners were reported to employ a variety of learning strategies. As for strategies for building up their vocabulary, they would like to use word processor, use the Internet to collect different categories of vocabulary; as for strategies used in reading activities, they prefer to read E-materials so as to increase the opportunity to encounter new vocabulary, use guessing and online dictionary during the reading; as for strategies used in listening activities, they would like to do listening practice with computer to learn some new words, download listening materials to review some vocabulary, listen extensively to encounter lots of new words, learning vocabulary when watching online movies and listen to online English news to familiarize hot vocabulary. However, learners respond negatively to the belief that words should be memorized, the computer assisted metacognitive strategy, and vocabulary learning in speaking and writing activities in CALL environment.

Second, there exists a certain correlation between vocabulary learning beliefs and strategies and their vocabulary learning achievements. The belief that "words should be learned through use" is positively correlated with vocabulary learning achievement. And the general belief that "the computer and the Internet are contributory to vocabulary learning" is also positively and very significantly correlated with vocabulary learning achievement. The computer assisted metacognitive strategy is not related to vocabulary learning achievement at significant level. Although learners take negative attitudes towards vocabulary learning in speaking and writing activities in CALL environment, the related strategies are correlated with vocabulary learning achievement very significantly. High achievers and low achievers are found to be significantly differentiated from each other in their adoption of VLS in CALL environment. High achievers tend to hold a stronger belief that "the computer and the Internet are contributory to vocabulary learning" and they are more inclined to use a variety of strategies, especially those strategies in reading activities, such as reading E-materials so as to have more chance to encounter new vocabulary, using guessing and online dictionary strategy when reading E-materials, getting familiar with hot words by reading English news, reading E-materials so as to have more chance to encounter new vocabulary. Apart from some strategies both groups prefer to adopt, high achievers would like to use computer to collect different categories of vocabulary, read English news on the Internet so as to familiarize hot vocabulary, record the new words making full use of the copy function of word processor, use computer to imitate the pronunciation, do online listening practice in order to familiarize the vocabulary they have learned and listen online English news to familiarize hot vocabulary, while lower achievers would like to listen intensively to encounter a lot of new words.

Third, although they are skillful in the operation of the computer in CALL environment, they lack confidence in computer assisted language learning. They are worried by some technological and unexpected problems of computers in the process of study or surfing on the Internet. 玩case these problems affect their normal learning, they would like to give up these ways. Comparatively speaking, they have little motivation to chat in chat rooms or communicate with others via QQ and MSN in English, and they are worried by some technological and unexpected problems of computers in the process of study or surfing on the Internet. Still, it is not very easy for most of them to learn new software for study.

311.4 Pedagogical Implications

In addition to the conclusions we have got, some pedagogical implications can also be elicited from the survey. First, it is noticed in the survey that students spend a lot of time in using computer and more than half of it in using computer to learn English. As an important and useful learning tool, the computer is also an instrument for entertainment, which inevitably unfolds itself as an amusement world full of distractions to learners. Therefore, how to strike a perfect balance between these two functions and how to integrate entertaining elements into vocabulary learning tasks are the top tasks of learners, teachers and researchers.

Second, positive beliefs on vocabulary learning via computer are helpful to learners' vocabulary developments. The teachers should encourage them to realize the importance and effectiveness of vocabulary learning via computer. In order to achieve that result, the teachers may create a forum on line, which acts as an information and communication channel between teachers and students. When they are designing English lessons, they may take different students' likes and dislikes into consideration, because that would develop students' interest and enthusiasm in computer assisted learning activities. Besides, on the one hand, the teachers should enlighten and assist students to make plans and set their aims in vocabulary learning; on the other hand, they should make the students sure that they should take more responsibility in the vocabulary learning. In a word, teachers should pay attention to students' negative factors and reduce or remove to a maximum degree so that they could become sensitive to vocabulary learning in CALL environment.

Third, teacher should give them more guidance in terms of computer literacy. Training and instructions are necessary to improve their computer knowledge and skill, and enhance their confidence in computer assisted language learning. Meanwhile, the hardware, such as computer centers and language labs, should be improved to provide students with more opportunities to fulfill their online English vocabulary study. A learning center can be made to provide students not only with computers but also various English learning materials. The materials can be disks, videos, courseware or other online materials. Students can get help from teachers in the center when they have problems on learning, choosing appropriated materials and even psychological problems.

Carthy (1990) claims that, at early stages of language development vocabulary instruction has been found to be more effective in building a fundamental vocabulary base than with contextual reading. As the subjects of the present study are the junior English majors, who can be considered English learners of higher level. Therefore, context-based vocabulary learning (e.g. extensive reading) should be more effective for them. As we know, in the new era that CALL takes a large coverage of knowledge sources, teachers should not ignore an important platform of the target language input. It is the very interactive and informative platform that creates many a good context for vocabulary learning. However, as the input is such enormous that teacher should pay attention to instruct or train students' ability of selecting the most appropriate materials for their vocabulary learning.

Forth, this survey reveals that computer assisted language speaking for vocabulary learning is a weak point despite of the popularity of CALL. This could be attributed to many reasons: first, for English learners, especially Chinese students, practicing oral English is a tough task. They would rather spend time in writing or reading repeatedly than using them in real situation via QQ or MSN. Second, for program developers, it is still a challenge to develop effective programs to facilitate English speaking. Consequently, for teachers and computer technicians, closer cooperation is required to create programs both compatible with computer function and geared to learners' needs. And for learners, they should try their best to alleviate computer anxiety, equip themselves with basic computer literacy, and be brave enough to try new learning methods, so as to find the best way of learning.

References

1. Anderson JP, Jordan AM (1928) Learning and retention of Latin words and phrases. J Educ Psychol 19:485–496
2. Atkinson RC (1975) Mnemonics in second language learning. Am Psychol 30:821–828
3. Atkinson RC, Raugh M (1975) An application of the mnemonic keyword method to the acquisition of Russian vocabulary. J Exp Psychol Hum Learn Mem 104(2):126–133
4. Avila E, Sadoski M (1996) Exploring new applications of the keyword method to acquire English vocabulary. Lang Learn 46:379–395
5. Bax S (2003). CALL–past, present and future. System 31:13–28
6. Beatty K (2003) Teaching and researching computer-assisted language learning. Longman, London
7. Bickel B, Truscello D (1996) New opportunities for learning: styles and strategies for computers. TESOL J 6: 15–19
8. Blake R (2001) What language professionals need to know about technology. ADFL Bull 32 (3):90–108
9. Brown TS, Perry FL (1991) A comparison of three learning strategies for ESL vocabulary acquisition. TESOL Q 4:655–670
10. Levy M (1997) Computer-assisted language learning: context and conceptualization. Oxford University, New York (in Press)
11. Luppescu S, Day R (1993) Reading dictionary and vocabulary learning. Lang Learn 43:263–287
12. Warschauer M, Kern R (eds) (2000) Network-based language teaching: concepts and practice. Cambridge University, New York (in Press)

Chapter 312
Bioinformatics Prediction of the Tertiary Structure for the Emy162 Antigen of *Echinococcus multilocularis*

Yanhua Li, Xianfei Liu, Yuejie Zhu, Xiaoan Hu, Song Wang, Xiumin Ma and Jianbing Ding

Abstract We wanted to determine the dominant epitopes of the Emy162 antigen, the secondary and the tertiary structure for the Emy162 antigen found in *Echinococcus multilocularis*. To do so, we analyzed the secondary structure and the tertiary structure of Emy162 protein. We used online software called Phyre2 Server to predict the secondary structure and 3DLigandsite for the tertiary structure of Emy162 protein. From the server we found that the random coil and the β-sheet accounted for approximately 40 % of secondary structure. After the bioinformatics analysis, the secondary and tertiary structures provided us important information for developing a vaccine using the dominant epitopes. This was an indication that it works as a potent dominant antigenic epitopes in Emy162 anatigen.

Keywords Emy162 · Secondary structure · Tertiary structure · Bioinformatics

Echinococcus multilocularis (*E.multilocularis*) is a kind of parasite. In their life cycles, foxes play a key role as definitive hosts and small mammals, mainly rodents (mouse, etc.) are the intermediate hosts. Accidentally humans can get infected and become aberrant hosts by ingesting *E. multilocularis* eggs. After oral uptake of eggs, a larva is released from the egg and transported through the blood and lymph vessels to other organs, where larvae can develop into metacestodes

Y. Li · X. Liu · Y. Zhu · S. Wang · J. Ding (✉)
National Clinical Research Base of Traditional Chinese Medicine of Xinjiang Medical University, 830000 Xinjiang, Urumqi, China
e-mail: djbing002@sina.com

X. Hu · J. Ding
College of Basic Medicine, Xinjiang Medical University, 830011 Xinjiang, Urumqi, China

S. Wang · X. Ma
State Key Laboratory Incubation Base of Major Diseases in Xinjiang and Xinjiang Key Laboratory of Echinococcosis, First Affiliated Hospital of Xinjiang Medical University, 830054 Xinjiang, Urumqi, China

(also known as alveolar hydatid). *Alveolar echinococcosis (AE)* [1], also known as alveolar hydatid disease, is a zoonotic helminthic disease caused by *E. multilocularis* larvae (alveolar hydatid) infection. AE is endemic and mainly confined to the cold regions of high latitude or tundra of the Northern Hemisphere [2]. In China AE infections are highly endemic over large areas of northwestern regions (such as Xinjiang and Gansu Provinces) [3, 4].

The initial stages of *E. multilocularis* larvae infection are always asymptomatic. Thus AE is usually diagnosed accidently when doing liver ultrasound in general check-ups and physical examinations. Therefore, *AE* are usually diagnosed at the advanced phase. Furthermore, when patients come to the hospital for treatment, more than 50 % of them have lost surgical cure opportunities [5]. Currently, there are several options for the treatments of AE. However these treatment methods and intervention measures are ineffective. Thus it is urgent to develop more effective prevention and treatment measures. One study found that immunizing the intermediate hosts with *Echinococcus granulosus* (*E. granulosus*) recombinant protein vaccine could protect against oncosphere infection. And the immune protective method was effective between 95–100 %. Therefore the immune prevention may be more effective measure to prevent the epidemic of hydatid disease. With the development of bioinformatics technology, epitope vaccine has become more and more important in immune prevention. Superior to traditional vaccines [6], vaccines based on epitopes are currently used as protective vaccines against infectious disease. A major challenge in the development of epitope based vaccines is to find out the most effective immunogenic sites of antigen [7]. Kouguchi [8] found that emY162 recombinant antigen could induce 74.3 % effectiveness in providing immunity within rats. Yoshinobu Katoh [9] suggested that the prevention of hydatid disease by molecular vaccine is feasible. 3DLigandSite is a web server for the prediction of ligand-binding sites, which automates the manual process we used for ligand-binding site prediction in the eighth round of the Critical Assessment of techniques for protein Structure Prediction(CASP8) [10]. They also mapped residue conservation onto the protein surface and made predictions combining data from both approaches. It also provides details of conservation information are not currently used in the prediction process.

In this study, based on Emy162 gene sequences we analyzed, the secondary and tertiary structures using computer technology and molecular biology software. Our results determined the dominant epitope of Emy162 antigen and provided experimental data for the preparation of epitope vaccine.

312 Bioinformatics Prediction of the Tertiary Structure

312.1 Materials and Methods

312.1.1 Amino Acid Sequence of Emy162 Protein

Based on the nucleotide sequence of Emy162 in GeneBank (GeneBank number: AB303298.1), the Emy162 protein is composed of 153 amino acid residues encoded by 5-466 regions of Emy162 mRNA. The amino acid sequence of Emy162 protein sequence was shown in Fig. 312.1.

312.1.2 Secondary Structure Prediction of Emy162 Protein

Secondary structure of Emy162 protein was predicted by online Phyre2 Server (http://www.sbg.bio.ic.ac.uk/phyre2/phyre2output/f7cdf21db59e6d02/summary.html). Steps in detail are as followed, Open this website, then input the sequence name in the blank of "Sequence name (optional):" Then paste protein sequence in "Paste a protein sequence below:" Output with to "70"; Modulate the primary parameters, say Number of conformational states: 4(Helix, Sheet, Turn, Coil), Similarity threshold: 8, Window width: 17. At last, press the "search" button.

MVLRFCLILLATSVIAEEVGVDPELIAKLTKKLQTTLPEHFRWIHVGSRSLEL
GWNATGLANLHADHIKLTANLYTTYVSFRYRNVPIERQKLTLEGLKPSTFY
EVVVQALKGDSEVYKYTGFIRTLAPGEDGADRAGGFALIFAMAGLLLLT

Fig. 312.1 Amino acid sequence of Emy162 protein Emy162 protein was encoded by mRNA (from 5 to 466 in the nucleotide sequence) and contained 153 amino acid residues

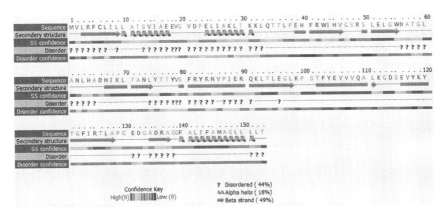

Fig. 312.2 The secondary structure prediction results of Emy162 protein

312.1.3 Tertiary Structure Prediction of Emy162 Protein

In order to know a tertiary structure of a protein, we can use online server 3DLigandsite. Paste a protein sequence into the sever. Predictive analysis of the Emy162 protein tertiary structure was conducted by online server 3DLigandsite (http://www.sbg.bio.ic.ac.uk). And the three-dimensional structure was compared by VAST.

312.2 Results

312.2.1 Secondary Structure Prediction Results of Emy162 Protein

After prediction by online Phyre2 Server software, the prediction results of Emy162 protein secondary structure were shown in Fig. 312.2. In the secondary structure, the proportion of α helix and extended strand (β fold) accounted for 18 and 49 %, respectively. The picture indicates that the regions which color close to blue represent the percentage of low possibility of epitopes in Emy162 protein. Regions with color close to red have a high possibility of dominant epitopes in Emy162 protein. The more extended strand and random coil the protein has the more likely it will form antigen epitope.

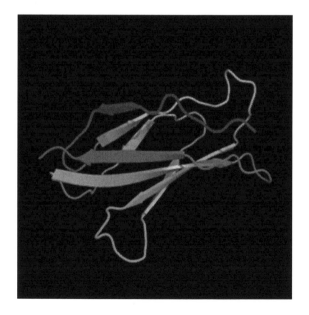

Fig. 312.3 The tertiary structure prediction results of Emy162 protein. Fold: Immunoglobulin-like beta-sandwich; Superfamily: Fibronectin type III; Family: Fibronectin type III (This image was created with 3DLigandsite)

312.2.2 Tertiary Structure Prediction Results of Emy162 Protein

The 3D Ligand site software was a useful tool for protein tertiary structure analysis. In this study, we obtained the tertiary structure of Emy162 protein by the 3D Ligand site software and compared the structure on VAST. The predicted conformational epitopes results were shown in Fig. 312.3. The figure shows us the overview of the 3DLigandSite algorithm. Epitopes of Emy162 antigen were predicted. The structural surfaces display the true epitopes in regions which color close to red. This figure was created with 3DLigandsite.

312.3 Discussion

Echinococcosis is severely harmful to human health and the development of social economy and animal husbandry [11]. At the advanced phase, the characteristic symptoms are liver failure, hepatic coma and portal hypertension complicated gastrointestinal bleeding, which could cause patients' death [12, 13]. Besides the liver, alveolar hydatid can also be transferred through the lymphatic or blood circulation to the lungs, brain and other parts of the body, creep the surface and parenchyma of organs and body cavity, like malignant tumor.

The research and development of epitope vaccine is a very difficult but highly targeted technology, which comprehensively utilizes molecular biology and immunology. A key step in the preparation of epitope vaccine is getting the epitope information. In recent years, with the development of bioinformatics, epitope prediction becomes much easier and more significant. Prediction with multi-parameter and multi-method analysis greatly improves the accuracy of epitope prediction. Protein secondary structure is closely related to epitope distribution. We first analyzed the secondary structure of Emy162 protein. Also the comprehensive analysis could improve the accuracy and specificity of epitope prediction. In the protein secondary structure, the structures of α-helix and β-pleated sheet are very regular and can't be deformed easily. Their structural stability is maintained by hydrogen bonds. However they are usually located inside the protein and are difficult for ligand binding. The β turn and the random coil regions are located on the surface of the protein. The surface structure of the protein could make appropriate changes to meet the functional needs. Therefore these structures are suitable for binding ligands and have a high possibility of forming epitopes. As analyzed by online Phyre2 Server software, the proportions of α helix and the extended area (β fold) were 18 and 49 %, respectively. This result indicates a good stability of the Emy162 antigen. The random coil and β turn, which were the potential epitope regions, accounted for around 40 %.

Protein tertiary structure, one of the higher-order structures of the protein, is a three-dimensional conformation of natural folded protein. Tertiary structure has a globular conformation formed by the further coiling and folding of the secondary structure. Therefore prediction of tertiary structure is a perfect supplementary to the prediction of Emy162 antigenic epitopes

The aim of this study is to obtain bioinformatics characteristics of Emy162 antigen. The online Phyre2 Server software and the 3DLigandsite were used to predict the secondary and tertiary structure of Emy162 antigen. The prediction results of secondary and tertiary structure suggest that there were potential epitopes in Emy162 antigen. These regions were the potential dominant epitopes of Emy162 antigen. Our findings provide experimental data for the identification and screening of epitopes, and further the development for safer and more efficient epitope vaccine. This will dedicate to better preventions and treatments of *AE*.

Acknowledgements This study was supported by the National Nature Science Foundation of China (81160378, 81160200, 81060135 and 30860263).

References

1. Jenkins EJ, Schurer JM, Gesy KM (2011) Old problems on a new playing field: Helminth zoonoses transmitted among dogs, wildlife, and people in a changing northern climate. Vet Parasitol 182:54–69
2. Eckert J, Schantz PM, Gasser P et al (2001) Geographic distribution and prevalence. WHO// OIE Manual on *Echinococcosis* in Humans and Animals: a public health problem of global concern 100–134
3. Craig PS (2006) Epidemiology of human *echinococcosis* in China. Parasitol Int 55:221–225
4. Nunnari G, Pinzone MR, Gruttadauria S et al (2012) Hepatic echinococcosis: clinical and therapeutic aspects. World J Gastroenterol 18:1448–1458
5. Kantarci M, Bayraktutan U, Karabulut N et al (2012) Alveolar echinococcosis: spectrum of findings at cross-sectional imaging. Radiographics 32:2053–2070
6. Ben YT, Arnon R (2005) Towards an epitope based human vaccine for influenza. Hum Vaccin 1:95–101
7. You L, Brusic V, Gallagher M et al (2010) Using gaussian process with test rejection to detect T-Cell epitopes in pathogen genomes. IEEE/ACM Trans Comput Biol Bioinform 7:741–751
8. Kouguchi H, Matsumoto J, Yamano K et al (2011) Echinococcus multilocularis: purification and characterization of glycoprotein antigens with serodiagnostic potential for canine infection. Exp Parasitol 128:50–56
9. Katoh Y, Kouguchi H, Goto A et al (2008) Characterization of emY162 encoding an immunogenic protein cloned from an adult worm-specific cDNA library of *Echinococcus multilocularis*. Biochim Biophys Acta 1780:1–6
10. Wass MN, Sternberg MJ (2009) Prediction of ligand binding sites using homologous structures and conservation at CASP8. Proteins 77:147–151
11. Rebmann T, Zelicoff A (2012) Vaccination against influenza: role and limitations in pandemic intervention plans. Expert Rev Vaccines 11:1009–1019
12. Grosso G, Gruttadauria S, Biondi A et al (2012) Worldwide epidemiology of liver hydatidosis including the Mediterranean area. World J Gastroenterol 18:1425–1437
13. Mandal S, Mandal MD (2012) Human cystic echinococcosis: epidemiologic, zoonotic, clinical, diagnostic and therapeutic aspects. Asian Pac J Trop Med 5:253–260

Chapter 313
IT in Education Application of Computer in Teaching Flavor and Fragrance Technology

Guangyong Zhu, Zuobing Xiao, Rujun Zhou, Yalun Zhu and Yunwei Niu

Abstract Fragrance and flavor play an important role in many fields. Fragrance and flavor technology is a core course for training the students whose major is light chemical engineering. This paper deals with the applications of computer in this course. The applications of Internet, flavor and fragrance computer software, electronic nose and electronic tongue in Flavor and Fragrance Technology were discussed. The Internet is widely used to gather information about flavors and fragrances. Flavor and fragrance creation computer software became an important tool for perfume development and expanding knowledge of perfumery raw materials. Electronic nose and electronic tongue are two devices controlled by computer and intended to detect odors and tastes respectively. They can avoid a number of drawbacks caused by human fatigue or stress.

Keywords Flavor and fragrance technology · Computer

313.1 Introduction

Fragrance and flavor play an important role and have been widely used in many products, such as perfume, soap, cream, lotion, shampoo, washing up liquid, food, wine, cigarette, etc. [1]. A fragrance or flavor is a mixture of fragrant essential oils or aroma compounds, fixatives and solvents used to give the human body, animals,

G. Zhu · Z. Xiao (✉) · R. Zhou · Y. Niu
Shanghai Institute of Technology, No. 100 Haiquan Road, Shanghai 201418, People's Republic of China
e-mail: zbingxiao@sina.com

Y. Zhu
School of Bioscience and Bioengineering, South China University of Technology, Guangdong, China

food, objects, and living spaces "a pleasant scent." Whether a particular product is called a fragrance or flavor substance depends on whether it is used as a perfume or a flavor [2].

Shanghai Institute of Technology offers four years of high-standard education in flavor and fragrance. Fragrance and flavor technology is a core course for training the students whose major is light chemical engineering. This course provides students with solid background in flavor and fragrance formulation, and flavor and fragrance application. The training goal is to become a perfumer or a flavorist. A perfumer is a trained professional who creates fragrances for household products, toiletries, cosmetics, and fine fragrances for men and women. A flavorist is someone who uses chemistry to engineer artificial and natural flavors. The training process to become a perfumer or a flavorist is intense and rigorous, spanning many years. The first task for a trainee perfumer or flavorist is to study hundreds of natural and synthetic materials, cataloguing and memorizing them according to their specific odors. Then, one must be able to create both simple and complex fragrances or flavor by combining and balancing these raw materials in creative and unique ways. This is a traditional training process.

A huge amount of excellent computer aided teaching flavor and fragrance technology already exists. A computer provides a practical approach to changes in information management, flavor and fragrance development, and analytical method. Applications of computer technology in flavor research were discussed in Ref. [3]. These applications included: sensory evaluation; computer system for handling and analysis of flavor and fragrance molecules; computer-based molecular design of artificial flavoring agents; mathematical approaches for quantitative design of odorants and tastants; use of computers for product optimization; economics of laboratory information management systems; instantaneous analysis of fragrances and flavors; multivariate and GC techniques in flavor research etc. [3]. In this paper, we focus on the new application of Internet, flavor and fragrance computer software, electronic nose and electronic tongue in Flavor and Fragrance Technology.

313.2 The Application of Internet in Flavor and Fragrance Technology

Usually, a textbook cannot possibly cover the field of flavor and fragrance in detail. Thus, it is deemed useful how to find information on flavors and fragrances. The important source of information in the flavor and fragrance area is the Internet. The Internet has brought us both convenience and a greatly expanded world of information. The Internet is widely used to gather information about flavors and fragrances and to communicate within or outside the flavor and fragrance company. A perfumer or flavorist may wish to find an individual with expertise in a given problem area. This can easily be done through Internet searches.

General information about the flavor and fragrance industry, such as current events in the industry, new chemicals approved, international legislation, can be found easily in the Internet. There is merit in doing searches to get this information. One of the most useful services of the Internet is the broad access to the literature. Retrieving patents or journals, either domestic or international, has been made easy via the Internet. It is possible to search and download complete patents or articles at no cost. In the development of fragrance and flavor, one of the challenges is to find suppliers of the numerous aroma chemicals needed. This is simplified by the power of search engines and corporate websites. The internet has made it possible to buy chemicals on a national and global basis. In a word, the Internet is very useful for new flavor and fragrance development.

313.3 The Application of Flavor and Fragrance Creation Computer Software

The perfumers and flavorist of today have at their disposal over 3,000 fragrance or flavor ingredients to choose from when creating a fragrance or flavor. These include natural oils, nature-identical materials and synthetic compounds [4]. Flavor and fragrance creation is one of main content in the course of Flavor and Fragrance Technology. Flavor and fragrance creation computer software has been developed and became an important tool for perfume creation. The software serves both as a password protected record keeping archive for flavor and fragrance formulas and as a flavor and fragrance development tool.

It enables trainee to keep thousands of formulas in a compact easy to search version with lots of easy to use tools to help the professional or complete beginner create better flavor or fragrance in less time. One of the important functions of this software is that we can learn new perfumery materials from it. It can help us expand our knowledge of perfumery raw materials.

More important is its ability to help us develop our formula by showing us, graphically, how it will smell when first applied and how its scent will evolve over time—minutes or even hours. We can observe this either on an animated pie graph or bar graph. Using this software, we can learn more about our formula.

Special bases and accords can assist in the creation of new fragrances. The software allows us to mix these elements, in whatever percentage we want, into a new creation. Using our favorite bases and accords in new creations can be done with the software.

One of the tools within software is the "Modify" tool. The "Modify the tone or balance tool" can suggest modifications of formula in eight categories: top note, middle note, bottom note, strength, freshness, "floweriness", depth and smoothness. The software can suggest modifications of each of these qualities in anywhere. Using the "Modify" tool to develop new flavor or fragrance is another important function of the software.

313.4 The Application of Electronic Nose in Flavor and Fragrance Technology

A challenging problem in the food and beverage processing industries is how to ensure the flavor quality of products. Traditionally, nose is used to evaluate quality parameters. However, this suffers from a number of drawbacks. For example, discrepancies can occur due to human fatigue or stress and clearly cannot be used for online measurements [5]. Thus the development of alternative methods is highly desirable.

An electronic nose is a device controlled by a computer and intended to detect odors or flavors. Figure 313.1 shows the electronic nose.

The electronic nose was developed in order to mimic human olfaction that functions as a non-separative mechanism: i.e. an odor/flavor is perceived as a global fingerprint. Essentially, the instrument consists of head space sampling, sensor array, and pattern recognition modules, to generate signal pattern that are used for characterizing odors. Electronic noses include three major parts: a sample delivery system, a detection system, a computing system.

The sample delivery system enables the generation of the headspace (volatile compounds) of a sample, which is the fraction analyzed. The system then injects this headspace into the detection system of the electronic nose. The sample delivery system is essential to guarantee constant operating conditions. The detection system, which consists of a sensor set, is the "reactive" part of the instrument. When in contact with volatile compounds, the sensors react, which means they experience a change of electrical properties.

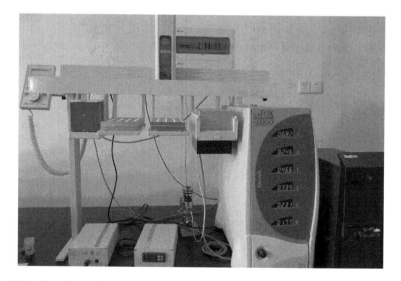

Fig. 313.1 The electronic nose

The adsorption of volatile compounds on the sensor surface causes a physical change of the sensor. A specific response is recorded by the electronic interface transforming the signal into a digital value. Recorded data are then computed based on statistical models. It is a very useful instrument in fragrance and flavor.

313.5 The Application of Electronic Tongue in Flavor and Fragrance Technology

The electronic tongue controlled by a computer is an instrument that measures and compares tastes. Figure 313.2 shows the electronic tongue.

Chemical compounds responsible for taste are detected by human taste receptors, and the seven sensors of electronic instruments detect the same dissolved organic and inorganic compounds. Like human receptors, each sensor has a spectrum of reactions different from the other. The information given by each sensor is complementary and the combination of all sensors' results generates a unique fingerprint. Most of the detection thresholds of sensors are similar to or better than those of human receptors. In the biological mechanism, taste signals are transducted by nerves in the brain into electric signals. E-tongue sensors process is similar: they generate electric signals as potentiometric variations. Taste quality perception and recognition is based on building or recognition of activated sensory nerve patterns by the brain and on the taste fingerprint of the product. This step is achieved by the e-tongue's statistical software which interprets the sensor data into taste patterns. Liquid samples are directly analyzed without any preparation,

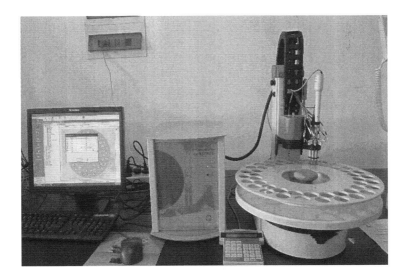

Fig. 313.2 The electronic tongue

whereas solids require a preliminary dissolution before measurement. Reference electrode and sensors are dipped in a beaker containing a test solution for 120 s. A potentiometric difference between each sensor and a reference electrode is measured and recorded by the E-Tongue software. These data represent the input for mathematical treatment that will deliver results. It is a very useful instrument for taste determination in flavor.

313.6 Conclusions

This paper concentrated on the application of computer in Flavor and Fragrance Technology. Internet, flavor and fragrance computer software, electronic nose and electronic tongue are important tools for flavor and fragrance studying. Their applications were discussed in this paper. The Internet is useful to obtain information about flavors and fragrances. Flavor and fragrance creation computer software became an important tool for perfume development and expanding knowledge of perfumery raw materials. Electronic nose and electronic tongue are two devices to determine odors and tastes respectively. They can avoid a number of drawbacks caused by human fatigue or stress. In a word, computer is very useful for flavor and fragrance studying.

Acknowledgments The authors thanks the National Natural Science Fund of China (21,276,157), International Cooperation Project of Shanghai "Mountaineering Plan" (11,290,707,600), and Project of Shanghai Institute of Technology (YJ2012-30) for financial support.

References

1. Zhu G, Xiao Z, Zhou R et al (2012) Fragrance and flavor microencapsulation technology. Adv Mater Res 535–537:440–445
2. Surburg H, Panten J (2006) Common fragrance and flavor materials, 5th edn. Wiley, New York
3. Warren CB, Walradt JP (1984) Computers in flavor and fragrance research. ACS, Wahington
4. Sell C (2006) The chemistry of fragrance, 2nd edn. RSC, London
5. Cole M, Covington JA, Gardner JW (2011) Combined electronic nose and tongue for a flavour sensing system. Sens Actuat B 156:832–839
6. Reineccius G (2006) Flavor Chemistry and Technology, 2nd edn. Taylor & Francis, Boca Raton

Chapter 314
Building an Effective Blog-Based Teaching Platform in Higher Medical Education

Bailiu Ya, Qun Ma and Chuanping Si

Abstract As an educational tool, blog is one of the user-friendly technological means that supports teaching and learning processes in higher education. There are many ways to use blogging in teaching and learning. In our university, we try to build a blog-based teaching platform for higher medical education. This platform provides a constructive and interactive learning environment where students and instructors negotiate, discuss, reflect and evaluate individual understandings of learning and teaching practice and experience. The use of this blog-based teaching platform has shown a positive impact on learning and professional developments. In our experience, what makes this process more meaningful and sustainable are active participation and high quality interaction which require collaboration and interaction together with commitment and support from students and instructors. In essence, this paper not only introduces the blog-based teaching platform building by our university, but also discusses the potential of blogs to support reflection and communication in higher medical education, and explores the strengths and weaknesses of current practice in order to build a more effective platform in the future.

Keywords Blog-based teaching platform · Higher medical education · Information technology · Blog

---

B. Ya · Q. Ma · C. Si (✉)
Jining Medical University, 272067 Shandong, China
e-mail: chpsi@163.com

B. Ya
e-mail: yabailiu@126.com

Q. Ma
e-mail: immunomotor@163.com

314.1 Introduction

Over the past few years there has been an increasing interest in the new generation of social media, especially Web 2.0 technologies. The users of internet have the opportunity to have a voice by means of Web 2.0, while they previously could only access to the information that the administrator of the site allows. In this way the users have begun to compose the content of the sites [1, 2].

As a Web 2.0 technology, the blog is a chronological publication in which personal thoughts and opinions are posted on websites [3]. Blogs help people to create, communicate, and publish online content more easily. Due to the ease of use, functionality and flexibility, they have become much more commonplace throughout the online environments. These attributes of the blog are also well suited to be used as teaching and learning media in higher medical education [1, 4]. Particularly in today's world it becomes impossible to think of an educational system without information and communication technology.

314.2 Blog-Based Teaching Platform Building in Higher Medical Education

A blog is an open system which receives all resources (e.g., video clips, photos, etc.), transforms them into desired outputs and sends these outputs back (e.g., permalink). Blogs have a visualization tool to enhance information retrieval and they are decentralized systems which don't require the need to intentionally visit a hub blog to communicate with others. In the field of education, blogs contribute to overcoming the limitations of current computer-mediated communication (CMC) technology, such as, causing difficulty in the management of communication, failing to provide a sense of ownership, causing anxiety, being instructor-centered, or having no archive capability [5].

Today's college students spend lots of time on the internet and engage instant messaging, blogging, downloading audio and video files, and online games in their daily lives. In other words, today's college students have grown up with these tools [6].

In the field of higher medical education, it is an inevitable trend for teachers to use blogs to assist teaching. Numerous teachers have realized the benefits of using blogs in educational contexts such as to improve their teaching effectiveness [2], enhance the communication environment between students and teachers [7], help promote more constructive and enthusiastic discussions [8] and enable students to better regulate and enhance their own learning [9].

Therefore, educators have tried to incorporate these online technologies into the classroom environments to increase student satisfaction and learning. We create a teaching blog-based platform, a platform to improve instructors and students teaching and learning process, our blog address: http://www.basicmed.com (Fig. 314.1).

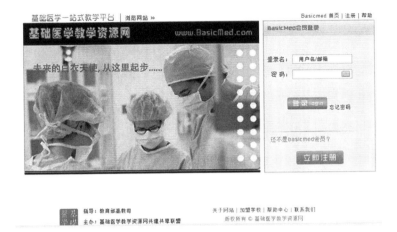

Fig. 314.1 The welcome page of the website

314.2.1 Experience of the Use of Blog-Based Teaching Platform

First of all, to improve the interactivity among instructors and students, instructors and students should be encouraged to allow other people to post comments on their own blogs. As a result, it is expected to increase the amount of feedback, which enhances self-motivation.

Second, because a blog is inherently designed to be compatible with other social software and websites, instructors and students are recommended to seek relevant information from other websites, regardless of information format, and share the information on a blog. The information could be text, video, or audio-based materials through other social software such as Podcast (Fig. 314.2).

Third, in our system, instructors are encouraged to be the primary contributor who is supposed to release qualified resources. The success of the system relies on instructors' capability of providing the resources. Bundled course materials are delivered by instructors through a system so that students could quickly find information (Fig. 314.3).

Fourth, as to solve the question of easy-to-find relevant information, our blog consists of multiple components such as entries, comments, tags, blogroll, permalinks, images, and so on, all of which includes a large number and variety of keywords. Thus, a single search query could result in many hits from the components (Fig. 314.4).

Fifth, as access to a wider audience than the traditional student–teacher relationship is more likely to reinforce collaboration and feedback, our blog is linked to similar other course blogs that belong to different schools across the states to help students find desired blogs and information. This facilitates the connection to wider audience (Fig. 314.5).

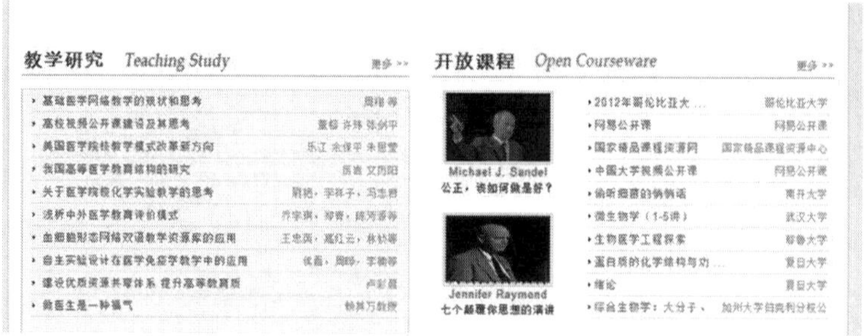

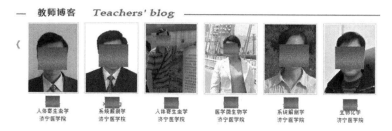

Fig. 314.2 Resources from other websites

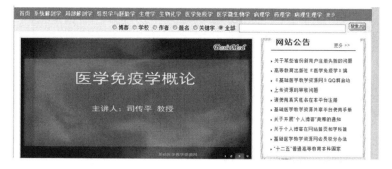

Fig. 314.3 The teachers' blog

Fig. 314.4 The search box

314.2.2 Limitations in Our Blog-Based Teaching Platform

There are still something to be done for our blog-based teaching platform building. For example, the RSS system is recommended to be embedded in a blog. In addition, instructors and students are required to learn how to use the RSS system. Students are more likely to satisfy with easy-to-use systems in which they are able to obtain information with fewer steps. RSS delivery might help students save time

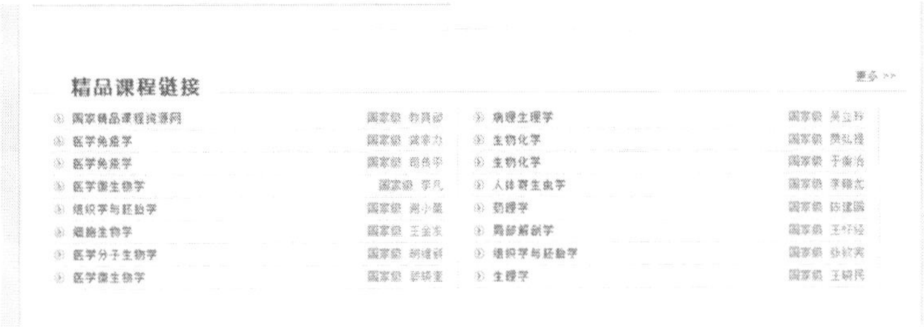

Fig. 314.5 The courses from other websites

and effort on retrieval information since RSS automatically informs students of ongoing discussions they are interested in. Additionally, numerous studies have been conducted to help Internet users find information in a short amount of time.

By using blogs, instructors possibly are afraid that it may attract criticism. Instructors have to spend extra time and effort to codify their knowledge. Moreover, after sharing knowledge, instructors lose the advantage of owning unique knowledge. Thus, some encouraging measurements should be taken to motivate instructors' decision to adopt teaching blogs.

314.3 Conclusion

Blogs are popular social networking tool that have risen out of web environments in the recent years. There are many advantages of using blogs in educational environments. Our experiences in using blogs have been overwhelmingly positive, which show that the use of blogs as a learning tool seems to be low-cost with high-returns in higher medical education. While student acceptance of technology in the classroom requires its perceived usefulness and ease of use, students do tend to learn best when they need information that they can put to use immediately. Blogs are an effective and efficient method of allowing students to access information as it is needed and to make connections between explicit knowledge from textbooks and tacit knowledge gained as students see how others can and are using the knowledge being shared. Blogs also introduce students to online learning communities so they can access and evaluate information, and construct new learning paradigms for themselves. Finally, effectively modeling ways to use blogs as a teaching and learning tool is a useful skill for our students to have as they embark on their journey of life-long learning.

While more research needs to be done as to how blogs can more effectively be used, it is a given that technology will continue to influence learning, and we will go on to explore the blog-based teaching platform in higher medical education.

References

1. Top E, Yukselturk E, Inan FA (2010) Reconsidering usage of blogging in preservice teacher education courses. Internet Higher Educ 13(4):214–217
2. Churchill D (2009) Educational applications of Web 2.0: using blogs to support teaching and learning. Br J Educ Technol 40(1):179–183
3. Chai S, Kim M (2010) What makes bloggers share knowledge? An investigation on the role of trust. Int J Inf Manage 30(5):408–415
4. Ellison N, Wu Y (2008) Blogging in the classroom: a preliminary exploration of student attitudes and impact on comprehension. J Educ Multimedia Hypermedia 17(1):99–122
5. Kim HN (2008) The phenomenon of blogs and theoretical model of blog use in educational contexts. Comput Educ 51(3):1342–1352
6. Roberts DF, Foehr UG (2008) Trends in media use. The future of children 18(1):11–37
7. Joshi M, Chugh R (2009) New paradigms in the teaching and learning of accounting: use of educational blogs for reflective thinking. Int J Educ Dev Using ICT 5(3)
8. Black L (2007) Blogging clicks with educators: online forums make assignments, ideas more accessible to students and parents. Knight Ridder Tribune Business New
9. Wang KT, Huang Y-M, Jeng Y-L, Wang T-I (2008) A blog-based dynamic learning map. Comput Educ 51(1):262–278

Chapter 315
Design and Implementation of Educational Administration Information Access System Based on Android Platform

Yifeng Yan, Shuming Xiong, Xiujun Lou, Hui Xiong and Qishi Miao

Abstract In order to help teachers and students to access the education management information system (EMIS) more conveniently, a client based on Android platform is designed and implemented in this paper. After logging, this client software can obtain user's education information from EMIS server using HTTP resolve mechanism, including basic personal information, student achievement, student course management and examination arrangement, etc. In development stage, regular expression which is an effective development method is applied to analyze complex data. The test results show that this client has perfect performance both in system compatibility and terminal compatibility. On one hand, it can adapt different mobile terminals' size and touch feature. On the other hand, it can adapt EMIS deployed in different colleges and universities due to its special design of universal data interface.

Keywords Android · Education administration information · Data access · Mobile terminal

---

Y. Yan · S. Xiong (✉) · X. Lou · Q. Miao
School of Computer Science and Telecommunication Engineering, JiangSu University, Zhenjiang, Jiangsu Province, People's Republic of China
e-mail: xsm@mail.ujs.edu.cn

Y. Yan
e-mail: yanephone@gmail.com

H. Xiong
Jingjiang College, JiangSu University, Zhenjiang, Jiangsu Province, People's Republic of China

315.1 Introduction

Educational administration is the core content of the colleges and universities daily management of the work [1]. It comes to teachers, students, administrators and discipline construction, and has been widely used in Web-based Educational Administration System [2]. At present, the university teachers and students tend to use a desktop computer to access the educational administration system, while accessing it with mobile terminals rarely. Because mobile terminals lack relevant application software to visit the educational administration system. Moreover, in spite of many smart phones can access the web through the mobile browser, the page of the Education system is mainly designed for desktop computer users. The use of mobile terminals exist resolution which is incompatible, display unsightly, inconvenient operation and many other inconvenience.

With the rise of mobile Internet, smartphone as the representative of the Android is becoming a mainly mobile application development platform [3]. Currently, there are a lot of researches and developments based on the Android platform. Gu et al. [4] proposed design of indoor LBS system based on Android platform and its implementation. They implemented the indoor information gathering and sampling, and accurate locate inside the house. Cheng [5] proposed an Android system design and implementation for Telematics services, which can be easily used in the places of daily life such as the bus, house and restaurant. These services make our lives much more convenient and productive. Zhu et al. [6] proposed a convenient and efficient library management design and its implementation. Geng et al. [7] able to log on and control a fixed terminal remotely through the smartphone. Tang proposed design and developing the communication helper based on Android [8]. It can be effective and humane management of the local phone address book. However, the market lacks educational administration information access to smartphone mobile applications currently. Therefore, we propose an educational administration information access system and its implementation. It develops smart phones educational administration information access platform with mobile communication technology. Besides, it can adapt different mobile terminals' size and touch feature, making users access to educational administration information instantly and conveniently.

315.2 Design of Communication Module

The system need to communicate with the server to get the information that we need. As a result, the system send the request packet containing the HTTP protocol to the server. Then the server return the query to the system. This system mainly uses the packages packaged by HttpClient [9] to implement the communication between the system and server.

315.2.1 Transport Mechanism of Data Package

Among all the network communication methods, the most frequently used is the Get method when the system needs to query some information from the server. The system sends the request to the server on the base of the URL address by using this method. The information sent to the server is started with the symbol of "?" and different information is distinguished by the symbol of "&". They will be sent to the server after all the information is added to the address of the web page. In addition, we need to add the access address of the previous level and the cookie produced during the visit in manual control. If we ignore this operation, the server will be mistaken for hot linking, leading to redirect the access address. As a result, we can't receive the needed information. The cookie produced is saved with static type the client during the interaction. In this way, once we submit the request to the server, the latest cookie will be added so that the verification will be passed.

Compared with the Get method, the method of Post is much safer. The method of Post submitted to the server with the type of Arrylist set, that is, params to send the data package to the server, rather than put the information on the URL. At the same time, the Post method also needs to add the access previous address and the cookie produced in manual control during the visit.

315.2.2 Communication Between System and Server

In order to get the information, the network needs to be accessed when the system is running. The process of communication between the system and server is showed in Fig. 315.1. At the beginning, we create the instance of the Handler and the HTTP Request to interact with the UI. Then we put the user's information into the data package. The client sends the request with the Get method or the Post method after packaging the requested data. The server is going to handle the information after the request, which comes from the client, is received successfully. Then the request returns to the client when the verification passes. The client resolves the valuable information from the data package and display the handled data on the screen after processing.

315.3 Design of Function Module

After analyzing the research on students, the system selects the five most frequently useful functions among all the students as Fig. 315.2 shows. As we can see, there are examination arrangements, curriculum, test scores, level examinations and selected courses. Besides, we also put the campus information related to our students' everyday life together with the previous five functions. The function

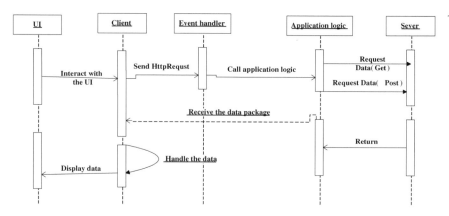

Fig. 315.1 Communication sequence of educational administration information access system

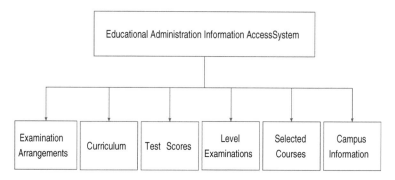

Fig. 315.2 Function module of educational administration information access system

of examination arrangements is used to search for recent examination information. The function of level examination is used to search for the test scores that the user has taken part in, such as CET and National Computer Rank Examination. The function of curriculum is used to look for the curriculum of this year. The function of test scores is used to search for the scores at different stages. The function of selected courses is used to search for the chosen courses of each semester. The function of campus information is to provide the latest campus developments. Then, we take the function of curriculum for example to explain the design process in detail.

First of all, TabView, which is used to represent date from Monday to Friday, is designed. Moreover, we have to add some mood pictures like this pretty black pig to represent each weekday. We can find class information of different period in the ListView under the TabView. Figure 315.3 shows us the design process of the curriculum searching. During the design process, the system sends request to the server at first. On the contrast, the server will return the necessary data package to the system after the server responds. However, the data package we recently get usually contains much content, most of which is useless or we don't care. As a result, we can get the curriculum that we need using the keywords <table> and </table>. Further, we can get every day's class information using keywords <tr> and </tr> and put the class information into a one-dimensional array. Then, we distinguish classes of different periods in a day by the keywords <td> and </td>. By far, we have got a two-dimensional array containing which week it is and which section it is. At last, we can split the information, such as teachers, classroom and the cycle of the class, by the keywords <br> and </br>. Through this series of processes, the valuable information can be extracted from the package and classified properly. In the end, the information we get has to be integrated before being bound to the adapter and displayed on the screen.

In order to beautify the user interface, we add a background picture to the ListView. However, we must transparent the ListView to prevent the whole screen from turning into black while dragging. Because of the limited UI in the mobile terminals, only can the class name be displayed on the ListView. So we need to touch off the Onclick event of the ListView to generate Activity that shows details. Besides, the detailed class information will be sent in the form of a string to a new Activity by the means of Intent, and be shown in classification on the EditView of the Activity.

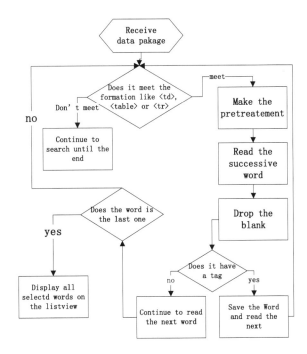

Fig. 315.3 Curriculum query design flow chart

315.4 Operating Environment and Experiment

After the system is designed, we developed an application example based on the Android platform. This section will explain how to implement the system with an application example in detail.

315.4.1 Running Environment of System

The running environment of the system is made up with the system Android smartphone, network, server and database. Figure 315.4 shows how the system debugs and runs in the network environment. The system uses the smartphone equipped with the Android operating system as its platform. Besides, it can run on smartphones of different model and resolution. The smartphone can get access to the Internet by 2G/3G networks or WIFI. And the mobile client will send request to the server of specified IP address. The server can interact with the mobile client so as to accomplish the task of data exchange in this process accordingly. The network is provided by the wireless carriers or broadband operators in the environment. The client communicates with server by specified IP address after the server gets a public IP address from the Internet.

Recently, the great majority of colleges have established server related with education information and implement the Web Service faced to browser basically. Therefore, we don't need to establish the server and the database repeatedly. As a result, we just need to know the IP address with the server, if we want to implement the communication between the client and the Server. There are two advantages: First, strengthening the portability of the system. Different universities can use this system by the means of modifying the server's IP address and the port

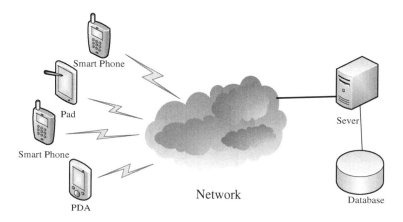

Fig. 315.4 Running environment of educational administration information access system

number written in the client. Second, improve the safety of the system. Before handling the data in the database, we need to pass the verification of the educational information database of different colleges. Second, different colleges always have different types of verification. The system we designed doesn't require the specific versification, so it provides a way of transparent access to the database.

315.4.2 Debug Running and Discussion of System

We have already developed educational information visiting system application based on Android operating system. The Android operating system is an mobile operating system [10] developed by Google based on the kernel of Linux 2.6 and its middleware, class Libraries and API are all compiled by C language. Android uses the Dalvik virtual machine with just-in-time compilation to run Dalvik, which is usually translated from Java byte code. The main hardware platform is the ARM architecture.

When the system is running, before clicking the Login button for submission the user name and password are filled in. Then, the system's main interface will display six main function of the system. Click the corresponding image button to open the corresponding function. Figure 315.5a shows the curriculum of Wednesday and Fig. 315.5b shows the test scores containing failed subjects in 2012–2013 the first school semester. Figure 315.5c shows some latest Campus Information including academic reports and so on. Click on the corresponding list item and the system will display the detail information on the screen. Figure 315.5d shows us the score of the subject of "Technical Training for Higher Teachers Vocational" in detail. As we can see, the information of semester, academic year, course code, score and grade point are displayed on the screen.

Multiple test experiments show that the system can search the educational administration information and campus information quickly and easily. Only if the

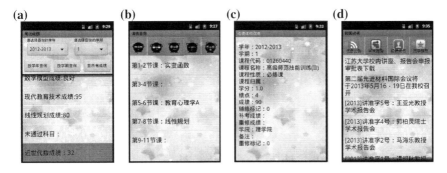

Fig. 315.5 Interface of **a** curriculum, **b** test scores, **c** campus information and **d** courses detail information

school server is running normally, no matter what time is it and where you are. At the same time, the school educational administration system can dock with the mobile platform perfectly without updating or modifying existing education administration system. Because of the openness of the Android operating system, any smart phone based on Android operating system can use the function of the system after the client application is downloaded and installed properly. Moreover, the platform has strong portability, thus developers can call existing platforms academic information access interface to develop their own local education visiting systems to meet the needs of different colleges.

315.5 Conclusion

This chapter is based on the Android platform, and it designed and implemented educational administration information access system. This system transfers HTTP protocol through Apache HttpClient, accessing to school educational administration system server to get the data, and makes use of regular expression on the data by further analysis, processing and handling. It can implement examination arrangements, curriculum, test scores, level examinations and selected courses without modifying the existing education management information system. With low-cost and wide range of applications, the system can all be customized and optimized according to different needs of the universities and colleges. It can also be integrated with library administration system or personnel administration system, making the range of further promotion. At the same time, the part of its function is able to rewrite, leading to the system applied to ordinary business or government authorities.

Acknowledgments This work is sponsored by undergraduate students scientific research projects Foundation of Jiangsu University under Grant No.11B007, Foundation of Jiangsu University under Grant No. 12JDG103 and College Students' Practice Innovation Training Program of Jiangsu Province under Grant No. 2012JSSPITP1256.

References

1. He XP, Li DP, Zhang T (2009) Algorithm and realization of classes merging in management of college physical education course selecting. Comput Eng Des 30(16):3859–3862
2. Meenakumari J (2008) Education and educational administration: a technological perspective. In: International conference on computer science and information technology. ICCSIT'08, pp 836–840
3. Meng X-W Hu X, Wang L-C, Zhang Y-J (2012) Mobile recommender systems and their applications. J Softw, pp 1–18
4. Gu C, Chen YQ, Liu JF, Zhou JY (2012) Design of indoor LBS system based on android platform and its implementation. Comput Eng Des 33(1):396–401

5. Cheng Y-H (2010) An android system design and implementation for telematics services. In: 2010 IEEE international conference on intelligent computing and intelligent systems (ICIS), pp 206–210
6. Zhu WJ, Zhang L, Wang YB, Zhao L (2011) Exploration on library smartphone application. New Technol Library Inf Serv 205(5):13–19
7. Geng DJ, Suo Y, Chen Y, Wen J, Lv YQ (2011) Design and implementation of Android phone based access and control in smart space. J Comput Appl 31(2):559–571
8. Tang M (2012) Design and developing the communication helper based on Android. Comput Sci 39(6A):573–576
9. Yao G-X (2007) Study and design of information integration model based on web data. In: IEEE international conference on control and automation. ICCA 2007, pp. 1385–1387
10. Khomh F (2012) Adapting Linux for mobile platforms: an empirical study of Android. In: 2012 28th IEEE international conference on software maintenance (ICSM), pp 629–632

Chapter 316
The Application of Information Technology and CBS Teaching Method in Medical Genetics

Yang Sun, Fang Xu, Yanjie Wang, Mingzhu Li, Ying Liang and Boyan Wu

Abstract Medical genetics is a fundamental course of preclinical medical education for undergraduate students of medical universities, which has important applications to clinical medicine, medical research and public health. It is important for medical students to identify genetic and genomic perspective on health and disease in their health professional's career. In this paper, a teaching method which combines advanced information technology (IT) with case-based study (CBS) method is proposed and carried out in the course of medical genetics. Two classes in the same grade are chosen as the comparable subjects. The teaching reform is put into practice in one class and the other one with traditional curriculum. Examination and questionnaire are performed and analyzed at the middle and end of the course. The results show that the new curriculum is more successful than the traditional one and the reform is welcomed by more than 80 % students. Furthermore, the students' motive of acquisition for knowledge has been inspired.

Keywords Information technology · CBS · Medical genetics

316.1 Introduction

With the rapid development of information technology (IT), medicine, education and lots of other fields have been promoted greatly and become inseparable with IT [1]. Medical genetics is of no exception. Thousands of genetic diseases could be

---

Fund project: Supported by Educational Research Fund of Heilongjiang University of Chinese Medicine and Foundation for Innovative Talents of Heilongjiang University of Chinese Medicine.

Y. Sun · F. Xu · Y. Wang · M. Li · Y. Liang · B. Wu (✉)
Heilongjiang University of Chinese Medicine, Harbin, China
e-mail: yangsun66@sina.com

diagnosed by the advanced IT. But most of the genetic diseases cannot be really cured. Patients may pass their illness on to their offspring. So it is important for medical students to know the language and concepts of human and medical genetics by take the course of medical genetics. But in most of the medical universities, the course has less hours compared with the contents. How to teach the course in the limited time is the problem, which instructors have to face in the current curriculum setting.

To resolve this issue, in this paper, network, multimedia communication and other information technologies are combined with case-based study (CBS) method to promote the teaching of medical genetics. The teaching reform is put into practice in two classes and evaluated by analysis of examination and questionnaire results.

316.2 Integration of IT and Curriculum

With the advanced teaching idea, the teaching reform is based on the integration of IT and curriculum. Computer and internet are the available methods for the students to cognize the medical genetic knowledge. It can also stimulate teachers and students' interest to search medical information. Teachers could transmit more information in the course to reduce the searching time with the application of IT. Simultaneity, teachers can update the knowledge conveniently. When IT is integrated completely in the course of teaching, it will become a useful and indispensable element in teaching. And construction of IT may improve the teaching level based on global optimization.

316.2.1 Combination of IT and CBS

Teaching method of CBS is also applied in the medical genetics course, which obtains obvious predominance based on IT. CBS is a teaching method, which connect problem-based learning (PBL) method with clinical medicine. Based on the clinical case, students are regarded as the core of the discussion in groups, which could strengthen their practical ability and improve their learning ability. During the discussion, teacher is not expected to answer the questions directly, but could give some prompts to the students. We combined CBS teaching method with IT and the method was applied to several classes.

316.2.2 The Process of the Teaching Mode

At first, the question or case should be introduced by the teacher. Secondly, the students investigate and search the answers by themselves by means of books, articles and internet. Thirdly, students are divided into several groups and discussion is made within each group. Then, a representative student is elected in every group to present their survey results with multimedia courseware. At last, the teacher will summarize and explain the case. The flow chart of the process is shown as Fig. 316.1. In practice, the mode could be diversified. For example, in our class, we let students get familiar with the question or case by videos or photos found from internet and other sources. Students explain the question or case by oral language and pictures with the help of multimedia. In the process, the interests of students on medical genetics are activated. Additionally, every case relates to the other subjects in fact. Though the focus of students' attention is a clinical case, knowledge of the related subjects will also be acquired. Therefore, the course is not limited to teach some known knowledge to students. More importantly, students have chances to grasp the method of learning and researching by themselves.

The following are cases.

There is a common chromosome disease, which is Down syndrome. Before we teach this part of content, we will show lots of photos of patients. We can let the students think why they look like each other. Students could sum the characters up by their own words. Most students are curious why parents who look normal could give birth to sick babies. The answer of the above puzzle could be found by searching books, articles, internet and other medias. After survey and discussion, they not only get a clear answer of this disease but also have a deep impression of chromosome diseases. In this phase, the students are eager to know the mechanism of the disease, which will promote the teaching quality.

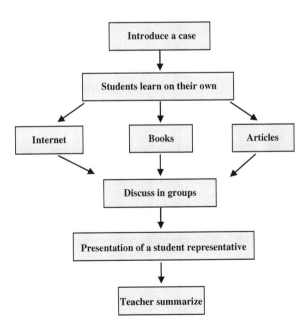

Fig. 316.1 The process of the teaching mode

Genetic counseling is more and more popular in China, now [2]. Long time ago, people neglected genetic disease and faced more genetic risks, which caused the higher rate of inherited diseases. When the counseling approached in China, there are more genetic cases that can be referenced in the medical genetic curriculum. There is a case that is from a family. A couple didn't have a baby for many years. They have several times of early habitat abortion. Then they divorced. The husband married the second wife, but the tragedy repeated. His first wife married again and born a healthy baby. We can discuss the case and let students think why they can encounter this kind of situation.

When talking about ecogenetics problems, we can ask them why the yellow race are drunk more easily than the white one. Usually, students are more interested in the question related with life. They are more willing to look through the information about the question by themselves.

316.2.3 Evaluation Paper

In the progress of the reform of this course, evaluation papers are used to survey and measure the feasibility of the proposed methods. In the paper, the question of whether you like the CBS with IT method is put forward to the students. Students could rate in four grades, which are A (very satisfied), B (satisfied), C (a little satisfied) and D (don't like). The number of choosing A accounts for 20 %. And the number of choosing B, C, D are 63, 17, 0 % respectively. It was found that most students considered CBS with IT method be useful for them.

316.2.4 Result Analysis

Two classes of undergraduate students of 2010 were chosen as comparable subjects. The class majored in Acupuncture and Tuina were taught using the traditional curriculum. The other class majored in Medical Psychology were selected to carry out the teaching reform. They took the same final-exam at the end of the course. Comparison of the exam result is as follows (Table 316.1). The two classes

Table 316.1 Comparison of two classes

	Acupuncture and Tuina			Medical psychology		
	Number	Average	Percentage (%)	Number	Average	Percentage (%)
100–90	6	92.80	10.91	6	93.00	14.29
89–80	22	84.63	40.00	29	84.55	69.05
79–70	17	75.67	30.91	7	75.43	16.67
69–60	10	62.86	18.18	0	0	0
Total	55	79.87		42	84.24	

were both sophomore undergraduate students, who had the same background knowledge and education experience. As shown in Table 316.1, the average score of Medical Psychology is higher than the other. There are more students between 100 and 80 in the class performing teaching reform. The rate between 70 and 79 was 16.67 % in the CBS with IT curriculum while 30.91 % in the traditional teaching curriculum. There are less students who score below 80 in Medical Psychology than the comparable class. It could be concluded that the class performing teaching reform gains the better result compared with the class of traditional curriculum.

316.3 Conclusion

(1) A teaching method which combines advanced IT with CBS method is proposed and carried out in the course of medical genetics.
(2) Examination performance and questionnaires indicate that reform class is more successful than the traditional class.
(3) Combination of IT and CBS could stimulate the motive of students to acquire knowledge by themselves, and is worth extending to other clinical courses.

References

1. Zhu X, Chen X (2012) The application of information push technology in clinical medicine education. Int Symp Inf Technol Med Educ, pp 539–540
2. Zhang Y, Zhong N (2006) Current genetic counseling in China. J Peking Univ 38(1):33–34

Chapter 317
Research on Practice Teaching of Law in the Provincial Institutions of Higher Learning

Haiying Zheng

Abstract Practice teaching is a breakthrough in improving quality of personnel training for law offered by the provincial institutions of higher learning. But there are many problems such as management system, evaluation system, teaching faculty, teaching environment for practice teaching in the provincial institutions of higher learning at present. On the problems aforesaid, we shall establish and improve evaluation system for practice teaching, strengthen building of the double-type teachers, increase investment in practice teaching of law and construct a convenient and practical base for practice teaching to enhance quality of practice teaching of law in the provincial institutions of higher learning through gradual realization of normalized management of practice teaching of law.

Keywords Provincial institutions of higher learning · Practice teaching · Evaluation system

317.1 Introduction

According to the related data statistics, there were over 600 law colleges in China by 2010, and about 400,000 enrolling law majors [1]. For most provincial law institutions, how to improve quality of law personnel training, to preserve own education features in fierce competition to fit in with severe employment situation and domestic demand for law higher learning, are problems required urgently to be solved now. Without question, provincial institutions should set personnel training

H. Zheng (✉)
Beihua University, Jilin, China
e-mail: zhenghyjl@163.com

H. Zheng
Civil and Business Law, Jilin University, Changchun, China

aim for application-oriented talents and strengthening practice teaching shall be taken as a breakthrough for its characteristic education.

317.2 Definition of Practice Teaching of Law and Main Teaching Methods

I rather agree with such a definition: practice teaching of law means teaching methods and concept consisting of concrete practice teaching in order to strengthen practicality and opening of law education, pay attention to cultivate legal and moral quality and law professional ability [2].

Methods mainly include: case teaching, court demonstration, moot court teaching, legal consultation, social investigation, legal clinic teaching, specialized probation, graduation practice and thesis and so on.

317.3 Present Condition of Practice Teaching of Law in the Provincial Institutions of Higher Learning

For cognition on importance of practice teaching of law, theorists have gotten to a common view presently. For various reasons, its development still has great differences.

Through investigation on practice teaching of law in more than ten institutions of Jilin Province, I found all of them adopted common mode in a way, but their forms were so simple and contents were so scattered. It still becomes a mere formality. The actual reasons are mainly listed as follows.

317.3.1 Mode of Practice Teaching of Law is Absent of Comprehensive Planning and is Not Integrated and is Immethodical

Currently, universal problem with establishment of practice course of law is lack of systematic training for students' vocational skills. There are not systematic cultivation plan, practice teaching program and materials in most of the provincial institutions of higher learning. Establishment and order of course and distribution of hours are all random.

317.3.2 Practice Teaching of Law is Lack of Evaluation System and Current Practice Teaching Shows a Mere Formality

Presently, for law majors, there are not concrete demands on date, times, contents, results of practice teaching that students participate in, also specific assessment standard are not set up, which make practice teaching just a formality.

317.3.3 Teachers that are Competent at Practice Teaching of Law are Limited

Teachers are direct implementers of teaching affairs of which ability for teaching will directly have a bearing on teaching quality and further impact quality of students that are brought up [3]. And yet now most teachers who are engaged in law teaching teach at school as soon as they graduated, they are usually short of judicial practical experiences which indicates practice teaching of law is an armchair strategist.

317.3.4 Investment in Practice Teaching of Law is Not Enough and Environment to Develop Practice Teaching is Poor

At present, many provincial institutions are short of teaching funds and investment in practice teaching is not enough, which make part of practice activities cannot be developed. The actualities restrict formation and development of diversified practice teaching of law.

317.4 Way to Raise Quality of Practice Teaching of Law in the Provincial Institutions of Higher Learning

317.4.1 Normalized Management of Practice Teaching of Law Will be Realized Gradually

To be specific, it is mainly indicated as follows:
Firstly, to lay down a ripe cultivation plan for practice teaching of law, I think cultivation plan for practice teaching of law shall be made of three modules. The first is basic ability module. The second is key ability module. The third is innovative

ability module. Specifically, skill cultivation of law shall be conducted ceaselessly for 4 years. Basic skill cultivation shall be emphasized in Grade 1 and Grade 2. Cultivation of key and innovative ability is stressed in Grade 3 and Grade 4.

Secondly, to institute a practice teaching program with theory teaching to science, on three modules requirements, practice teaching program shall arrange course hours scientifically, specify teaching aim and task and further define teachers' responsibilities, which will make each practice teaching connect with theory teaching, mode that theory and practice go side by side will be established.

Thirdly, to strengthen construction of practice teaching materials of law, law institutions may organize teachers to compile practice teaching materials with external senior lawyers, lawyers according to characteristic of practice. The teaching materials shall accord with three modules requirements and comply with teaching program.

317.4.2 To Establish and Improve Evaluation System of Practice Teaching of Law

We should build a relatively independent evaluation system equivalent to traditional theory teaching, separate practice teaching from general theoretical teaching, calculate credits and hours independently, thus deserved status of practice teaching of law could be ensured and sequence of practice teaching be stabilized and final aim for practice teaching be accomplished [4].

317.4.3 To Strengthen Construction of Double-Type Teachers Team

So-called double-type teachers are that they master in not only law theories but also law practice. This requires that provincial institutions of higher learning must keep their eyes open for double-type teachers when they bring in teachers; furthermore, training on the original teachers shall be strengthened. Teachers may be appointed to departments of legal practice for practice exercises; justicers, procurators can be employed to teach practice course.

317.4.4 To Increase Investment in Practice Teaching of Law and Build Convenient and Practical Bases for Practice Teaching

Firstly, our state finance shall establish special appropriate to base construction of practice teaching of law, and provincial institutions are required to provide relevant funds according to proportion for construction of practice base in school.

Secondly, school shall actively contact all departments of legal practice, sign agreement on construction of actual training base with them and build bases for practice teaching of law outside school.

317.5 Conclusion

Law undergraduate education in China undertakes dual task of quality and vocational education. Key to accomplish the dual task is to develop practice teaching of law, to combine practice teaching with theory teaching effectively, to train students for application-oriented law practitioners with good grounding, broad view and high quality that will satisfy the needs of market economics and legal system construction.

Acknowledgments The thesis is a research result of major teaching and research project of Beihua University "research on practice teaching of law" and a result of staged research on Education and Scientific Research Project (GH12063) of Jilin Province Education and Science Research Leading Group.

References

1. China Law Society (2011) Annual Report on China's Judicial Construction
2. Shao W (2008) Construction and operation of system of practice teaching of law undergraduate education of in china. Shandong Normal University, Jinan, 8
3. Gu Y (2011) Research and practice of system of practice teaching of law. Higher Corres J (Philosophy, Society, and Science Edition) 12:12
4. Li K, Zhao Q (2001) Difficulty and way out for practice teaching of law in the local instituions of higher learning. Legal Syst Soc 2: 225–227

Chapter 318
Path Selection for Practice Teaching of Law in Institutions of Higher Learning

Rongxia Zhang

Abstract Law education is a type of vocational education, so practice teaching link must be adopted correctly. In recent years, practice teaching of law in our institutions of higher learning has been paid more attention and some good achievements have been obtained, but there are still so many problems. To bring practice teaching into full play in law education, teaching concept must be changed on the basis of present condition of law education: a reasonable curriculum system for practice teaching must be set up, practice teaching mode of law applicable to Chinese actual conditions must be created and quantification index in the light of each practice teaching link must be concretely worked out. By using information technology, management system for practice teaching of law shall be perfected and scientific assessment evaluation system shall be formulated; practical ability of teachers from institutions of higher learning shall be enhanced to provide practice teaching with qualified teaching faculty.

Keywords Law education · Practice teaching · Path selection

318.1 Introduction

Development of market economy and construction of legal society make a real demand on training of application-oriented law personnel with high quality, which decides that nowadays aim for law personnel training in institutions of higher learning should be oriented towards society and practice. However, general observation on status quo of law education in China, practice teaching link is seriously deficient and systematic practice teaching can not be established, which

R. Zhang (✉)
Jilin University, Changchun, China
e-mail: zhangrx55@163.com

made that student could not fit in with the needs of practice work at all after they graduated from school. So it is a very important task for present law education to strengthen our law practice in institutions of higher learning in China and it has become imperative to establish a feasible system for practice teaching.

318.2 Connotation of Practice Teaching of Law in Institutions of Higher Learning

Practice teaching of law is object to theoretical teaching of law in concept. Generally thinking, practice teaching means that teaching link is specially offered to support theoretical teaching of law and to foster students to analyze and solve problems and to intensify training of law practice ability of students. Its connotation is so rich, mainly covers the following listed from viewpoint of type: in-class and outside-class practice teaching link. For the former, for example, mock teaching such as classroom case discussion, debating, moot court and so on are made subject to different courses; for the latter, varieties of opportunities to practice are given to the students that they could unite theory with practice, for instance, applied teaching such as cognition practice, graduation practice that students are organized to participate in and practice activities such as law aid and law clinic that students are specially arranged to attend combining with law science characteristic [1]. A complete recognition on concept of practice teaching of law in institutions of higher learning presently has not come into being in China, some practice teaching links were established by institutions of higher learning according to its own actual situation, in general, the development is greatly lack of balance.

318.3 Problems Existing in Practice Teaching of Law in Our Institutions of Higher Learning

Although practice teaching of law in institutions of higher learning certainly has been taken seriously in recent years, most of the law schools and departments increased practice teaching link and achieved an effect in varying degrees. All in all, there are still a series of problems in current practice teaching of law. For example, Position of aim for law education is not definite; Practice teaching link of law is lack of systematicness and standardization; Management system for practice teaching of law is not perfect and is short of scientific evaluation system; Condition backing to practice teaching of law is not enough.

318.4 Path Selection for Practice Teaching of Law in Our Institutions of Higher Learning

In view of existing problems in practice teaching of law in our institutions of higher learning, some train of thoughts are put forward to improve further development of practice teaching link of law in our institutions of higher education, and aim for law education will be realized ultimately.

318.4.1 To Define Aim for Law Education and to Change Teaching Concept

Aim for law education personnel training shall be various. Among law majors, some of them may be lawyers, judges, prosecuting attorneys and part of them may be engaged in theoretical research, and some of them will work at government authorities, cultural organizations or company enterprises in charge of direct or indirect work concerning law affairs [2]. So, "prominent tendency for law education shall be placed on professional law education, basic occupational education and application-oriented personnel mode" [3]. Law education is also a type of vocational education, so training aim for law education that we must make clear is to foster high quality application-oriented law personnel with professional law theory and vocational skills. On the one hand, importance of practice teaching of law must be completely realized and change from overweight theoretical teaching to having practice teaching treasured will be achieved gradually. On the other hand, students are the principal part in practice teaching that shall be specified and practical ability to analyze and solve problems of students shall be fostered and enhanced. During all practical trainings, transformation from teaching mode that teachers are the main body to teaching mode that students are the main part will be realized to make students change from receiving listeners to active behavior subjects.

318.4.2 To Set Up Reasonable System for Practice Teaching of Law

318.4.2.1 To Set Up a Reasonable Curriculum System for Practice Teaching

To cultivate students' practical ability and to advance law practical skills are mostly determined by design and concrete implementation of curriculum system for practice teaching of law. As a result, the first task is to draw up a systematic workable plan for practice teaching to develop practice teaching of law, varieties of practice teaching courses will be established reasonably and practice teaching shall be forcibly entered in teaching program. Teaching materials applicable to practice teaching shall be planed and constructed, teaching content, teaching aim and teaching plan shall be specified to make practice teaching systematize and standardize. It is very necessary to set up a curriculum system for practice teaching of law that will give so much importance to practice teaching and to enter law practice in teaching program, which could strengthen the understanding of the importance of practice and guarantee the quality of practice teaching activities of law.

318.4.2.2 To Work Out Quantification Index in the Light of Each Practice Teaching Link

We take law clinic course as cardinal line, social practice as foundation, and establish practice mode that court auditing, practice with law affairs departments, law aid and moot court, three-gradation cultivation mode of practice teaching will be worked up progressively. The 1st gradation, in grade 1 and grade 2, on the basis of theoretical knowledge of law, case teaching and others as approaches, combining means such as court auditing and probation, students' legal consciousness and perceptual knowledge of law will be fostered; the 2nd gradation, in grade 2 and grade 3, through moot court, law clinic course, experimental teaching is carried out to train students' professional ability; the 3rd gradation, in grade 3 and grade 4, for the duration of holiday practice, students will participate in law aid activities to improve thought and communication skills of students and to build sense of social responsibility and enterprise of students. By such three-gradation cultivation mode of practice teaching, combining inside school with outside school, long term with short term, practical law affairs with legal business training, students' association with vocational study are achieved and a plat will be built for students to study law during practice [4].

318.4.2.3 To Work Out Quantification Index in the Light of Each Practice Teaching Link

In order to really ensure hours and quality that students attend practical activities, it is necessary to draw up a rather reasonable system for practice teaching of law and lay down a series of evaluation index, which requires specific quantification index shall be worked out in the light of each practice teaching link, for instance, moot court teaching credits, practice teaching hours, evaluation items and evaluation grading standard and so on shall be quantified to make practice teaching of law evaluable and then aim for enhancing students' practical skills will be accomplished finally.

318.4.3 To Perfect Management System for Practice Teaching of Law and to Formulate Scientific Assessment Evaluation System by Using Information Technology

318.4.3.1 To Perfect Management System for Practice Teaching of Law

All regulations and rules on management of practice teaching of law shall be established and improved, system for stimulation and restriction on practice teaching teachers shall be built by schools to motivate teachers and students to take part in practice teaching. To energize the administration on each practice teaching link to ensure stable order of practice teaching and to advance quality of practice teaching of law. Furthermore, during practice teaching management, the advantage of information technology is fully utilized to establish scientific management system and thus modernization of practice teaching management of law will be accomplished.

318.4.3.2 To Formulate Scientific Assessment Evaluation System for Practice Teaching of Law

Whether assessment evaluation system for practice teaching is scientific or not determines quality control and quality security of practice teaching, so building of evaluation system for practice teaching must be scientific, reasonable and feasible and the system must be overall and objective, not only covers methods of evaluation on teachers but also standard of evaluation on students, furthermore, includes evaluation index such as whether establishment of practice teaching course is reasonable or not, operation is orderly or not, etc. We can make full use of modern information technology to formulate assessment evaluation system, and will achieve enhancement of effect on practice teaching on this account. For evaluation check on teachers, performance shall be the criterion on which title promotion and allowances are based to motivate enthusiasm in practice teaching. Especially for assessment on students' participation in practice teaching, quantified assessment shall be carried out, for example, it shall be stipulated that students have a not less than 2 months cognition practice each year and practice report must be completed with evaluation achievement, etc. by faculty advisor to ensure hours and effect what students participate in practice teaching.

318.4.4 To Increase Investment and to Build Supporting System for Practice Teaching

Smooth development of practice teaching of law needs support and coordination given by us in many ways. Comparing with class teaching, practice teaching has a higher demand on venue condition, faculty advisor team, equipment and so on. To enhance quality of practice teaching must entirely depend on laboratory, laboratory equipment, practice base, specialized practice teaching instructor, moot court and adequate funds, etc. that are perfect. Firstly, capital investment in practice teaching of law shall be increased to provide stable material security for practice teaching. Secondly, a steady practice base shall be built to guarantee that practice teaching link is developed smoothly. Thirdly, to enhance practical ability of teachers from institutions of higher education provides qualified teachers for practice teaching.

318.5 Conclusion

To sum up, we should squarely face the problems that arise in law education in institutions of higher learning. While traditional theoretical instruction is given to students, practice teaching link is developed and reform of law education is promoted actively, thus aim for law practitioners training that satisfy the needs of the society is realized finally.

Acknowledgments The thesis is a result of staged research of education and scientific research project of Jilin Province Education and Scientific Research Leading Group "Research on Building and Operation of Practice Teaching of Undergraduate Law Education in the Provincial Institutions of Higher Learning" (Project No. GH12063) and a research result of major teaching and research project of Beihua University "research on practice teaching of law".

References

1. Lei Y, Sun S (2007) Necessity and connotation of practice teaching of law in institutions of higher learning. Educ Prof (32):157
2. Huo X (2005) Rethinking the positioning of legal education. Law Educ (2):4
3. Jun S (2004) Research on aim and mode of personnel training of law education in institutions of higher learning at the new period. Law Rev (5):148
4. Shao W (2011) Building and operation of practice teaching of undergraduate law education. Chin Adult Educ (8):124

Chapter 319
Inhibition Effects of Celery Seed Extract on Human Stomach Cancer Cell Lines Hs746T

Lin-Lin Gao, Chang-Xiang Zhou, Xiu-Feng Song, Ke-Wei Fan and Fu-Rong Li

Abstract The inhibition of tumor cell growth without toxicity in normal cells has attracted attention as an important target in cancer therapy. As a food and drug, Celery Seed Extract (CSE) has been shown its anti-tumour effect by inhibition of tumor promotion and inducement of tumor cell apoptosis, but its mechanism and relation with the expression of gap junction protein is still not well known. The present study was designed to evaluate the relationship between inhibition of expression of gap junction protein Connexin 43 (Cx43) and anti-tumor effect of CSE on human stomach cancer cell lines Hs746T. Methods: The human stomach cancer cell line Hs746T was used in the study. The effects of CSE on Connexin 43 were examined by RT-PCR, western blot and immunofluorescence; cell growth and proliferation was examined by the 3-(4,5-dimethylthiazol-2-yl)-2,5-diphenyl-tetrazolium bromide (MTT) assay; cell apoptosis was determined by apoptosis related protein bcl-2 and bax. Results: CSE inhibited the growth and proliferation on Hs746T; CSE increased the expression of Cx43 mRNA and protein; CSE decreased Bcl-2 and increased Bax on Hs746T cells. Conclusion: This study firstly shows that CSE can increase Cx43 expression in mRNA and protein level, and exerts its anti-tumour effects on stomach cancer Hs746T cells via inhibiting cell proliferation and inducing cell apoptosis.

Keywords Celery seed extract · Connexin 43 · Apoptosis · Tumour · Proliferation

There is significant evidence that GJIC is important in at least some prodrug/suicide gene systems by augmenting the bystander effect (BE). GJIC is made up of connexins (Cxs), among which Cx43 is present in most tissues. Stomach cancer is one of the most frequent digestive system cancers and the leading cause of death among malignancies in most of country in the world [1]. Recent evidence suggests

L.-L. Gao (✉) · C.-X. Zhou · X.-F. Song · K.-W. Fan · F.-R. Li
Atherosclerosis Institute, Department of Pathology and Pathophysiology, Taishan Medical University, Taian, People's Republic of China
e-mail: dejia99@126.com

that apoptosis of cells is closely related to the occurrence, progress and metastasis of tumors [2]. Study of the mechanisms of apoptosis in tumor cells is an important field of tumor therapy and molecular cancer biology [3, 4]. Celery or Apium graveolens L (Fam. Umbelliferae), is widely grown in the temperate zone as a garden crop, and its leaf stalks are used as a popular vegetable in most of Asian countries and extract of celery has been recommended in Chinese herbal medicine as a remedy for hypertension and the "cleansing" of blood [5]. Gap-junctional intercellular communication (GJIC) is an important mode for cell-to-cell communication. Dysfunctional GJIC is exhibited in most cancer cells. GJIC is made up of connexins (Cxs), among which Cx43 is present in most tissues [6]. Most of cancer cell express low level of Cx43 and the restoration of the Cx43 can significantly inhibit the tumor cell growth and proliferation. Therefore Cx43 is a potential target for cancer therapy. The present study shows that CSE can increase Cx43 and inhibit the growth and proliferation partly by the reduction of Bcl-2 and increase Bax on human stomach cancer cell lines Hs746T.

319.1 Meterials and Methods

319.1.1 Reagents and Chemicals

RPMI-1640 medium, fetal calf serum and trypsogen were purchased from GIBCO (Canada). 3-(4,5-dimethylthiazol-2yl)-2,5-diphenyl tetrazolium bromide (MTT), penicillin, streptomycin, and trypsin were purchased from Amresco Chemical Co. Ltd. (USA). Propidium iodide (PI) was purchased from Sigma (USA). The Annexin V/PI-FITC apoptosis detection kit was purchased from BD Biosciences (USA). The primary antibodies for Bcl-2, Bax, β-actin and the secondary antibody were acquired from Cell Signaling Technology (USA), and all chemicals were of analytical grade and were obtained from Tianjin Chemical Reagents Co. Ltd. (Tianjin, China).

319.1.1.1 Preparation of Celery Seed Extract

The supercritical fluid extraction (SFE), was scaled-up 100-fold using a preparative HA221-50-06 SFE system (SITEC Co. Ltd., Switzerland). A 350 g amount of sample was placed in the extraction vessel with a 1,000 mL capacity, and extracted statically for 1.5 h and then dynamic extraction for 2.5 h by flowing liquid CO_2 at a rate of 40 L h-1. The pressure and temperature in the extraction vessel was 25 MPa and 45 °C respectively, and which changed to 6 MPa and 35 °C in the separate vessel. The extract in supercritical fluid was depressed directly into separate vessels. The crude extract obtained was brown grease and some semisolid (98 g). This extracts were named CSE and dissolved in RPMI 1640 medium in the required amount stored in a refrigerator at 4 °C until used.

319.1.1.2 Cell Cultures

Cells were obtained from the Chinese Type Culture Collection (Shanghai Institute of Cell Biology, Chinese Academy of Science, Shanghai, China), cultured in RPMI 1640 medium supplemented with 10 % heat-inactivated fetal bovine serum, penicillin (100 U/mL) and streptomycin (100 μg/mL) at 37 °C in a humidified atmosphere of 95 % air and 5 % CO_2; the medium was changed every other day. When the cultures were 75–90 % confluent, the Hs746T cells were collected and re-plated onto 96- or 24-well plates at an appropriate density according to experiment.

319.1.1.3 MTT Assay

Cell viability was measured using the MTT assay, Confluent cells were treated with various concentrations of CSE or vehicle for 24 h. The cells was incubated for 4 h 37 °C in fresh serum-free RPMI-1640 medium, which contained MTT at a final concentration of 0.5 mg/ml, then cells from each well were solubilized with 100 μl DMSO for optical density reading at 570 nm. Cell viability was expressed as the percentage of MTT counts of treated cells relative to those of the control (% of control).

319.1.1.4 Reverse Transcription PCR

Expression of the Cx43 gene in the Hs746T cells was measured by a reverse transcription-polymerase chain reaction (RT-PCR) assay. Total RNA was extracted from the Hs746T cells with a TRIZOL reagent (Invitrogen) according to the manufacturer instruction. Synthesis of cDNA from mRNA transcript was performed with Reverse transcriptional kit (TAKARA, Shimon-Ku, Japan). The PCR reactions of Cx43 (primer forward 5-GATGAGGAAGGAAGAGAAGC -3, reverse 5- TTGTTTCT-GTCACCAGTAAC-3) and $β$-actin (primer forward 5- ′ GATGCA-GAA GGAGATCACTG -3, reverse 5- GGGTGT AACGCAACTAAGTC-3′, consisted of a hot start (5 min at 94 °C), 35 cycles of 30 s at 94 °C, 30 s at 55 °C, and 40 s at 72 °C, followed by final extension step at 72 °C for 10 min.

319.1.1.5 Western Blot

Cells were rinsed once with PBS and then scraped off with lysis buffer (Pierce, USA), added protease inhibitor cocktail tablets (Roche, Switzerland). Total protein concentrations were determined using the Bicinchoninic Acid (BCA) Protein Assay Kit (Pierce, USA). Primary antibody Cx43, Bcl-2, Bax and tubulin are pursued from (Santa Cruz, CA, USA). Western blot analysis was carried out as described previously.

319.1.1.6 Immunofluorescence Staining

Cells were plated on glass slides in the 24-well plates. When cells reached 50 % confluence, they were treated with 0.1 % DMSO (V/V) vehicle control for 24 h. The Cells were fixed with 4 % paraformaldehyde and permeabilized with 1 % Triton X-100. Then blocked with 10 % goat serum, the cells were reacted with anti-mouse monoclonal Cx43 antibody followed by FITC-conjugated goat anti-mouse antibody (Sigma, USA) diluted in PBS-Evans blue. Fluorescence was visualized using fluorescent microscope.

319.1.1.7 Statistical Analysis

All experiments were repeated at least three times. The values reported the mean of triplicates (±SD). Statistical analysis was performed using the statistical software package SPSS 13.0 (SPSS). A p–value of 0.05 (two-sided) was considered statistically significant.

319.1.2 Result

319.1.2.1 Cytotoxic Activity of CSE on Hs746T Cells

The cytotoxic activity of CSE was evaluated in the Hs746T cells. As a test to confirm the cytotoxicity of CSE, the cells were treated with (0 ∼ 500 μg/ml) of CSE. The Hs746T cells were incubated with CSE, and their morphological alterations were verified via a phase- contrast microscope. After 24 h of incubation with various concentrations of CSE, many cells exhibited cytoplasmic shrinkage, and either detached from each other or floated in the medium. In order to clarify these results further, we performed the MTT assay. The cell viability of Hs746T cells treated with 50, 100 and 300 μg/ml CSE for 24 h decreased in a dosed dependent manner (Fig. 319.1). The highest inhibition in this study was determined as 23.1 % at a concent ration of 300 μg/ml of URE, whereas cells treated with CSE exhibited neither cytoplasmic shrinkage nor either detached from each other, under a phase contrast microscope.

319.1.2.2 CSE Induce Cx43 Expression

As showed previously, CSE inhibited the Hs746T cells growth and proliferation, however the mechanism of the CSE anti-cancerous effect was not clear. Most of the gastric cancer cell lines have low level of Cx43. Hs746T cells are highly metastatic human gastric cancer cell line, which express barely detected level of Cx43 and do not form functional gap junction. We used it as a model to test

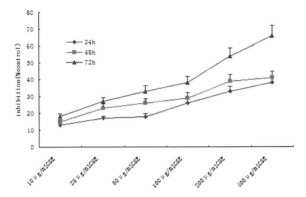

Fig. 319.1 CSE inhibited the viability of Hs746T cells. Hs746T cells were treated with CSE at the indicated concentrations for 0-72 h. Cell viability was then determined by MTT assay and expressed as the mean ±SD, n = 3. The OD value at 570 nm is proportional to the number of cells with CSE

whether CSE induced the Cx43 expression and displayed anticancer effect. According the MTT assay results, Three different concentrations of CSE were selected to treat the Hs746T cells. Semi-quantitative RT-PCR (Fig. 319.2), Western blot analysis and immunofluorescence (date not show) revealed an increase in endogenous Cx43 mRNA and protein expression following by CSE treatment, especially on 25 μg/ml CSE. However higher concentration of CSE, such as 100 μg/ml, did not induce higher level of Cx43 (data not show).

319.1.2.3 CSE Down-Regulate Bcl-2 and Up-Regulate Bax Expression

Now CSE upregulated the Cx43 mRNA and decreased the cell survival on Hs746T cells. We next detected the anti-apoptotic and pro-apoptotic family member Bcl-2 and Bax, to figure out whether it was involved in apoptotic pathway. We examined the Bcl-2 and Bax protein following the CSE treatment on Hs746T cells by Western blotting. The result showed that CSE treatment decrease the Bcl-2 level, especially on 100 μg/ml, and stable express of Cx43 gene on Hs746T cells showed the similar result (Fig. 319.3); We also found that apoptotic protein Bax exhibited the inversed result (Fig. 319.3), which showed that Bcl-2 and Bax played an important role on the CSE involved anticancer effect in Hs746T cells.

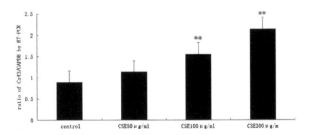

Fig. 319.2 CSE induced Cx43 mRNA and protein expression on Hs746T cells. * $P < 0.05$ versus vehicle treated and ** $P < 0.01$ versus vehicle treated

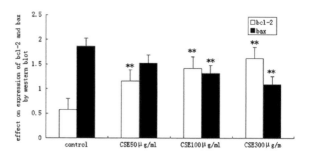

Fig. 319.3 CSE treatment down-regulated Bcl-2 and upregulated Bax expression. * $P < 0.05$ versus vehicle treated and ** $P < 0.01$ versus vehicle treated

319.1.3 Descussion

It has been shown that normal human gastric tissue express Cx43 and Cx26 [7]. Here, we have shown that the gastric slightly expressed Cx43 (Fig. 319.3). However, most of the other normal cell lines exhibit low or no expression of Cx43 and Cx26. The mechanisms by which the expression of a Connexin gene in tumors are not known. The attempts to determine whether specific mutations of Connexin genes occur in tumors have failed, suggesting that other mechanisms regulating Connexin expression are involved. RT-PCR analysis indicated that this regulation was at the transcriptional level, because no Cx43mRNA was detected in some other cell lines. So far, the underlying mechanisms of the pharmacological effect of celery seed in cancer therapy have been unclear, and this study examined the effect of CSE and its underlying mechanisms on inhibition of tumor cell proliferation. In the present study, CSE also has been shown to inhibit the growth on human gastric cancer Hs746T cells. However, the antitumor effects of CSE on gastric cancer cells through gap junctional mechanism have not been investigated. This study provides the first evidence that CSE induces the Cx43 mRNA and protein expression and exhibits its growth inhibition on Hs746T cells.

Most of the gastric cancer cell is lost or impaired of Connexins comparing with the normal gastric epithelial cell, which suggest that the Connexins is related to the gastric carcinogenesis. Some studys also showed that Connexins is involved in the gastric cancer progression [8]. The raise of Connexins can inhibit the growth of gastric cancer cells and have the synthesis effects of chemical treatments. A number of studies showed that Connexins can exert its anti-tumor effects by forming gap junctional intercellular communication (GJIC), therefore increase Connexins and improved GJIC may establish a new, effective therapy for gastric cancer [9]. However, transfection of Cx43 gene into gastric cancer Hs746T cells reversed the transformed phenotype without enhancing the activity of GJIC, which suggest that independent function of Connexins also play an important role on cell growth, tumorigenicity and differentiation.

Most previous studies on the relationship between GJIC and carcinogenesis have been carried out with experimental model systems, in which an inverse relationship between the levels of GJIC and the expression of transformed phenotypes was often observed [10]. In human carcinogenesis, such a good correlation is not generally found. Gastric cancer Hs746T cells expressed low levels of Cx43 which were used as the model to examine the effects of CSE on Cx43 by RT-PCR, western blot and immunofluorescence. The data showed that CSE induced Cx43 expression either in mRNA or in protein level, and both stable expression also had growth suppressive effect on Hs746T cells. Thus Cx43 played an important role on CSE induced growth control. It has been reported [11] that clinicopathologic outcome of abnormal expression of Cx43 showed prognostic significance in human gastric squamous cell carcinoma, in accord with this study which Hs746T cell displayed a upregulation of Cx43 by the treatment of CSE. The results showed that CSE induced the expression of Cx43 on Hs746T cell, and Cx43 is contributed to the anti-tumor effect of CSE.

Apoptosis plays a critical role in embryogenesis, carcinogenesis and virally infected cell death. And in this study, in order to determine whether the cytotoxic activity of CSE was due to apoptosis, the Hs746Tcells were treated for 24 h with various concentrations of CSE. We also conducted Western blot analysis in order to determine the level of the bcl-2 and Bax, two important hallmark of apoptosis. CSE displayed the inhibition in growth and proliferation on Hs746T cells. Bcl-2 family member Bcl-2 and Bax were involved in the apoptosis induced by CSE of Hs746T cell. Interestingly, previous studies showed that Cx43 served as an anti-tumor gene, one of the mechanism was that it could reduce the Bcl-2. The data showed that CSE treatment not only decreased the Bcl-2, increased Bax, but also had growth inhibition by exogenous expression of Cx43 in Hs746T cell. The results indicated that the anti-proliferative effect of CSE on Hs746T cells was attributable to apoptosis associated with Bcl-2 family activation.

Therefore, our results suggest that CSE can increase the Cx43 gene expression, this cell growth inhibition partly by the reduction of Bcl-2 and increase of Bax. However the mechanism which CSE elicits Cx43 upregulation is still unclear, further research will be needed.

Acknowledgments This research was financially supported by the Department of Education of Shandong Province (No J12LM02) and Plan Projects of Taian Science and Technology Bureau (No 20113024).

References

1. Jemal A, Siegel R, Xu J et al (2010) Cancer statistics, 2010. CA Cancer J Clin 60:277–300
2. Hung JH, Lu YS, Wang YC et al (2008) FTY720 induces apoptosis in hepatocellular carcinoma cells through activation of protein kinase c signaling. Cancer Res 68:1204–1212
3. Zhang Y, Chen AY, Li M et al (2008) Ginkgo biloba extract kaempferol inhibits cell proliferation and induces apoptosis in pancreatic cancer cells. J Surg Res 148:17–23
4. Decrock E, Vinken M, De Vuyst E et al (2009) Connexin-related signaling in cell death: to live or let die? Cell Death Differ 16:524–536
5. Chang CY, Huang ZN, Yu HH et al (2008) The adjuvant effects of Antrodia camphorate extracts combined with anti-tumor agents on multidrug resistant human hepatoma cells. J Ethnopharmacol 118:387–395

6. Decrock E, Vinken M, De Vuyst E et al (2009) Connexin-related signaling in cell death: to live or let die? Cell Death Differ 16:524–536
7. Boban M, Ljubicic N, Nikolic M et al (2011) Lack of prognostic significance of connexin-43 labeling in a series of 46 gastrointestinal stromal tumors. Int J Biol Markers 26:124–128
8. Loncarek Jadranka, Yamasaki Hiroshi, Levillain Pierre et al (2003) The expression of the tumor suppressor gene Connexin 26 is not mediated by methylation in human esophageal cancer cells. Mol Carcinog 36:74–81
9. Oyamada M, Oyamada Y, Takamatsu T (2005) Regulation of expression. Biochim Biophys Acta 1719:6–23
10. LiuY, Zhang X, Li ZJ et al (2010) Up-regulation of Cx43 expression and GJIC function in acute leukemia bone marrow stromal cells post-chemotherapy. Leuk Res. 34:631–640
11. Hirschi KK, Xu C, Tsukamoto T (1996) Gap junction genes Cx26 and Cx43 individually suppress the cancer phenotype of human mammary carcinoma cells and restore differential potential. Cell Growth Differ 7:861–870

Chapter 320
Research on the Practice of Teaching Auto Selective Course While China Stepping into Automobile Society

Zhang Tiejun and Guan Ying

Abstract With China's rapid evolution into car society, environmental and social problems with traffic in the city are concerned by people. For lack of car culture in China in compared with U.S., it has practical significance to publicize and popularize the knowledge of car among the undergraduate students major in non-vehicle engineering. These subsistent problems were analyzed and discussed, the author put forward some countermeasure and advices, and also the selective course "car and her culture" for students, which intended to educate them about the negative impact of cars on quality of life and on the environment. According to the objective need combined years of teaching experience, the authors present the main teaching contents and ideas, programs of instruction and innovated teaching mode of this course. Then lists out the teaching guidelines, put it into teaching practice by means of multimedia, internet and campus car culture festival etc. It has obtained good teaching and practice effect. Meanwhile, it can enhance the students learn cars comprehensive knowledge and broaden their horizons.

Keywords Car society · Car culture · Selective course · Education

320.1 Introduction

The love affair with the automobile is not purely an American phenomenon. Across the world, consumers are racing to buy more and bigger cars. Between 2000 and 2009, car sales went up ninefold in China. China surpassed the United State to take the first place among auto sale and manufacturer nations, which has advanced 9–10 years than our expectations. By the end of last year, the auto

Z. Tiejun · G. Ying (✉)
Chongqing University of Arts and Sciences, 402160 Chongqing, China
e-mail: ztj1965@tsinghua.org.cn

production and sale is more than 19 million vehicles and the total number of civil motor vehicles had reached 120 million, which have risen to the second place in the world. Now, the country sees 1,000 new cars on its streets every day.

According to the international standard, if 20 % family owns car in one country, this country will step into auto society. The newest statistics this year showed that China has entered a car society. Car culture was born in the United States long long time ago, in 1976 a professor from MIT has written a book "car culture" and 1990 another book "the machine that changed the world" was published, In no other country does the automobile have sway over the national psyche. But are we prepared in mind by now? The first quarter of this year, private car owners broke 1 billion, and at this rate, 10 years later, 60 % family will have cars in China.

320.2 The Situations of Traffic and Environments

Nowadays, China is facing the most serious new crisis car culture deprivation. So, the author put forward the selective course "the auto and her culture" for students, and enhancing to promote competence education for car culture. It caters to quality education for auto society and should be and has been greatly promoted. With the coming of auto society, a series of problems appears in bigger cities in China. For example, traffic jam, poor oil standard with too much sulphur in it, haze weather, high traffic accident death rate, less dominant public transport systems, official cars abuse and the excessive reliance on private cars, parking area, street and road downtown are becoming very crowd, petroleum resources limited so on. How to solve the development China car social damage to the environment, imperfect traffic management and weak awareness of safety, it is all must face the challenge. There is a serious need for top-down design for China car society the government, the public and the environmentalists [1, 2].

320.2.1 The Situations in Chinese Big Cities

The auto industry in Chongqing keeps ahead in China. Last year, cars made in Chongiqng were sold 11.4 vehicles per minute. Too many cars have created a lot of serious problems in our city. Besides congestion, accidents and fast fuel consumption, cars are responsible for a good part of air pollution with a speed from 18 to 23 km/h during rush hours. All the time, they are pumping huge amounts of waste gases into the atmosphere. These gases are very harmful, causing disease and even death [3].

In China big cities, such as Beijing (the No.1 Blocking), Chongqing became "the No.1 Blocking" in the southwest of China. The public is puzzled by parking, traffic jam car accident-prone, high levels of PM2.5 and other car negative issues.

Therefore, elementary auto training system and related courses setting must be developed to publicize and popularize the knowledge of automobile to eliminate "illiterates and semi-illiterates" citizens on car.

320.2.2 Air Pollution, Car Problem and Some Countermeasure

Air pollution and problems with urban commuting are of great concern to people today. European surveys have shown that over six people in ten say that traffic in the city is unbearable. Nine out of ten people believe that increasing public transport is a priority in combating air pollution and seven out of ten say they support a ban on car traffic in the centre of cities on certain days. However, at the same time, the number of cars and urban traffic is constantly increasing, eroding the quality of life of urban dwellers with the increase in air pollution, stress, etc.

One possible solution is to design and develop clean cars and clean fuels. In Chongqing, some of the public buses begin to run on natural gas, which does not give off as much carbon dioxide as the petrol. But it may take years for the new models of clean cars completely replace the traditional ones. Another solution is to develop modern public transportation systems and restrict the use of private cars. If the price of petrol rises constantly and the public vehicles are efficient and convenient enough, most people will not buy private cars. And the total number of cars in big cities will reduce greatly. On the whole, the elimination of air pollution needs the collective efforts from the government, the public and the environmentalists [4]. It is high time to we had new urban planning top-down designed, developed countries also provided us successful experience for reference, such as introduction of high-rise automatic parking garage in Germany.

320.2.3 Environmentally Urban Transport Experiences

In European countries, Car Free Day is an international festival of environmentally sensitive transport. The day is part of an approach aimed at reclaiming cities and represents an important chance for dialogue. It focuses on raising the awareness of urban dwellers with respect to nuisances caused by the use of private cars in the city (air pollution, noise, etc.). It also stresses the rights of pedestrians and cyclists, the need for more and better public transport, and helps people rediscover their local architectural heritage. The idea is to reconsider urban transport with the prospect of sharing streets more efficiently. Over 2,000 towns and cities around the world are taking part in this activity.

320.3 China's Unhealthy and Unhappy Car Culture

For many Chinese people, owning a car has become a symbol of success and of personal freedom. We would never argue that private cars don't provide a measure of convenience and control over one's daily life. More importantly, the spike in car ownership is not simply a response to underserved transportation needs. Car ownership is also a status symbol for the new capitalist class. For example, sales of SUVs went up by 40 %. Size matters. People want to have a car that shows off their status in society. No one wants to buy small. Luxury producers such as Rolls-Royce, say sales to China's new rich are soaring.

While automobiles are a critical part of any transportation system, car culture makes it difficult to create sustainable urban transport. When consumer demand calls for size and horsepower—not mobility or sustainability—fuel efficiency is quickly sacrificed. Moreover, when cars become so culturally valued, rather than simply functionally important, necessary reforms for sustainable transport become difficult. Reclaiming space from cars for bicycles, buses or pedestrians, for example, incurs predictable complaints from car drivers who feel that their mode of transportation is specially privileged over all others.

Cars are heavy polluters, spewing both greenhouse gases and local particulate pollution into the air. Car accidents are also major causes of death in China. In 2011, there were more than 60,000 traffic-related fatalities with 9.8 million cars on the road.

Let's start with the basics: traffic. Take Beijing as an example. Much of Beijing was built before the massive explosion of private car ownership, with street area ratio less than 25 %. The infrastructure is simply not designed to carry as many as more than 5.19 million vehicles are present today, leading to average car speed of 20 km/h. Anyone who has spent any amount of time can comment on the horrible traffic jams that have made getting around a stressful, time-wasting chore.

Certainly the pollution cars create is a serious issue—in Shanghai, for example, some 70 % of urban air pollution comes from car exhaust. The impact this has on public health is severe and profound.

But we'd like to address a more fundamental truth: When cities are built to accommodate cars, they are no longer designed to accommodate people. "Green travel" is being promoted in many cities around China. The authors appealed to the government and the crowd to improve the poor's traffic condition, and improve car awareness and knowledge of the community.

320.4 Main Teaching Contents, Guidelines and Mode

Vehicle and motorcycle driving training schools place much emphasis on driving skillfully, while ignoring car cultural education for short-term training. Learners Crammed for their driving tests to learn some new traffic regulations. Only few university and some vocational college having automobile specialty. The former give lesson about car culture but its beneficiaries are few, the latter pay close attention to automobile detection examination maintenance and repairing, giving little attention to car cultural education. China was cut off herself from the outside world, the car industry was the Cinderella, and people's consumption desire were restrained for far too long, hence lack of car culture.

Our school is a comprehensive college, and has no professional course on vehicle engineering before. Car and culture form good interaction, health concept of consumption, and build a good car culture environment, constructing the harmonious society is the premise of the car. To speed up the development of modern city car society construction, establishes the car social external environment support system, in the social development process, the government play the leading role, constructing the harmonious society is the foundation of the car. So, the authors sets this automobile selected course which give 700 students a systematic training on car each year.

320.5 Conclusions

Through applying various teaching tools and resources, students are interested in learning, and also their learning abilities are enhanced. This course intended to educate students on the negative impact of cars on quality of life and on the environment, aiming to make students aware about the use of public transport, cycling, walking, car and other alternative methods of transportation.

Students can keep abreast of the times with the car development, and they also can understand the car deeply and clearly. So students can change their conceptions about cars from the ignorant and confused into clear. The student's knowledge and learning abilities have been expanded and improved, so they understand the relationships among cars, society, and environment more deeply.

References

1. Xiao S, Shen G, Liu S (2009) Reflection on structuring harmonious automobile society. J Hubei Automo Indus Inst 23(1):77–80
2. Hu X (2010) Auto-society and the evolution of urban governance pattern. Urban Prob 9:67–71
3. Guo H, Zhang T (2011) Automobile using and management, 1st edn. Beijing University Press, Beijing, 248–254
4. Wen Y et al (2013) LNG vehicles technology development and its prospect of popularization and application. Chem Eng Oil Gas 1:1–5

Chapter 321
An Integrated Research Study of Information Technology (IT) Education and Experimental Design and Execution (EDE) Courses

Guoying Wang and Yunsheng Zhang

Abstract This article discusses an integrated research study of Information Technology (IT) Education and Experimental Design and Execution (EDE) courses. Based on analyses of the disjunction between current information technology education and how education is delivered in students' majors, the authors investigated a revolutionary idea of integrating information technology education into experimental design and execution courses, with the goal of strengthening medical student IT education from the perspectives of IT awareness, IT abilities and IT morality. Through combining experiment content with teaching methods, harmonizing students' abilities with teachers' duties and similar measures, the authors explored the best approach and methods to integrate Information Technology (IT) and Education and Experimental Design and Execution (EDE) courses. This research corrects the previous impression of IT education as being theoretical and useless to medical study, makes IT education practical to students and plays a critical role in the major courses of students. This approach thus both facilitates the implementation of IT education and improves teaching quality in students' major courses.

Keywords Information technology education · Experimental design and execution (EDE) courses · Integration

As the core supplier of innovative scientific education and training, universities play a significant role in cultivating creativity in students [1]. With educational models now changing from "biology-medicine" to "biology-psychology-social

G. Wang
The Medical College of Henan University, The Medical College, New Campus of Henan University, Kaifeng 475004 Henan Province, China
e-mail: medwgy@163.com

Y. Zhang (✉)
The Nursing School of Henan University, The Nursing School of Henan University, New Campus of Henan University, Kaifeng 475004 Henan Province, China
e-mail: zhangyunsheng@henu.edu.cn

medicine", the primary educational goal has also transformed from simply imparting knowledge to instead cultivating a student's abilities, especially medical student creativity. Meanwhile, with the Internet's rapid development, information technology-based education is playing an increasingly important role in nurturing creative and talented students. Therefore, our research is an important first step. Through educational reform, IT-assisted education becomes integrated into medical education and forms a key component of major courses. In this paper, an integrated research study into information technology education and Experimental Design and Execution (EDE) courses was conducted in a course titled Disease Etiology. In this research we tested several trial approaches and obtained some very encouraging and satisfying results.

321.1 Problems Existing in the Current Information Technology Education Approaches

There is one primary problem in existing course design, namely IT-based education is disconnected from professional education. Medical students are asked to take compulsory courses in basic computer knowledge, reference searching and related information education courses. However, because the professors teaching these courses are computer majors they lack a medical education background and are not familiar with medical information systems. Consequently these courses are limited to giving medical students general computer knowledge and do not produce an integration of IT-based knowledge with the major courses in medicine. In practice, students need not only fundamental computer knowledge, but also a familiarity of the application of IT education to medical study [2, 3].

There are several problems existing among students, the primary one being that many students pay little attention to acquiring IT-based knowledge. A considerable proportion of students believe that IT courses are less important than their major courses and aren't closely connected and relevant to their majors in medical studies [4]. In daily studies, they seldom use IT-based knowledge to enhance their medical studies and are inept at utilizing IT resources online. Secondly, students are often unskillful in singling out useful information. Indeed, many students pay close attention only to their textbooks and very few undergraduate students are familiar with the highly-ranked academic journals in the field of medicine. When asked to do research on their own, they often feel lost facing so many seemingly useful resources but having difficulty in choosing the best ones. Thirdly, students in general are not good at analyzing and evaluating information. Quite a few students report that they encounter difficulty in ignoring useless and even misleading information in an effort to select truly helpful information. Fourthly, students demonstrate weak abilities in properly and effectively utilizing information. The most common problem is that students don't know how to optimize their findings when presenting them in written form, and they have challenges successfully integrating strong background research work with their own individual, original thoughts and analyses [5].

321.2 Some Revolutionary Thoughts on Integration of Information Technology Education and EDE Courses

With the aimed of addressing the above mentioned problems, a redesigned teaching plan was carefully designed. Combined with EDE courses, medical student IT assisted education was strengthened by promoting IT awareness, IT familiarity and good IT judgment. Through integration of IT-based education and medical courses, a new teaching model was established to facilitate the delivery of IT-assisted education and to improve medical courses' teaching qualities, as well as to reinforce the cultivation of students' creativity.

321.3 The Content of Integration of IT Education and EDE Courses

321.3.1 Cultivating IT Awareness

To effectively cope with and cure continually arising new diseases, new therapeutics and pharmaceuticals must be explored, and our medical technology must be updated. In short, medical development is surprisingly rapid. For medical students, the major courses at school merely give them a basic foundation. In our information-based society, only by accepting IT-assisted education, mastering information technology, and constantly searching for information can one fulfill the need for lifelong learning and keeping up with a constantly advancing society. In fact, the ability to search for knowledge is more important than mastering knowledge itself [6]. IT-assisted education benefits students' self-study abilities and creativity, and is therefore indispensible for future individual development of these students. In this course, students were introduced to such awareness and encouraged to actively explore new knowledge and search for new information, in order to improve and enhance their IT familiarity [7].

321.3.2 Cultivating IT Familiarity

Before starting the EDE courses, students were asked to fill out a questionnaire, which was designed to evaluate student abilities for collecting, selecting, evaluating and utilizing information. By analyzing student feedback, a detailed and appropriate teaching plan was designed. According to the teaching goals, the teaching content, and the students' IT knowledge levels, IT competence training was integrated into EDE courses through multiple teaching methods, step by step and from simple to complex. Only by introducing IT education into the major courses can a stable IT education basis be engendered [8].

The Disease Etiology experiments had four sequential components, from a replication experiment to a comprehensive experiment, to a design experiment and finally to a creative experiment. According to each component's function, the corresponding IT incorporation ability cultivation goal was established.

321.3.2.1 Replication Experiment

Experiments of this category mainly cultivated the students' experimental execution skills and validated the theories learned in class. Such experiments are comparatively easy, and have fixed content. Each experiment program was independent of the others. As to the period for conducting replication experiments, we set specific target goals for a student's IT abilities. Students were expected to get familiar with the common techniques for searching for academic information, acquiring basic searching competence, being able to read academic papers and to select useful and pertinent information. Meanwhile, we summarized the teachers' responsibilities. Teachers were to combine experiment content, to introduce the frequently-accessed medical databases, professional websites, academic journals and major reference books to students, so as to get students exposed to these professional information resources. Then, by illustration, teachers were instructed to help students develop basic and effective searching methods. After that, some experiment assignments were given to students for after-class practice and for reinforcing their abilities. For example, while teaching about a specific parasite's epidemic status, each student was asked to search for 10 related papers, then read them and write a brief summary of the papers.

321.3.2.2 Comprehensive Experiment

Students independently conducted comprehensive experiments, to practice varied kinds of disease etiology diagnostic techniques. In addition, the content of comprehensive experiments was connected with the results from previous replication experiments; experiment teaching was connected with clinical diagnosis; and students gained hands-on experience and improved their comprehension mastery. During this period, the goals of students' IT abilities were to become familiar with the frequently-accessed medical databases, professional websites, academic journals and major reference books, and to acquire proficient searching abilities. Students were expected to be able to quickly locate and accurately select required academic information. Correspondingly, the teachers' responsibilities were to demonstrate to students how to distinguish between a "broad search" and an "accurate search", and to train students to master the methods of extending and narrowing the reference scales. In brief, students should learn to improve their accuracy rate and hence efficiency in searching for related papers [9]. For example, there are three disease etiology diagnostic methods to identify a parasite. By reading related academic references, students became familiar with each method's application scope and accuracy, compared their own experiment results to their acquired knowledge, and then wrote a short essay. In that way, the students' information acquiring abilities were gradually integrated with their experimental abilities.

321.3.2.3 Design Experiment

Students were divided into groups and then teammates cooperated to design experimental plans. Based on previously researched information and thorough reading, they analyzed, proposed questions, chose topics and designed their plans. The goals for advancing students' IT abilities were to improve their IT competence for searching references and of utilizing information comprehensively. Meantime, the teachers' focus shifted from developing students' proficiency in searching references to improving students' abilities for analyzing and evaluating researched information. Through practice, students were able to acquire reliable, advanced and practical information by thorough analyses and evaluation, and were able to adopt implicit knowledge from researched information as well [10]. Based on the major studies, by searching, analyzing and evaluating information, and designing experiment plans, IT knowledge and major knowledge were well integrated and better understood. Students also changed their studying style from accepting knowledge passively to exploring knowledge actively.

321.3.2.4 Creative Experiment

With the aim of teaching the solving of specific problems, creative experiments concentrated on fostering students' creative awareness and creativity by modifying and innovating experiment skills and methods. During this period, students were expected to reach specific goals, namely by referencing previous studies in their majors and IT education, students could reconstruct their knowledge system, efficiently utilize available resources and information, dare to question learned knowledge and through experiments validate their assumptions. By that point, these undergraduate students indeed had obtained a certain level of research ability, which is normally assumed of graduate students. In this period, the teachers' duties were helping students reconstruct the new knowledge system by analyzing, evaluating and summarizing major knowledge with researched knowledge, to ensure the last step of transformation from knowledge to abilities. In the end, IT education and EDE courses were well integrated.

321.3.3 Developing Good IT Judgment and Morality

IT morality consists of the restriction and rules of regulating information production and information transformation, as well as the standards of correctly employing IT awareness and IT abilities [11]. Students were educated to observe and respect social morality and laws, exploit information logically and legally, reject harmful information and repudiate information crime.

321.4 Implementation of the Integration of IT Education and EDE Courses

This study was done in the second year of a five-year-long program. Among the 25 classes, we selected 12 classes (532 students in total) as the experimental group to implement the teaching reforms, while the other 13 classes didn't receive any related instruction and therefore were considered as a control group.

The 12 classes exposed to teaching reform gained a lot. Students independently designed 98 experiments; by conducting experiments, students published 10 papers in total; and students applied and were given two College Student Innovative Experiment Programs, a national one and a provincial one. The control group, the 13 classes not exposed to teaching reform produced no research results.

The final results of our study revealed that by implementing teaching reform employing Integrated Research Study of Information Technology (IT) Education and Experimental Design and Execution (EDE) courses, students improved their awareness of utilizing information technology to facilitate study in their major, strengthened their abilities for selecting, analyzing, evaluating and utilizing information, and had a deeper understanding of information and academic morality.

321.5 Conclusion

An EDE course is a significant component of medical teaching. In this research study, IT education was well integrated into the EDE courses, which strengthened information technology's application in the field of medical study. This approach restructured the previous situation in which IT education was general and unrelated to major courses, broke down the barriers between theory and application, and made it possible to internalize knowledge into abilities. Meanwhile, IT education and EDE courses cooperated well, and played an advantageous role in cultivating creative students. Through this integrated research study, we explored a new educational approach to teaching medical students, modified the traditional teaching model, realized the transformation from imparting knowledge to developing abilities, and established a new EDE course model.

References

1. Wang W (2009) Innovation and development: retrospection and prospection of medical information education in China. J Med Inform 30(12):1–5, 11
2. Qin YB, Zhao WH (2012) Reform and practice of information education in traditional Chinese medicine college. J Liaoning Univ Tcm 14(4):271–272
3. Wang LW, Cao JD, Wang W (2010) Supply and demand differences of medical information talents in health informationization domain. China High Med Educ 8:1–5
4. Sun FM, Wang Q (2009) Survey of and strategy for medical college student's information literacy. J Shandong Normal Univ (Humanit Soc Sci) 54(2):81–84
5. Wu JZ (2008) Talking about the present situation of and countermeasures for information literacy of today's university students. Scitech Inf Dev Econ 18(12):179–180
6. Yang XM, Zhang F, Hou LL (2011) Status quo of information literacy education for medical students and information literacy training. China Med Educ Technol 25(3):249–252
7. Lin XH (2011) Discussion on the college students' information consciousness. J Jiangsu Teachers Univ Technol 17(3):82–84
8. Qin F, Zhang L (2004) Information age is greatly in need of developing college student's information accomplishment. J Sichuan Coll Educ 20(1):69–70
9. Gao YX (2010) Information literacy of medical personnel under informatization environment. J Med Inform 31(4):81–84
10. Hu H, Zhao WL, Li CL (2007) To strengthen information analysis and evaluation competency. Res Med Educ 6(5):399–400, 423
11. Du ZY (2008) Developing information literacy of undergraduate students of pharmaceutical universities. Northw Med Educ 16(3):446–447, 456

Chapter 322
Empirical Study of Job Burnout Among Higher Vocational College Teachers

Cheng Wang

Abstract Long working hours, frequent multitasking, and relatively high burden coming from the nature of higher vocational college teachers' job make them tend to suffer from job burnout. Job burnout usually quenches teaching passion, threats teachers' mental and physical health, and thus slow down the development of education. This work compares job burnout situations in three higher vocational colleges of different quality, trying to explore new ways to control job burnout among higher vocational college teachers.

Keywords Job burnout · Higher vocational education · Intercollegiate comparison

322.1 Introduction

Higher vocational college teachers, who play a key role in nurturing highly skilled workers, are faced with an increasing amount of unprecedented opportunities as well as challenges arising in the current development and reformation of higher vocational education system. Job Burnout is a major factor in the fatigue and underperformance of higher vocational college teachers. It has a direct influence on teachers' mental health, thus essentially wastes the limited education resources in our country. Therefore, job burnout among higher vocational college teachers requires sufficient attention of us concerning teachers' physical and mental balance as well as the development of higher vocational education in China.

American psychologists Maslach and Pines took social psychological approach in the study of job burnout. They proposed that emotional exhaustion, depersonalization and reduced personal accomplishment are the three components that

C. Wang (✉)
Department of Foreign Language, Anqing Vocational and Technical College, Anqing, China
e-mail: Walt2009@aqvtc.cn

characterize the mental state of job burnout Emotional exhaustion, which has been shown to be the core component of job burnout, is characterized by the overwhelming feelings of being emotionally overextended and drained. Prolonged feelings of exhaustion will lead to negative emotions and a tendency to react to clients in an overly passive and impersonal way, which is depersonalization. A reduced sense of personal accomplishment refers to the loss of feelings of self-efficacy and a growing negative judgment of one's efforts. Recent researches into the job burnout among higher vocational college teachers in China mostly concern general phenomena. However, in-depth theoretical analysis and empirical discussion are still lacking.

322.2 Methods

322.2.1 Sample

The targeted population was set in three vocational and technical colleges in Anhui Province. They were Anhui Vocational and Technical College (National Model College), Anqing Vocational and Technical College (Provincial Model College) and Xuancheng Vocational and Technical College (ordinary college). Two hundred and ten questionnaires were mailed to teachers in those three colleges (45 in Anhui Vocational and Technical College, 124 in Anqing Vocational and Technical College and 41 in Xuancheng Vocational and Technical College). A total of 201 questionnaires were returned, of which 170 were effective (40 from Anhui College, 95 from Anqing College and 35 from Xuancheng College). The effective response rate was 84.6 %. In all, 47 male teachers with average age 31.3 ($SD = 8.0$) and 119 female teachers with average age 30.2 ($SD = 6.1$)—four had missing sex data—participated. Numbers of teachers teaching in the first semester to the sixth semester are 33 (19.4 %), 31 (18.2 %), 22 (12.9 %), 28 (16.5 %), 31 (18.2 %), 25 (14.7 %). The mean number of teaching hours was 13.5. The mean number of years of teaching experience was 10 years. Number of unmarried teachers was 59 (34.7 %).

322.2.2 Measures

The MBI used in the traditional educators' job burnout measure comprises three dimensions: emotional exhaustion (E), depersonalization (F) and personal accomplishment (G). Taking the Chinese culture background and current vocational education situation into consideration, we add two more dimensions based on an extensive investigation. They are research exhaustion (H) and skill confusion (I).

Our job burnout scale for higher vocational college teachers is following:

- E1 My job puts too much stress and burden on me
- E2 I feel frustrated by my job
- E3 I feel used up at the end of the workday
- F1 I am afraid that teaching makes me detached to people
- F2 I feel impossible to reach teaching goals on some students
- F3 I feel no passion in teaching and facing with students
- F4 I don't' like my colleagues
- G1 I don't think being a vocational college teacher is valuable to society
- G2 I feel unsatisfied with my job
- G3 I feel incapable of handling problems in teaching and issues about students
- G4 I work harder than before but cannot achieve what I expect
- G5 My job is neither challenging nor intriguing
- G6 I feel no motivation in teaching
- H1 Research puts too much stress on me
- H2 I feel doing research is just for promotion
- H3 I will not work on a research project if I am not asked to do that
- H4 Research is meaningless to vocational college teachers
- I1 I feel technical skills are too complicated
- I2 I find no effective way to enhance my technical skills
- I3 I don't know how to deal with different standards in technical skills
- I4 I cannot see the future trend in the development of my technical area

Table 322.1 Mean and standard deviation of each item

Item	Number of responses	Mean	SD
E1	170	3.43	0.904
E2	170	3.33	1.024
E3	170	3.43	0.904
F1	170	2.83	1.010
F2	170	3.87	0.978
F3	170	2.36	0.807
F4	170	2.75	1.063
G1	170	4.16	0.635
G2	170	3.53	0.755
G3	170	3.83	0.774
G4	170	3.28	0.970
G5	170	3.60	0.902
G6	170	3.57	1.027
H1	170	2.93	1.100
H2	170	3.77	0.971
H3	170	2.46	0.907
H4	170	2.85	1.033
I1	170	2.85	1.080
I2	170	3.67	0.968
I3	170	2.57	0.817
I4	170	2.81	1.043

Table 322.2 Mean and standard deviation of the general level of job burnout and its five subscales

	Number of responses	Mean	SD
Job burnout	170	3.3357	0.42694
Emotional exhaustion	170	3.3954	0.90361
Depersonalization	170	2.9491	0.62416
Personal achievement	170	3.6496	0.37373
Research exhaustion	170	3.1844	0.57921
Skill confusion	170	2.8976	0.60987

322.2.3 Data Analysis

Effective returned questionnaires were indexed. SPSS 13.0 was used in managing and analyzing data.

322.3 Results

322.3.1 General Job Burnout Situation Among High Vocational College Teachers

Tables 322.1 and 322.2

322.3.2 Comparison of Job Burnout Situation Among Colleges of Different Quality

See Table 322.3

322.4 Conclusion

Mean value of every item exceeds 2 (Table 322.1), which shows a significant job burnout situation among teachers in the three higher vocational colleges.

Mean values of three subscales—emotional exhaustion, personal achievement and research exhaustion—exceed 3 (Table 322.2), which shows higher vocational college teachers often suffer problems of emotional exhaustion, low achievement and research strain.

All but one of the items associated with depersonalization and skill confusion have a mean value less than 3. This demonstrates that depersonalization and skill

Table 322.3 Mean of job burnout and five subscales in three colleges of different quality

	Anhui vocational and technical college (N = 40)	Anqing vocational and technical college (N = 95)	Xuancheng vocational and technical college (N = 35)
Job burnout	3.3325	3.3059	3.4203
Emotional exhaustion	3.4117	3.3536	3.4903
Depersonalization	2.8116	2.9649	3.0634
Personal achievement	3.6258	3.6942	3.5557
Research exhaustion	3.0836	3.2252	3.1889
Skill confusion	2.9769	2.841	2.9604

confusion are minor problems among higher vocational college teachers compared with emotional exhaustion, low personal achievement and research exhaustion.

To help higher vocational college teachers to overcome job burnout, first, we have to promote their social status by introducing more investments into higher vocational education and drawing the society's attention to the importance of this form of education. Secondly, colleges should provide better work environment and more opportunities of high level academic exchange and skills promotion. Thirdly, we should help teachers to keep their own mental and physical balances and release job pressures. In the end, intercollegiate cooperation should be strengthened, helping good experiences in fighting job burnout to be shared.

References

1. Maslach C, Jackson SE (1982) The Measurement of experienced burnout. J Occup Behav 2:99–115
2. Pines M (2005) The Burnout measure short version. Int J Stress Manag 12(1):78–88
3. Gold Y (1984) Burnout: a major problem for the teaching profession [J]. Education 104(3):271–274
4. Fleming DS, Barton GV Stannek (1998) Teacher burnout: how to keep the flame burning Teaching Elementary Physical Education 9(2):8–9
5. Xu FM, Zhu CS, Shao LC (2005) Relations in job burnout and other factors in primary school teachers. J Psychol Sci 28(5):1240–1242
6. Huang Q (2006) Relation between job pressure and job burnout in higher vocational college teachers. J Huangzhong Univ of Sci and Technol
7. Zeng LJ (2004) Predict Job burnout in primary school teachers based on job pressure. J Educ Dev 3:79–81
8. Wang F, Xu Y (2004) Relation between job exhaustion and social support in primary school teachers. Acta Psychologica Sinica 5:568–574
9. Wang XC, Zhang Y, Gan YQ, Zhang YW (2005) Job burnout scales in primary school teachers. Chinese J Appl Psychol 2:170–175
10. Xu FM, Zhu CS, Huang WF (2005) Job burnout, job pressure and self-esteem in primary school teachers. Psychol Explor 1:74–77
11. Shao LF, Gao FQ (2005) Social support and job burnout in primary school teachers. J Shandong Normal Univ 4:150–153

Chapter 323
Appeals on College Moral Education: Based on Open Environment of Laboratories Under Campus Network

Jun-Yan Zhang

Abstract As the main content of high education reform, the open environment of laboratories under campus network is an effective way to cultivate practical and creative abilities, moralities and faiths and values for students. Within such environment, college moral education faces both favorable opportunities and severe challenges and presents new appeals different from traditional ones.

Keywords University laboratory · Open environment · Campus network · Moral education · Appeals

Experiences have proved that the openness of the laboratories provides favorable conditions for the personnel training in the colleges and universities, which will not only help college students to enter the scientific research fields and build proper knowledge structure before their graduation, but also promote integrated development in their wisdom, diathesis and abilities. Nevertheless, with the booming of campus network, various information will irresistibly extend the space and time of teaching and learning and broaden the way of learning of the students and alter the teaching strategies and thoughts, which will put forward new requirements on the moral education of college students. As the main part of education reform, the openness of the laboratory based on the campus network is an effective way to promote the practical ability and creativity and to build the moral belief and the values of students. In this mode, the campus education faces both favorable opportunities and tough challenges. Judging by the condition, campus network, which is free, imaginary, offers an entirely new environment to moral education. However, it is easy for the students to forget responsibilities and moral requires in the real world. Since the cyber world is open and covert, students

---

Chinese Book Classification Code: G641, G482 Document Identifier Code: A

J.-Y. Zhang (✉)
Department of Education, Nanyang Institute of Technology, 473000 Nanyang, China

are easily misled and abandon their pursuit of science. Therefore, appeals for moral education with open environment of laboratories under campus network have entered the vision. I hope to provide some referential experiences for the campus moral education through my treatise.

323.1 The Opening Construction of Laboratory Under Network

In the open mode, besides the routine experimental teaching task to be performed, the laboratory should also share the information and resources with the outside world, so as to let the students choose experimental project by themselves. In the meantime, teachers can keep track of the process of the experiment and also maximize the cyber effect of laboratory.

323.1.1 To Share Laboratory and Cyber Resources with Information Technology

Laboratories in the universities possess a large amount of material and information resources, which are the fundamental condition for high-standard teaching and research. With stream-line findings of teaching and research, the storage and variety of the information in the laboratories has been dramatically enlarged. In order to take advantage of available resources and reduce the configuration for repeated resources, new management procedures should be established in the open mode. In the process of network sharing, all kinds of resources (material and information included) in the fields of university teaching, scientific research and community service could be made use of. Thus resources-using rate could be improved and the configuration of resources would be more appropriate and the share of resources for universities and society could be realized. It is also convenient for the students and teachers and people of all walks to have an access to the distribution of resources, functional structure and method. And in this process, social school-running benefits would increase.

323.1.2 To Promote the Standardized Management of Laboratory with Information Technology

The informatization of education and management has been an important guarantee to various works in college. As one of the weakest links, the informationlization for the lab has been a task of top priority. In fact, the information construction built on colleges high standard campus network system is maturing. Massive open-ended materials are gathering on the network platform. Compared with the network system for other organizations, it is nearly perfect. College personnel training has been gaining informational support from this network system. At the same time, universities and all the departments have been able to operate courseware, net course and distance learning on the internet. Through this channel, students can learn knowledge from their own needs. Besides, because of the popularity and openness of the network, no matter students or teachers, individuals in it may have some kind of dependence on it. Objectively speaking, the needs for internet accelerate the information construction of the labs. However, in the open mode, the regulatory lacunae of net platform would bring new problems to the moral education in universities. Therefore, it appears to be a necessity to normalize the lab management by relying on information technology.

323.2 New Challenges and Opportunities from Open Laboratory Network

323.2.1 The Pluralism of Cyber-Culture in the Campus Brings Challenges Towards Moral Education

In the open mode of the laboratories, different and even contradictory ideas would be spreaded and collided on the network platform. How difficult it would be to judge a multidimensional and varied question in an exclusive manner could not be calculated. Under such circumstances, traditional moral education will be deeply impacted. As the students have more access to information, they will get in touch with more complicated views. Consequently, this group can hardly comprehend the information in the way moral educators have assumed. When they collect various views and change their thoughts into reality, the multidimensional thinking will cause qualitative changes in their behavior and consciousness, which will have negative effect on their worldview, values, lifeview to some extent. With the uncontrolled spread of multidimensional thoughts, the authority of moral educators is broken up. How to guarantee the place for moral educators in universities remains an issue to be solved. Though tradition tells us that teacher is respected and plays an important role in their life. Because of the development of the internet, students no longer obtain their whole knowledge from the old ways. The original mode has been broken up. Internet, the fourth generation of mass media, has taken the place. The status of the moral educators has been abased. Furthermore, the knowledge structure of some moral educators is obsolete. Since they know little about computer and network, they could not effectively take control of the information among the students and conduct their behavior. Scarcely could they be adapted to the moral work under the internet.

There is a great clash between the widely-used modern network and traditional teaching mode in university moral education. The latter is being replaced by open-functioned network media. In the open laboratory mode, by taking advantage of the platform from the students' needs, creative thinking will be integrated with open-space teaching and the freedom as well as the fun for learning will be acquired in the accurate learning content at proper learning time. While in the "no boundaries" new teaching mode, we should promote students' learning environment and learning effect with the aid of the network and gradually build new a teaching structure based on students' autonomous learning and personalized teaching method. But it is not the fact, the requirements of the times calls college moral educators. The moral teaching content, teaching materials, teachers' quality is still in the adaptation and adjustment stage, the serious lag effect makes the realization of this goal within sight but beyond reach.

323.2.2 Universal Adaptability of the Campus Network Offers Favorable Platform for Moral Education

In the open mode of laboratory, to ensure the timeliness and universality of moral education for colleges and universities means more direct and deeply work effect and the efficiency and effect of moral education will be promoted. As mentioned above, the limitation of time and space for moral education will be infinite widened by the open network. Traditional moral education and practical activities are no longer restricted by number of people, time and place. Country, society, family and school will work as a whole in the field of moral education. The strength in the same direction together will form a powerful educational force, which will extend originally limited space of moral education field into an infinite open education space that is common to the society. Therefore, the school moral education department should constantly convey relevant information to students through the campus network and collect the student's thoughts through the network, in order to give accurate guidance timely.

Laboratory network open mode has two basic functions, one is to realize the self–education of the student, the other is to build favorable campus culture. With full respect for the educates, the former function will help them to participate in moral education of their own free will and give full play to their potentials initiativity. Needless to say, the openness of the network is able to guarantee the individuality of students, since any one subject of network will seek materials through network from personal interests. Through their expression, comment and discussion on the ideas with others, self-education will be realized unconsciously. In addition, the open network environment can promote the formation of a good campus culture, which will influence students' thoughts and behavior. The campus network is the embodiment of the campus culture in the network world. Campus network with rich information and favorable culture will fully exhibit the excellence of school and can provide high quality service for the community through the campus network, promoting the construction of the style of study and the school spirits.

The network is universally applicable, which attracts the favor of students and complies with the principle of guidance for moral education work, so the actual effect is easy to see. Especially in the laboratory open mode, the development of network provides new opportunities for the campus moral education, which is mainly reflected in that laboratory information network also provides material resources as well as information resources for the network users beyond the limitation of time and space. The time and distance among network subjects (teachers and students) are also greatly expanded (extended). Therefore, the moral educators should take advantage of this platform, paying close attention to students' network learning, network consumption, network communication and so forth. They should face up to the situation in a positive way: Not "blocking", but "leading"–that is to make full use of the students' interest in network and guide it to the right direction. Then the effect of moral education is apparent.

323.3 Open Network Platform to Strengthen Laboratory Management, Promoting Moral Education Reform

323.3.1 To Strengthen the Organization and the Guidance to the Students with an Open Laboratory Management

In the open mode of laboratory, we should not wipe out the openness and freedom of campus network. If our supervision is too meticulous or not flexible enough as the real world, it will run counter to our desire. Therefore, on the basis of laboratory opening, supervision of campus network should be based on students' self-discipline and self-rule. The teachers are responsible for the overall supervision and guidance. This ensures the freedom and openness of the network and trains the students' ability in self-discipline and self-rule and can also guarantee the healthy growth of students. In addition, the way of open management under the condition of network of differs from that of traditional moral work. It expands students' learning space out of classroom. It enables students to accept moral education in practice rather than in the classroom. In this way, good network morality and social morality was formed.

323.3.2 To Strengthen the Supervision of Open Network

Today, to ensure university moral education work goes on smoothly, it is necessary for staff and students together to create a healthy and upward culture environment. Therefore, the construction for an excellent campus website becomes the inevitable requirement. In the open model of laboratory, there will be a certain number of college students lost themselves in the internet world and gradually their social communication and interpersonal skills are lost, too. They escape from real life and cut themselves from society. At this point, various functions of campus network are revealed. Not only can it be used as the party's propaganda fronts, timely and accurately delivering the call of the party, but will the attract students interests to healthy campus culture under the guidance of university governor. Eventually it contributes to the formation of a green campus and green network to ensure the healthy development of students.

323.3.3 To Develop Network Moral Education Software

Up to now, the development of moral education software in China is relatively backward. How to make the moral education work into the operational procedures and combine various disciplines of knowledge with the moral education work has become a pressing matter of the moment. Therefore, the university moral education workers should take the laboratory opening as an opportunity and make full use of modern science and technology through the network carrier to develop and utilize of the network moral education software for moral education. In addition, universities should also combine legal education, revolutionary education, national education, science and technology education and industry standard education to make the Internet moral education more practical and feasible.

323.3.4 Open up New Network Approach to Establish a New System of Moral Education

In order to cater more for appeals of the network moral education in colleges and universities, the scientificity of network should be fully made use of and new system of moral education network should be built. For example, online resources of moral education together with moral education practice can be combined to maximize excellent resources and to endow moral education work with distinct characteristics. Besides, with the combination of classroom and online teaching, a set of teaching material and courseware was provided on the unique network platform for college moral education. Thus the network education effect is strengthened; at the same time, corresponding network management regulations should be developed to prevent the adverse information among students so that a healthy Internet environment of moral education shall be built.

323.4 Conclusion

At present, our colleges and universities are mostly confined to moral teaching, working range is limited to within the campus, coupled with outdated ways of working, so that moral education in a relatively isolated closed state, moral effect is not ideal. In open mode, the laboratory network management is not only able to update moral philosophy, moral reform the traditional model, build a healthy and active network moral education environment, improve the management level, but also make full use of existing resources and dynamic student development resources to maximize the laboratory open mode network education effectiveness for the college moral education services, improve the quality of moral education in universities and promote healthy growth of students.

References

1. Bai Z (2010) Reform and construction of laboratory management system. Res Explor Lab (8):22–24
2. Gao B, Wang Z (2006) Discussion on open laboratory management mode based on the network environment. Exp Technol Manag (9):123–126
3. Gu Y (2009) Moral dilemma and path selection of campus network culture. J Liaoning Admin Inst (1):94–95
4. Li X, Wei G (2011) The positive effects of network on moral education in colleges and universities. Extracurricular Educ China (7):6
5. Li X, Zhu Y (2010) Campus network construction and moral education in colleges and universities. Theory Union Pract (6):84–86
6. Li Z (2011) A brief talk on the network teaching resources construction. Coll Lab Res (6):108
7. Liu G (2007) Discussion on the laboratory construction planning. Res Explor Lab (5):61–63
8. Pan H (2010) Discussion on the open mode of laboratories in colleges and universities. J Guangzhou Sports Univ (5):12–14
9. Sang Y (2009) On the construction and reformation of laboratory. J Anhui Univ Technol (3):87–89
10. Shi R, Yu X, Liu Y, Li L (2010) Exploration of the opening management mode of laboratory in universities. Exp Technol Manag (4):164–166
11. Song W (2008) On the application of the campus network in the harmonious network in ideological and political education. Educ Explor (8):111–112
12. Wang F (2008) Discussion on open laboratory management mode in colleges and universities. Sci Technol Manag Res (9):152–153
13. Wang J (2011) Improve the management level of the laboratory. Coll Phys Exp (2):56–57
14. Wang Q (2008) The rise of campus network culture and moral education in colleges and universities. J Henan Bus Coll (2):117–118
15. Yang Y, Gao G, Qiu X, Jiang W, Cai F (2010) Research on countermeasures of nursing laboratory resource utilization. Nurs Res (11):90–91
16. Yi X, Liu W (2010) On the construction of moral education system of campus network. J Hunan Ind Polytech (3):119–120
17. Zeng K, Cao F, Cao X (2009) Utilize campus network to carry out moral education work. Exp Teach Apparatus (12):53–54
18. Zhong Z, Li X, Chen Y (2010) Construction of campus network and ideological and political education. Sci Technol Dev Enterp (24):139–141

Chapter 324
Intercultural Pragmatics Research on Written Emails in an Academic Environment

Su Zhang

Abstract As an important part of information technology, email is now pervasive in our everyday lives. In western universities, email is widely used in the academic environment. Although it functions as a modern communication tool, email is also a good channel for students to practice their second language. However, how to write an appropriate email in an academic environment is seldom taught to English as a foreign language (EFL) and English as a second language (ESL) students. In this research study, through analyzing 30 feedbacks from EFL, ESL and English as native language (ENL) students, some linguistic differences were identified, analyzed and discussed. It is apparent that some linguistic features are instinctive to ESL learners while others are more obscure and therefore hard to acquire. Email, because of its special linguistic features and wide application should be given more attention in English education in China.

Keywords Email · English · ESL, EFL, ENL students · Pragmatics

324.1 Introduction

With the rapid development of the Internet in the past 5 years, email has become more and more widespread. Email is an interesting form of communication because the language of email has characteristics of both written and spoken language [1]. Emails in an academic environment, such as emails from students to professors, because of the power distance are slightly inclined to be a bit formal while still retaining some informal characteristics. Communicating by email between professors and students is very common in the US, but is less common in

S. Zhang (✉)
College of Foreign Languages, Henan University, Minglun Street, Kaifeng 475001, Henan Province, China
e-mail: zszhangsu@gmail.com

China. Among the limited academic emails in China, only a small portion is written in English. According to Li's survey, many Chinese students "find it hard and prefer to do it in L1 (Chinese)" when emailing their professors (Li 2010). Besides that, how to write an English email is seldom taught in English classes in China. In some ESL courses or seminars in the US, writing emails is treated as an explicit learning object. For example, at Carnegie Mellon University there is a seminar titled "Email for Academic Purposes". However, because of their heavy course load and seating restrictions, only a limited number of students can actually take advantage of such seminars. For similar reasons, although writing academic emails is also taught in some ESL books like *Academic Interactions–Communicating on Campus* [1] and *Academic Writing for Graduate Students* [2], it is not clear how many Chinese students who study in the US actually read them. Therefore, learning how to write academic emails is usually acquired naturally through daily email exchanges.

Based on the information mentioned above, a research study related to pragmatics acquisition in writing emails in an academic environment was designed and conducted. Following are the research questions of this study:

1. What pragmatics characteristics are revealed in the academic emails written by Chinese students in China who study English as a foreign language (EFL students), by Chinese students at an American university who study and acquire English as a second language (ESL students) and by English native speakers (ENL students)?
2. How well have ESL students acquired the ENL's pragmatics characteristics in writing academic emails? How did they acquire such skills? Which aspect is easier to acquire and which aspect is harder to acquire?

324.2 Methods

324.2.1 Participants

There were three groups of participants in this study and each group was comprised of ten students. Participants in group one (ENL) were all English native speakers, nine of whom were American undergraduate or M.A students and the other one, a Canadian Ph.D. student. Most of the American students were students at Carnegie Mellon University, in varied disciplines. Participants in group two (EFL) were all Chinese students in China, who had not been abroad. These students were all English majors at Henan University, including both senior students and MA students. During their undergraduate studies, they would have had American native English speakers as language instructors for 2 years, usually one class of about 45 min per week. It is uncommon for such students to write English emails, either to their Chinese professors who teach English or to their language instructors. However, since they were English majors, their English competence should have been better than non-English-major students. Participants in group three (ESL) were all Chinese students studying in the US at the time of the survey. Among those ten students, there were seven MA students in different majors at various universities, an undergraduate student and two Ph.D. students. The length of these students' stay in the US ranged from 7 months to 6 years. Since they had been immersed in the American academic environment for more than 7 months, they should have become familiar with writing academic emails by the time they answered the questionnaire.

324.2.2 Instrumentation

A questionnaire was carefully designed for this study. The questionnaire consisted of two parts—background information and a writing email task. The background part asked participants to state where they came from, where they were living and how long they had been in the US if they were ESL students. In the writing email part, participants were provided the task stated below:

> Suppose in one of your courses your professor asks you to give a presentation in class on the following Tuesday on a certain chapter of a textbook, but you don't hear clearly whether he says chapter one or chapter two. What's more, you want to ask him whether there are any specific requirements for the presentation. Please compose a short email to your professor to try to get answers to your questions (If you are female, please use the name Anne; if you are male, please use the name Tom. Thank you!).

In this study, a participant might accomplish three things in total, namely, apology, request and expressing thanks. In fact, the latter two appeared in all feedback while only one group of participants' feedback included an apology.

The reason to choose such a topic was because since EFL students hadn't been exposed to the western education system, they might be unfamiliar with some western academic topics, such as asking for an extension or having a personal meeting with a professor and thus they could very likely have problems understanding the task and composing an email, although they would have the experience of giving presentations in everyday study. Therefore, all three groups should have been able to comprehend this task, while EFL students lacked the experience of writing English emails and could therefore be regarded as similar to a control group and reflecting the original status of ESL students before they came to the US.

324.2.3 Data Collection

First, a questionnaire was designed as mentioned above. Second, this questionnaire was sent to author's friends who belonged to these three categories of students and these friends were also asked to forward the questionnaire to their friends.

All participants were asked to send their feedback to a certain email address. Third, feedbacks were collected and all of those participants who didn't fit into any of the three groups were rejected. For example, emails from students who were studying in Australia and in Britain were eliminated, because British English may differ slightly from North American English in the preferred writing styles.

324.2.4 Data Analysis

All 30 responses from the three groups were analyzed and then the differences within the three were divided into two categories, style and content. The 'style' part included title, position of complimentary close and name and content of complimentary close. The 'content' included five subcategories: greeting, self-identification, apology and explanation, request and thank you. These individual items will be explained in details in the Results section. After that, through analysis, some characteristics for each subcategory were identified. Some of them are related to pragmatics; for example, there are both direct and indirect speech acts in requests. However, some have little relation to pragmatics, such as for the position of the complimentary close and name: while most participants wrote it on the left, some participants wrote it on the right.

After statistical analysis, the findings were discussed by the author and a native English speaker and an ESL student. With the native speaker, reasons for the big differences in some characteristics between ENL and EFL were discussed. As to the ESL student, she was showed the analytical results and asked a few questions related to how she acquired certain pragmatic characteristics of native speakers. These two short interviews gave the author much inspiration and the interviewees also found the differences interesting.

324.3 Results

324.3.1 Style

In the system of analysis, style comprised three parts—title, existence of complimentary close and position of complimentary close and name are shown in Table 324.1.

"Title" refers to the very beginning of an email, how one addresses the recipient of the email. In this study, all ENL students used the title "Professor". For EFL students, 80 % used the title "Professor" while 20 % students used "Sir" or "Mr.", neither of which is commonly used to refer to a professor in a western university. This finding was similar to Li's finding (Li 2010). Among ESL students, 90 % of students chose to use "Professor" while only one student used

Table 324.1 Summary of the data of the three groups' feedback on style

	Title		Position of complimentary close and name		Complimentary close	
	Professor (%)	Other (%)	Left (%)	Right (%)	Have (%)	Don't have (%)
ENL	100	/	100	/	30	70
EFL	80	20	50	50	70	30
ESL	90	10	100	/	70	30

"Dr.", which is acceptable as well but maybe sounds slightly formal. However, none of the ESL students still used "Sir" or "Mr.", which means they were aware of how they were expected to address their professors in emails.

"Complimentary close" refers to short phrases usually written above the writer's name at the end, which is used to show politeness. Common complementary closes are "Yours sincerely", "Best", "Regards" and so on. Complimentary closes are more frequently used in formal letters and email, like business letters. In this study, only 30 % ENL students used a complimentary close. In contrast, 70 % of both EFL and ESL students used a complimentary close. The interesting thing is EFL and ESL students both seemed to prefer especially one of two complimentary closes, "Yours sincerely" and "Sincerely". When later interviewed, an ESL student explained that she had never thought of its formality. She did so just because she considered it as an indispensible part of an email, just like title and name. The reason she chose "sincerely" was because the word looked complex and cool. This result shows that the formality of the complimentary close is not that salient to ESL students and they tend to take it as formulaic.

As to the "position of complimentary close and name", all ENL and ESL students chose left justification, while 50 % of EFL students chose right justification. Right justification is usually used in traditional letters and formal email. It is very uncommon to right justify the complimentary close and name in everyday emails. From this result we can see that this characteristic must be very salient to ESL students for they all acquired it.

324.3.2 Content

'Content' consisted of five subcategories, "greeting", "self-identification", "apology", "request" and "thank you".

324.3.2.1 Greeting

In this study, "greeting" refers to sentences which appeared at the very beginning of the email, to greet the professor, such as "I hope this message finds you well".

Results show 30 % of ENL students used a greeting. The percentages for EFL students and ESL students were 20 and 10 %. Three greetings of ENL students were "I hope this message finds you well", "I hope your week has been going well", "Hope you are doing well", which all showed their good wishes. Two Chinese students wrote "How are you" and one wrote "Hello". In the interview, a native speaker revealed that although "how are you" wouldn't be considered wrong, it doesn't abide by customs for this sort of email. However, in Chinese custom, it is a habit to write "how are you" at the very beginning of the letter, regardless of the relationship between writer and receiver. So it is assumed that these two Chinese students just transformed this from their first language directly to second language.

324.3.2.2 Self-identification

"Self-identification" refers to sentences like "This is Tom" and "My name is Anne. I am a student in your XXXX class". As shown in Table 224.2, for ENL students, only one participant wrote "This is Tom." Three ESL and seven EFL students identified themselves. The obvious difference is presumably caused by the class sizes and relationships between professors and students in American versus Chinese academic environments. In the US, classes tend to be smaller and a professor is more likely to know every student in his or her class soon after the semester starts. However, to the contrary, classes in China are usually large and therefore it is difficult or impossible for a professor to know every student in his or her class. Thus, EFL students felt the need to self-identify first. For ESL students, after they came to the US and soon were aware of this new situation, they then would gradually feel at ease skipping self-identification. The original question intentionally gave no hint as to whether the class the student was in was large or small, but given the fact that the students were being told to give a presentation in the next class, it would be implied that the class had to be fairly small.

324.3.2.3 Apology

Not all students wrote apologies in their email. The portions of students who apologized didn't differ much within the three groups, with percentages of

Table 324.2 Summary of self-identification frequency in the three groups' emails

	Self-identification	
	Have (%)	Don't have (%)
ENL	10	90
EFL	70	30
ESL	30	70

ENL (30 %), EFL (50 %) and ESL (30 %). However, the content of their apology differed conspicuously.

A typical ENL student's apology was "I'm sorry for taking up your time." A typical EFL or ESL student would apologize with something like "I am sorry that I didn't hear clearly about the requirement in the class".

One of Leech's politeness maxims is called "the modesty maxim", summarized as "minimize praise of self" and "maximize dispraise of self" [3]. Paired with "the modesty maxim" is "the maxim of approbation", which is summarized as "minimize dispraise of other" and "maximize praise of other" [3]. Both the modesty maxim and the maxim of approbation explain the EFL's and ESL's apologies. Their apologies maximized the dispraise of themselves and minimized dispraise of professors. It may be in fact that the professor didn't explain clearly, or that the professor spoke too quietly such that students couldn't hear him or her clearly, but no matter what the real situation was, Chinese students would write it was their fault and not their professor's so that they didn't hear clearly. They used such a method to save the professor's face. In comparison, ENL students seemed not to care whose fault it was and their apologies in fact tended to sound more like "thank you for your time". It is not clear whether this difference was caused by value focus in different cultures, because while saving face is very important in Chinese culture, sharing time beyond one's duty time is obviously something that requires gratitude to be shown in the American culture.

324.3.2.4 Request

In all of the 30 responses, there were five kinds of requests, four belonging to direct speech and one to indirect speech.

For indirect speech, an example sentence was "I am not sure whether I will be presenting information from Chap. 1 or Chap. 2." In this case, the participant displays the "Face Threatening Act" [3] off record, expressing his or her question indirectly.

For direct speech, there are four variations in total. Each kind will be illustrated with a real example. The first type is "interrogative", which means students ask directly in the form of a question, for example, "Would you also be able to remind me of the specific requirements for the presentation?" As shown in Table 324.3, this kind of request was the most frequently used. The second type is "imperative", which means

Table 324.3 Linguistic categories of request speech in feedbacks

Request speech	Direct				Indirect
	Interrogative	Imperative	Declarative	Chinese characteristic directive	
ENL	7	0	3	0	4
EFL	7	2	1	4	2
ESL	6	0	4	0	4

students use an imperative sentence to request, for example, "Please tell me so I can prepare my presentation much better". Because imperative sentences can sound like an order, it is usually considered less polite [4]. The third type is "declarative", meaning students express their question in a declarative sentence, for example, "I want to ask whether there are any specific guidelines that I should adhere to during my segment". One point that needs to be clarified is that this type of request is different from an indirect request, though both of them are declarative sentences. Direct declarative sentences usually include words such as "ask", "want to know", "want to clarify" to express a clear request while indirect speech only mentions the participants' confusion but without an apparent request. The fourth type was only shown by EFL students and therefore is called "Chinese characteristic directive". Such a request first starts with indirect speech and then adds one direct declarative or direct imperative. A good example is this passage "I'm wondering next Tuesday which chapter my presentation will focus on, chapter one or chapter two. Besides, I also want to know what requirements about the presentation you have given to us. Would you please email the answers to me so that I could make the presentation more successful?"

ENL students are used to indirect speech, which is more implied. However, that seems quite "unsafe" to Chinese students, who are worried about their own English level and are afraid professors wouldn't understand them and therefore prefer an explicit request. Maybe that can explain the reason for the "Chinese characteristic directive", why EFL students feel the need to add one direct speech request after an indirect speech one. As shown in Table 324.3, ESL students didn't make such types of request and used more indirect speech than EFL students did, which reveals that ESL students were becoming familiar with a native speakers' indirect request style.

As mentioned above, imperative can be considered less polite. Apparently, ESL students noticed this point and didn't use that form any longer. Another interesting discovery was that ESL students seemed to acquire the direct declarative request, which is also preferred by ENL students but seldom used by EFL students.

324.3.2.5 Thank You

Note the sentence pattern "thank you for +N". As shown in Table 324.4, ENL students used only "thank you for your time", which tends to be formulaic.

Table 324.4 Categories of "Thank you" in the feedback

	Top two most frequent used "thank you" patterns	Times used
ENL	Thank you for your time.	4
	Thank you very much.	4
EFL	Thank you very much.	4
	Thank you for +N (consideration, help, answer, patience).	4
ESL	Thanks/Thank you.	3
	Thank you for +N (time, your elaboration, consideration).	3

However, when it comes to EFL students and ESL students, the N varies. A native speaker explained that although words like "consideration" are not wrong, they are not what native speakers would say. "Thank you for your time" tends to be a fixed formula. The only ESL student who wrote "thank you for your time" was my roommate. When asked whether she just acquired this phrase from emails she received or she learned it somewhere explicitly, she said she had read something somewhere explicitly mentioning that this phrase is the standard saying.

324.4 Discussion

From the Results section we can see that Chinese students studying in the US (ESL students) have acquired some characteristics of native English speakers, which is related to their experience studying abroad. However, while some points seem to be quite easy to acquire, such as the position of the complimentary close and name, some points are harder to adopt, such as the content of an apology.

Previous studies that examined the role email exchanges played in EFL teaching were usually longitudinal studies under a researcher's instruction. In Ndemanu's research [5], "An online epistolary project" between some Cameroonian French-speaking students and Canadian English-speaking students, it was found that over more than 1.5 years of email exchanges, Cameroonian students showed "incremental gains" in their "English-language acquisition". Another report of related research is Liu's semester-long email exchange activity [6] focusing on "power perceptions and negotiations". In that research, Liu discussed the power differentials in the email exchanges and how Taiwanese students "adopted varied discursive and non-discursive strategies to negotiate the power differentials." As with these two research studies, the present research also discovered that email exchanges with ENL students can improve the ESL writing skills of students. But in contrast with the aforementioned longitudinal researches, the research presented here proposed a specific email topic and used a control group (EFL) and a comparative group (ENL) to pinpoint what pragmatic characteristics ESL students had acquired.

This study has produced some very interesting results and encourages further studies. However, the research reported here had its limitations. Because all of the EFL students were English majors it meant that their English competence would almost certainly be better than the original abilities of the ESL students and therefore they were not the optimal choice as a type of control group. So in a future study, having participants who share similar background experiences would make the study more precise. What's more, a future study could explore more about the differences among ESL students based on how long they have lived in the US.

324.5 Conclusion

From this research, we see that although natural acquisition can help improve a person's second language pragmatics competence, it is far from sufficient if one wants to be close to a native speakers' level. Explicit teaching and pinpointing are very effective and therefore should be given attention in academic language teaching. As for EFL students, their English professors should encourage them to communicate more in English by email so that they can actually apply English in everyday, real life contexts.

References

1. Feak CB, Reihart SM, Rohlck TN (2009) Academic interactions—communicating on campus. The University of Michigan Press, Michigan
2. Swales JM, Feak CB (2004) Academic writing for graduate students—essential tasks and skills. The University of Michigan Press, Michigan
3. Cutting J (2009) Pragmatics and discourse. Routledge, New York
4. Hartford BS, Bardovi HKT (1996) At your earliest convenience: a study of written student requests to faculty. In: Pragmatics and language learning. Monograph Series vol 7, pp 55–69
5. Ndemanu TM (2012) The contribution of email exchanges to second language acquisition: a case of cross-cultural communication between Africa and North America. In: The reading matrix vol 12, Number 1, Apr 2012
6. Liu YC (2011) Power perceptions and negotiations in a cross-national email writing activity. J Second Lang Writ 20(2011):257–270
7. Shujing L (2010) An email-assisted mode of teaching college English. In: Language learning and new technologies: proceedings of the 2nd international conference on language learning at Peking University. Peking University Press, Beijing

Chapter 325
Construction of a Differentiated Embryo Chondrocyte 1 Lentiviral Expression Vector and Establishment of its Stably Transfected HGC27 Cell Line

Rui Hu, Yun-Shan Wang, Yi Kong, Pin Li, Yan Zheng, Xiao-Li Ma and Yan-Fei Jia

Abstract Human differentiated embryo chondrocyte 1 (DEC1), has been suggested to play key roles in immune regulation, cell differentiation, proliferation and apoptosis, circadian rhythms, hypoxia response and carcinogenesis. However, the role of DEC1 in gastric cancer have not been well established. Lentiviral vectors are widely used for the stable expression of genes and currently under development for clinical use in gene therapy. Therefore we intended to construct a lentiviral DEC1 expression vector and then establish a gastric cancer cell line with stable expression of DEC1. The coding sequence of gene was amplified using PCR and cloned into pGV218 vector. 293T cells were transfected using Lipofectamine 2000 and packaged for the recombinant lentivirus particles. When the cloned sequence was identified to be right, the recombinant lentivirus particles were amplified in a large quantity. The titer of virus was determined by real-time PCR. Subsequently, we collected the lentivirus venom to infect the HGC27 cells and establish a stable, overexpressed cell line named GFP/DEC1-HGC27. This study will provide a new cell model for further study of the role of DEC 1in the pathogenesis of gastric cancer.

Keywords DEC1 · Lentiviral expression vector · Gastric cancer · HGC27

R. Hu · Y.-S. Wang · Y. Kong · P. Li
Shandong University School of Medicine, Jinan, Shandong 250012, China

Y.-S. Wang · Y. Zheng · X.-L. Ma · Y.-F. Jia (✉)
Central Laboratory, Jinan Central Hospital, Affiliated to Shandong University,
Jie fang road 105, Shandong, Jinan, China
e-mail: jiayanfei_@126.com

325.1 Introduction

Human differentiated embryo chondrocyte 1 (DEC1), a basic helix-loop-helix (bHLH) transcription factor, has rat and mouse orthologs named enhancer of split and hairy related protein-2 (SHARP-2) and stimulation of retinoic acid 13 (Stra13), respectively [1]. Overexpression of DEC1 has been reported to contribute to cell differentiation, proliferation and apoptosis, circadian rhythms, hypoxia response and carcinogenesis [1–4]. High levels of DEC1 expression are also detected in a variety of cancer cell lines including leukaemia, colon and lung adenocarcinoma, gliomas and breast cancer [5–7] indicating it play a pivotal role in carcinogenesis. We have previously shown that DEC1 mRNA and protein were upregulated significantly in gastric cancer tissue [4]. Importantly, the increased DEC1 expression was correlated with poor differentiation of gastric cancer, suggesting that DEC1 may play an important role in the differentiation and progression of gastric tumors. However, the function and mechanism of the DEC1 gene is not completely understood, so it is necessary to build an efficient and simple approach for studying the effect of DEC1 in vitro.

In this study, we successfully constructed a lentiviral expression vector that can over-express DEC1 and establish human gastric caner cell lines stably expressing DEC1, providing a foundation for further studies on the function of DEC1 in gastric cancer.

325.2 Materials and Methods

325.2.1 Vectors and Cells

Lentiviral expression vector pGV218 and envelope helper vectors pHelper 1.0 and pHelper 2.0 were produced by Genechem (Shanghai, China). E. Coli DH5a used in subclone, 293T cells used in envelope were conserved by Genechem. The human gastric carcinoma cell line, HGC27 (from Cell Bank of Chinese academy of sciences), was cultured in DMEM medium (Invitrogen) supplemented with 10 % FBS (Invitrogen), 1 % antibiotics. They were incubated at 37 °C in 5 % carbon dioxide–humidified air.

325.2.2 Construction and Identification of Recombinant DEC1 Lentivirus Vector

Referring to GenBank gene sequences, the software Premier 5.0 was used to design DEC1 primers. The upstream primer was: 5′GCCACCATGGAGCGG ATC CCCAG3′. The downstream primer was: 5′ATCTTGCAGCATTCACAAA3′.

The total RNA was extracted from cancer cell line MGC803 and then got the DEC1 cDNA by RT-PCR. DEC1 was obtained using the cDNA as a template and the primers above by Landing type PCR. The PCR products were separated by agarose gel electrophoresis and the DEC1 coding region fragment DNA was extracted and purified using DNA gel extraction kit (Promega) and DNA recovery kit (Promega) separately. The purified DEC1 fragment and gene plasmid were digested separately with AgeI (Takara). The two recovered products were ligated using In-Fusion kit (Genechem) and the ligated product was used to transfect E. coli DH5. The E. coli clones were cultured in LB medium containing AMP and the plasmid was extracted by plasmid extraction kit (QIAGEN). The correct transformant was identified by PCR analysis and DNA sequencing.

325.2.3 Packaging, Concentration and Titration of Recombinant DEC1 Lentivirus Vector

Purified pGV-DEC1, pHelper 1.0 and pHelper 2.0 plasmid transfected 293T cells were used to produce lentivirus. The supernatant of cell culture were harvested after 48 h cultures. Then virus was purified with plus-20 kit (Millipore, USA) and storage at −80 °C. The production of control virus enveloping pGV followed the same protocol, meanwhile. The titer of recombinant lentivirus was determined by real-time PCR. The viral concentration mentioned above was served as stock solution and a 10-fold dilution series was performed until dilution fold reached 10–5. The six samples were used to transfect 1×105 293T cells respectively. 4 d later, the total cellular RNA of each group was extracted using Trizol according to the manufacturer's instructions. 20 μl cDNA was obtained after reverse transcription and 1 μl cDNA was taken to perform real-time PCR using SYBR Master Mixture (Takara).

325.2.4 Gastric Cancer Cell Transduction with Recombinant Lentivirus and Selected by Puromycin

The day before transduction, HGC27 cells were seeded into 96-well cell-culture plates at a density of 5×10^3 cells per well. On the day, they were transduced with 200 μl of the already described virus-containing supernatant. At 24 h post transduction, the mix was replaced with fresh cell-culture medium. 48 h post transduction, the cells were collected for protein isolation and western blot analysis. In order to produce stably transduced cells 48 h post transduction, 5 μg/ml of puromycin (Sigma) were added to the medium, as a means of selecting clones containing the insert. The puromycin cotaining medium was replenished every 3 days. The cells remained in the selective medium for 2 weeks. 2-fold serial dilutions of puromycin were prepared in a preliminary test, 5 μg/ml of puromycin being considered as the final selective concentration. After 12 days, puromycin-resistant HGC27 cell pools were established.

325.2.5 Western Blotting Analysis

After the transfection of HGC27 cells, the cells were rinsed with PBS and lysed with SDS–PAGE protein loading buffer containing 5 % 2-mercaptoethanol. For western blot analysis, total protein was separated on 10 % SDS-PAGE and transferred onto nitrocellulose membranes (0.45 μm, Millipore, Billerica, MA, USA), which were incubated for 24 h at 4 °C with the antibodies for DEC1 (1:500, Santa Cruz Biotechnology), then horseradish peroxidase-conjugated anti-mouse IgG antibody (Santa Cruz Biotechnology) after a final wash. Reactions were developed with use of 4-chloro-1-naphthol (Sigma) and H_2O_2. Signals were detected with use of an enhanced chemiluminescence kit (Amersham Pharmacia, Buckinghamshire, UK). GAPDH level was an internal standard.

325.2.5.1 Statistical Analysis

All the experiments were performed in triplicate. Data were analyzed with the SPSS 13.0 Student t test to evaluate the significance of differences in gene expression. The results were expressed as mean ±STD. The level chosen to define whether treatments were significantly different from mock controls was $p < 0.05$.

325.3 Results

325.3.1 Construction of Recombinant Lentiviral Vectors of DEC1 Gene

Entire DEC1 cDNA sequence was obtained by PCR reaction (Fig. 325.1). AgeI digested DNA was linked to pGV 218 and produced pGV-DEC1 vector. The positive clones were identified by PCR (Fig. 325.2) and the result of DNA sequencing further confirmed that the inserted fragment was consistent with our target sequence. The recombinant lentiviral vector was packaged in 293T with a viral titer of 2×10^8 Tu/ml.

Fig. 325.1 Fragment containing entire DEC1 cDNA sequence, F: products of PCR reaction

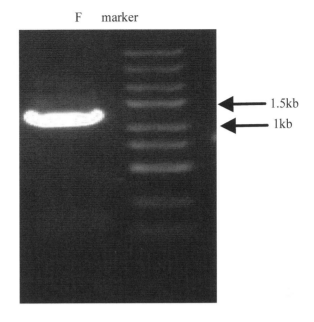

Fig. 325.2 Colony PCR tests of transformed DH5a. Samples 1–6: Products of PCR reaction with boiled DH5a cells as templates ①:ddH2O; ②: negative control; ③: GAPDH; ④: marker; ⑤–⑩: sample 1–6; The samples 3–6 were positive

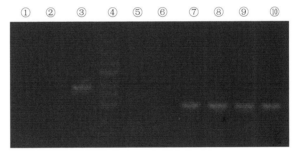

325.3.2 Lentivirus-Mediated Expression Vector Integrate into Genome and Provide Stable DEC1 Overexpression in HGC27

In the present study we chose gastric cancer cell HGC27 for transduction with DEC1. Transduction with GFP served as a control. The DEC1 and the GFP transduced cells can show green fluorescence confirmed by immunofluorescence staining (Fig. 325.3). The western blotting analyses confirmed DEC1 expression in stable DEC1-transduced cells but not in GFP-transduced cells (Fig. 325.4). These data confirmed the establishment a stable gastric cancer cell line of expression of DEC1 protein.

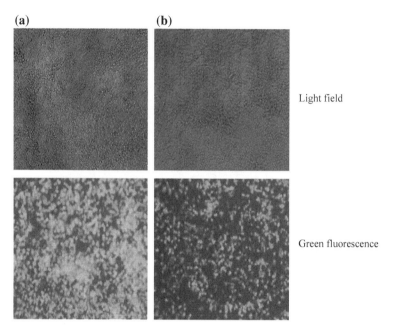

Fig. 325.3 The GFP expression of HGC27 cells after being infected by pGV and pGV-DEC1 (**a**: pGV, **b**: pGV-DEC1)

Fig. 325.4 Western blotting analysis of pGV-DEC1 transfected HGC27 cells. ① PGV (GFP-transduced cell); ② PGV-DEC1 (DEC1 and the GFP transduced cells)

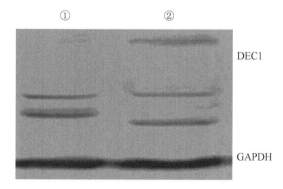

325.4 Discussion

Among gene delivery systems, lentiviral vectors derived from human immunodeficiency virus type 1(HIV-1) have gained considerable status in a variety of applications by their capacity to achieve stable infection, maintain long-term transgene expression, transducer both dividing and nondividing cells [8–10] and have a promising future in clinical applications [11, 12]. Severals surveys have show that overexpression of DEC1 affected the expression of apoptosis related-factors such as Bcl-2, Fas, Bax, c-Myc, survivin and vascular endothelial growth factor (VEGF) as well as caspases in some tumor tissues [13–15]. It will be easier to study the function of DEC1, if the gene can be expressed in target cells via an effective vector. Furthermore, if expressed alongside certain apoptotic factors, the DEC1 gene may be a good target gene for gene therapy.

In this study, we constructed the DEC1 recombinant lentiviral expression vector. Using molecular cloning techniques such as PCR and DNA sequencing, the human DEC1 lentiviral expression plasmid was successfully constructed and high titer viral particles were obtained after plasmid transfection in packaging cells. HGC27 cells were successfully infected and stable expression of DEC1 was confirmed by Western blotting. This will allow for a detailed examination of the mechanism of DEC1, including its relationship to apoptotic and proliferative genes.

Acknowledgments This work was financially supported by National Natural Science Foundation of China (NSFC No. 81000869 and NSFC No. 81272588), 973 Project grant (2012CB966503 and 2012CB966504).

References

1. Shi XH, Zheng Y, Sun Q, Cui J et al (2011) DEC1 nuclear expression: a marker of differentiation grade in hepatocellular carcinoma. World J Gastroenterol 17(15):2037–2043
2. Wu Y, Sato F, Bhawal UK, Kawamoto T, Fujimoto K et al (2011) Basic helix-loop-helix transcription factors DEC1 and DEC2 regulate the paclitaxel-induced apoptotic pathway of MCF-7 human breast cancer cells. Int J Mol Med 27(4):491–495
3. Bode B, Shahmoradi A, Taneja R, Rossner MJ, Oster H (2012) Genetic interaction of Per1 and Dec1/2 in the regulation of circadian locomotor activity. J Biol Rhythms 27(2):180
4. Zheng Y, Jia Y, Wang Y, Wang M, Li B, Shi X, Ma X et al (2009) The hypoxia-regulated transcription factor DEC1 (Stra13, SHARP-2) and its expression in gastric cancer. OMICS 13:301–306
5. Li Y, Zhang H, Xie M, Hu M et al (2002) Abundant expression of Dec1/stra13/sharp2 in colon carcinoma:its antagonizing role in serum deprivation-induced apoptosis andselective inhibition of procaspase activation. Biochem J 367:413–422
6. Zhang L, Li QQ (2007) Embryo-chondrocyte expressed gene 1, downregulating hypoxia-inducible factor 1 alpha, is another marker of lung tumor hypoxia. Acta Pharmacol Sin 28(4):549–558
7. Chakrabarti J, Turley H, Campo L, Han C, Harris AL, Gatter KC, Fox SB (2004) The transcription factor DEC1 (stra13, SHARP2) is associated with the hypoxic response and high tumour grade in human breast cancers. Br J Cancer 91:954–958
8. Santhosh CV, Tamhane MC, Kamat RH, Patel VV, Mukhopadhyaya R (2008) A lentiviral vector with novel multiple cloning sites: stable transgene expression in vitro and in vivo. Biochem Biophys Res Commun 371:546–550
9. Ravet E, Lulka H, Gross F, Casteilla L, Buscail L, Cordelier P (2010) Using lentiviral vectors for effcient pancreatic cancer gene therapy. Cancer Gene Ther 17:315–324
10. Trobridge GD, Beard BC, Gooch C et al (2008) Effcient transduction of pigtailed macaque hematopoietic repopulating cells with HIV-based lentiviral vectors. Blood 111:5537–5543

11. Wang H, Tan SS, Wang XY, Liu DH, Yu CS, Bai ZL et al (2007) Silencing livin gene by siRNA leads to apoptosis induction, cell cycle arrest and proliferation inhibition in malignant melanoma LiBr cells. Acta Pharmacol Sin 28:1968–1974
12. Thomas M, Greil J, Heidenreich O (2006) Targeting leukemic fusion proteins with small interfering RNAs: recent advances and therapeutic potentials. Acta Pharmacol Sin 27:273–281
13. Li Y, Xie M, Yang J, Yang D et al (2006) The expression of antiapoptotic protein survivin is transcriptionally upregulated by DEC1 primarily through multiple sp1 binding sites in the proximal promoter. Oncogene 25:3296–3306
14. Peng Y, Liu W, Xiong J, Gui HY et al (2012) Down regulation of differentiated embryonic chondrocytes 1 (DEC1) is involved in 8-methoxypsoralen-induced apoptosis in HepG2 cells. Toxicology 301:58–65
15. Wu Y, Sato F, Bhawal UK, Kawamoto T, Fujimoto K et al (2011) Basic helix-loop-helix transcription factors DEC1 and DEC2 regulate the paclitaxel-induced apoptotic pathway of MCF-7 human breast cancer cells. Int J Mol Med 27(4):491–495

Chapter 326
Construction of Expression Vector of miRNA Specific for FUT3 and Identification of Its Efficiency in KATO-III Gastric Cancer Cell Line

Yong-Hong Xin, Yan-Fei Jia, Qiang Liu, Hong Zhang, Hai-ning Zhu, Xiao-li Ma, Yong-Jun Cai and Yun-Shan Wang

Abstract Human blood group Lewis antigen, which is fucosylated glycoconjugates involved in the development of several pathologies. Fucosyltransferases are enzymes that add fucose to precursor glycan structures: FUT3 catalyze the addition of fucose to the α 1-3, 4 position and are detected in epithelial cells. As the expression of Lewis a is mainly controlled by FUT3, which can influence Lewis a'S synthesis, we choose FUT3 as our target gene to silence. In our study, we constructed FUT3-specific miRNA expression vector successfully. It showed in the experiment that FUT3—specific miRNA expression vector could actively inhibit FUT3'S expression in mRNA level in KATO—III gastric cancer cell1 line, and decrease Lewis antigen'S synthesis as weII growth. From this experiment, we obtain the best mi RNA sequence of FUT3, which may serve as a new strategy for investigating the mechanism of molecular glycol—pathology of gastric cancer targeted tumor gene therapy.

Keywords FUT3 · Lewis antigen · Gastric cancer · miRNA · KATO-III · RNAi

---

These authors Yong-Hong Xin, Yan-Fei Jia are contributed equally to this paper.

Y.-H. Xin · Y.-J. Cai
Department of Blood Transfusion, Fourth People's Hospital of Jinan,
Taishan Medical College, Jinan, Shandong, China

Y.-F. Jia · X. Ma · Y.-S. Wang (✉)
Shandong University, Central Laboratory, Jinan Central Hospital, Jie fang road 105, Jinan, Shandong, China
e-mail: sdjnwys@163.com

Q. Liu
China National Heavy Duty Truck Group Corporation Hospital, Jinan, Shandong, China

H. Zhang
Clinical Laboratory, Jinan No. 6 People's Hospital, Jinan, Shandong, China

H. Zhu
Zi Bo Municipal Center For Disease Control and Prevention, Zibo, Shandong, China

326.1 Introduction

Lewis antigens are fucosylated oligosaccharides carried by glycoproteins and glycolipids in the terminal position of carbohydrate chains. These antigens, biochemically related to the ABH blood groups, are synthesized by the sequential action of specific glycosyltransferases (FUT). FUT protein family is involved in the synthesis of cell surface antigen through catalyzing the transfer of GDP-Fucose to the N-acetylglucosamine residue of glycoproteins. The FUTs family is divided into four subfamilies, a-1, 2, a-1, 3/4, a-1, 6, and protein O-FUT. In the a-1,3/4 FUT subfamily, at least eight members have been discovered (FUT3, FUT4, FUT5, FUT6, FUT7, FUT9, FUT10, and FUT11 [1–7].

FUTs have been shown to be involved in various biological processes, including cell adhesion, lymphocyte homing, embryo-fetal development and tumor progression [8, 9]. FUT3, the Lewis enzyme, predominantly synthesizes a4- and to a lesser extent a 3-fucosylated oligosaccharides with the resulting products Lea, Leb, sLea, Lex, sLex, Ley [10]. Furthermore, increases of sialyl-Lewisa was also found to be associated with disease progression and bad prognoses. The expression of these FUTs in cancer tissues has been exhaustively studied. However, the relationships between FUT expression and sialyl-Lewis antigen expression have never been in depth analyzed on human gastric cell lines. To confirm the role of FUT3, we used a RNAi strategy by expressing FUT3—specific miRNA expression vectors in the gastric cancer cell line, which expresses a significant amount of endogenous FUT3, an a [1, 4] Fuc-T activity, and harbors the sialyl-Lewis a(sLea) cell surface antigens. We have shown that the inhibition of FUT3 expression in human gastric cancer cells resulted in the decrease of sialyl-Lewis a antigen expression.

326.2 Materials and Methods

326.2.1 Cells and Culture Conditions

Gastric cancer cell line KATO-III cultured in Dulbecco's modified Eagle's medium (DMEM) supplemented with 10 % fetal bovine serum (FBS) and incubated at 37 °C in a humidified atmosphere with 5 % CO_2.

326.2.2 Design of miRNAs and Construction of Plasmids

Two different miRNAs targeting different parts of the FUT3 gene were designed: 5′-AACTGCAGCAGGAATCCAGGT-3′; 5′-AACCCATACAGTGAATCCATT-3′. This included sequences that contain a GC ratio ranging from 40 to 60 %, sequences without 3 successive Ts, and sequences specific only to the targeted gene as confirmed by basic local alignment search tool (BLAST) against the human gene database. The two sequences were individually incorporated into a pair of oligonucloetides (produced by Shanghai Invitrogen Biotechnology) where the target sequence appears as antisense followed by sense orientations separated by a 9-nucloetide spacer sequence. The annealed oligonucleotides were cloned into pcDNAU6. 2-GW/EmGFP-miR expression Vector (Invitrogen) according to the manufacturer's recommendations.

326.2.3 Transient Transfection of Plasmids

One day before transfection, 100,000 cells per well were plated in a 6-well plate without antibiotics so that cells would be 90 % confluent at the time of transfection. The cells were transfected with 2 μg/4 μg/8 μg of Vector FUT3 miRNA1/2 and empty plasmids, using 5 μl/10 μl/20 μl of Lipofectamine 2000™ (Invitrogen). Media were changed at 6 h after transfection and replaced with 1 ml of fresh complete medium.

326.2.4 Reverse Transcript-Polymerase Chain Reaction Analysis

Human FUT3 PCR primers used in experiments are 5′gcaaggcttagaccagttcg3′ and 5′aaaggccatgtccatagcag3′. Human GAPDH primers are 5′attcaacggcacagtcaagg3′ and 5′caccagtggatgcagggat3′. Total RNA was isolated from the cells by TRIzol (Invitrogen) after transfection. RNAs were reversely transcribed into cDNAs using RNA PCR Kit (AMV) Ver.3.0 (Takara) according to the manufacturer's instructions. The reactions were performed on ABI PRISM®5700 sequence detection system (Applied Biosystem). The mRNA expression level of FUT3 was normalized to the mRNA expression level of the reference gene GAPDH.

326.2.5 Flow Cytometer

sLea antigens were determined by immunofluorescence staining followed by flow cytometric analysis with the FACS Calibur flow cytometry with Cell quest software and associated software (Becton–Dickinson, Lysis II). The cells were incubated with anti-sLea antibody (CHEMICON) for 30 min at RT. After washing thoroughly with PBS, the cells were stained with a FITC-labeled anti-goat antibody for 30 min at 4 °C. Nonspecific staining was determined by using a control goat Ig.

326.2.6 Statistical Analysis

The data were represented as mean ± SD. The data was analyzed with statistical software of SPSS11.5. Student's *t* test was used to assess differences between the treatment group and control group. $P < 0.05$ was considered statistically significant.

326.3 Results

326.3.1 DNA Sequencing

DNA sequencing showed targeting miRNA oligonucleotides were correctly inserted into the pcDNAU6. 2-GW/EmGFP-miR expression Vector without base mutation (Fig. 326.1).

326.3.2 Transfection with FUT3-specific miRNA down-regulated FUT3 mRNA levels to silence FUT3 gene

According to the results of quantitative real-time PCR (Fig. 326.2), no significant difference ($P > 0.05$) was detected in the levels of FUT3 mRNA between blank control group and empty vector group. The mRNA expression of miRNA group were significantly lower than that in empty vector group ($P < 0.05$), respectively. These data suggested that FUT3 mRNA levels in KATO-III cells decreased significantly after transfection with FUT3 miRNA. Transfection with FUT3-specific miRNA could result in FUT3 mRNA degradation to silence FUT3 gene.

326.3.3 Transfection with FUT3-specific miRNA inhibited sLea protein expression in KATO-III

FACS analysis showed that, the levels of sLea protein expression in the miRNA group were significantly lower than that in blank control group and empty vector group, respectively ($P < 0.05$; Fig. 326.3), while the difference between blank control group and empty vector group was not significant ($P > 0.05$). These data indicated that FUT3-specific miRNA silencing mRNA could significantly reduce the levels of sLea protein expression in KATO-III cells.

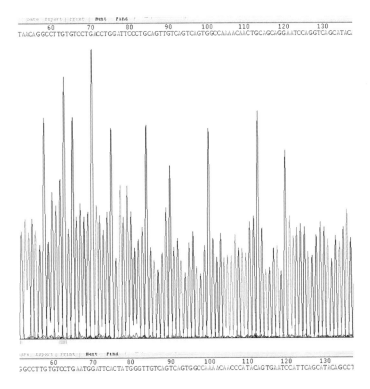

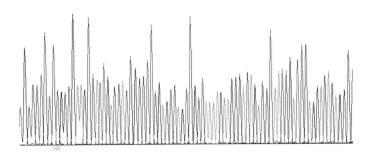

Fig. 326.1 The result of sequencing of the insert

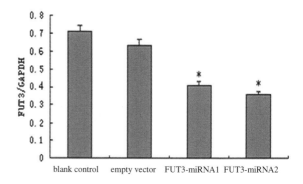

Fig. 326.2 qRT-PCR was performed to analyze the mRNA expression

326.4 Discussion

In our cell line model, we confirmed that sLea antigen was related to the levels of FUT3 gene expression. In fact, both at basal conditions and after decreasing FUT3 mRNA levels with FUT3-specific miRNA expression vector, sLea antigen levels were correlated with FUT3 mRN As sLea are the major terminal carbohydrate structures that bind to selectins and interfere in tumor cells rolling and metastasis

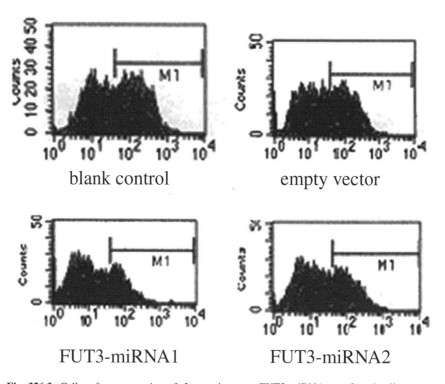

Fig. 326.3 Cell surface expression of sLea antigens on FUT3-miRNA transfected cells

[11], it is fundamental to understand the biosynthesis of these sialyl-Lewis antigens and their regulatory mechanisms. Biosynthesis of sLea antigens is dependent upon the addition of fucose in a-1,3 or a-1,4 linkage to sialylated precursors by an a-1,3 or a-1,4 FUT. FUT3 is highly detected in normal gastric epithelium [12], and has α-1,3 and α-1,4 fucosyltranferase activity. To identify the endogenous fucosyltransferase species responsible for the synthesis of these cell surface antigens, we used a RNAi approach by transfecting the KATO-III cells with a FUT3-specific miRNA expression vector. The data presented here showed, for the first time in gastric cancer cells, that the decrease of FUT3 expression by the transfection of FUT3-specific miRNA expression vector results principally in a decrease of sLea antigen expression on cell surface.

Therefore, the expression of sLea antigens in gastric cancer seems to be controlled by FUT3 expression. The impairment of sLea antigen expression could become a good challenge in the development of antiadhesion treatments for gastric cancer metastasis. FUT3 seems to be essential in the regulation of the expression of sLea s antigens on the cell surface and appears as an important target to develop novel anti-adhesion therapies for gastric cancer based on specific miRNA expression vector as therapeutic molecules.

References

1. Kukowska-Latallo JF, Larsen RD, Nair RP, Lowe JB (1990) A cloned human cDNA determines expression of a mouse stage-specific embryonic antigen and the Lewis blood group alpha(1, 3/1, 4)fucosyltransferase. Genes Dev 4:1288–1303
2. Lowe JB, Kukowska-Latallo JF, Nair RP (1991) Molecular cloning of a human fucosyltransferase gene that determines expression of the Lewis x and VIM-2 epitopes but not ELAM-1-dependent cell adhesion. J Biol Chem 266:17467–17477
3. Weston BW, Nair RP, Larsen RD, Lowe JB (1992) Isolation of a novel human alpha (1,3)fucosyltransferase gene and molecular comparison to the human Lewis blood group alpha (1, 3/1, 4)fucosyltransferase gene. Syntenic, homologous, nonallelic genes encoding enzymes with distinct acceptor substrate specificities. J Biol Chem 267:4152–4160
4. Weston BW, Smith PL, Kelly RJ, Lowe JB (1992) Molecular cloning of a fourth member of a human alpha(1,3) fucosyltransferase gene family. Multiple homologous sequences that determine expression of the Lewis x, sialyl Lewis x, and difucosyl sialyl Lewis x epitopes. J Biol Chem 267:24575–24584
5. Sasaki K, Kurata K, Funayama K et al (1994) Expression cloning of a novel alpha 1,3-fucosyltransferase that is involved in biosynthesis of the sialyl Lewis x carbohydrate determinants in leukocytes. J Biol Chem 269:14730–14737
6. Kudo T, Ikehara Y, Togayachi A (1998) Expression cloning and characterization of a novel murine alpha1, 3-fucosyltransferase, mFuc-TIX, that synthesizes the Lewis x (CD15) epitope in brain and kidney. J Biol Chem 273:26729–26738
7. Roos C, Kolmer M, Mattila P, Renkonen R (2002) Composition of Drosophila melanogaster proteome involved in fucosylated glycan metabolism. J Biol Chem 277:3168–3175
8. Cailleau-Thomas A, Coullin P, Candelier JJ (2000) FUT4 and FUT9 genes are expressed early in human embryogenesis. Glycobiology 10:789–802
9. Smithson G, Rogers CE, Smith PL (2001) Fuc-TVII is required for T helper 1 and T cytotoxic 1 lymphocyte selectin ligand expression and recruitment in inflammation, and

together with Fuc-TIV regulates naive T cell trafficking to lymph nodes. J Exp Med 194:601–614
10. Kukowska-Latallo JF, Larsen RD, Nair RP (1990) A cloned human cDNA determines expression of a mouse stagespecific embryonic antigen and the Lewis blood group(1,3/1,4)fucosyltransferase. Genes Dev 4:288–1303
11. Dimitroff CJ, Lechpammer M, Long-Woodward D, Kutok JL (2004) Rolling of human bone-metastatic prostate tumor cells on human bone marrow endothelium under shear flow is mediated by E-selectin. Cancer Res 64:5261–5269
12. Lopez-Ferrer A, de Bolos C, Barranco C, Garrido M, Isern J, Carlstedt I, Reis CA, Torrado J, Real FX (2000) Role of fucosyltransferases in the association between apomucin and Lewis antigen expression in normal and malignant gastric epithelium. Gut 47:349–356

Chapter 327
Molecular Cloning, Sequence Analysis of Thioesterases from Wintersweet (*Chimonanthus Praecox*)

Li-Hong Zhang, Qiong Wu, Xian-Feng Zou, Li-Na Chen, Shu-Yan Yu, Chang-Cheng Gao and Xing Chen

Abstract A coding region of wintersweet cDNA was cloned via screening a wintersweet cDNA library. The *CpFATB* cDNA is 1110 bp in length with an open reading frame (ORF) of 1107 bp encoding a protein of 369 amino acids. Molecular weight and isoelectric point of the protein is 41.72 kD and 7.72, respectively. Bioinformatics analysis shows that a signal peptide with 49 amino acid residues and Protein Localization Sites exists in the chloroplast stroma. This classifies the protein as stable.

Keywords Thioesterases · Bioinformatics · Wintersweet

327.1 Introduction

Fatty acyl–acyl carrier protein thioesterases (FAT) was initially identified in the Escherichia coliand has been found to be widespread in eukaryotes, bacteria, and archea and to be involved in a range of cellular processes including fatty acid biosynthesis [1]. Two different classes of FATs have been described in plants, based upon their amino acid sequence and substrate specificity, namely FATA and FATB [2]. The FATA thioesterases have the highest in vitro activity for 18:1-ACP substrates and exhibit a much lower activity for saturated acyl-ACP substrates [3]. Conversely, FATBs prefer saturated acyl group substrates, but also have activity for unsaturated acyl-ACPs [4]. In the current study, a putative acyl–acyl carrier protein thioesterase cDNA (CpF ATB) was cloned by screening a cDNA library of wintersweet (*Chimonanthus praecox*). The Bioinformatics Toolkit is a platform that integrates a great variety of tools for CpFATB sequence analysis to predict the possible functions, inquiry this protein properties.

L.-H. Zhang (✉) · Q. Wu · X.-F. Zou · L.-N. Chen · S.-Y. Yu · C.-C. Gao · X. Chen
Key Laboratory of Agricultural Products Processing, Changchun University, Changchun, People's Republic of China
e-mail: zhlh2005@sohu.com

327.2 Methods

327.2.1 CpFATB Cloning and Analysis

A wintersweet cDNA library was constructed using a SMART™ cDNA Library Construction Kit from wintersweet corolla material (Sambrook et al. 1989). The coding region of CpFATB was amplified by PCR from the wintersweet cDNA library using the following primers

sense primer: 5'-GCTCTAGAACCATGGCCGCTACT,
anti-sense primer: 5'-CCGCTCGAGTCTTTCATTCATTC ATCACAA.

Thirty thermal cycles were carried out, each consisting of 45 s at 95 °C, 1 min at 54 °C, and 90 s at 72 °C in an automatic thermal cycler. PCR products were separated on a 1 % agarose gel and visualized under UV light.

327.2.2 Bioinformatics Analysis

Physicochemical properties and molecular features of CpFATB were predicted by bioinformatic approaches including physical and chemical properties analysis, hydrophobicity analysis, domain analysis, phylogenetic tree analysis and subcellular localization analysis. Homology search using the program BLAST (Basic Local Alignment Search Tool) from NCBI (National Center for Biotechnology Information, Washington, D.C.). BLAST can be used to infer functional and evolutionary relationships between sequences as well as help identify members of gene families. Protein Secondary Structure Prediction using SOPMA from http://npsa-pbil.ibcp.fr/. The Hydrophobicity profile predicted of FAT amino acid sequence by DNAMAN and MEGA4x1 software. SignalP server predicts the presence and location of signal peptide cleavage sites in amino acid sequences. PSORT software predicts protein subcellular location.

327.3 Results

327.3.1 Cloning and Characterization of CpFATB cDNA Sequence

A coding region of wintersweet cDNA (CpFATB) was cloned via screening a wintersweet cDNA library. The CpFAT cDNA is 1107 bp form a single open reading frame, predicting a 369 amino acid polypeptide (Fig. 327.1). Sequence homology was investigated using NCBI-BLAST provided by the National Center

Fig. 327.1 The ORF nucleotide sequence and putative amino acid sequence of CpFATB

```
  1  M S M I A S S V G A A F F P A Q G I I K
 21  S K P A G L H V K A N G R A S P S I D G
 41  P K V T V G L E G T N A S S T R K F M N
 61  L L P D W S M L L A A F T T I F E K Q K
 81  V V V D Q F R F G H D R L V Y S E N F T
101  I R S Y E I G A D Q T A S I E T V M N L
121  L Q E T G I N C F R S L G L L L D G F D
141  S T V E M C K R D L I W V V T R M Q V I
161  V D H Y P S R G D T V E V E T H C G A Y
181  G K H G H R R E W L I R N S K T G Q I L
201  T R A T S V L V V M N K R T R R L S I L
221  P D E V R R E L E P Y F M E N L S V M K
241  D Q G R K L P K V D H S I A D Y V R Q G
261  L T C Q W S D L D I N Q H V N H I K Y V
281  K W I F E S V P V S I L E S H E I S S M
301  T L E F K R E C G K D S M L Q S L T A V
321  V S G R R V D G S V E E T D V E F Q H L
341  L Q L E D G P E V M R G T T K W R P K S
361  T L F P N S I S H *
```

for Biotechnology Information. Sequence analysis showed that the gene had typical characteristics encoding FAT protein family, the gene was named as CpFATB (Fig. 327.2).

327.3.2 CpFAT Conservative Regional and Phylogenetic Tree

Use of NCBI (http://www.ncbi.nlm.nih.gov/Structure/cdd/wrpsb.cgi) this gene encoding amino acids are conservative regional analysis, CpFAT belongs the plant acyl–acyl carrier protein (ACP) thioesterases (TEs). Acyl-ACP thioesterase,This family consists of various acyl–acyl carrier protein (ACP) thioesterases (TE) these terminate fatty acyl group extension via hydrolysing an acyl group on a fatty acid (Fig. 327.3).

A simple phylogenetic tree to show the relatedness of CpFATB to other FATs also indicates the protein from wintersweet belongs to FATB class (Fig. 327.4). These results suggest that CpFATB may have similar function with B class members in plant.

Q9SQI3.1	RecName: Full=Myristoyl-acyl carrier protein thioesterase, chloropl...	409	409	97%	3e-112
ABU96744.1	chloroplast acyl-ACP thioesterase [Jatropha curcas] >gb|ACT09360...	407	407	97%	7e-112
ADA79524.1	chloroplast acyl-ACP thioesterase [Macadamia tetraphylla]	406	406	95%	2e-111
XP_002284850.1	PREDICTED: hypothetical protein [Vitis vinifera]	404	404	95%	6e-111
CBI28125.1	unnamed protein product [Vitis vinifera]	404	404	95%	1e-110
AAD01982.1	palmitoyl-acyl carrier protein thioesterase [Gossypium hirsutum]	403	403	96%	2e-110
AAB71729.1	acyl-ACP thioesterase [Myristica fragrans]	400	400	97%	1e-109
ACO57189.1	acyl acyl-carrier-protein thioesterase type B [Camellia oleifera]	399	399	97%	3e-109
ACO57188.1	acyl acyl-carrier-protein thioesterase type B [Camellia oleifera]	398	398	97%	7e-109
XP_002515564.1	palmitoyl-acyl carrier protein thioesterase [Ricinus communis] >gbl...	397	397	91%	1e-108
AAD42220.2	palmitoyl-acyl carrier protein thioesterase [Elaeis guineensis]	397	397	99%	1e-108
ACO63293.1	acyl acyl-carrier-protein thioesterase [Camellia oleifera]	397	397	92%	1e-108
ACO57190.1	acyl acyl-carrier-protein thioesterase type B [Camellia oleifera]	396	396	97%	2e-108
CAN81819.1	hypothetical protein [Vitis vinifera]	393	393	90%	2e-107
ABC47311.1	FATB [Populus tomentosa]	393	393	97%	2e-107
ABD83939.1	palmitoyl-ACP thioesterase [Elaeis guineensis]	391	391	99%	6e-107
ABK96561.1	unknown [Populus trichocarpa x Populus deltoides]	390	390	97%	9e-107
XP_002324952.1	predicted protein [Populus trichocarpa] >gb|EEF03527.1| predicte...	389	389	97%	2e-106
ABO38856.1	acyl ACP-thioesterase [Arachis hypogaea] >gb|ABO38557.1| acyl A...	389	389	92%	4e-106
AAB71581.1	acyl-acyl carrier protein thioesterase [Cuphea calophylla subsp. m...	388	388	97%	5e-106
ABO38555.1	acyl ACP-thioesterase [Arachis hypogaea]	388	388	92%	5e-106
ABO38554.1	acyl ACP-thioesterase [Arachis hypogaea]	388	388	92%	6e-106
ABO38558.1	acyl-acyl carrier protein thioesterase [Arachis hypogaea]	386	386	92%	2e-105
XP_002309244.1	predicted protein [Populus trichocarpa] >gb|EEE92767.1| predicte...	384	384	93%	7e-105
XP_002309243.1	predicted protein [Populus trichocarpa] >gb|EEE92766.1| predicte...	383	383	93%	2e-104

Fig. 327.2 Aligment of the *CpFATB* gene amino acid sequence in GenBank

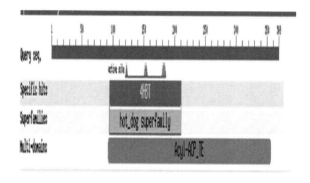

Fig. 327.3 Analysis of conserved domain

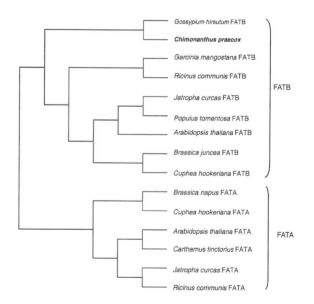

Fig. 327.4 Phylogenetic tree analysis of *Fat*

327.3.3 Fundamental Properties of Protein

Use http://www.expasy.ch/tools/ Primary structure analysis, A coding region of wintersweet cDNA was cloned via screening a wintersweet cDNA library. The CpFATB cDNA is 1110 bp in length with an open reading frame (ORF) of 1107 bp encoding a protein of 369 amino acids. Molecular weight and isoelectric point of the protein is 41.72 kD and 7.72, respectively. Formula is $C_{1843}H_{2934}N_{520}O_{548}S_{18}$. Extinction coefficients are in units of $M-1$ $cm-1$, at 280 nm measured in water. The N-terminal of the sequence considered is M (Met). The estimated half-life is 30 h (mammalian reticulocytes, in vitro), >20 h (yeast, in vivo), >10 h (Escherichia coli, in vivo). The instability index (II) is computed to be 38.27. This classifies the protein as stable. Aliphatic index is 86.29.

327.3.4 Protein Secondary Structure Prediction and Analysis of Hydrophobicity

Protein secondary structure prediction using SOPMA. The gene containing 40.33 % Alpha helix (Hh), 4.63 % Beta bridge (Bb) 14.99 % Extended strand (Ee), 40.05 % Random coil (Ee) (Fig. 327.5).

The software of DNAman are applied to analyze to these FATs in clustering (Fig. 327.6). The hydrophobic protein of the gene expression of the maximum value of 2.91, is located in 205 bp, the minimum value is −3.60, located in 211, 18 bp as the hydrophobic region.

327.3.5 Chloroplast Transit Peptides and Protein Localization Sites

Use http://www.cbs.dtu.dk/services/, The ChloroP server predicts the presence of chloroplast transit peptides (cTP) in protein sequences and the location of potential cTP cleavage sites. The predicted length of the presequence is 49 bp.

Fig. 327.5 Secondary structure prediction of *CpFATB*

```
          10        20        30        40        50        60        70
           |         |         |         |         |         |         |
MIASSVGAAFFPAQGIIKSKPAGLHVKANGRASPSIDGPKVTVGLEGTNASSTRKFMNLLPDWSMLLAAF
eehhhhhhhhhhhhheeecccccccccttcceeeecccceeeccccccccchhhhhccthhhhhhhh
TTIFEKQKVVVDQFRFGHDRLVYSENFTIRSYEIGADQTASIETVMNLLQETGINCFRSLGLLLDGFDST
hhhhhhhhhhhhhheccccceecteeeeeeeecccccchhhhhhhhhhhhhhhhhhheecctcccch
VEMCKRDLIWVVTRMQVIVDHYPSRGDTVEVETHCGAYGKHGHRREWLIRNSKTGQILTRATSVLVVMNK
hhhhhtheeeehhhheeetccccccceeeeeeehccttccccccceeeeectttcheeehhccheeeehh
RTRRLSILPDEVRRELEPYFMENLSVMKDQGRKLPKVDHSIADYVRQGLTCQWSDLDINQHVNHIKYVKW
hhhhhhccchhhhhhccccccccccccccccccccchhhhhhcccccccccccccccchhhhhhh
IFESVPVSILESHEISSMTLEFKRECGKDSMLQSLTAVVSGRRVDGSVEETDVEFQHLLQLEDGPEVMRG
hhhhccchhhhhhhhhhhhhhhhcccchhhhhhhhccccccccccccchhhhhhhhhttcceeeh
TTKWRPKSTLFPNSISH
cchecccccccccccc
```

Fig. 327.6 Analysis of Hydrophobicity

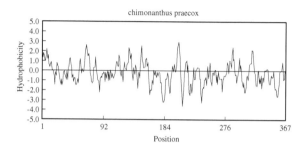

Name	Length	Score	cTP	CS-score	cTP-length
Sequence	369	0.543	Y	2.303	49

PSORT—Prediction of Protein Localization Sites. The possibility exists in the chloroplast stroma reached 50.3 %

Final Results:

chloroplast stroma—Certainty = 0.503 (Affirmative) < succ>

mitochondrial matrix space—Certainty = 0.432 (Affirmative) < succ > chloroplast thylakoid membrane—Certainty = 0.255 (Affirmative) < succ > microbody (peroxisome)—Certainty = 0.245 (Affirmative).

327.4 Conclusion

A full-length complementary deox-yribunucleic acid (cDNA) of a fatty acyl–acyl carrier protein thioesterase (CpFATB) was isolated from a *Chimonanthus praecox* (wintersweet) cDNA library. Wintersweet is a hardy shrub native to Chinese montane regions and is known to be tolerant to many biotic and abiotic stresses including cold, drought, and avariety of plant pathogens [5]. Bioinformatic analysis also demonstrated that CpFATB contains the hotdog fold/domain [6]. The cDNA is 1, 110 nucleotides in length, of which 1, 107 bp form a single open-reading frame, predicting a 369 amino acid polypeptide. Molecular weight and isoelectric point of the protein is 41.72 kD and 7.72, respectively. Bioinformatics analysis shows that a signal peptide with 49 amino acid residues and Protein Localization Sites exists in the chloroplast stroma.This classifies the protein as stable. This gene may be of use in the production of drought-tolerant crops pecies and, as such, is worthy of further characterization and investigation.

References

1. Ohlrogge JB, Kuhn DN (1979) Subcellular localization of acyl carrier protein in leaf protoplasts of Spinacia oleracea. Proc Natl Acad Sci USA 76:1194–1198
2. Voelker TA, Jones A, Cranmer AM, et al (1997) Broad-range and binary-range acyl–acyl–carrier protein thioestera sessuggest an alternative mechanism for medium-chain production in seeds. Plant Physiol 114:669–677
3. Dörmann P, Voelker TA, Ohlrogge JB (2000) Accumulation of palmitate in Arabidopsis mediated by the acyl–acyl carrier protein thioesterase FATB1. Plant Physiol 123:637–643
4. Salas JJ, Ohlrogge JB (2002) Characterisation of substrate specificity of plant FATA and FATB acyl-ACP thioesterases. Arch Biochem Biophys 403:25–34
5. Zhang SH, Wei Y, Liu JL, et al (2011) CpCHT1 an apoplastic chitinase isolated from the corolla of wintersweet (Chimonanthuspraecoxcommunis L.) exhibits both antifungal and antifreeze activities. Biol Plantarum 55:141–148
6. Dillon SC, Bateman A (2004) The Hotdog fold: wrapping up a superfamily of thioesterases and dehydratases. BMC Bioinforma 5:109

Chapter 328
Effects of Bodymass on the SDA of the Taimen

Guiqiang Yang, Liying Zhang and Shaogang Xu

Abstract Specific Dynamic Action (SDA), the metabolic phenomenon resulting from the digestion and assimilation of a meal, is generally influenced by body mass. The effects of body mass on SDA of taimen (*Hucho taimen*, Pallas) was evaluated, by measuring the temporal pattern of the oxygen consumption rates of taimen with body masses, 38, 31, 24, 17, 10 g, after feeding, at 17.5 °C, Factorial scope of peak VO_2, Duration and SDA_E had a tendency to decrease with reduced body mass.

Keywords Specific dynamic action · Bodymass · Taimen

328.1 Introduction

Feeding causes an increase of metabolic rate, which initially escalates rapidly, reaches a peak value and then gradually declines to the pre-feeding rate. This phenomenon, termed "Specific Dynamic Action" (SDA) [1, 2], reflects the energy requirements of the behavioral, physiological and biochemical processes that constitute feeding, including capture, handling, ingestion, digestion, the assimilation of prey and the increased synthesis of proteins and lipids associated with growth [3–5].

The parameters that are usually used to describe SDA include Standard Metabolic Rate (SMR), Peak VO_2, Factorial scope of peak VO_2, Duration, SDA_E (energy expended on SDA, kJ • kg^{-1}) and SDA coefficient [3, 6]. These parameters of the SDA depend on the species [6, 7], meal size [7, 8], meal type [6, 8, 9],

---

G. Yang (✉) · L. Zhang · S. Xu
Beijing Fisheries Research Institute, Beijing 100068, China
e-mail: ygqheb@yahoo.com.cn

feeding frequency [10], temperature [11] body mass [12], and composition of the diet [13].

Results from earlier studies suggest that SDA is dependent on body mass in some ectotherms [6]. However, only a limited number of studies have evaluated on the effects of body mass on SDA were related to fish [14]. No previous study, as far as is known, has reported the influence of body mass on SDA response in taimen.

Taimen are the largest specie in the Salmonidae family and the distribution of taimen has been seriously diminished by dams, water diversion, pollution and overfishing [15]. As a result of its decline, the taimen is now listed as a threatened species throughout its native range, and is being considered for listing in the International Union for Conservation of Nature's (IUCN) red list [16]. The relationship of the metabolic rates of this unfed fish with body mass has been studied by Kuang [17]. But no studies have explored the effects of body mass and body mass on the SDA responses of taimen. There were two major objectives of the present study: (1) to determine whether this taimen responds to increasing body-mass by increasing SMR and Peak VO_2; (2) to document Duration, SDA_E and SDA coefficient of this taimen.

328.2 Introduction Materials and Methods

Taimens were obtained from Yudushan Coldwater Fishery Base of Beijing Fisheries Research Institute and acclimated to the diets (produced by Beijing Hanye science and technology Co. Ltd) in a rearing system for 2 weeks prior to the metabolism experiment. During this period, the fish were fed with their diet twice per day (at 10:00, 16:00). The ingredients of the experimental diets are listed in Table 328.1. The oxygen content was kept above 5 mg $\bullet$ L^{-1}, the pH ranged from 7.3 to 8.0 and ammonia-N was kept below 0.025 mg $\bullet$ L^{-1} during the experimental period. A 12/12-h (light/dark) photoperiod was used to simulate natural light cycle.

The SDA response was measured with five different body masses (10, 17, 24, 31, 38 g) using fish (3 ~ 14 fish per group, three repeated groups in each body mass level). The oxygen consumption rate (OR) was measured continually during this period for three repeated groups per body mass level. Three groups of taimen were given the approximate 0.8 % ration of diet using five different body mass

Table 328.1 Proximate composition of the diet

Ingredient	Percent dry mass (%)	Ingredient	Percent dry mass (%)
Protein	46.0	Lysine	2.6
Lipid	12.0	Total phosphorus	0.9
Carbohydrate	5.0	Calcium	1.0
Ash	14.0		

levels (10, 17, 24, 31, 38 g): 10 g, 14 per group; 17 g, 9 per group; 24 g, 6 per group; 31 g, 5 per group; 38 g, 3 per group. At body mass, 3 ~ 14 fish were acclimated individually in perforated plastic cages with a surface area of 1500 cm^2 and a water volume of 60 L. Each cage was put in a recirculating system, and the temperature was controlled at 17.5 ± 0.5 °C. Then the fish were acclimated for 2 weeks prior to the experiment. Oxygen consumption for several fish (3–14) as one group was measured using a 4-chamber (3.15 L) continuous flow respirometer. A feeding opening was installed at the front of the respirometer chamber in order to feed the fish. The faces were siphoned using a tube mounted at the rear of the chamber.

For each metabolic trial, several variables were quantified, as described by Jobling [3] and Stephen [6]: (1) Standard Metabolic Rate (SMR); (2) Peak VO$_2$; (3) Factorial scope of peak VO$_2$; (4) Duration; (5) SDA$_E$, and (6) SDA coefficient (%). The oxygen consumption was converted to energy using a conversion factor of 13.56 J mg O$_2^{-1}$ [18]. A monofactorial variance analysis was performed using SPSS16.0 to compare the variables among different levels. $P < 0.05$ was considered significant. All data are presented as mean ± S.E. Non-linear estimation was also used when necessary. Figures were drawn by Microsoft Excel software.

328.3 Results

There was no significant difference in meal size ($n = 15$, $P = 0.394$) among different body mass groups (Table 328.2). With each body mass level, metabolic rate increased significantly 1 h after feeding, peaked at 2–4 h post-feeding, and then decreased gradually to the fasting level (Figs. 328.1, 328.2). With the approximate meal size but different body mass, both SMR and Peak VO$_2$ had a tendency to increase with reduced body mass (SMR, $n = 15$, $P < 0.001$; Peak VO$_2$, $n = 15$, $P < 0.001$) (Table 328.2). The relationship between SMR (mg • kg^{-1} • h^{-1}) and body mass (W, g) was described as: SMR = 615.15 W$^{-0.4341}$, ($R^2 = 0.9910$, $n = 15$, $P < 0.001$). The relationships between Peak VO$_2$ (mg • kg^{-1} • h^{-1}) and body mass (W, g) was described as: Peak VO$_2$ = 551.98 W$^{-0.2632}$, ($R^2 = 0.9982$, $n = 15$, $P < 0.001$).

Just the contrary, factorial scope of peak VO$_2$, Duration and SDA$_E$ had a tendency to decrease with reduced body mass (factorial scope of peak VO$_2$, ANOVA, $n = 15$, $P = 0.047$; Duration, $n = 15$, $P < 0.001$; SDA$_E$, $n = 15$, $P < 0.001$) (Table 328.2). The relationship between factorial scope of peak VO$_2$ and body mass (W, g) was described as: factorial scope of peak VO$_2$ = 0.0126 W + 1.2247, ($R^2 = 0.426$, $n = 15$, $P = 0.047$). The relationship between Duration (h) and body mass (W, g) was described as: Duration = 0.1462 W + 6.1576, ($R^2 = 0.9601$, $n = 15$, $P < 0.001$). The relationship between SDA$_E$ (kJ • kg^{-1}) and body mass (W, g) was described as: SDA$_E$ = 0.1093 W + 4.2406, ($R^2 = 0.9539$, $n = 15$, $P < 0.001$). SDA coefficient decreased from 33.61 ± 1.24 to 26.42 ± 0.91 as body mass decreased from

Table 328.2 Effects of body mass on several variables of SDA in taimen

Variables	Body mass (g)				P
	38	31	24	17	10	
Body mass (g)	37.33 ± 0.98[a]	30.90 ± 1.74[b]	24.67 ± 0.74[c]	16.44 ± 0.67[d]	10.64 ± 0.42[e]	<0.001
SMR (mg · kg^{-1} · h^{-1})	124.20 ± 6.36[a]	141.06 ± 7.72[b]	156.71 ± 8.25[c]	181.61 ± 8.04[d]	218.72 ± 9.26[e]	<0.001
Meal size (% of body mass)	1.78 ± 0.03	1.66 ± 0.04	1.58 ± 0.04	1.63 ± 0.05	1.60 ± 0.02	0.394
Peak VO$_2$ (L/min)	214.29 ± 7.02[a]	223.07 ± 8.83[ab]	235.60 ± 6.03[b]	265.18 ± 9.43[c]	296.38 ± 9.73[d]	<0.001
Factorial scope of peak VO$_2$	1.73 ± 0.15[a]	1.58 ± 0.15[a]	1.50 ± 0.12[ab]	1.46 ± 0.11[b]	1.36 ± 0.10[b]	0.047
Duration (h)	11.33 ± 0.58[a]	11.00 ± 0.00[a]	10.00 ± 0.50[b]	8.17 ± 0.29[c]	7.83 ± 0.29[c]	<0.001
SDA (kJ/kg)	8.33 ± 0.08[a]	7.88 ± 0.11[b]	6.63 ± 0.10[c]	5.83 ± 0.10[d]	5.65 ± 0.12[d]	<0.001
SDA coefficient (%)	25.46 ± 1.24[a]	17.74 ± 0.64[b]	17.23 ± 0.92[b]	14.63 ± 0.93[c]	14.41 ± 0.91[c]	<0.001

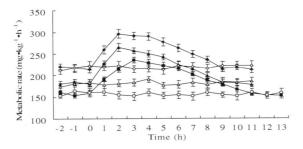

Fig. 328.1 The metabolic rate (mg • kg^{-1} • h^{-1}) in taimen with different body masses (●: with body mass 10 g at a meal size of 1.60 %; ○: with body mass 10 g and unfed; ▲: with body mass 17 g at a meal size of 1.63 %; △: with body mass 17 g and unfed; ■: with body mass 24 g at a meal size of 1.58 %; □: with body mass 24 g and unfed)

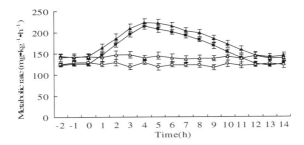

Fig. 328.2 The metabolic rate (mg • kg^{-1} • h^{-1}) in taimen with different body masses (▲: with body mass 31 g at a meal size of 1.66 %; △: with body mass 31 g and unfed; ■: with body mass 38 g at a meal size of 1.78 %; □: with body mass 38 g and unfed)

37.33 ± 0.98 to 10.64 ± 0.42 g (Table 328.2). The SDA coefficient of body mass 17, 10 g were lower than that of the other body mass levels. No significant relationship was found between SDA coefficient and body mass.

328.4 Discussion

Factorial scope of peak VO$_2$ were 1.36–1.73 in taimen (Table 328.2), depending on body mass, a similar order of magnitude to that found in other fishes. Factorial scope of peak VO$_2$ were 1.12–2.22 in juvenile cod with a wet body mass of 0.45–4.20 g [19], 1.2–2.0 in juvenile *Melanogrammus aeglefinus* with a dry body mass of 0.115–4.493 g. Jobling listed values of relative peak VO$_2$ from the literature from many species of fishes and found that peak SDA range between 1.6 and 2.6 times the standard or low routine metabolism [3]. Values of factorial scope of peak VO$_2$ from this study thus fall within the range of other published values.

Duration increased with decreasing body mass and ranged from 7.83 ± 0.29 to 11.33 ± 0.58 h (Table 328.2). The shorter duration of SDA in small juvenile cod may be due to a higher rate of digestion needed to fuel a higher mass-specific metabolism and higher growth rates compared to larger taimen. Small fish digest a meal faster than larger fish. Similar to other studies [19], SDA_E increased with increasing body mass and significant effect of body mass on the SDA was found in the present study (Table 328.2). Further experiments with even higher body weights than used here may be more informative since this taimen can be reach 50 kg.

Acknowledgments This study was supported by the major projects of Agriculture Ministry (201003055-05), Beijing major projects (D121100003712002); major projects of Agriculture Ministry (99124120); Beijing project (SCSYZ201211-4).

References

1. Xie XJ, Sun RY (1991) Advances of the studies on the specific dynamic action in fish. Acta Hydrobiol Sinica
2. McCue MD (2006) Specific dynamic action: a century of investigation. Com Bio Phys A Mol Integrat Physiol
3. Jobling M (1981) The influences of feeding on the metabolic rate of fishes: a short review. J Fish Biol
4. Jobling M (1993) Bioenergetics: feed intake and energy partitioning. In: Rankin JC, Jensen FB, (eds) Fish ecophysiology. Chapman & Hall, London
5. Wells MJ, Odor RK, Mangold K, Wells J (1983) Feeding and metabolic rate in *Octopus*. Mar Freshwater Behav Physiol
6. Stephen MS, Jessica AW (2007) Effects of meal size, meal type, and body temperature on the specific dynamic action of anurans. J Comp Physiol B
7. Jobling M, Davis PS (1980) Effects of feeding on metabolic rate, and the specific dynamic action in plaice. J Fish Biol
8. Secor SM, Faulkner AC (2002) Effects of meal size, meal type, body temperature and body size on the specific dynamic action of the marine toad, *Bufo marinus*. Physiol Biochem Zool
9. Pan ZC, Xiang J, Lu HL, Ma XM (2005) Influence of food type on specific dynamic action of the Chinese skink *Eumeces chinensis*. Comparat Biochem Physiol A
10. Guinea J, Fernandez F (1997) Effect of feeding frequency, feeding level and temperature on energy metabolism in *Sparus aurata*. Aquaculture
11. Robertson RF, Meagor J, Taylor EW (2002) Specific dynamic action in the shore crab, *Carcinus maenas* (L.), in relation to acclimation temperature and to the onset of the emersion response. Physiol Biochem Zool
12. Beaupre SJ (2005) Technical comment: ratio representations of specific dynamic action (mass-specific SDA and SDA coefficient) do not standardize for body mass and meal size. Physiol Biochem Zool
13. Peter T (2000) Relationship between specific dynamic action and protein deposition in calanoid copepods. J Exp Mar Biol Ecol
14. Brodeur JC, Calvo J, Johnston IA (2003) Proliferation of myogenic progenitor cells following feeding in the sub-antarctic notothenioid fish *Harpagifer bispinis*. J Exp Biol
15. Holcik J, Hensel K, Nieslanik J (1988) The eurasian huchen *Hucho hucho*: largest salmon of the world. Kluwer Academic Publishers, Hingham

16. Matveyev AN, Pronin NM, Samusenok VP, Bronte CR (1998) Ecology of Siberian taimen *Hucho taimen* in the Lake Baikal Basin. J Great Lakes Res
17. Kuang YY, Yin JS, Jiang ZF, Xun W, Li YF (2003) The correlation between oxygen consumption of *Hucho taimen* and body weight, water temperature
18. Elliott JM, Davison W (1975) Energy equivalents of oxygen consumption in animal energetics. Oecology
19. Soren LH (2003) Scope for activity, specific dynamic action and growth in early juvenile stages of Atlantic Cod. B S Roskilde University, Denmark

Chapter 329
Effects of Temperature on the SDA of the Taimen

Guiqiang Yang, Ding Yuan and Shaogang Xu

Abstract The effects of temperature on SDA of taimen (*Hucho taimen*, Pallas) was evaluated, by measuring the temporal pattern of the oxygen consumption rates of taimen, after feeding, at four constant temperatures, 11.5, 14.5, 17.5, 20.5 °C. Peak VO_2 increased linearly as temperature increased. Two peaks were observed during the SDA response at 11.5 °C, and it may be mainly resulted of mechanical SDA and biochemical of SDA when temperature was low enough. SDA_E increased slowly to the maximum at 17.5 °C, and then decreased at 20.5 °C. The relationship between SDA_E (kJ · kg^{-1}) and temperature (t, °C) was described as: $SDA_E = -0.1163t^2 + 3.771t - 22.467$, ($R^2 = 0.9999$, n = 12, $P < 0.001$). The result showed that the optimum growth temperature of taimen occurred at 17.5 °C.

Keywords Specific dynamic action · Temperature · Taimen

329.1 Introduction

Specific dynamic action (SDA) is the metabolic phenomenon resulting from the digestion and assimilation of a meal [1, 2]. This phenomenon reflects the energy requirements of the behavioral, physiological and biochemical processes that constitute feeding and the increased synthesis of proteins and lipids associated with growth [3–5].

The parameters that are usually used to describe SDA include SMR, Peak VO_2, factorial scope of peak VO_2, Duration, SDA_E and SDA coefficient [3, 6]. These parameters of the SDA depend on the species [6, 7], meal size [7, 8], meal type [6, 8, 9], feeding frequency [10], temperature [11] body mass [12], and

G. Yang (✉) · D. Yuan · S. Xu
Beijing Fisheries Research Institute, Beijing 100068, China
e-mail: ygqheb@yahoo.com.cn

composition of the diet [13] (Table 329.1). Results from earlier studies suggest that SDA is dependent temperature in some ectotherms [6]. However, only a limited number of the studies that have evaluated the effects of temperature on SDA have been carried out on fish [14]. No previous study has reported the influence of temperature on SDA response in taimen.

Taimen (*Hucho taimen*, Pallas) are the largest specie in the Salmonidae family and the distribution of taimen has been seriously diminished by dams, water diversion, pollution and overfishing [15]. As a result of its decline, the taimen is now listed as a threatened species throughout its native range, and is being considered for listing in the International Union for Conservation of Nature's (IUCN) red list [16]. The relationship of the metabolic rates of this unfed fish with temperature has been studied by Kuang [17]. But no studies have explored the effects of temperature on the SDA responses of taimen. There were two major objectives of the present study: (1) to determine whether this taimen responds to increasing temperature by increasing SMR and Peak VO_2; (2) to document factorial scope of peak VO_2, Duration, SDA_E and SDA coefficient of this taimen.

329.2 Materials and Methods

Experimental fish: Taimens were obtained from Yudushan Coldwater Fishery Base of Beijing Fisheries Research Institute and acclimated to the diets in a rearing system for 2 weeks prior to the metabolism experiment.

Experimental protocol: The SDA response was measured at four temperature levels (11.5 ± 0.5, 14.5 ± 0.5, 17.5 ± 0.5, 20.5 ± 0.5 °C) using 15 fish (five fish per group, three repeated groups in each temperature level). At each temperature, five fish were acclimated in perforated plastic cages with a surface area of 1500 cm^2 and a water volume of 60 L. Each cage was put in a recirculating system, and the temperature was adjusted to experimental temperature at a rate of 1 °C per day. Then the fish were acclimated for 2 weeks prior to the experiment. The oxygen consumption rate (OR) was measured continually during this period for three repeated groups per temperature level. After 24 h fast, the fish were placed in the chamber and allowed to acclimate for 24 h without food. OR was measured one time at 1 h intervals and used as standard metabolic rate. Then a 0.8 % ration of experiment diet was offered to the experimental fish. After the fish finished the diet, the chambers were closed immediately, and the OR was

Table 329.1 Proximate composition of the diet

Ingredient	Percent dry mass (%)	Ingredient	Percent dry mass (%)
Protein	46.0	Lysine	2.6
Lipid	12.0	Total phosphorus	0.9
Carbohydrate	5.0	Calcium	1.0
Ash	14.0		

monitored. The duration was determined by a pilot experiment and guaranteed the postprandial metabolic rate returning to the prior status. Energy content of the diets was determined by bomb calorimetry (CN61 M/1B, Beijing zhongxi taian Co., Ltd. China). Dissolved oxygen concentration was measured at the outlet of the chamber by an oxymeter (YSI 550A, YSI Incorporated, USA).

For each metabolic trial, several variables were quantified, as described by Jobling [3] and Stephen [6]: (1) Standard Metabolic Rate (SMR); (2) Peak VO_2; (3) Factorial scope of peak VO_2; (4) Duration; (5) SDA_E, and (6) SDA coefficient (%). The oxygen consumption was converted to energy using a conversion factor of 13.56 J mg O_2^{-1} [18]. A monofactorial variance analysis was performed using SPSS16.0 to compare the variables among different levels. $P < 0.05$ was considered significant. Figures were drawn by Microsoft Excel software.

329.3 Results

Neither body mass nor meal size differed significantly among different temperature levels (n = 12, P > 0.05) (Table 329.2). At 14.5, 17.5, and 20.5 °C, metabolic rate increased significantly 1 h after feeding, peaked at 4–5 h post-feeding, and decreased gradually to the fasting level (Fig. 329.1, Fig. 329.2). The temperature strongly influenced SMR (n = 12, $P < 0.001$) and Peak VO_2 (n = 12, $P < 0.001$) (Table 329.2). SMR and Peak VO_2 both increased linearly as temperature increased from 11.5 to 20.5 °C.

The temperature also had a significant effect on Duration (n = 12, $P < 0.001$), SDA_E (n = 12, $P < 0.001$), and SDA coefficient (n = 12, $P < 0.001$) (Table 329.2). Duration for 11.5 °C was significantly higher than that of the other temperature levels. SDA_E of 14.5 and 17.5 °C were significantly higher than that of 11.5 and 20.5 °C. The relationship between SDA_E (kJ • kg^{-1}) and temperature (t, °C)

Table 329.2 Effects of temperature on several variables of SDA in taimen

Variables	Temperature (°C)				P
	11.5	14.5	17.5	20.5	
Body mass (g)	31.10 ± 0.50	29.10 ± 0.66	30.90 ± 1.74	29.9 ± 0.73	0.139
SMR (mg · $kg^{-1} \cdot h^{-1}$)	89.10 ± 4.82^a	115.97 ± 5.98^b	141.06 ± 7.72^c	186.83 ± 4.96^d	<0.001
Meal size (% of body mass)	1.74 ± 0.01	1.63 ± 0.02	1.66 ± 0.04	1.66 ± 0.02	0.093
Peak VO_2 (L/min)	131.38 ± 6.42^a	196.16 ± 7.97^b	223.07 ± 8.83^c	252.74 ± 6.86^d	<0.001
Factorial scope of peak VO_2	1.47 ± 0.15^a	1.69 ± 0.16^{ab}	1.58 ± 0.15^{ab}	1.35 ± 0.07^b	0.075
Duration (h)	16.00 ± 0.50	12.33 ± 0.29	11.00 ± 0.00	9.83 ± 0.29	<0.001
SDA (kJ/kg)	5.51 ± 0.07^a	7.77 ± 0.08^b	7.88 ± 0.11^b	5.95 ± 0.07^c	<0.001
SDA coefficient (%)	12.33 ± 0.47^a	19.90 ± 0.61^b	17.74 ± 0.64^c	14.49 ± 0.65^d	<0.001

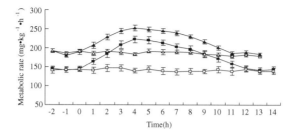

Fig. 329.1 The metabolic rate (mg kg^{-1} h^{-1}) in taimen at different temperatures (▲: fed with experimental diet at a meal size of 1.66 % body mass at 20.5 °C; △: unfed at 20.5 °C; ■: fed with experimental diet at a meal size of 1.66 % body mass at 17.5 °C; □: unfed at 17.5 °C)

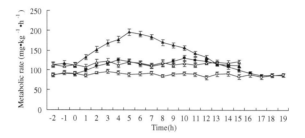

Fig. 329.2 The metabolic rate (mg kg^{-1} h^{-1}) in taimen at different temperatures (▲: fed with experimental diet at a meal size of 1.63 % body mass at 14.5 °C; △: unfed at 14.5 °C; ■: fed with experimental diet at a meal size of 1.74 % body mass at 11.5 °C; □: unfed at 11.5 °C)

was described as: $SDA_E = -0.1163t^2 + 3.771t - 22.467, (R^2 = 0.9999, n = 12, P < 0.001)$.

329.4 Discussion

Several studies that examined the effects of temperature on SDA have shown that the Peak VO$_2$ increased with temperature, whereas the Duration decreased with temperature in ectotherms [11, 19]. A similar trend was found in the taimen in the present study (Table 329.2). Studies attempting to elucidate the relative contribution of the various components of digestion to SDA have divided SDA into "mechanical SDA" and "biochemical SDA" [9]. Mechanical SDA represents the cost of physical processing of food, whereas biochemical SDA is the postabsorptive cost of assimilation. As temperature decreased, the metabolic rate of ectotherms decreased as well as the rate of biochemical action. As a result, two peaks were observed during the SDA response at a lower temperature, which might be due to a rapid startup of the mechanical process with a lag of the biochemical process [20]. In the present study, the metabolic rate of taimen at 11.5 °C has two peaks (Fig. 329.2).

With the approximate body mass but different temperatures, the meal size (% of body mass) could reach to 1.2 ~ 1.5 % as temperature increased from 11.5 to 17.5 °C. However, at 20.5 °C, the highest meal size (% of body mass) was only 0.83 %, and taimen were aversion to diets. In the present, with the approximate meal size but different temperatures, SDA_E increased slowly to the maximum (7.88 ± 0.11 kJ · kg^{-1} · h^{-1}), and then decreased drastically to the lower state (5.95 ± 0.07 kJ · kg^{-1} · h^{-1}) (Table 329.2). The possible reason is that 20.5 °C was out of optimum growth temperature, and physiological functions of the related tissues and organs were limited to some extent. As a result, the optimum growth temperature of taimen is 17.5 °C.

Acknowledgments This study was supported by the major projects of Agriculture Ministry (201003055-05), Beijing major projects (D121100003712002); major projects of Agriculture Ministry (99124120); Beijing project (KJCX201101004).

References

1. Xie XJ, Sun RY (1991) Advances of the studies on the specific dynamic action in fish. Acta Hydrobiol Sinica
2. McCue MD (2006) Specific dynamic action: a century of investigation. Com Bio Phy- A: Molecul Integrat Physiol
3. Jobling M (1981) The influences of feeding on the metabolic rate of fishes: a short review. J Fish Biol
4. Jobling M (1993) Bioenergetics: feed intake and energy partitioning. In: Rankin JC, Jensen FB, (eds) Fish ecophysiology. Chapman & Hall, London
5. Wells MJ, Odor RK, Mangold K, Wells J (1983) Feeding and metabolic rate in *Octopus*. Marine Freshwater Behaviour Physiol
6. Stephen MS, Jessica AW (2007) Effects of meal size, meal type, and body temperature on the specific dynamic action of anurans. J Comp Physiol B
7. Jobling M, Davis PS (1980) Effects of feeding on metabolic rate, and the specific dynamic action in plaice. J Fish Biol
8. Secor SM, Faulkner AC (2002) Effects of meal size, meal type, body temperature and body size on the specific dynamic action of the marine toad, *Bufo marinus*. Physiol Biochem Zool
9. Pan ZC, Xiang J, Lu HL, Ma XM (2005) Influence of food type on specific dynamic action of the Chinese skink *Eumeces chinensis*. Comparative Biochem Physiol A
10. Guinea J, Fernandez F (1997) Effect of feeding frequency, feeding level and temperature on energy metabolism in *Sparus aurata*. Aquaculture
11. Robertson RF, Meagor J, Taylor EW (2002) Specific dynamic action in the shore crab, *Carcinus maenas* (L.), in relation to acclimation temperature and to the onset of the emersion response. Phy Bio Zool
12. Beaupre SJ (2005) Technical comment: ratio representations of specific dynamic action (mass-specific SDA and SDA coefficient) do not standardize for body mass and meal size. Physiol Biochem Zool
13. Peter T (2000) Relationship between specific dynamic action and protein deposition in calanoid copepods. J Exp Mar Biol Eco
14. Brodeur JC, Calvo J, Johnston IA (2003) Proliferation of myogenic progenitor cells following feeding in the sub-antarctic notothenioid fish *Harpagifer bispinis*. J Exp Biol
15. Holcik J, Hensel K, Nieslanik J (1988) The eurasian huchen *Hucho hucho*: largest salmon of the world. Kluwer Academic Publishers, Hingham

16. Matveyev AN, Pronin NM, Samusenok VP, Bronte CR (1998) Ecology of Siberian taimen *Hucho taimen* in the Lake Baikal Basin. J Great Lakes Research
17. Kuang YY, Yin JS, Jiang ZF, Xun W, Li YF (2003) The correlation between oxygen consumption of *Hucho taimen* and body weight, water temperature
18. Elliott JM, Davison W (1975) Energy equivalents of oxygen consumption in animal energetics. Oecol
19. Beaupre SJ (2005) Technical comment: ratio representations of specific dynamic action (mass-specific SDA and SDA coefficient) do not standardize for body mass and meal size. Physiol Biochem Zool
20. Luo YP, Xie XJ (2008) Effects of temperature on the specific dynamic action of the southern catfish, *Silurus meridionalis*. Comparative Biochem Physiol A

Chapter 330
Wireless Heart Rate Monitoring System of RSS-based Positioning in GSM

Hongfang Shao, Jingling Han, Jianhua Mao and Zhigang Xuan

Abstract Due to the uncertainty of patient's location, the outbreak of cardiovascular disease (CVD) will result in unnecessary delays for rescue. We present an encouraging system that works in real time to monitor the heart rate data. The location of mobile terminal (MT) can be obtained with lower cost based on RSS positioning approach in GSM. According to definite priority, location information, together with heart rate data is sent to the monitoring center. As the cardio tachometer, small and suitable to be worn, is wirelessly connected to the MT in the proposal. It offers convenience to users if they go outside. Implemented by auto-reminding and cooperating with emergency center, the system can save valuable time to rescue patients.

Keywords Heart rate data · Location information · GSM · RSS positioning

330.1 Introduction

Fast pace in modern life has greatly changed people's habits. It also caused many chronic diseases, including the cardiovascular disease (CVD). According to some surveys, the cardiovascular disease has ranked the first among deaths of over 40, 60 % of which occurred at home or in the community. Furthermore, the proportion of death has still been increasing every year [1, 2]. If patients with the CVD, who fell in a dangerous situation, can be found and treated in time, the probability for

---

H. Shao (✉) · J. Han
Information Centre, Yixing People's Hospital, Yixing, Jiangsu 214200, People's Republic of China
e-mail: Shuangshuang868@sina.com

J. Mao · Z. Xuan (✉)
The 359 Hospital of PLA, 212001 Zhenjiang, China
e-mail: 277150355@qq.com

their survival should be in the vicinity of 70 ~ 80 %. Generally, suffering from the CVD, they could hardly take care of themselves, causing great economic burden to the family. One promising way is to render them early prevention, duly detection, and comprehensive treatment.

The apparatus of previous electrocardiogram monitoring was wired with the data memory unit and the display unit. Technological advancement now makes it possible to monitor remotely a patient's heart rate signal, in both wire and wireless connection, and send the data from the monitoring device to the server. Many telecardiology real-time monitoring systems, e.g. proposed in literature [3, 4], have transmitted the data to monitoring center through the combination of GPS and GPRS. Some are complex in the structure or inconvenient for patients to go out. And others take on poor real-time. All of these techniques cannot determine indoor location accurately when patients need first-aid.

We present a real-time monitoring system of heart rate data, based on RSS positioning method in GSM. In this way, the user's location can be obtained with low cost. According to definite priority, location information, together with heart rate data is sent to the monitoring center, which is essential in urgency for patients. As the cardio tachometer, suitable to be worn, is wirelessly connected to the MT. It offers convenience to users if they go outside.

330.2 Overall Structure of the System

Figure 330.1.shows that the system consists of three units: heart rate data acquisition unit, data remote transmission unit and real-time heart rate management system at the monitoring center.

330.2.1 Heart Rate Data Acquisition

The unit of heart rate acquisition, a detection device worn by the user's wrist or finger, is responsible for collecting human heart beating signal. The signal is acquired through the piezoelectric transducer or the infrared sensor. After being amplified, filtered, and shaped, the signal is sent to the remote data transmission unit by the Bluetooth (BT) module.

330.2.2 Data Remote Transmission

This unit is to transmit the data sent from the BT to the monitoring center. There are three parts in the unit, i.e. the GSM communication networks and SMS gateway, Internet, and the server. MT is a special device which is designed to send

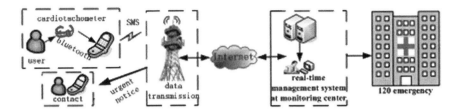

Fig. 330.1 Overall structure of the proposed design

the data to the server through the GSM module. The platform in the monitoring center includes server software and SMS module, feeding back diagnostic information to the users and their contacts.

330.2.3 Geographic Location Positioning

In order to duly find the users when they need first-aid, users' geographic location unit provides real-time positioning parameters for remote monitoring center. For the sake of reducing the cost both for the network and the MT, positioning method is achieved by reading RSSs [5] from the base stations (BSs) to the MT in GSM network, and adopting location algorithm.

330.2.3.1 Principle of RSS-Based Positioning

RSS positioning method uses the geometric properties to estimate the target location. For simplification, we consider the location only in a two-dimensional plane. Let the true location of MT is $[x_s, y_s]^T$, and the coordinate of the ith BS is $[x_i, y_i]^T$, $i = 1, 2, \ldots N$. The distance between MT and the ith BS, denoted by d_i, is given by [6]

$$d_i = \sqrt{(x_s - x_i)^2 + (y_s - y_i)^2}, \quad i = 1, 2, \ldots N \quad (330.1)$$

There is the noise or range error n_i in the process of realistic measurement. We assume that the measurement errors $\{n_i\}$ are zero mean Gaussian variables with known variance σ^2. Hence, formula (1) is rewritten as follows:

$$r_i = d_i + n_i = \sqrt{(x_s - x_i)^2 + (y_s - y_i)^2}, \quad i = 1, 2, \ldots N \quad (330.2)$$

From the viewpoint of the geometry, MT lies on the circle radius by the distance r_i, centered at the corresponding BS. The circles are indicated by equations

Fig. 330.2 Principle of geometric positioning

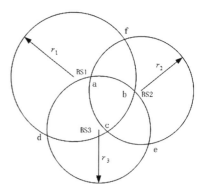

$$(x_s - x_i)^2 + (y_s - y_i)^2 = r_i^2, \quad i = 1, 2, \ldots N \tag{330.3}$$

Our algorithm uses three circles for location calculation, which means that N = 3. As shown in Fig. 330.2, the estimation of location as MT can be obtained through seeking the optimum solution among the intersection region of all three circles.

330.2.3.2 Positioning Algorithm

Figure 330.3 shows the algorithm [7] proposed flowchart. GSM system constantly monitor and measure RSSs from multiple BSs to ensure cell handover for MT successfully. As the location of BS is fixed, the location of MT can be estimated on the basis of reading RSSs from the BSs. Then, the data processing unit of the MT performs the algorithm every 1 min. Calculation result will be saved in the memory unit of it.

Fig. 330.3 Flowchart of the proposed algorithm

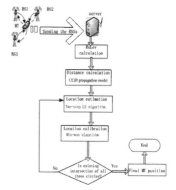

330.2.4 Real-Time Heart Rate Management

Similar to common information management systems, the MS has increased different features—the unit of diagnostic advice from the CVD specialists, information feedback unit and the function of alarm and alerts in emergency. Heart rate data sent from the GSM is compared with a given threshold. Thus the MS need to make corresponding decision as:

(1) Within the given threshold. Data would be stored for future check-up.
(2) Greater than the given threshold. Sending warning messages e.g. go to hospital as soon as possible to the MT and the contact.
(3) Be in cardiac arrhythmia. Call the emergency center immediately, providing the information of user's location to avoid the occurrence of life-threatening accidents.

330.3 Conclusion

A part of mobile telemedicine systems, the wireless heart rate monitoring system has been long developed overseas and fulfilled some achievements. But research of the field in our country was relatively afterwards. The suggested system is advantageous in low-cost, convenience and real-time. Our approach can cooperate with the emergency center to rescue people's life. It outperforms regarding applicable prospect and actual value.

References

1. Wu YL, Lei MJ (2010) The relationship between aging and cardiovascular disease. Chin J Gerontol 30(8):1164–1167
2. Moshui Chen (2007) Effect of resting heart rate on the prognosis of patients with cardiovascular diseases. Heinan Medicine 18(3):14–15
3. Eyal Dassau, Louis.J, Francis J.Doyle,III(2009) Enhanced 911/Global Position System Wizard: A Telemedicine Application for the Prevention of Severe Hypoglycemia—Monitor, Alert, and Locate. J Diabetes Sci Technol, 3(6):1501–1506
4. Peng Sheng-hua.Yu Xiao-e.Lai Sheng-sheng(2012) Design of a remote medical monitoring alarm system based on GPS and GPRS. Chinese Journal of Tissue Engineering Research, 16(13):2328–2331
5. Ni WW, Wang Zongxin (2004) An indoor Location Algorithm Based on the Measurement of the Received Signal Strength. Natural Science 43(1):72–76
6. Peter Brida.Peter Cepel, Jan Duha(2005). Geometric Algorithm for Received Signal Strength Based Mobile Positioning. Radioengineering 14(1):1–7
7. Wang X, Wang Z X, O Dea B(2003) A TOA based location algorithm reducing the errors due to non-line-of-sight propagation. IEEE Trans Veh Technol 52(1):112–116

Chapter 331
Research of Separable Polygraph Based on Bluetooth Transmission

Zhan-ao Wu, Tingting Cheng, Jianhun Mao and Feifei Wang

Abstract Currently, the collector and the receiver of medical polygraph are usually in wired connection form, thus unsuitable for patients to wear and affecting the correct collection of their physiological data. To solve this problem, this paper has developed a separable polygraph to improve the traditional polygraph by means of Bluetooth piconet communication technology. We use Bluetooth short-range wireless communication module instead of cables of the traditional polygraph. The separate polygraph is flexible to operate and can collect patients' physiological data without affecting their repose. It has a favorable application foreground.

Keywords Separable polygraph · Physiological data · Bluetooth technology · Wireless data transmission

331.1 Introduction

Polygraph (also known as polysomnogram analysis system) refers to collect physiological data (such as EEG, ECG, snoring, pulse, pulse wave, breathing rate et al.) under the sleeping condition of patients, which is inputted to the recorder after being processed and kept in disks or other recording medium for analysis [1]. By combining with the existing automatic sleep analytic software, medical staff can get sleep structure, process and sleep cardiovascular function diagram of

Z. Wu (✉)
The 359 Hospital of PLA, Zhenjiang 212001, China
e-mail: staff236@yxph.com

F. Wang
Dental of the Fourth People's Hospital, Zhenjiang 212001, China
e-mail: 277150355@qq.com

patients, search for the abnormal EEG and sleep-related breathing disorder, and analyze the types and severity through recording and analyzing for patients' physiological data and then get correct diagnostic conclusions for the diseases related to sleep disorder, sleep apnea and hypoventilation syndrome, reduce the mistakes in the process of diagnosis and treatment as far as possible.

At present, the medical polygraph in the market adopts wire connection between the collector and the receiver. It is not convenient for the patients to wear them. The equipments of wire connection may make the patients rest poorly, so the normal collection of their physiological data may be affected. Some patients cannot sleep well in strange beds (beds in hospital), which also can affect the data collection.

To solve these problems, this paper comes up with separable medical sleep polygraph, which segregates the collector and the receiver into two parts. The wireless collector is portable, so it will not affect patients' normal rest. The patients can collect physiological data related to sleep breathing at their own house and send the collected data through the short-range wireless communication device then keep the data in SD cards and take the SD cards to hospital for doctors to diagnose. The frequency hopping mechanism of Bluetooth is based on the master's address and clock sequence, and its output frequency spot sequence has uniformity, periodicity and good hamming correlation features [2, 6]. Hence, this paper adopts Bluetooth communication technology for wireless data transmission to achieve the separation of collection device and receiving device. However, due to the openness of radio channel, there is also some data transmission interference in the direct use of Bluetooth wireless technology. On the basis of the Bluetooth frequency-hopping technology, this paper insures the secure transport of wireless data through fixing Bluetooth wireless data transmission channel. That is to say, the hopping sequences of Bluetooth master device are to be divided into five subsequences, which will be improved and assigned to Bluetooth devices to eliminate communications interference between piconets. This separate equipment is easy to operates and cost-effective. It is convenient for patients to collect physiological data without affecting their rest and the measured data is more accurate. Thus it also helps medical staff to diagnose the patients' symptoms correctly, cure the patients' diseases earlier and it has a contribution to reducing medical accidents and disputes. Therefore, it has a broad application foreground.

331.2 Structure of Separable Sleep Polygraph

The separable polygraph is mainly realized the separation of the data collector and the data receiver. It changes the wire connection into wireless connection, and mainly consists of physiological data collector, data recorder and data analysis system. Physiological data collector is used to collect physiological data related to sleep breathing and is kept in the collector temporarily. It will be transmitted through Bluetooth device when the data recorder send a data transmission request;

Fig. 331.1 Structure of separable sleep polygraph

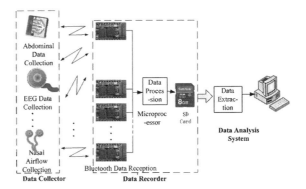

the data recorder is used to receive the data transmitted by physiological data collector and keep the data as a file in SD card; data analysis system analyzes the data in the SD card with the aid of international PSG system and generates comprehensive sleep analysis report. The functional structure of the separable sleep polygraph is presented in Fig. 331.1.

331.2.1 Physiological Data Collector

Patients suffering from obstructive sleep apnea (OSA) should be treated according to their own conditions, so polygraph needs to record sleep breathing parameters like EEG, ECG, EOG, EMG, snoring, pulse, oxygen saturation, pulse wave and breathing rate. These physiological data are signals induced by the sensor and then output them after amplification process. For example, the heart rate data collector amplifies, filters and reshapes the collected heart rate signal of the body, and then transmits the data through Bluetooth module [3]. Figure 331.2 is the functional structure of the heart rate data collector.

When monitoring the sleep breathing physiological data, the data recorder distinguish the data source and then keep them in a specified data file of corresponding data forms. In addition, the separable polygraph needs several collecting devices which integrated Bluetooth module to transmit data. In order to distinguish these devices, this paper is going to add a unique identification code before the Bluetooth module transmits the data. Then the data source and forms will be identified by the identification codes once the data recorder receives the data and they will be saved in corresponding files.

Fig. 331.2 Functional structure diagram of heart rate data collector

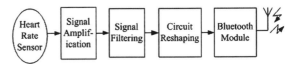

331.2.2 Data Recorder

The data recorder is used to receive the data transmitted by the physiological data collector and save the data in memory locations. It is mainly composed of data receiving portion, microprocessor, and storage device.

The data receiving section is to realize wireless communication between the Bluetooth transmitter module and receiver module in piconet [4]. But there are data collisions both in Bluetooth modules of data collector and data recorder since the open of the wireless channel. The collisions will become interference source of each other, and affect the smooth transmission of data. To avoid the interference and data collisions, the microprocessor distributes a frequency channel for every Bluetooth module of the physiological data collector for data transmission [5]. However, the frequency channel at this time is random, and the disturbance between each Bluetooth module is big. To resolve this interference problem, this paper re-programs the frequency channel of the transmission of data.

Bluetooth frequency hopping sequence has many advantages: it has ideal uniform spectral characteristics and a very long cycle that cannot be cracked easily by smart jammer; it can generate a lot of hopping sequence with good hamming correlation properties which is useful in a multiple access communication. In addition, its hardware implementation is also relatively simple and easy. So this paper makes a series of improvement for channel number sequence based on Bluetooth hopping frequency selection mechanism. Divide the first 160 frequency spots of FH sequences, generated by the Bluetooth master device, equally into five subsequences with cycle length of 32, and carry on reverse order arrangement and redundant filling to part of the sequences. And then distribute to five Bluetooth modules separately. Thus change the random channel message transmission into fixed channel message transmission. For the hamming correlation characteristics of the 5 subsequences simulated with MATLAB, it will be find that the largest value of Hamming correlation is 3, and there is only one value of 3, the other values usually are 0 and 1. The Hamming correlation characteristics between each subsequence are very good. And it will achieve good anti-jamming ability. The simulation results are presented in Fig. 331.3.

331.2.3 Data Analysis System

At present, several companies have developed several automatic sleep analysis softwares combined with sleep experts throughout the world. These softwares have powerful functions and excellent performance. If provided with the data interfaces conform to the analysis softwares, they can provide clear and accurate analysis report.

By extracting the data in SD cards and transforming into corresponding data forms, the automatic sleep analysis system can display the complete

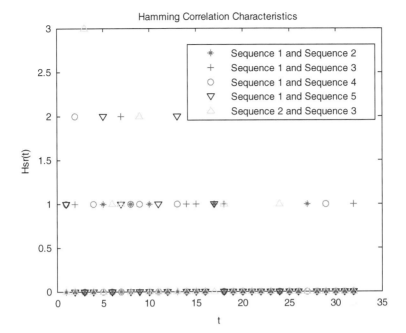

Fig. 331.3 Correlation characteristics of subsequences after improvement

electrocardiogram and other ECG physiological indicators of the patient while the sleep apnea event happens. And then the doctors can judge whether the patient suffers from OSA, provide scientific and exact clinical diagnosis for patients, and prepare for the next necessary treatment.

331.3 Conclusion

With the improvement of people's living standards, more and more people become obese and there is a trend of younger age. It is surveyed that the proportion of overweight people's sleeping apnea is three times higher than the normal people, and even severe cases may lead to sudden death overnight. The separable polygraph proposed in this paper is based on the Bluetooth transmission technology, in which Bluetooth module for wireless transmission replaces the traditional polygraph cable transmission. It is flexible and easy operation, so that patients can go to the hospital to apply for such a device to acquire the sleeping physiological data at home, for early detection of sleeping apnea syndrome and then get early treatment before it threatens their life.

References

1. Hou X, Liu H, Wang (2004) Bao-hua. Design of the multichannel physiology recorder. Chin J Med Instrum, 28(1):5–11
2. Bluetooth Special Interest Group (2007) Specification of the Bluetooth System-Core v2.1 + EDR. November 4
3. Smith D, Solem K, Laguna P, Sornmo L (2009) Model-based detection of heart rate turbulence using mean shape information. Biomed Eng, August 25
4. Tabassam AA, Heiss S, Hoiing (2007) Bluetooth device discovery and hop synchronization by the eavesdropper. Paper presented at emerging technology, November 12–13
5. F Guo (2007) Bluetooth data transmission performance enhancement technology research. Paper presented at the Xi'an Institute of microelectronics and solid electronics, Xi 'an University, May 2007
6. Qi Yan (2012) Design of bluetooth intelligent wireless control system based on android. Intell Ident Tech 20:95–96

Chapter 332
The Design of Intelligent Medicine Box

Jianhua Mao, Xiubin Yuan and Hongfang Shao

Abstract In order to avoid delaying and emitting the execution of doctor's advice, this article puts forward the scheme of intelligent medicine box based on WinCE technology. The intelligent medicine box has the functions of time to remind and managing the doctor's advice and it can ensure that doctor's advice can be implemented timely and accurately. The intelligent medicine box not only contributes to rapid recovery of patients but also reduces medical accidents and disputes and it will have a good prospect of application.

Keywords Intelligent medicine box · Time reminding · Management system of doctor's advice

332.1 Introduction

Timeliness and accuracy of doctor's advice implementation will be directly related to rapid recovery issue of patients. The correct implementation of doctor's advice can reduce medical errors and harmonize relations of doctor and patient. The incorrect implementation of doctor's advice will affect rehabilitation of patients in the gently condition or lead to dead accidents in the severe condition. Thus, to implement doctor's advice correctly and effectively is an important guarantee to harmonize the relations between doctors and patients and to ensure the life safety of patients [1].

J. Mao (✉) · X. Yuan
General Hospital of Nanjing Military Region, 212001 Nanjing, China
e-mail: 277150355@qq.com

H. Shao
Information Centre, Yixing People's Hospital, 214200 Yixing, Jiangsu, China
e-mail: shuangshuang868@sina.com

Implementation procedure of conventional doctor's advice is to read, check, confirm and print the implementation sheet, implement it and observe curative effect and adverse reaction. Doctor's advice is mainly sequentially implemented by nurses in order of priority. In order to ensure accuracy of doctor's advice implementations, the nurses need to read implementation sheet carefully, to sort them in order of priority and the category of doctor's advice and then to implement doctor's advice according to the sequence. This method will not only cause the waste of time and human resources, but also lead to emission and wrong execution when nurses handle the schedule [2].

In recent years, medical disputes shows ascendant trend year by year [3]. In the implementation process of doctor's advice, the phenomena, such as delayed or omitted implementation, even wrong medication and wrong injection are often happen [4]. In order to take medicine without error and the timely implementations doctor's advice, this article puts forward the intelligent devices (hereinafter referred to as IMB) attached to the medicine box that can receive and send information automatically and have the function of time to remind. The IMB can wirelessly receive the doctor's advice information sent from the doctor's duty room, sort the doctor's advice information according to time and carry out the time reminding for doctor's advice. After the doctor's advice is implemented, it can observe the reactions of patients, improve work efficiency of hospitals and avoid medical disputes, which will have a good application prospect.

332.2 Composition and Function of the Intelligent Medicine Box

The IMB can wirelessly receive and send the information from the doctor's duty room, sort doctor's advice and manage doctor's advice. After the doctor's advice is implemented, it can observe the reaction of patients, pass back the doctor's advice to the backstage management system of doctor's advice in the doctor's duty room. The function diagrammatic sketch of this intelligent medicine box is as showed in Fig. 332.1.

The IMB is composed of three parts of doctor's advice information receiving, time remind network and doctor's advice management system [5].

The IMB finishes doctor's advice information receiving, sorting, acousto-optic warning when the implementation time of doctor's advice arrives, information collection and query of information after doctor's advice is implemented and passing back the implemented doctor's advice to the backstage management system of doctor's advice in the doctor's duty room. Some minutes (for example 10 min) before the implementation time of doctor's advice arriving, the IMB will send out a warning sound and remind the nurses that the implementation time of doctor's advice will arrive.

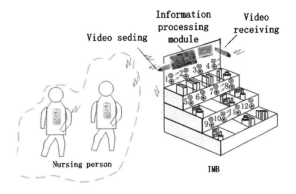

Fig. 332.1 Function diagrammatic sketch of intelligent medicine box

332.2.1 Doctor's Advice Receiving

The doctors will issue the doctor's advice after the wards are checked in everyday. And these doctor's advices will be input into the computer management system of doctor's advice in the doctor's duty room, which will regularly send the doctor's advice information to the IMB in the nursing room. The IMB receives the doctor's advice information sent from the doctor's duty room through the receiving module of radio frequency identification and converts the doctor's advice information in txt format into that in the text format that can be identified by SqlCE database.

The system firstly gets a doctor's advice after conversion and compares it with the doctor's advice information in the local management system of doctor's advice. If it already exists, this doctor's advice will be discarded. Otherwise, it will be inserted into the management system of doctor's advice. It is reciprocated like this and all the received information of doctor's advice will be inserted into the management system of doctor's advice through comparison.

332.2.2 Time Reminding Network

The design of time reminding network is the design key of IMB. Usually, after the IMB receiving the doctor's advice information, the nurses will draw medicines and articles needed by the implementation of doctor's advice from the pharmacy according to the content of received doctor's advice and put them into the IMB respectively according to the patients [6]. The execution of doctor's advice is triggered in real time. The management system of doctor's advice will query the doctor's advices in the entire databases of doctor's advice in every fixed period of time (for example 10 min). After the today's doctor's advices are obtained, they will be showed on the screen of IMB according to the time sequence and the name of patients. Five minutes before the implementation time of doctor's advice arrives, the backstage management system of doctor's advice in the doctor's duty

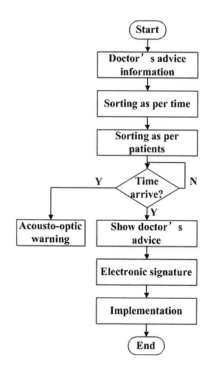

Fig. 332.2 The flow chart of implementation network of this doctor's advice

room will send out a message to the mobile of nurse and remind the nurse that the implementation time of doctor's advice will arrive. When the implementation time of doctor's advice arrives, the IMB will send out the warning sound and flashing light and the screen of intelligent medicine box will show the patients and the doctor's advice information that will be implemented, remind and make it convenient for the nurses to check the information of patients, the content of doctor's advice that will be implemented etc. The reminding sound will continue till the nurses carry out the electronic signature, input the signature password and press down the button of implementation. And then, it will end. At the same time, the information of implementation time and implementation person of this doctor's advices will be stored in the local databases of intelligent medicine management system so as to prepare for the necessary query. The flow chart of implementation network of this doctor's advice is as shown in Fig. 332.2.

332.2.3 The Management System of Doctor's Advice

The management system in the IMB has the functions to manage patient information, nurse's information and implemented doctor's advice information, pass back the implemented doctor's advice information to the backstage management system of doctor's advice in the doctor's duty room.

Patient information management is helpful for the nurses to check the patient information such as name, gender, age, admission time etc. when the doctor's advice is implemented. By this way, the error rate of implementing doctor's advice will be reduced.

The nurse information is input into the databases in advance and it can reduce the amount of keyboard click. When the nurses carry out the electronic signatures, they choose the pull-down menu. It rapidly increases the speed of electronic signature of nurses and greatly improves the accuracy of information.

Because information on doctor's advice, nurses and implementation time has been stored at any time in the process of implementing doctor's advice, the research, classification and statistics can be carried out on the implemented doctor's advice, patients' information and nurses' working capacity, etc.

The IMB also provides the function to pass back the implemented doctor's advice to the backstage management system of doctor's advice in the doctor's duty room. This function can effectively add up the implementation situations of doctor's advice. When the implementation of doctor's advice is wrong, the responsibilities are explicit. All the doctor's advices during the hospitalization of this patient can be printed for the patient to view them.

332.3 Conclusion

The timely and accurate implementation of doctor's advice is the largest guarantee for the rapid recovery of patients. At the same time, it is also the important foundation to reduce medical disputes. The IMB put forward in this article realizes the intelligence and informatization in implementing doctor's advice. It can contribute to improving the quality of hospital care and helping the patients rapidly recover, prevent and reduce medical accidents and medical disputes and contribute to building the harmonious relations between doctors and patients. Therefore, this system has a good of prospects in application.

References

1. Xu F, Wang Y (2007) Practice and experience of preventing medical disputes. SE China Natl Defence Med Sci 9(1):120–125
2. Cheng W (2006) Status of clinical care information construction and Thinking. SE China Natl Defence Med Sci 8(2):142–143
3. Revere L, Black K, Zalila F (2010) RFIDs can improve the patient care supply chain. Hosp Top 88(1):26–31
4. Cao W (2010) Thinking of accelerating the digital hospital construction and development. SE China Natl Defence Med Sci 12(6):I0002–I0003
5. Wang H, Shi Y, Dan Z (2011) Automatic reminder system of medical orders based on Bluetooth, WICOM2011 Wuhan. 25–27 Sep 2011
6. Mao JH, Zheng Y, Wu Z-A, Zhang Y (2012) Doctor perform based on Bluetooth technology automatically alert management system. SE China Natl Defence Med Sci 14(1):78–79

Chapter 333
The Questionnaire Survey about the Video Feedback Teaching Method for the Training of Abdominal Examination in the Medical Students

Liu Juju, Ma Huihao, Xie Yuanlong, Qin Lu and Jian Daolin

Abstract To investigate the effect of video feedback teaching method on skilling training for physical examination of abdomen in the medical students. A small class, 50 students of clinical medicine specialty in medical college in China Three Gorges University, was randomly selected and video feedback teaching method was used for replacing the traditional teaching method. Each student received a questionnaire survey 2 weeks after the skill experimental class. The student accepted video feedback teaching method to a large extent and thought that video feedback teaching method can raise the student's interest, enable students to gain more. There is more advantage in raising the student's study efficiency, aggressive and independence than traditional teaching method. However, video feedback teaching method requires the students to spend more extra-curricular time for the skill training. The video feedback teaching method is an applicable teaching method for medical students' clinical skills training. This method can more enhance the students' motivation and enthusiasm and more improve training efficiency compared with the traditional teaching method.

Keywords Abdominal examination · Clinical skills · Video feedback teaching method

---

L. Juju · M. Huihao · X. Yuanlong · Q. Lu · J. Daolin (✉)
The Second Clinical Medical College of Three Gorges University, Yichang, 443001 Hubei, People's Republic of China
e-mail: 976760430@qq.com

L. Juju
e-mail: 286051889@qq.com

333.1 Introduction

The traditional clinic skills training teaching method mainly adopts the form that teachers give students a demo and they practice themselves after class, then assess students by examination. This method can't ensure the correctness of students' operation. To solve this problem, the foreign educationist first proposed to use the video feedback teaching method into clinic skills training. The video feedback teaching is a skill that records students' operation by video equipment, and students can compare themselves' video with normal video to find the deficiencies in their operation after class, thus improve the clinic skills training. This survey applies the video feedback teaching to the medical students' skilling training for physical examination of abdomen and conducts a questionnaire survey about acceptance and application of the students' effect for this teaching method.

333.2 Subjects and Methods

Take 50 students of class 4 grade 2009 in medical college in Three Gorges University as the subjects. During experimental class of skilling training for physical examination of abdomen in diagnostics, teacher first explains operation steps and correct operation technique, and then gives students a demo of clinic skills operation. Secondly, the students should acquaint themselves with the contents and requirements of physical examination of abdomen, and record the operation process with mobile phone, camera or video camera when students take the skills training. Furthermore, the teacher randomly selects part of the video, taking a playback of the selected video, commends and finds mistakes in these video. Students are required to adopt various ways to review and analysis video feedback. 3 weeks after the first time experimental class, each student should be asked to submit a copy of the most satisfied video of abdominal operation training by themslef. Moreover, 2 weeks after the end of experiment class, students are asked to fill in unified and completely open questionnaire, which is the self-made and the content of the questionnaire are shown in Table 333.1. The questionnaire is amended according to the preliminary survey feedback, and questionnaire survey is conducted by trained investigators on respondents. The recycled questionnaires should be filtered strictly, and unqualified questionnaires are weeded out to ensure the quality of investigation.

333.3 Results

50 questionnaires were given out, and we recycled 46 questionnaires answered anonymously, of which 20 were male (43.5 %) and 26 were female (56.5 %). All the 50 students handed in a copy of their most satisfied abdominal operation training video on time.

333 The Questionnaire Survey about the Video Feedback Teaching Method

Table 333.1 The survey questionnaire about the video feedback teaching method applied in the clinic skills training of the medical students

Male ☐	Female ☐
1 The form you have used in the video feedback analysis	
Analyzing by comparing with the normal video	☐
Analyzing through self review	☐
Analyzing by discussing among groups	☐
Analyzing online through remote network	☐
Analyzing under the guidance of teachers	☐
Other ways	☐
2 Through teaching video feedback, how is your master in the abdominal examination practice now?	
3 Do you gain something in the video feedback? What is the biggest aspect of harvest?	
4 Are you interested in the video feedback teaching? Please state your reasons.	
5 What is the advantage and disadvantage of video feedback method do you think?	

Notes: The video feedback is a method that makes use of video equipment recording operation, and it is also a new teaching method that improves students' operation skills and cognitive abilities by information analysis and feedback. In order to evaluate the effectiveness of this method, we design this survey questionnaire and hope to get cooperation with you. Please answer the following questions carefully and truthfully, thank you!

The way of analysing the video feedback adopted by students. Thirty-two students (70 %) analyzed the video by comparing themselves' video with the standard video, then practiced and studied about the experiment by reviewing and analyzing video feedback. Ten students (21 %) adopted discussion between groups. Three students communicated with teachers and studied under the guidance of teachers. Only one studied by reviewing books.

Students' master degree for physical examination of abdomen after the video feedback teaching method. With the video feedback teaching method, students' master degree for abdominal examination operation is shown as Table 333.2.

Students' achievements from video feedback teaching. About achievements from video feedback teaching, 42(91 %) of students felt fruitful. The main achievmants are mainly composed of the following: Thirteen (31 %) of them thought that this method could make them more clearly about their shortcomings and defects in the physical examination operation. Eight (19 %) thought it could improve self-regulated learning skills. Seven (17 %) believed that the method improved learning their motivation. Nine (21 %) said that it could improve the students' operation standardization and coordination of clinical skills. Five (12 %)

Table 333.2 Master degree of the students for abdominal examination operation

Master degree	Number	Ratio (%)
Basic	21	45.68
More than basic	6	13.04
Good	16	34.78
Excellent	3	6.52

Table 333.3 Advantages and disadvantages of the method

Advantages	Disadvantages
Improving the students' learning efficiency (15, 32.61 %)	It is waste time of making video (19, 41.30 %)
Improving the enthusiasm of students' autonomous learning (12, 26.09 %)	Currently teaching resources are insufficient (14, 30.43 %)
Making students more clearly about their advantages and disadvantage (8, 17.39 %)	Reducing the direct communication between teachers and students (7, 15.22 %)
Cultivating the students' interest (5, 10.87 %)	Students are lack of initiative and enthusiasm (3, 6.52 %)
Improving the students' own requirements (3, 6.52 %)	Students are difficult to maintain high enthusiasm for studying (2, 4.35 %)
Making the teacher know more about each students' learning situation (3, 6.52 %)	To seek for video effects, students may hide mistakes intentionally in operation (1, 2.17 %)

thought that it could be in favor of students to collaborate together and improve the team cooperation spirit of students. Because of lacking initiative, only four students thought that they gain nothing.

Students' interest in video feedback teaching method. Only four (9 %) of the students though it was a waste of time, and they were not interested in video feedback teaching method, while there were 42 (91 %) of the students being interested in this kind of teaching method, of which 13 students believed that video feedback teaching method was innovational and impressive. Ten students (24 %) believed that the new method could improve the students' enthusiasm and initiative; nine students (21 %) thought it could make students more clearly about their shortcomings; six students (14 %) considered it to combine theory with practice; Four people (10 %) thought that it could improve the students' learning efficiency.

The advantages and disadvantages of the video feedback teaching method. The advantages and disadvantages of the video feedback teaching method which is mentioned in questionnaires by students are shown as Table 333.3.

333.4 Discussion

The video feedback teaching is a method of recording the process of students' clinic skills training by video equipment and then making the students gaining information feedback on the recorded video in many ways, in order to improve the effect of teaching skill training. Students compare themselves' video with normal video. Then they are guided by teachers, discussing with each other, or reviewing by themselves to analyze the video. Thus they can find their mistakes in operation and correct them, forming a kind of loop learning model which needs constant practice and feedback. Ultimately achieve the goal of improving students' clinical skills.

Reliability and accuracy of the results. In the process of questionnaire survey, we adopted a secret ballot system for all the respondents that answered questionnaires. It made sure students have no hesitation to express their own opinions and suggestions. The recovery and effective ratio of the questionnaire reached to 92 %. After recycling questionnaire, the video group counted and checked the questionnaires, then summarized the results of the questionnaires. It ensured integrity, authenticity and accuracy of the survey information, and achieved the purpose of this questionnaire survey. To a great degree, it also truly reflected students' evaluation on that video feedback teaching method applied to the skills training for physical examination of abdomen.

Application of the video feedback teaching method in the clinical skills training. In some west countries, the video feedback teaching method have been widely researched and used in skills learning and training teaching for clinicians [4], residents [5], medical students [6] and nursing students [7]. This teaching method mainly focuses on self assessment [8]. It through open self-evaluation of advantages and disadvantages, or assessing in half authentication way by designing questionnaire. Of course, it also can take use of the feedback information, obtained from the communication between teachers and students, to finish assessment. Our results of the questionnaire survey showed that 70 % of the students compared their own video with the normal video. Then they analyzed and reviewed by themselves to study, and evaluated the strengths and weaknesses of this method in an open way. Only 7 % of the students did the feedback assessment by communicating with teachers. Therefore, the video feedback teaching method greatly improves the enthusiasm of the students' autonomous learning. And the percentages of students who rely on communicating with teachers to study greatly reduced.

It has been confirmed that the video feedback teaching method can combine students' theory with practice to improve students' interest on learning. As a new teaching form, the video feedback teaching method is quite attractive to students. Recording video is the basis of video feedback teaching method. The video recorded is a kind of very objective data, and it also can be preserved for a long time. Compared with the traditional teaching method, it gives students a chance to allocate study time by themselves. And it isn't confined that the teacher points out the students' deficiencies in operation only in class. Using the Internet, the students and teachers are convenient to discuss on the operation video after class. Moreover, compared with the traditional teaching which describes by words, the operation video is more specific, vivid and flexible, it also can improve the students' enthusiasm and initiative. In traditional teaching, classmates or the manipulators observe the process of the operation from a certain angle, thus the correctness of the students' operation is judged. But the recorded video can reflect the details of the students' operation from different angles. Let the students be more aware of their deficiencies and the details of the clinical skills operation. Video feedback teaching requires other student to help records video while a student is conducting clinical skills training. After video shooting,the students can discuss with each other and analysis by comparing their own video with the normal video, then they can find their deficiencies in operation. The whole process is conducted in the form of team, it can greatly improves the students' team consciousness and ability to collaborate. Our results also showed that the majority of students were interested in video feedback teaching method. They fully affirmed the harvest that the method brought to them, and they supported that this kind of teaching method could be extended to more skills training.

The advantages and notable problems of video feedback teaching method once it is applied to the clinical skills training. Video feedback teaching method has its own advantages. Compared with traditional teaching method, the biggest difference is that the video feedback teaching method can record the students' operation by video equipment, so the students have no limit on the time of studying. In addition to communicate with the teacher in the classroom, the students can allocate study time by themselves after class. It not only improves the students' enthusiasm, but also the learning efficiency of novices [12]. In the process of recording video, students will concentrate more energy on personal operation. And the effect of training can be improved. The video feedback can show the same details of the same operator from different angles, thus the operator can observe and analysis their operation more carefully, and they can correctly distinguish their operation and know the location nonstandard. Compared with the normal video, the video feedback teaching method can improve the requirements of the students for their own operation video, and then improves the requirements of the students for their own clinical skills training. In addition, the video of the students' clinical skills operation can also be fed back to the teachers. More entirely do the teachers know the practice and mastery level of the students for clinical skills operation. Teachers needn't inspect the operation of students on the spot in the laboratory as they were before. It not only saves time but also makes teachers more fairly and entirely evaluate on the grades of students, therefore teachers can more rationally make a formative assessment on the achievement of students.

Of course, to achieve the good effect of the video feedback teaching method, some problems are worthy of note. First, the comprehensive study and education of the video teaching method should be strengthened between teachers and students, and they can understand the advantages and disadvantages of the method. So they can better apply this method to the teaching of clinical skills training. The core of the video teaching feedback method is self analysis and independent evaluation, and this method focuses on comparing the operation of students with the normal operation. The communication between students and teachers may be reduced. Some students worry about that this method may reduce the experience passed on by teachers to them. Therefore, in order to achieve better results, the video feedback teaching needs close cooperation between teachers and students. Second, how to arouse and keep the enthusiasm or interest of students by applying this teaching method. Although the students generally expressed great interest in the teaching method and benefited from it, but how to improve the evaluations approach of students' academic performance by submitting a video operation, making the video feedback teaching method achieve better effects. To prevent the video feedback teaching method becoming meaningless, attention should be paid to avoiding the students deliberately hiding some mistakes when the video are being shot. Third, shooting video may distract the operator's attention, but this process has educational value. At last, in order to ensure the quality of the shoot of video operation, the video equipments should be equipped completely as more as possible, and the opening hours of the skills training center should be more enough. At present, the students can only use their own mobile phones and cameras to record video or make the video outside skills training centers, both which may result in lengthy and poor quality video, so the video is analyzed more difficultly, and it requires more time [15].

In conclusion, compared with traditional teaching method, the video feedback teaching method takes more time, and it may also face the problem that the lack of teaching resources. But this method can improve students' interest, mobilize the enthusiasm of the students to take skills training consciously, improve learning efficiency of the students and make the students distinguish their operation and know the location nonstandard more clearly. Therefore, students widely accept to apply the video feedback teaching method in the teaching of clinical skills operation. In order to make this kind of teaching method achieve the best effect as it is applied in the skills training. It is necessary to research and evaluate this teaching method in depth. So as to improve the service quality of clinical skills teaching.

References

1. Hannah AC, Millichamp J, Ayers KA (2004) Communication skills course for undergraduate dental students [J]. J Dent Educ 68(9):970–977
2. Pinsky LE, Jcyce E (2000) A picture is worth a thousand words use of videotape in teaching [J]. J Gen Inrern Med 15(11):805–810
3. Sharp AJH, Platts RJH, Drocqedu MH (1989) An assessment of the value of video recordings of receptionists [J]. J R Coll Gen Pract 39(327):421–422
4. Scherer LA, Chang MC, Meredith JW et al (2003) Videotape review leads to rapid and sustained learning [J]. Am J Surg 185(6):516–520
5. Olsen JC, Gurr DE (2000) Video analysis of emergency medicine residents performing rapid-sequence intubations [J]. J Emerg Med 18(4):469–472
6. Bowden T, Rowlands A, Buckwell M et al (2012) Web-based video and feedback in the teaching of cardiopulmonary resuscitation [J]. Nurs Educ Today 32(4):443–447
7. Minardi HA, Ritter S (1999) Recording skills practice on videotape can enhance learning-a comparative study between nurse lecturers and nursing students. J Adv Nurs 29(6):1318–1325
8. Crook A, Mauchline A, Maw S et al (2012) The use of video technology for providing feedback to students: Can it enhance the feedback experience for staff and students [J]. Comput Edu 58(1):386–396
9. Zick A, Granieri M, Makoul G (2007) First-year medical students' assessment of their own Communication skills: A video-based, open-ended approach [J]. Patient Educ Couns 68(2):161–166
10. Yoo MS, Son YJ, Kim YS et al (2009) Video-based self-assessment: implementation and evaluation in an undergraduate nursing course [J]. Nurs Educ Today 29(6):585–589
11. Wieling MB, Hofman WHA (2010) The impact of online video lecture recordings and automated feedback on student performance [J]. Comput Educ 54(4):992–998

12. Xeroulis GJ, Park J, Moulton C et al (2007) Teaching suturing and knot-tying skills to medical students: A randomized controlled study comparing computer-based video instruction and (concurrent and summary) expert feedback [J]. Surgery 141(4):442–449
13. Cardoso AF, Moreli L, Braga FTMM et al (2012) Effect of a video on developing skills in undergraduate nursing students for the management of totally implantable central venous access ports [J]. Nurse Educ Today 32(6):709–713
14. Kardash K, Tessler MJ (1997) Videotape feedback in teaching laryngoscopy [J]. Can J Anesth 44(1):54–58
15. Mackenzie CF, Xiao Y, Hu FM et al (2007) Video as a tool for improving tracheal intubation tasks for emergency medical and trauma Care [J]. Ann Emerg Med 50(4):436–442

Chapter 334
Correlation Analysis on the Nature of Traditional Chinese Medicine

Zhang Pei-Jiang

Abstract Based on the textbooks as data source, such as "Chinese Pharmacopoeia", "Traditional Chinese Pharmacology", "Pharmacy" (reference), "The Traditional Chinese Medicine Herbal Essence", "Pharmacology of Traditional Chinese Medicine" and "New Traditional Chinese Medicine", etc. We try to find the correlation between the traditional Chinese medicine nature, we built the Chinese Medicine database which include the data of Traditional Chinese Medicine nature, functions and indication. We found the closely frequent itemsets from the experiment results, which can provide a reference for the research of Traditional Chinese Medicine.

Keywords Traditional Chinese medicine · Nature · Frequent itemsets · Correlation analysis

334.1 Introduction

The Traditional Chinese Medicine nature can also be known as Traditional Chinese Medicine property, which conclude four properties, five flavours, channel tropism, promotion and demotion, toxicity, etc. Each performance of Traditional Chinese Medicine was derived by the drug apply to the body in the long-term medical practice [1, 2]. In recent years, the researchers have more and more study on the traditional medicinal properties from the literature, experiment and clinical practice, they provide a good foundation for the traditional medicinal properties to further development. However, the complexity [3] of the medicinal theory lead to the main researchers focus on single or double combination in the traditional

Z. Pei-Jiang (✉)
Henan University of Traditional Chinese Medicine ZhengZhou, Jinshui Road NO. 1, Zhengzhou 450000, China
e-mail: zpj@hactcm.edu.cn

Chinese medicine nature, then the results can easily lead to the limited understanding on this basis.

Data mining [4, 5] has become the important technology in the field of pharmaceutical research, which can found the implied data and regular knowledge from the mass data. We can use data mining technology to mining the valuable data from the data of traditional Chinese medicine. Mi Zhou [6] use data mining to research the missing medicinal medicine based on the decision tree algorithm. More and more experiments [7–10] show that data mining techniques can reveal many implicit relationship in the traditional Chinese medicine, and it not only conducive to traditional Chinese medicine information structured, but also help promoting the standardization of traditional Chinese medicine, which is an important part of the modernization of Chinese medicine.

In this paper, we build the database based on the mass data of traditional Chinese medicine nature with its function and indications. We found the closely frequent itemsets and the valuable regular rule through analyzing the experiment result, which provide the support data for the traditional Chinese medicine.

334.2 Data Collected and Methods

The nature of traditional Chinese medicine play an important role in the study of the attributes of traditional Chinese medicine. In this paper, we build the database which data source from the authority text books, such as "Chinese Pharmacopoeia", "Traditional Chinese Pharmacology", "Pharmacy"(reference), "The Traditional Chinese Medicine Herbal Essence", "Pharmacology of Traditional Chinese Medicine" and "New Traditional Chinese Medicine", etc.

For the four properties of traditional Chinese medicine, the traditional record concludes four kinds of *"cold, hot, warm and cool"*. In this paper, we expand the four properties of traditional Chinese medicine to nine properties, which concludes *"flat, warm, cool, hot, cold, slightly cold, big chill, big hot, slightly warm"*. For the five flavours of traditional Chinese medicine, the traditional record concludes five kinds of *"sour, salty, sweet, bitter, acrid"*. In this paper, we expand the five flavours to fifteen kinds, which concludes *"tasteless, sweet, sweet-acrid, bitter, astringent, sour, slightly sweet, slightly bitter, slightly astringent, slightly sour, slightly acor, slightly salty, slightly acrid, salty, acrid"*. For the channel tropism of traditional Chinese medicine, we conclude the twelve parts of the body based on the text book of "Chinese Pharmacopoeia". However, parts of traditional Chinese medicine don't belong to the single part of body, such as the channel tropism of "A Jiao" maybe conclude *"lung, liver, kidney"*, In this paper, we reorganize the channel tropism of "A JIAO" to *"lung, liver, kidney"*, we also reorganize the channel tropism of "A WEI" to *"spleen and stomach"*.

For the function of traditional Chinese medicine, we extracting and cleaning the data that from the textbooks, in this paper, we have collected the three hundred ninety-six kinds of function, such as "soothe the nerves, tocolysis, tonifying lung", etc. On the other hand, each kinds of traditional Chinese medicine conclude different functions,such as the function of "A JIAO" is "hematinic, moistening, hemostasis, nourishing yin", the function of "AI YE" is "dispelling cold, relieve pain, hemostasis".

For the indications of traditional Chinese medicine, in this paper, we have collected one thousand one hundred fifty-nine kinds of content, which included "ai qi, bai dai, bai hou, bai ri ke", etc. Meanwhile, each kinds of traditional Chinese medicine include more indications, such as the indication of "A JIAO" is "uterine bleeding, hematochezia, egersis, Coughing phlegm-heat type", etc. which include sixteen kinds of indications.

334.3 Research Results

Based on the data from the textbooks, after collecting and cleaning the data of traditional Chinese medicine, we build the database of SQL Server, which include the property, flavour, channel tropism, function, indication of traditional Chinese medicine. On this experiment, we analyzed the single part of traditional Chinese medicine, based on the results of frequent itemsets, do the loop processing with connections and pruning processing until the strong association rules be found.

334.3.1 The Nature Theory of Traditional Chinese Medicine

After analyzed the data of database, we found the different traditional Chinese medicine has quit large distribution, the nature of "cold, cool, flat" share a larger number in the seven hundred seventeen kinds of traditional Chinese medicine, while the nature of "hot, big cold, big hot" very few in number, the Fig. 334.1 shown the data distribution of traditional Chinese medicine nature, Fig. 334.2 shown the data distribution of flavour.

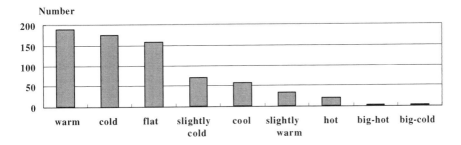

Fig. 334.1 Data distribution of traditional Chinese medicine nature

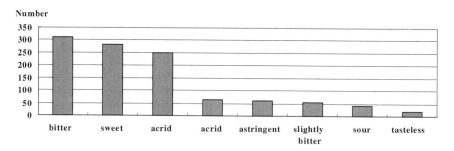

Fig. 334.2 Data distribution of traditional Chinese medicine flavour

From the figure we can found the flavour of "bitter, sweet, acrid" share a large number in the data distribution, while the number of "slightly astringent, slightly sour, slightly salty" share few.

334.3.2 The Function and Indication of Traditional Chinese Medicine

In the database of traditional Chinese medicine, the function of "clearing heat, detoxify, relieve pain, detumescence" has a large number, such as the function of "qing re" related one hundred seventy-one traditional Chinese medicine. While the function of "YiYin, GongJi" has few number, such as the function of "clearing heat" related one traditional Chinese medicine, which named "Dehumidity". The Fig. 334.3 shown data distribution of function and Fig. 334.4 shown data distribution of indication.

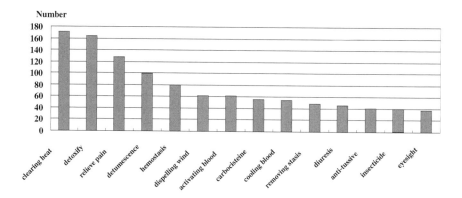

Fig. 334.3 Data distribution of traditional Chinese medicine function

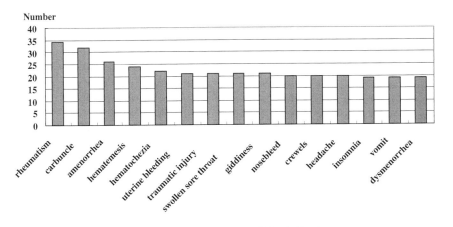

Fig. 334.4 Data distribution of traditional Chinese medicine indication

Table 334.1 Frequent itemsets in nature-flavour-channel tropism

Nature	Flavour	Channel tropism	Support	Support rate (%)
Warm	Acrid	Spleen	62	20.81
Cold	Bitter	Liver	48	16.11
Warm	Acrid	Liver	45	15.10
Warm	Acrid	Stomach	44	14.77
Warm	Acrid	Lungs	43	14.43
Flat	Sweet	Liver	40	13.42
Cold	Bitter	Lungs	39	13.09
Flat	Sweet	Lungs	38	12.75

Table 334.2 Frequent itemsets in nature-flavour-channel tropism-function

Nature	Flavour	Channel tropism	Function	Support	Support rate (%)
Cold	Bitter	Liver	Clearing heat	30	1.72
Cold	Bitter	Liver	Detoxify	27	1.55
Cold	Bitter	Lungs	Clearing heat	24	1.38
Cold	Bitter	Lungs	Detoxify	23	1.32
Cold	Bitter	Large intestine	Clearing heat	21	1.20
Warm	Acrid	Spleen	Relieve pain	21	1.20
Warm	Acrid	Liver	Relieve pain	21	1.20

334.3.3 Correlation Analysis in the Nature

The association rule is an important branch of data mining, which reflect the correlation between the objects. In this database, we found two hundred ninety-eight frequent itemsets, and the nature of "warm" has the strong relationship with the flavour of "acrid" and the channel tropism of "spleen", which related the sixty-two kinds of traditional Chinese medicine, such as "A WEI, AI YE, BA JIAO HUI XIANG, BAN XIA", etc. Table 334.1 shown the closely relationship in nature flavour and channel tropism. Table 334.2 shown the closely relationship in nature flavour and channel tropism and function.

334.4 Conclusions

Association rule is an important tool in the data mining, which also can provide the technique for the fields of traditional Chinese medicine. In this paper, we build the database with data from the textbooks, after collecting and cleaning, we count and analyzed the experiment results and found the strong relationship in the natures of traditional Chinese medicine.

References

1. Gao XM (2007) Science of Chinese pharmacology.China Press of Traditional Chinese Medicine, Beijing, pp 69–87
2. National Pharmacopoeia Committee (2010) Pharmacopoeia of People's Republic of China. The medicine science and technology press of China, Beijing
3. Wang L, Peng JS, Yang YS (2010) Philosophical analysis of the Chinese herb property theory. Med Philos 52–53
4. Tian L (2005) The application of data mining in the field of traditional Chinese Medicine. Chin J Basic Med Tradit Chin Med 710–712
5. Han JW, Micheline K (2010) Data mining: concepts and techniques, 2nd edn. In: Fan M, Meng XF (Trans.). China Machine Press, Beijing
6. Zhou M, Wang Y, Qiao YJ (2008) Yanjiang: predict the preliminary study of Chinese medicine lack of potency based on data mining. Chin J Inf Tradit Chin Med 93–94
7. Zhang B, Lin ZJ, Zhai HQ (2008) A research of traditional Chinese medicine property based on "three elements" hypothesis. Chin J Tradit Chin Med 221–223
8. Jin R, Lin Q, Zhang B (2011) A study of association rules in three-dimensional property-taste-effect data of Chinese herbal medicines based on Apriori algorithm. J Chin Integr Med 794–803
9. Zhang H, Fan XS (2009) Research on association rules on asthma medication regularity between ancient and modern. Chin J Inf Tradit Chin Med 94–95
10. Li H, Cai ZH (2003) Application of association rules in medical data analysis. Microcomputer development,13:94–97

Chapter 335
The Classification of Meningioma Subtypes Based on the Color Segmentation and Shape Features

Ziming Zeng, Zeng Tong, Zhonghua Han, Yinlong Zhang and Reyer Zwiggelaar

Abstract This paper proposed an automatic method for the classification of meningioma subtypes based on the unsupervised color segmentation method and feature selection scheme. Firstly, a color segmentation method is utilized to segment the cell nuclei. Then the set of shape feature vectors which are calculated from the segmentation results are constructed. Finally, a k-nearest neighbour classifier (kNN) is used to classify the meningioma subtypes. Experiment shows that the classification accuracy of 85 % is achieved by using a leave-one-out cross validation approach on 80 meningioma images.

Keywords Meningioma · Segmentation · Classification · Color · Shape features

335.1 Introduction

Meningiomas are a diverse set of tumors generated from the meninges and the membranous layers surrounding the central nervous system. According to the world health organization (WHO), the majority of benign WHO Grade I

Z. Zeng (✉) · Z. Han
Information and Control Engineering Faculty, Shenyang Jianzhu University,
Liaoning, China
e-mail: zengziming1983@gmail.com

Z. Zeng · R. Zwiggelaar
Department of Computer Science, Aberystwyth University, Aberystwyth, UK

Z. Tong
School of Management, Shenyang Jianzhu University, Shenyang, Liaoning, China

Z. Han · Y. Zhang
Shenyang Institute of Automation, Chinese Academy of Science, Shenyang,
Liaoning, China

meningioma can be categorized into four subtypes: fibroblastisch, meningotheliomatoes, psammomatoes and transitional. Computerized image analysis may enable an objective, standardized, and time-saving assessment of these prognostic features. Several automatic meningioma classification methods are proposed. Qureshi et al. [1] proposed a method based on discriminant wavelet packets (DWP) and learning vector quantization (LVQ) to classify the meningioma subtypes. In [2], an adaptive discriminant wavelet packet transform and local binary patterns (LBP) is utilized for meningioma subtype classification. In [3], a multi-resolution analysis technique is introduced to resolve the issue of intra-class texture variation on the basis of stability of adaptive discriminant wavelet packet transform (ADWPT). However, most methods on meningioma classification fail to consider the features of the shape of the regions of interests (ROI). In this paper, an automated classification method is presented to classify the meningioma subtypes based on an unsupervised segmentation scheme and shape features.

335.2 The Proposed Method

The proposed method contains two steps. In the first step, the density inhomogeneity in the gray level images is corrected and the density of cell nuclei is enhanced. Then a color segmentation scheme is utilized to segment the ROI. In the second step, a ten dimensional feature vector for each image is calculated by using the segmentation results. Subsequently, a k-nearest neighbor classifier [4, 5] is used to classify the meningioma subtypes.

335.2.1 Region of Interests Segmentation

As a preprocessing, the original color image (such as Fig. 335.1a) is converted into $L^* a^* b^*$ color space. Then the a channel (such as Fig. 335.1c) after image inverting is convolved by using a Gaussian kernel. Subsequently, the generated image (such as Fig. 335.1d) is subtracted with L channel (such as Fig. 335.1b) in order to enhance the cell nuclei and correct the density inhomogeneity of the background. An example of the enhanced result see Fig. 335.1e.

In the first step, the color information is used to segment the ROI. Specifically, due to the fact that the cell nuclei exhibits lower intensity compared with other tissues in the density enhanced image (such as Fig. 335.1e), a low threshold is used to segment ROI in order to make sure the segmentation results are true positives. Then the segmentation results (such as Fig. 335.1f) are used as masks to extract the corresponding color pixels in the original color image. Then the AE (the color difference in $CIEL^* a^* b^*$ color space) is calculated for every pixel in the image between that pixel's color and the average $L^* a^* b^*$ color within the mask region:

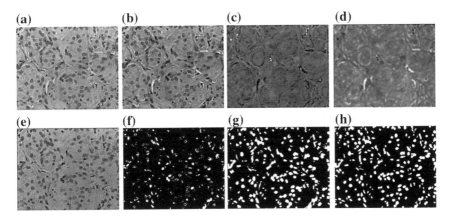

Fig. 335.1 An example of color segmentarion scheme. **a** original image, **b** L channel, **c** a channel, **d** a channel after image inverting convolved by a gaussian kernel, **e** density enhanced image, **f** thresholding by using a small value, **g** color segmentation result, **h** ground truth given by a human expert

$\Delta E = \sqrt{(L - L_{mean})^2 + (A - A_{mean})^2 + (B - B_{mean})^2}$, where L, A and B are the pixel color values for each channel. L_{mean}, A_{mean} and B_{mean} are the mean values in the mask region for each channel. Subsequently, we use the mask region $Mask$ to calculate the threshold $T_{tolerance}$:

$$T_{tolerance} = mean(\Delta E \times Mask) + 2 \times std(\Delta E \times Mask), \qquad (335.1)$$

where $mean(\cdot)$ and $std(\cdot)$ denote the mean and standard deviation values, respectively. Then we use the $L^* a^* b^*$ color in the corresponding region to estimate all other similar color regions. The acquired values (L_{mean}, A_{mean}, B_{mean}) are used to calculate AE for all the pixels in the original color image. Each color pixel value is calculated in a 3×3 window, if $k = i$ $AE/9 < T_{tolerance}$, the pixel will be segmented as ROI. Finally, some small gaps within the ROI are filled by using the morphology method. An example of the segmentation result is shown in Fig. 335.1g.

335.2.2 Feature Selection and Classification

In the second step, we extract eight local features and two global features. For the local features, we label the previous binary segmentation results (assuming each label as a ROI). For each label, eight features are calculated according to the shape of each ROI. In addition, two additional features are extracted from the whole image. All the feature details are shown as Table 335.1.

Table 335.1 The features of meningioma subtypes

Label	Methods	Description
1	Area	The number of pixels in each label
2	Major axis length	The major axis length of the ellipse region which has the same standard second-order central moment in each label
3	Minor axis length	The minor axis length of the ellipse region which has the same standard second-order central moment in each label
4	Perimeter	It is computed by calculating the distance around the boundary of each labelling region
5	Eccentricity	The eccentricity of the ellipse region which has the same standard second-order central moment in each label
6	Extent	The proportion of the pixels in each labelling region and the minimum bounding rectangle of this labelling region
7	Equivalent diameter	The diameter of a circle which have the same area with the labelling region
8	Convex area	The number of pixels within the minimum convex polygon of each label
9	Opacity	The proportion of the number of pixels within all the cell nuclei region and the number of pixels in the whole image
10	Label number	The total number of cell nuclei in the image

For each label, we extract features vector which is instituted from 1 to 8 in Table 335.1. Then the average of the eight features is calculated as a single vector. The global features from 9 to 10 on the whole ROI labels are also extracted. The eight dimensional features and two additional global features can generate a ten dimensional feature vector which is used for modelling and testing in this work. The k-nearest neighbor classification [4, 5] is a statistical pattern recognition method. In this step, it is used to assign samples (as ten dimensional vectors) to one of the meningioma subtypes (fibroblastisch, meningothelioma- toes, psammomatoes and transitional) by searching for samples in a learning set with similar values in a predefined feature space. The learning set consists of pre-classified samples, which are added to the feature space according to their feature values. A vector extracted from a new image is classified by comparison with the K learning samples that are closest in terms of Euclidian distance to it in the feature space. The most frequent class among the K learning samples is assigned to new image. According to the meningioma shape features which are extracted from the meningioma segmentation results, the meningioma subtypes can be modelled by using kNN.

335.3 Experiments

To evaluate the cell nuclei segmentation method, the 80 meningioma images (resolution 1300 × 1030 pixels) are used to evaluate the proposed classification method. The meningioma datasets are obtained from neurosurgical resections at

Table 335.2 Confusion matrices for training sets $(K = 5)$, with the overall classification accuracy equal to 85 %

	Meningioma subtypes	Truth				Classification accuracy (%)
		F	M	P	T	
Predicted	F	19	0	0	1	95
	M	0	17	0	3	85
	P	1	0	17	2	85
	T	1	2	2	15	75

Table 335.3 The accuracy of the meningioma subtype classification

Technique	Classifier	F(%)	M(%)	P(%)	T(%)	Avg(%)
DWP and LVQ [1]	ANN (LVQ)	90	75	80	75	80
ADWPT and LBP [2]	SVM (Gaussian)	90	85	85	75	83.75
Our method	kNN	95	85	85	75	85

the Bethel Department of Neurosurgery in Bielefeld, Germany. It contains four different kinds of meningioma subtype: fibroblastisch, meningotheliomatoes, p- sammomatoes and transitional. Each subtype includes 20 images. The microtome sections were stained with haemalaun and eosin, dehydrated and cover-slipped mounting medium. The meningioma images were required by using Zeriss Axio-Cam HRc color camera at standardized 3200 K light temperature.

To evaluate the classification result, four subtypes (fibroblastisch, meningotheliomatoes, psammomatoes and transitional) are used, including all the 80 meningioma images in the meningioma dataset. In the first, the color information is used to segment all the images. Then ten dimensional feature vector is extracted from each image. Subsequently, the Euclidean distance in a kNN classifier was used to measure the similarity between feature vectors and leave-one-out cross validation was used for evaluation. Specifically, all the extracted feature vectors from the datasets which contain 80 meningioma images are divided into eighty parts. Then the seventy-nine parts is used to train by turn and left one part as test data. The mean of eighty times estimation will be regard to the algorithm accuracy. Table 335.2 shows the confusion matrix of classification by using the local and global features. Our classification accuracy is 85 %. Table 335.3 shows the classification accuracy for each subtypes as well as the overall mean. In [1], the classification accuracy of 80 % is achieved by using discriminant wavelet packets (DWP) and learning vector quantization (LVQ). In [2], the overall agreement is equal to 83.75 % by using local binary pattern (LBP) and adaptive discriminant wavelet packet transform (ADWPT) features. Comparing with [1, 2], our result shows improvement in the overall mean (Avg).

335.4 Conclusion

This paper presents an automatic meningioma classification approach. The proposed method has the following advantages. Firstly, this color segmentation scheme and feature selection method can achieve the purpose of unsupervised classification of the different meningioma subtypes. Secondly, according to the classification results, our method is more robust than some state-of-the-art methods. In the future, some observed issues will be addressed on three aspects. Firstly, the multi-scale feature based on the size of the cell nuclei will be investigated. Secondly, the application on the other kinds of cell nuclei by using the proposed method will be further investigated. Thirdly, more state-of-the-art methods will be used to compare with the proposed method.

References

1. Qureshi H, Rajpoot N, Masood K, Hans V (2006) Classification of meningiomas using discriminant wavelet packets and learning vector quantization. In: Proceedings of medical image understanding and analysis
2. Qureshi H, Sertel O, Rajpoot N, Wilson R, Gurcan M (2008) Adaptive discriminant wavelet packet transform and local binary patterns for meningioma subtype classification. In: Proceedings 11th medical image computing and computer-assisted intervention. Lecture notes in computer science, vol 5242, pp 196–204
3. Qureshi H, Rajpoot N, Nattkemper T, Hans V (2009) A robust adaptive wavelet- based method for classification of meningioma histology images. In: Proceedings of MICCAI workshop on optical tissue image analysis in microscopy, histopathology and endoscopy
4. Friedman J, Baskett F, Shustek L (1975) An algorithm for finding nearest neighbors. IEEE Trans Comput C-24:1000–1006
5. Warfield S (1996) Fast kNN classification for multichannel image data. Pattern Recogn Lett 17:713–721

Chapter 336
An Extraction Method of Cerebral Vessels Based on Multi-Threshold Otsu Classification and Hessian Matrix Enhancement Filtering

Xiangang Jiang and Yunli Qiu

Abstract An integrated cerebral vascular enhancement method based on the multi-threshold Otsu classification for gray voxels relative to cerebral vessels and the multi-scale Hessian feature for the tubular object enhancement is presented. It implements the multi-threshold Otsu classification to get the cerebral vascular gray voxels, and exploits these voxels' geometric characteristics by Hessian matrix. And Hessian matrix's eigenvalues and eigenvectors are used to form a tubular object response function which would be used for further mathematical morphology processing to smooth and mend vessels' region. Compared with other tubular object enhancement methods, it behaves higher accurateness with stable robustness.

Keywords MRA image · Cerebral vessels · Multi-threshold Otsu classification · Hessian matrix · Morphology

336.1 Introduction

The diameter and curvature of cerebral vessels are important indicators in diagnosing relevant diseases. MRA is commonly used in angiography imaging technology, however, which is of low contrast along with random noise. Therefore, it's necessary to explore the enhancement technology for thin vessels with few voxels lost. The reason why to enhance cerebral vessels is that we want to emphasize

X. Jiang (✉) · Y. Qiu
School of Basic Science, East China Jiaotong University, Nanchang, Jiangxi (province), China
e-mail: jxg_2@tom.com

Y. Qiu
e-mail: qeros@qq.com

vascular structural form and restrain the non-critical image background like grey matter, skull, scalp, hydrocephalus or noises which can be ignored at the same time. With non-linear diffusion image filtering methods, Catte et al. applied different scale coefficients to make the image smooth without making the margin obscured on the edge. Orkisz suggested using the median filtering along the direction of vessels to make the vessels region enhanced. Frangi found that using multi-scale similarity measurement based on Hessian matrix to analyse vessels can get a better enhancement effect.

In order to wipe out impurities, the multi-threshold Otsu classification special for vascular objects, as well as vascular enhancement filtering and mathematical morphology which are based on Hessian matrix, is probed to enhance and mend cerebral vessels. The eigenvalues and eigenvectors of Hessian matrix are used to form the response function of cerebral vessels. Experiments show that the method of integrated extraction and enhancement is of high accuracy and robustness, which meets the clinical needs of analysis of cerebral vascular image.

336.2 Image Segmentation Methods for Cerebral Vessels

Image segmentation is a processing of partitioning a digital image into multiple clustering data with specified features. The goal of segmentation is to simplify and change the representation of an image into a state that is more meaningful and easier to be analyzed. The common used methods contain thresholding methods, clustering methods, region-growing methods and split-and-merge methods. Grey thresholding method is the most common used method because of its simple calculation and high efficiency. Therefore, the Ostu classification combined with Hessian matrix enhancement is applied to the extraction of cerebral vessels in the project.

336.2.1 Initial Segmentation of Relative Voxels of Cerebral Vessels via the Multi-Threshold Otsu Classification

A human brain MRA image contains cerebral vessels, as well as the skull, the gray matter and other tissues. In a MRA image, the cerebral vessels' intensities are always in high gray level, while the intensities of background and the gray matter are in low gray level. Fig. 336.1 is the gray histogram of a human brain MRA image. The intensities of cerebral vessels mainly distribute within the region $(C, 255]$, while that of the image background distributes within the region $[0, A)$, and that of the gray matter and cloud-like impurities distribute within the region (A, C).

The multi-threshold Otsu classification is developed from the single-threshold Otsu method. It separates the image into multiple clustering gray voxels by

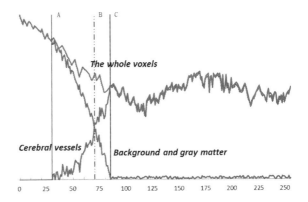

Fig. 336.1 The gray histogram of a human brain MRA image

maximizing the variance which indicates the difference between classes to minimize the wrong probability. The main procedures are as follow:

1. Count the number n_i of each gray level i, set the total number $N = \sum_{i=0}^{255} n_i$, and the probability of each gray level would be $p_i = n_i/N$;
2. Let m and $T = \{t_0 = -1, t_1, t_2, \ldots, t_m, t_{m+1} = 255\}$ ($t_i < t_j$, $i < j$) be the number of thresholds and the vector of thresholds ($t_1, t_2, \ldots, t_m$ are thresholds while t_0 and t_{m+1} are the endpoints of the domain);
3. Compute probabilities $p_{t_i t_{i+1}}$, gray averages $\omega_{t_i t_{i+1}}$, and variances σ_T corresponding to all possible T;

$$\begin{cases} p_{t_i t_{i+1}} = \sum_{j=t_i+1}^{t_{i+1}} p_j \\ \omega_{t_i t_{i+1}} = (\sum_{j=t_i+1}^{t_{i+1}} j p_j)/p_{t_i t_{i+1}} \\ \sigma_T = \sum_{i=0}^{m} p_{t_i t_{i+1}} \omega_{t_i t_{i+1}} \end{cases} \quad (336.1)$$

4. Select the best vector of thresholds $T_{best} = \{t_1, t_2, \cdots, t_m\}$ such that $\sigma_{T_{best}} = \max_T \sigma_T$;
5. Reset all voxels' intensities $I(x, y, z)$ in the 3D MRA image according to Eq. (336.2).

$$I(x, y, z) = t_i \quad t_{i-1} < I(x, y, z) \leq t_i, 1 \leq i \leq m+1 \quad (336.2)$$

After the above five procedures being finished, the intensities of 3D brain image are partitioned into m classes and they include only m colors or intensities. In this paper, m is 3 so there are four classes of gray voxels. The first one $[0, A)$ mainly contains gray matter, the second one (A, B) is a transition region containing both gray matter and some cerebral vessels in low gray level, the third one (B, C) is also a transition region containing both gray matter and some cerebral vessels in high gray level, and the last one $(C, 255]$ mostly contains cerebral vessels. Since the first class hardly contains cerebral vessels, it is abandoned directly in the follow-up processing. The second and the third classes containing cerebral vascular voxels should be further discriminated by their geometric characteristics.

336.2.2 The Tubular Enhancement Filtering Based on Hessian Matrix

Background region, cerebral vascular region and two transition regions are sorted out via the multi-threshold Otsu classification. The enhancement filtering based on Hessian matrix is implemented to enhance vessels region and remove non-vessel voxels which are wrapped with other organs' gray intervals. Hessian matrix is formed by the image differential of high order and reflects orientation feature of image. As a matter of fact, the maximum eigenvector shares the same orientation with tubular objects. Considering the diverse scales of the diameter of cerebral vessels, Gaussian function is introduced to the tubular enhancement filtering based on Hessian matrix and change the standard offset to adapt the filtering for different scales. According to the convolution properties, derivative of spatial scale I_{ab} is obtained by computing the convolution of the image and the second derivative of Gaussian filtering.

$$\begin{cases} I_{abc} = I \otimes \dfrac{\partial^2 G(x,y,z;\sigma)}{\partial a \partial b \partial c} \\ G(x,y,z) = \dfrac{1}{2\sigma^2} e^{\frac{-(x^2+y^2+z^2)}{2\sigma^2}} \end{cases} \quad (336.3)$$

In a 3D image, Hessian matrix is constructed from the second derivative of each voxel.

$$H = \begin{bmatrix} I_{xx} & I_{xy} & I_{xz} \\ I_{yx} & I_{yy} & I_{yz} \\ I_{zx} & I_{zy} & I_{zz} \end{bmatrix} \quad (336.4)$$

In Eq. (336.4), I_{xx} is the second partial differential along x direction, I_{xy} is the second partial differential along two directions of x and y. It is believed that the second partial differential with the maximum module is always perpendicular to orientation tubular objects such as cerebral vessels. λ_1, λ_2 and λ_3 in ascending order of their magnitudes are the eigenvalues of H.

The filtering would output the maximum value if and only if the spatial scale σ of Gaussian function is appropriate to the real diameter of the vessels according to the property of Gaussian function. This method could take account of both ideal vessels structure and the fuzziness of medical image of vessels. The half width of local windows always equals to 3σ, and the diameter of vessels is less than the width of windows in current scale, so bright vessels in dark background satisfies the conditions: $\lambda_2, \lambda_3 < 0$, $|\lambda_1| \approx 0$ and $|\lambda_1| << |\lambda_2| \approx |\lambda_3|$. Three composite variables are defined as Eq. (336.5) composed of the three eigenvalues as the adapted response factors of tubular objects between them.

$$R_A = \frac{|\lambda_2|}{|\lambda_3|}, R_A = \frac{|\lambda_1|}{\sqrt{\lambda_2 \lambda_3}}, S = \|H\|_F = \sqrt{\sum_{i=1}^{3} \lambda_i^2} \quad (336.5)$$

In a current scale, the response function of cerebral vessels is defined as Eq. (336.6).

$$V(\sigma, I) = \begin{cases} 0 & \text{if } \lambda 2 > 0, \lambda 3 > 0 \text{ or } f(x,y) < IT_A \\ \exp(-\frac{2c^2}{|\lambda 2|\lambda 3^2})(1 - \exp(-\frac{R_A^2}{2\alpha^2}))\exp(-\frac{R_B}{2\beta^2})(1 - \exp(-\frac{S^2}{2\gamma^2})) \end{cases} \quad (336.6)$$

In Eq. (336.6), α and β are used to distinguish linear objects from non-linear objects, γ and c are smoothing parameters for the whole region consideration. In this paper, we define the parameters in the ranges: $\alpha \in [0.3, 1]$, $\beta \in [0.3, 1]$, $\gamma \in [20, 50]$ and $c \in [10^{-6}, 10^{-5}]$. $V(\sigma, I)$ would reach its maximum if and only if the width of searching cube windows matches the diameter of vessels where $\sigma \in [\sigma_{min}, \sigma_{max}]$, and $V(I)$ is defined as follow.

$$V(I) = \max_{\sigma\min \leq \sigma \leq \sigma\max} V(\sigma, I) \quad (336.7)$$

The spatial scale σ varies from σ_{min} to σ_{max} by a small step each time. The less σ is, the smaller vessels will be enhanced, while the greater σ is, the bigger vessels will be enhanced. With regard to the response function with variable scales, the larger the range is and the smaller the step length is, the more sizes will be considered. In order to check out the effects with different spatial scales, four tests will be carried out with single selected σ with 0.3, 1, 2 and with a range of [0.3, 2] in a step length being 0.4 respectively, and the relevant response results are as follow.

The results reveal that a given scale only works well for the vessels with a special diameter. The relevant vessels are only enhanced while other non-linear objects are hardly affected. Small vessels are enhanced with a small σ shown in Fig. 336.2a, while medium vessels are enhanced shown in Fig. 336.2b, c. The vessels with multiple diameters are enhanced with a changeable σ shown in Fig. 336.2d, while the former 3 examples in which the scales are fixed only affect the vessels with special diameters.

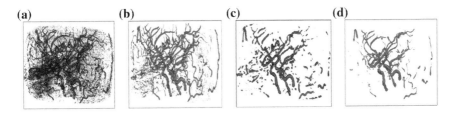

Fig. 336.2 The response results of the filtering with single-scaleand multi scale σ, **a** $\sigma = 0.3$, **b** $\sigma = 1$, **c** $\sigma = 2$, **d** $\sigma \in [0, 3, 2]$, step=0.4

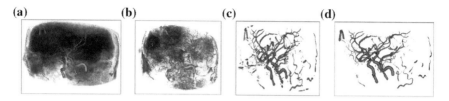

Fig. 336.3 The cerebral vascular extraction procedures, **a** The original image, **b** Processed by Otsu classification, **c** Processed by the filtering, **d** Restored by tophat operator

It costs much more time if the filtering based on Hessian matrix is applied to all voxels in the whole 3D image. Considering the region $[0, A)$ mainly containing dark background, so the filtering processing will spend less time while being only applied to the region (A, C).

336.3 Results and Analysis

In the experiments, the software environment is Delphi 7 and the hardware environment is a desktop computer with AMD Athlon 2 X4 610e CPU and 4 GB memory. The experiments include 5 procedures. Firstly input an original 3D slice data as Img0 shown in Fig. 336.3a; secondly process Img0 by the multi-threshold Otsu classification and obtain segmented data as Img1 shown in Fig. 336.3b; thirdly process Img1 by the filtering based on Hessian matrix and obtain voxels which only contain cerebral vessels with special diameter as Img2 shown in Fig. 336.3c; fourthly recuperate Img2 by Tophat operator which is a morphological operator and obtain Img3 as Fig. 336.3d; finally merge original image (gray) with tubular objects (red) shown as Fig. 336.4 with different angles. The original MRA image is a spatial reference to cerebral vessels in the 3D simulation model.

In Fig. 336.3, a clearer outline of brain vessels appears after being processed via the multi-threshold Otsu classification, and a 3D brain vessels image which is

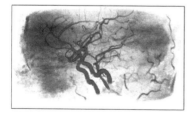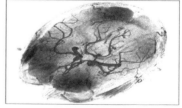

Fig. 336.4 The final result by merging original 3D image (*gray*) with tubular objects (*red*) in different projecting angles

Table 336.1 The effects of different methods in the two aspects of tubular extraction and smoothness

Methods	Tubular extraction (%)	Smoothness (%)
Median filtering	66	73
Non-linear diffusion filtering	75	92
Hessian filtering	91	81
Hessian filtering and anisotropic diffusion	91	92

only related to tubular elements stands out through being enhanced via the Hessian-based filtering. It is showed up in different projecting angles shown in Fig. 336.4, which merge the original 3D image with the cerebral vessels smoothed and recuperated by a morphological operator and filled with red color. It shows clearly the global hierarchical relation between brain vessels and other organs.

Different methods have different impacts of tubular extraction and smoothness on 3D data. Table 336.1, from which the method (Hessian filtering and anisotropic diffusion) proposed in this paper obviously has a better integrated effect than the other three methods in the two aspects of tubular extraction and smoothness, is the statistical result of different methods.

336.4 Conclusions

In this paper, firstly classifies the gray levels of 3D human brain MRA images by the multi-threshold Otsu algorithm and extracts all voxels which completely contain brain vessels, secondly filters cerebral vessels via multi-scale linear filtering based on Hessian matrix, thirdly effectively restores the discontinuous vessels by self-adapted Tophat operator to which the response function with linear structures is applied, fourthly implants the smooth vessels into the original 3D brain data which benefit the analysis of diseases and the simulation of operations. The system achieves a better robustness within the same accuracy, and the further research will be focused on the quick Hessian eigenvector extracted method with template representations of Hessian operator and the non-linear anisotropic diffusion.

Acknowledgments This work was supported by National Natural Science Foundation of China (61262031) and Jiangxi Province Graduate Innovation Fund Project (YC2012-S081).

References

1. Kao Y-H, Teng MMH, Zheng W-Y et al (2010) Removal of CSF pixels on brain MR perfusion images using first several images and Otsu's thresholding technique. Magn Reson Med 3:743–748
2. Lesage D, Anglini ED, Bloch I et al (2009) A review of 3D vessel lumen segmentation techniques: models, feature and extraction schemes. Med Image Anal 13(6):819–845

3. Zhang W, Ling H, Prummer S et al (2009) Coronary tree extraction using motion layer separation. Med Image Comput Assist Interv 12(1):116–123
4. Koller TM, Gerig G, Szekely G et al (1995) Multiscale detection of curvilinear structures in 2-D and 3-D image data. In: Proceedings of ICCV vol 2, pp 864–869
5. Hesser J, Männer R, Braus DF et al (1996) Real-time direct volume rendering in functional magnetic resonance imaging. Magn Reson Mater Phys Biol Med 2:87–91
6. Dzyubak OP, Ritman EL (2011) Automation of hessian-based tubularity measure response function in 3D biomedical images. Int J Biomed Imaging 2011:1–16
7. Liu S-P, Chen J (2010) Enhancement method for retinal images based on Gabor filter and morphology. J Optoelectron Laser 21(2):318–322
8. You J, Chen Bo (2011) New approach to retinal image enhancement based on hessian matrix. J Comput Appl 31(6):1560–1562

Chapter 337
Architecture of a Knowledge-Based Education System for Logistics

Dianjun Fang and Xiaodu Hu

Abstract Nowadays the technologies develop so fast that people cannot keep pace with the increasing logistics knowledge. In order to provide a professional platform of learning modern logistics, moreover, to shorten learning time and improve the learning efficiency, this paper introduces a knowledge-based education system which provides different user groups with well-formed learning contents. The architecture of the system as well as its four main modules is the focus of the paper. Additionally, the learning strategies and the mechanism of formulating learning plan are interpreted. It is a good foundation for the future knowledge-based education system in the logistics and supply chain management.

Keyword Education system · Logistics · SCM · Knowledge base · Knowledge-based education system

337.1 Introduction

Nowadays, the economics develops increasingly fast and the demand on goods exchange grows also quickly. In order to adapt to different application environment in practice, logistics systems with more advanced technologies are deployed, algorithms with higher complication are used for the planning of logistics systems and numerous logistic strategies emerge. Under this circumstance, the data and information as well as the knowledge and experiences in the area of logistics increases continuously day by day.

Whilst data and information are surely without effort to be stored, the knowledge and experience differing from people are hardly to keep. A DIKW

D. Fang · X. Hu (✉)
CDHK of Tongji University, Siping Road 1239, Shanghai 200092, China
e-mail: felix.hxd@gmail.com

Chain is mentioned in [1] to reveal the differences between data, information, knowledge and experiences. Thus, it is necessary to find a proper solution to maximize the utilization of knowledge and experiences. In such sense, the knowledge-based system (KBS), which can collect, store and manage organized knowledge, is appropriate to support the purpose. In [2], several relevant technologies for modeling, managing and representing knowledge in KBS are investigated and presented.

The application of KBS has many successful examples in the area of medicine, agriculture and manufacturing already. In this paper, however, it focuses more on applying KBS in education. Knowledge and experiences should not merely be kept and used. More important, they should be passed on to the next generation. In [3], architecture of an E-learning system in manufacturing industry is introduced. With manufacturing training materials, scenario case base and problem solving methods being provided, the system educate the employees to ensure their continuous competence in handling their task. In addition, an educational system based on semantic web technology is written in [4]. This technology provides more adaptability, robustness and richer learning environments in building KBS. Moreover, a Web-based education system with the purpose of creating Web learning environment is proposed in [5]. The integrated tools with Web Services have a characteristic of powerful adaptability for management, authoring, delivery and monitoring of learning content. Furthermore, KBS is also applied in logistics. A knowledge-based logistics strategy system referred in [6] is designed for supporting the logistics strategy development stage by retrieving and analyzing useful knowledge and solutions.

However, there exists little research on applying KBS as educational system for logistics. Combined with the idea of customizing learning contents and process, as described in [7, 8], we strive to put forward a kind of KBS which serves to educate people with personalized logistics knowledge. Firstly, we focus on depicting the architecture of the knowledge-based education system for logistics in Sect. 337.2. Then in Sect. 337.3, the application process of the system will be elaborated with an illustration. Afterwards, characteristics of this system will be portrayed. At last, results of applying KBS with a case will be presented, in order to verify the feasibility of the system.

337.2 Knowledge-Based Education System for Logistics

The purpose of building Knowledge-based Education System for Logistics (KESL) is to educate different user groups with logistic knowledge. Based on a Knowledge Base (KB), which contains full of educational materials of logistics, we strive to organize these materials strategically and then present the knowledge in a way that learners can assimilate them on their best performance.

337.2.1 Architecture of KESL

The architecture of KESL consists of four modules and the system is divided into three layers, as illustrated in Fig. 337.1. Firstly, the internal layer is responsible for supporting the learning activities of interactive layer by obtaining, maintaining and organizing data and formulating instructional learning strategy. Additionally, the interactive layer mainly relates to user's actions during learning. Moreover, the external layer is an indispensable ingredient, in which stand the system designer and supporting information from the Internet.

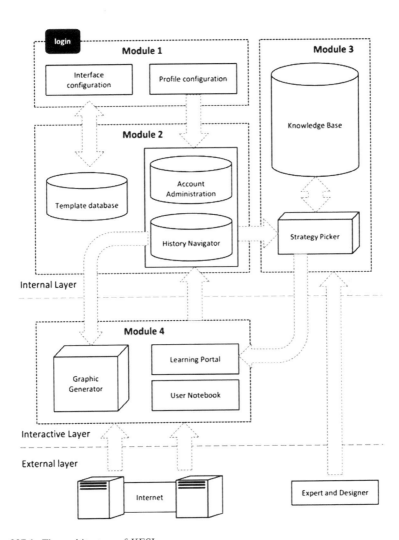

Fig. 337.1 The architecture of KESL

337.2.1.1 Module 1 Entrance

By Entrance, users can login and start their learning journey. In the first time, users will be asked to input their profiles. The configuration of their inputted information is the only identification for every individual. Consequently, the information will be saved in the Account Administration and used for formulate personalized learning plan. The required information from users is listed in Table 337.1.

337.2.1.2 Module 2 User Management

In this module, the Account Administration acts like a transit depot between users and message processing. On the one hand, it receives profile configurations from module 1 and obtains users' feedbacks from module 4; on the other hand, it delivers feedbacks to Strategy Picker every time users add some feedback during learning. This operation repeats continuously and it forms a closed-loop feedback system, so that the Strategy Picker could be immediately updated and always ready to formulate an adapted learning plan. Moreover, to achieve effective knowledge storage, a multi-dimensional database (MDB) technology could be used, which is proposed in [9]. It facilitates the knowledge representation, navigation and maintenance with a high performance level. Furthermore, the process of storing knowledge is also a process of establishing clusters. It enables data mining for potential usage.

The History Navigator in this module relates to record the learning process for every user. These recordings are stored in personal account. They will be utilized afterwards in the process of reviewing at the beginning of the next round of learning.

Additionally, the Template Database stores kinds of interface styles. Users can define their own style and it will be saved in personal account.

Table 337.1 Options and attributes for classifying different groups of people

Attributes	Options
User groups	Student, teacher, company personnel, manager, specialist, common people, ...
Ages	<18, 18–24, 24–30, 30–50, > 50
Be engaged in	Economics, finance, journalism, engineering mechanics, material science, supply chain management, ...
Previous experience	No foundation, common knowledge, broad vision, specialized in (), ...
Purpose of learning	Interests, brief understanding, basic skills, additional knowledge for main major, practical knowledge for work, teaching, know-how, ...

337.2.1.3 Module 3 Knowledge Center

The Knowledge Center is composed of Strategy Picker and Knowledge base. It receives different information from other modules as constraints and according to them then formulates the appropriate learning strategy and pick up the corresponding educational materials.

Knowledge Base

The Knowledge Base (KB) consists of a database and its structure, by which different domains and layers of logistic knowledge are revealed, as illustrated in Fig. 337.2. In database, knowledge is collected from various ways: Encyclopedia for logistics, logistic Handbook, technical drawing and documents from logistic projects, scientific articles, curriculums provided by university, literatures, PowerPoint from internet and so on. Furthermore, all these collected knowledge are divided into five layers, as is shown in Table 337.2 and Fig. 337.2.

Additionally, in order to make sure that all the knowledge objects can be picked out appropriately, they must be assigned several attributes. These attributes are previously given by the knowledge base designer and will be matched with constraints from users. They can describe the location of every educational material, reveal a fuzzy relationship between knowledge objects or indicate the abstraction level of a knowledge object and so on.

Strategy Picker

Strategy Picker is actually an inference engine. It is responsible for formulating the most appropriate instructional learning plan. As already mentioned in former text, module 3 receives different information from other modules which contains constraint conditions. After the Strategy Picker has received those constraints, it starts to search for a basic learning strategy at first and then to collect needed knowledge through the basic learning strategy. According to different users, there are primarily three basic learning strategies applicable:

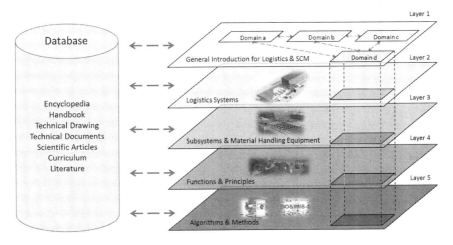

Fig. 337.2 Structure of the knowledge base

Table 337.2 Layers of the knowledge base and contents in each layer

Layer	Knowledge examples
General introduction	Terms about logistics and SCM, PPT and PDF files.
Logistics systems	Explanation of logistics systems with picture, video, 3D-animation., planning procedure, Best practices
Subsystems and equipment	Container and pallets, rack system, forklift, conveyors, sorter etc.
Functions and principles	FIFO, LIFO, location management, route control, transport regulations and roles, layout plan principles
Algorithms and methods	Performance calculation, dimensioning, simulation etc.

- Expanding Learning: The learner learns the knowledge, which is distributed in the same layer, to broaden his horizon. The mechanism of searching learning material is to find the knowledge whose location label contains the same layer index.
- Top-down Learning: The learner learns the knowledge in a specific domain from basis to proficiency. The mechanism of searching learning material is to find the knowledge whose location label contains the same domain index.
- Knowledge-centered Learning: Having learned a specific knowledge, the learner start to study other related knowledge in order to strengthen the comprehension of the centered-knowledge. The mechanism of searching learning material is to find the knowledge which have a better fuzzy correlation with the focused knowledge and whose location label can be in any domain.

Applying a type of learning strategy indicates a definitive knowledge retrieval path. Based on the location label and fuzzy relationship, the knowledge retrieval process is performed by inductive indexing approach and the nearest neighbor algorithm along with the researching path. Since the search direction and connection between knowledge have been determined, a series of educational materials will be selected out after traversal.

337.2.1.4 Module 4 Learning Platform

The users can learn knowledge audiovisually from Learning Platform. The learning process consists of reviewing and learning.

In this article, we suggest that a reviewing process being introduced. According to Ebbinghaus forgetting curve, people forget more than 60 % of their learning things after 1 day. It is of little significance when people learn the knowledge only once. Therefore, we bring in an interactive process during learning activities, namely, the feedback from users about how difficult they feel about the content and how confident they feel they had understood the knowledge. The knowledge with higher difficulty or with lower score of understanding is prior to be reviewed.

There are three ways of using the system. Users can determine how to learn by themselves:

- Passive learning
  - Receive knowledge material on screen
  - Go along with the instruction till to the end
- Positive learning
  - Knowledge Map: well-constructed knowledge links in a graph on which man can select whatever he wants to learn.
  - Search Engine: always ready to retrieve knowledge
- Interactive learning
  - Scoring: the user marks a knowledge unit with a score in certain area, so that the system response to modify its operation
  - Notebook: the user takes note for the learned knowledge and writes it on the board, in order to recall the memories by reviewing in the next round of learning. In this way, the efficiency of learning improves obviously.

337.3 Application Process

As illustrated in Fig. 337.3, the flow chat shows the system application process. Firstly, the user must open an account and configures his profile information. After logging in, the system will check user's learning history. If the latest learning history exists, a review process will be organized by the system and the user could choose to review or deny. Then the Strategy Picker forms an instructional learning plan and selects appropriate knowledge materials out according to the user's initial settings. Consequently, the educational contents will be provided in front of the learner. However, the learner could choose to learn things positively, to browse the knowledge freely and study whatever he wants; or to follow the learning instruction step by step. In both of the two learning processes the learner could have interactive activities. These activities as feedback will be sent back to Strategy Picker in real-time. Thus, the learning material and instructional plan could always be updated and personalized until the user has finished the learning activities. At last, the learning history and feedbacks in this round of learning will be stored and be prepared to serve the next round of learning.

337.4 Result Analyses

At first, the users input their profile information into the system by Entrance, which is not illustrated in this paper. The options of user profile are presented in Table 337.1. For every user, the profile configuration can only load in the first

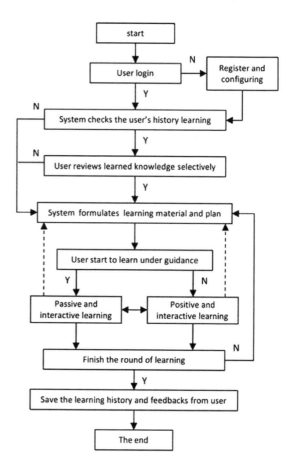

Fig. 337.3 Application process of the system

time, this process is not necessary later. In this case, the name of the learner is Wang Jianguo, the age 29 years old and so on.

Having received the entered user profile, KBS will determine the learning strategy and provide the learner with appropriate materials intelligently, according to user's group, age, job, previous experience and purpose of learning. In this case, Jiang Jianguo is forklift driver and has little knowledge about logistics. The only knowledge he was familiar with is the forklift truck. Therefore, the system decides to use the knowledge-centered learning strategy. We can judge from the Fig. 337.4 that the user has already learned once at last time. As we can see, the knowledge in learning history provided by KBS is appropriately assigned. For instance, the classification of material handling equipment is firstly recommended, then the details of counterbalanced forklift, reach truck and later so on. The learner chooses one option of the learning history, namely the typical transmission organ of counterbalanced forklift truck. It shows that Jiang has given an understanding score with 3.5 point to this knowledge during latest learning. It means that he has

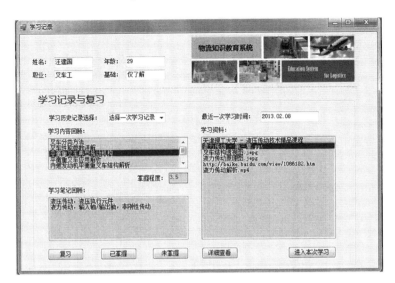

Fig. 337.4 Page of learning history

to review it in time after learning, so that he can get a better learning performance. On the right side, some provided learning materials are listed for this knowledge. On the bottom side, the latest learning notes for this knowledge are shown in the box. They are helpful for the learners to recall their memories and to improve their learning performance.

After reviewing, as shown in picture Fig. 337.4, we choose to enter the next page to start a new learning. as picture Fig. 337.5 depicts, in this round of learning, the KBS provides not only the learning materials of counterbalanced forklift, but

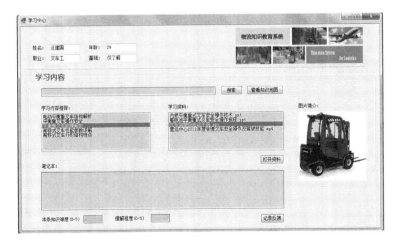

Fig. 337.5 Page of learning center

also the knowledge of reach truck. The available materials are also listed on the right side which concludes summarized document and video. Besides, the user can feedback his learning feelings by noting or scoring on the bottom of learning platform page. What are learned in this round will be recorded and shown as reviewing contents in the next round of learning.

337.5 Conclusions

KESL works with several characteristics. Knowledge materials in KBS can be added, maintained and updated to adjust to changes. Meanwhile, the learning strategy is well calculated and can be optimized by users' feedback continuously. Different from a traditional educational system, KESL has also a review process which could improve the efficiency and effectiveness of user's learning. In addition, the capability of customizing the learning interface could provide the users with good learning experience and keep them from the impression of boring learning. Furthermore, a direct-viewing demonstration of learning outcome could deepen their understanding of their efforts.

KESL is a professional frame for the further development of the knowledge-based education system in the logistics and supply chain management. The new knowledge can be easily integrated. The next development steps could be the application for smart phones and smart TV.

References

1. Sajja, Akerkar (eds) (2010) Knowledge-based systems for development. In: Advanced knowledge based systems: Model, applications and research. TMRF e-Book, vol. 1, pp 1–11
2. Li BM, Xie SQ, Xu X (2011) Recent development of knowledge-based systems, methods and tools for one-of-a-kind production. Knowl-Based Syst 24:1108–1119
3. Ma X (2009) Design of a flexible E-learning system for employee's education in manufacturing industry based on knowledge management. In: IEEE international symposium on it in medicine and education doi: 10.1109/ITIME.2009.5236228
4. Bittencourt II et al (2009) A computational model for developing semantic web-based educational systems. Knowl Based Syst 22:302–315
5. Peredo R, Canales A, Menchaca A, Peredo I (2011) Intelligent web-based education system for adaptive learning. Expert Syst Appl 38:14690–14702
6. Chow HKH, Choy KL, Lee WB et al (2005) Design of a case-based logistics strategy system. Expert Syst Appl 29:272–290
7. Qing Y, Yang Y, Chen J (2004) Goal-oriented platform based on knowledge-point: a new model of distance education system. In: Proceedings of the 18th international conference on advanced information networking and application (AINA'04), vol 2, pp. 528–531
8. Huang XL (2011) Study of personalized e-learning system based on knowledge structural graph. Proc Eng 15:3366–3370